Third Edition

MANAGEMENT OF HEARING HANDICAP
Infants to Elderly

DEREK A. SANDERS
State University of New York at Buffalo

Prentice Hall, Englewood Cliffs, New Jersey 07632

Library of Congress Cataloging-in-Publication Data

SANDERS, DEREK A.
  Management of hearing handicap : infants to elderly / Derek A.
  Sanders.—3rd ed.
      p. cm.
  Previously published under title: Aural rehabilitation.
  Includes bibliographical references and index.
  ISBN 0-13-051194-3.
      1. Hearing impaired—Rehabilitation. 2. Deaf—Rehabilitation.
  3. Audiology. I. Sanders, Derek A. Aural rehabilitation.
  II. Title.
  RF297.S35   1993
  362.4'28—dc20   92-30171

Acquisition editor: *Julie Berrisford*
Editorial/production supervision and interior design: *Edith Riker*
Cover design: *Ray Lundgren Graphics, Ltd.*
Prepress buyer: *Kelly Behr*
Manufacturing buyer: *Mary Ann Gloriande*
Editorial Assistant: *Nicole Signoretti*

Previously published as *Aural Rehabilitation: A Management Model*

© 1993, 1982, 1971 by Prentice-Hall, Inc.
A Simon & Schuster Company
Englewood Cliffs, New Jersey 07632

Printed in the United States of America

10 9 8 7 6 5 4 3

ISBN 0-13-051194-3

Prentice-Hall International (UK) Limited, *London*
Prentice-Hall of Australia Pty. Limited, *Sydney*
Prentice-Hall Canada Inc., *Toronto*
Prentice-Hall Hispanoamericana, S.A., *Mexico*
Prentice-Hall of India Private Limited, *New Delhi*
Prentice-Hall of Japan, Inc., *Tokyo*
Simon & Schuster Asia Pte. Ltd., *Singapore*
Editora Prentice-Hall do Brasil, Ltda., *Rio de Janeiro*

Contents

Preface: To My Reader

The concept of management, which is central to the discussion in this book, at first may appear to be too business oriented, inimical to the personal humanistic image most of us have of our work with people. However, it is only as effective managers that we are likely to succeed in improving the lives of those persons with impaired hearing. Each limitation imposed upon a person's ability to meet the demands of his or her lifestyle results in a decrease in the capacity to function optimally.

As the ability to meet demands decreases, unmet needs arise; life becomes progressively more difficult and more restricted both for the individual and for the important people in his or her life. At some point this becomes unacceptable and our help is sought. Our task is to understand the needs which the hearing impairment has created, to identify the demands, and to marshall and manage effectively the additional resources necessary to optimize a person's function in all aspects of life.

I stress, therefore, that it is the management of resources on behalf of the person that must be our focus. Just as a financial consultant helps us to manage our money to maximize its return according to our individual needs so must we work in consult with our client to invest available resources in the most profitable manner.

The task we confront requires a cooperative model involving the child or adult and others significant in his or her life in a close planning and working relationship with several professionals. The otologist and audiologist are primary in diagnosis of the problem. The audiologist is the expert on the technological resources of amplification and assistive listening and alerting devices. The audiologist also may assume the major management responsibility for all aspects of adult rehabilitation. More commonly this role is assumed by a speech-language pathologist once hearing aids have been fit. Other professionals, including the family physician, social worker, psychologist, and nursing home staff, may be involved. The primary management professional must coordinate the resources these professionals can provide.

The management of the resources needed by children and their families is far more complex. Because hearing impairment in childhood affects language and speech, social development and education, it will be the speech-language pathologist or teacher-of-the-hearing impaired who will play the major role. He or she must work closely with the audiologist, psychologist, classroom teacher, specialist teachers, school nurse, and administrator. The relationship with the parents must be paramount if success is to be maximal.

Because of the varied and ever changing needs of the child and the family each professional at some time will be turned to for assistance, thus I address the book to all who participate in the total management process. Each of you will draw different information from it which I hope will facilitate your relating to the problem.

In writing this book I have been the primary assessor of the needs and manager of resources. Yet the notion of a single-authored text is a misnomer, for the end product derives from the utilization of many resources. I owe a particular debt to two persons, my wife Cynthia, who typed all my handwritten copy, and Dee Sciandra who meticulously produced the computer copy which went to the publisher. Without these two persons there would have been no book. I own much to a number of others, my copy editor, Linda Pawelchak, whose care, patience, and insight greatly enhanced the final copy; my three prepublication reviewers, Harold L. Bate, Western Michigan University, Sharon A. Lesner, University of Akron, and James McCartney, California State University, whose comments and guidance were invaluable; and my photographer, Jim Ulrich, who is also involved in my books. Finally, I thank in advance you, my reader, for maintaining an open mind as you read, for evaluating every concept critically, and for your willingness to acknowledge that I, like you, know only a small part of the whole. Nevertheless, we each endeavor to make at least a small contribution to the enormously rewarding task of helping others.

Derek A. Sanders
Buffalo, New York

MANAGEMENT OF HEARING HANDICAP

1

The Challenge of Management

My intent in this first chapter is to provide a broad perspective of the task of helping children and adults to overcome the problems that come from having hearing difficulties. It is frightening to be confronted for the first time with a client who has a particular kind of communication disorder. You believe that the client expects you to have all the knowledge to "cure" the problem, or at least to teach him/her to function normally again; you know that you cannot. Over the years I have come to terms with this problem. It is crucial to realize right at the beginning of your professional education that there is no perfect solution, no proven method that works for everyone, no packaged plan of intervention to use with persons with impaired hearing anymore than there is for persons with aphasia or stuttering problems. Of course our profession, through research, clinical experience, and trial and error, has accumulated considerable wisdom. Your education, in part, is intended to allow us to pass on this knowledge to you. However, the knowledge will not provide you with clear-cut solutions to problems, nor will you know exactly what to do for each client. Education is about teaching you how to think; it develops in you the skills necessary to observe, to analyze, and to evaluate situations. Education, to be effective, must teach you to see the same problem from different perspectives, to observe similarities and differences among problems, and to identify available resources and use them appropriately in a problem-solving format.

1

Most of all, education should stimulate your creativity and encourage you to be flexible.

Our first goal, therefore, is to take a holistic look at the task that confronts us, to see it in its broadest perspective. We will examine the components of the communication process in general terms to see how they relate to each other, and we will consider how we can break down the task of working with persons with impaired hearing. Once you have an idea of the whole task, we can afford to examine each component in some detail, always keeping in mind its place in the larger picture.

THE PROBLEM OF UNDERSTANDING HEARING IMPAIRMENT

It is very difficult for those of you who have normal hearing to imagine what it is like to be deprived of part of that sense. You can plug your ears with cotton and observe the difficulties you have hearing everything people say, but that experience no more simulates a permanent hearing problem than closing your eyes makes you blind. The partial and temporary deprivation of auditory acuity that you experience differs from hearing impairment in five important ways:

1. Although the sound you received is reduced in loudness, it is distorted only minimally.
2. Unlike the hearing-impaired person, you have a normal auditory system with which to process the sounds you do hear.
3. You still can monitor your own speech with minimal difficulty.
4. You can remove the plugs at any time, so you will not experience the psychological effects of feeling different, inadequate, or stigmatized at school, work, or in social situations.
5. Your family, friends, and other important people in your life will know it is a game; they will go along with it for the length of the project.

For the hearing-impaired person, the hearing problem is permanent, though its effects may change with age, with changing circumstances, or we hope through our intervention procedures. To be maximally effective in helping these children and adults, we first must acknowledge that no matter how much we learn about hearing impairment, we do not know what it is like to be hearing impaired. Few of us even know what it is like to live with a hearing-impaired person on a daily basis. I was shocked to find how little of what I know exerted a positive influence on my feelings and behaviors during a period in which my wife had a significant hearing impairment. From that experience I learned directly the difference between knowing about something and actually experiencing it. I learned how great an impact even a temporary hearing impairment can have on personal relationships and how negative the effects of adaptations family members unwittingly make to the changed circumstances can be.

Diagnostic versus Management Perspectives

If you have been educated in the diagnostic procedures we use in audiology, you will have been taught to seek objective data. Emphasis in the diagnostic stage is on quantitative results and accurate assessment of the auditory system. As far as possible, our goal is to rule out subject variability, that is, the differences that make people individuals. We attempt to standardize test conditions and procedures, to use techniques such as immittance measures and evoked response audiometry that do not require active participation by the client. We use a heavily scientific medical model with a modest amount of subjectivity very successfully at this stage.

The reverse is true when we are faced with the task of assessing and reducing the impact of the hearing impairment on the life of the individual and the family. The management stage must involve the client maximally; the procedures are highly individualized and the knowledge base is shared—although you know the general case, the client experiences the particular. This is not to say that there is no body of scientific data to draw upon, no technology to assist us, nor a structure within which to work, for without these, this book could not be written. What it does mean is that management demands a partnership in which you and your client share different kinds of expertise in seeking the common goal of improving the quality of the client's life. In the chapters to come, we will examine the information that we have about the effects a hearing impairment usually has on the ability of an individual to function as he/she would wish. In the case of a child, we will examine the influence hearing impairment has upon developmental processes and upon the child's ability to fulfill the parents' normal aspirations. I have stressed that the problem of impairment of hearing is a family problem, not simply that of an individual, so we will consider together the total impact of the impairment. This is important because the model of intervention is based upon identification of needs of different kinds and upon the identification and utilization of various available resources to meet those needs.

THE IMPORTANCE OF TERMINOLOGY

When we speak together about hearing impairment, we use various terms that are descriptive of the condition. Many of these terms are used when we explain or discuss hearing impairment with adults or with the parents and teachers of children. As professionals we assume that we all share a common understanding of what each term labels, and we tend to use such terms without giving a great deal of thought to them. Yet a term is the indicator of a whole concept and all the ramifications that accompany that concept. Unfortunately, it is not possible to transmit a concept or idea from one person to another, a highly important fact to which we will pay much attention in our discussion of the nature of human communication. The terms we use do not *convey* ideas; they only *evoke* them in the listener. Thus the definition or concept that a term evokes is that held by the person who hears it. This often is a rather different concept from the one held by the person who uses it. Much interference to the learning process occurs when the meaning attributed to a term by the listener differs from that intended by the speaker. Even more serious are the associated implications and assumptions that the listener correctly or incorrectly makes on the basis of a term or label. To be effective in communicating with each other, we must make every effort to ensure that we attribute equivalent meanings to terms we use. We must be equally careful that those we counsel also understand what we mean by the terms we use and that we encourage clients to share with us their understanding as well as the concerns and feelings that a particular label evokes for them. As we progress in our discussion of information relative to the management of the problems caused by impaired hearing, I will attempt to explain carefully each new term. At this point, consider some terms we use often in discussing hearing deficiency.

Hearing Impairment

Hearing impairment is an all-inclusive generic term. It encompasses all types and degrees of hearing deficiency, congenital and acquired, in children and adults. The term *hearing impairment* says that hearing is not normal, that there is a physical/physiological auditory problem, but it says nothing more. Similarly one can describe persons with impaired hearing as being *hearing impaired*. To do so tells us nothing about how severe the impairment is nor how it affects the individual. The terms *hearing deficient/deficiency* are synonymous with hearing impairment. I try to avoid referring to "the hearing impaired." It is dehumanizing to lump together everyone with a disorder: "stutterers," "aphasics," "dysarthrics," "cleft palates," or "the hearing impaired." I prefer to refer to "persons/individuals with impaired hearing."

It is important to be able to differentiate between the actual physiologic/neural deficit as evidenced by threshold measures and the practical or "functional" effects of the deficit on the person's ability to attain or maintain a normal life-style. The terms *audiometric* and *functional* allow us to do this. These adjectives qualify two categories of hearing impairment, namely *hard-of-hearing* and *deaf*.*

Hard-of-Hearing

The term *hard-of-hearing* categorizes a person in terms of how he/she functions communicatively. Children or adults who are hard-of-hearing use hearing as their primary mode of communication. Vision, more often than not, provides an essential secondary source of information in communication situations. Children in this category learn to speak primarily through the use of residual hearing, assisted by a hearing aid. Adults who lose part of their hearing continue to use oral communication. It should be noted, however, that there is a growing interest among young persons who are hard-of-hearing in learning at least some sign language. This interest generally is motivated by a desire to learn more about and to be able to relate to

---

* Hard-of-hearing means a hearing-impairment, whether permanent or fluctuating which adversely affects a child's educational performance but which is not included under the definition of "deaf" in this section. 34CFR 300.5(B)(3)

"Deaf" means a hearing-impairment which is so severe that the child is impaired in processing linguistic information through hearing, with or without amplification which adversely affects educational performance. 34CFR 300.5(B)(1)

their more severely hearing-impaired peers who are deaf. This increasing interest in sign language is one of the most positive indications in many years of the breaking down of barriers between the two groups.

In the past, most persons who were hard-of-hearing studiously avoided association and identification with those who were deaf. Being hard-of-hearing allowed one to identify with the normal-hearing orally communicating population; deafness was considered a stigma. However, a progressive liberalization of attitudes toward minority group members in general and toward those who are disabled has occurred among the general population over the past 20 years. This has been reflected in an increased awareness and interest in the population of people who are deaf and in acknowledgment of the richness of the language they use. Deafness is not quite the stigma it used to be.

Deaf

The word *deaf* identifies an extremely complex cluster of meanings. It defines, of course, the severity of the sensorineural hearing deficit, but it identifies also a matrix of effects that result from the sensory deprivation. Also implied by the term is a language behavior, a distinctive culture with its own folklore, theater, and a growing body politic, as well as a perception of the world different in many ways from our own. The narrowness or breadth of our understanding and use of the term *deaf* has significant implications for how we perceive persons born deaf. It affects how we relate to them, what we expect of them, and our appreciation of the ramifications of both congenital and acquired deafness on their lives. When we work with children who are deaf, our interpretation of the term will influence our philosophy regarding communication systems for their education and the counsel we give to parents. We also must be cautious about how we understand and accept the body of information encompassed by the psychology of deafness that has been developed by professionals. We must be careful that this information not blind us to explanations of behavior within a normal model of psychology (Goffman, 1969). Reflect on the fact that the psychology of exceptionality asks us to see persons who are deaf as psychologically different from us, rather than as individuals behaving as we would were we confronted by the same circumstances.

We must evaluate these influences that the semantics of the term *deafness* have on us, for we are responsible for a holistic management of the problems created by hearing impairment—not simply with improving communication function.

Audiometric Classification of Deafness. Even audiometric classification of deafness is not simple. Medically the differentiation is made on the basis of a 90dB average pure tone deficit in the speech frequencies (500 1K 2K 4K) of the better ear (AA00, 1965). Audiograms, however, are prone to misinterpretation due to the variety of ways in which they can be categorized (Erber, 1981). Even more important is the fact that pure tone thresholds tell us nothing of a person's ability to process speech with residual hearing, an ability that varies even within a category of hearing deficiency (Erber, 1981).

Erber (1981) has stated that although a person who is deaf can perceive intensity changes in speech occurring as a function of time, he/she has little or no appreciation for frequency. Coupled with this is poor pitch discrimination for such frequencies as are audible. As a result auditory speech discrimination is extremely poor in most cases of deafness (90 + dB HL). Thus a further characteristic that clearly separates the deaf from hard-of-hearing category is that persons who are deaf are unable to rely on the auditory system as their primary channel for communication and learning even with amplification (Ross, 1977). Complicating our interpretation of the term *deaf* is the fact that the degree of sensorineural hearing deficit in infancy is not the only determinant of potential for development of spoken language when appropriate amplification and parent guidance is provided at an early age. It has been emphasized (Ling, 1976; Ling & Ling, 1978) that many, if not most, children with deficits of 90dB HL and even greater can achieve acceptable oral communication skills given appropriate training. These children not infrequently exhibit linguistic and academic skills superior to some children with moderately severe impairment (Knauf, 1978).

The recent development and application of cochlear implants in children will add a further significant factor in our concept of what is meant by the term *deaf*. Cochlear implant technology recognizes the absence of cochlear function but to some degree surmounts this deficiency by stimulating the cochlear nerve fibers directly. Simply stated, the acoustic speech signal is decoded by a microprocessor worn like a body aid. A simplified version of the signal is then fed as a patterned electrical stimulus along a fine wire that has been inserted surgically into the cochlea. At points along the cochlear, the wire makes contact with the cochlear nerve endings. In this way a very reduced pattern of the acoustic information is fed to the auditory system. The results have proven very promising. The long-term results with young prelinguistically deafened children have yet to be reported. The potential for allowing very young children to receive information about the acoustic signal appears to be great given further knowledge and technical advancement. If it becomes possible to provide significant amounts of speech information to a young child in this pseudohearing form, we may well have to significantly reconceptualize our definition of a *deaf child*.

Persons who are hearing impaired do not readily fit neatly into the categories of hard-of-hearing or deaf. Thus the adverbs *audiometrically* and *functionally* or *behaviorally* become essential when describing hearing impairment.

Audiometric/Audiometrically

The terms *audiometric/audiometrically* imply that the statement we are making about a child or adult refers to the severity of hearing impairment only as defined by audiometric measures. The information, thus labeled, deliberately excludes any reference to the effect upon the child's or adult's ability to function. When a person's average thresholds in the speech frequency range 500–2000 Hz exceed 90dB, we classify him/her as "audiometrically" deaf (Stark, 1974). By the same criterion, a deficit of less than 90dB would classify someone as hard-of-hearing. This classification is of only limited value. It tends to be helpful in referring to a person's demonstrated performance as exceeding, being compatible with, or falling short of what we know those classified as audiometrically deaf usually are able to achieve. Remember, such expected standards are as much a function of present technology and teaching effectiveness as they are of the person who is deaf. However, one should be extremely cautious when using audiometric classifications to predict what a young child can be expected to achieve either in terms of communication or education. Our concern in management must focus on the measured or potential ability to function.

Functional Effects

Functional effects is an extremely valuable term, for it refers to how the individual behaves or functions in language, communication, and learning situations. Many factors, which we will consider later in some detail, contribute to and influence a person's functional ability. For example, a child with a 70dB hearing impairment before fitting with hearing aids and before communication education may well function as a deaf child. Even though she is audiometrically hard-of-hearing, her communication and language may resemble closely that of a deaf child. After hearing aid use and appropriate management procedures, in a face-to-face situation in a quiet room at a distance of four feet from the teacher, the same child may function normally when the teacher is talking about familiar content material. However, in a large classroom when she must look at a text illustration being explained by a teacher whose face she cannot see, she functions as a hard-of-hearing child.

Allied to the differential categories of functional and audiometric are the terms *disability* and *handicap*. The term *hearing disabled* is the legal term used to identify all children shown to have impaired hearing. It replaces the term *hearing handicapped* used in earlier legal documents (20 USC 1401 (1) 15 300.5). Personally I find a need to conceptualize two different entities as directed by those terms. For the purpose of this text, I will use the term *disability* to refer to the actual physical/physiologic or sensory condition. *Handicap* identifies the limiting effects of the disability. Correct use of these terms does much to keep clear in our minds, and in the minds of the parents, spouses, and other persons important to management, the physiological reality of the disabling condition, and the degree to which the attitudes and efforts of all concerned are able to mitigate its handicapping effect on function. Significant hearing impairment is always a disability, while the handicap, that is, the degree to which that disability limits a child or adult in life, is a variable over which we can exert much control. It is the prevention or minimizing of a handicap, the improvement of the functional behavior of persons with impaired hearing, that this book is about. This is the challenge that we and our clients share—to overcome or reduce the handicap that, without intervention, would be imposed by the disability.

EXAMINING THE EFFECTS OF HEARING IMPAIRMENT

The Acoustic Signal

To understand the nature of hearing impairment and its effects, it will be necessary to approach the topic from many angles. The whole problem, of course, derives from the fact that damage to the organ of hearing means that any sound, environmental or speech, is distorted by the ear. To understand what this means, we will need to review the nature of the acoustic signal, particularly the speech signal, to determine the ways in which the distortion occurs. Remember, it is not just speech that is distorted, but all sounds, so we need to seek a common denominator that will allow us to understand what distortion means. That denominator, we will see, is *information*. The word *information* as used here does not refer to meaning. "Bits" of information are analogous to pieces of a jigsaw puzzle. No one piece conveys anything meaningful on its own; each contributes information to the ultimate recognition of what the puzzle represents, that is to say, what the picture represents or means. The most important puzzles we solve daily are those involving ideas. The most valuable pieces in that puzzle are speech patterns. We use these to identify which of all possible ideas is being referred to. Since the speech puzzle must be put together before the ideas are recreated, we need to pay particular attention to the acoustic characteristics of speech and the ways that hearing impairments distort these acoustic patterns and thus remove valuable information that they convey.

Distortion of speech patterns is not, however, a phenomenon entirely attributable to hearing deficiency. Since speech patterns are transmitted from speaker to listener by molding the vocal acoustic stream, the speech signal will be subject to the effects of the environment through which it must travel. Acoustic distortion in the form of reverberation and noise exerts a serious effect on the quality of the signal, smearing the pattern and thus making it harder to recognize. Room acoustics are important to all of us, but they often are critical for the person with impaired hearing. The information removed from the speech signal by poor room acoustics will lower the total amount of information that passes through the defective cochlea to the hearing-impaired person's brain. Often it is reduced below the critical amount necessary to reconstruct the intended idea or message. Intervention to combat the negative effects of room acoustics on the fidelity of the speech signal becomes an important goal in assisting hearing-impaired children and adults in communication situations. The human system always seeks to adapt to changed circumstances. When information from one source is reduced, other sources become more valuable. The visual signal is one of those sources.

The Visual Signal

The reduction in the performance of one sensory modality causes a person to seek compensatory enhancement of the use of the remaining unimpaired systems. Vision is an important communication modality in its own right. The whole field of the visual arts depends upon vision as the medium of its existence. Hearing impairment obviously does not affect the quality of the visual signal. What is does is to place far greater emphasis upon information available in the visual channel than is true for those of us with normal hearing. The integrity of the visual system is thus crucial for the person with a deficiency of hearing. Unfortunately conditions that cause hearing impairment frequently also affect vision. To emphasize the importance of optimizing visual acuity, we will examine why persons with impaired hearing often are more likely than the population in general to have a visual defect. We will consider also the most common visual defects and the influence they have on the processing of the visual signals relevant to communication. One of the primary goals in management is to maximize resources that can augment the total information available to a hearing-impaired person in a communication situation. The visual signal constitutes an excellent source of information relevant to, but different from, that contained within the acoustic signal. To maximize the use of the supplementary visual channel, you need to be familiar with the nature of the visible information available in a communication environment, and in particular with the visual cues generated when we communicate. When you are familiar with this resource, you will be able to design educational tasks to modify the communicative behavior of the person with impaired hearing in ways that maximize his/her use of visual information. It would be convenient if vision could compensate completely for the deficiencies of hearing. Unfortunately there are limitations to the amount of information that can be extracted from visual stimuli. Some of these limitations are within the environment itself, some in the physical relationship of the person to the environment. To the extent that we know what these are and how they operate, we can teach the person who is hearing impaired to exert greater control over them, thus reducing the effect of the limitations. Always we are seeking to manage situations to the greater advantage of our client.

The visible information generated by the act of speech itself is not amenable to direct control. Nevertheless it is important to know how much information one can expect a person to derive from visible speech patterns under varying conditions. This knowledge will influence directly how we perceive the process of visible speech recognition, the degree of emphasis we place upon attempting to improve a client's ability to use the skill, and how we go about teaching a person to make greater use of visual cues to the spoken message.

THE PROCESS OF COMMUNICATION INTERACTION

The root cause of the difficulties experienced by persons with impaired hearing lies in the disruption that the disability causes to the normal processes of interacting with others. Although a hearing deficiency affects a person psychologically, educationally, and socially and often affects work performance as well, problems in each of these areas originate in the reduced ability of the person to meet normal communication demands.

A Communication Model

Human communication takes many forms, but communication through verbal language is the dominant method. Many theoretical models exist that attempt to depict the components and processes involved in verbal communication. Some models have been used to develop computer systems that allow communication between individuals and computers using speech. Nevertheless, no theory or model exists that replicates the complexity of the human communication process. We may never reach the point where we fully understand how it works. Meanwhile, you will be confronted with the problem of improving the communication performance of a person with impaired hearing. Even though you cannot know the intricacies of communication, you must have a conceptual model in order to develop an intervention approach that makes sense to you and your client. It would be unwise to expect a text to present you with a highly structured way of looking at the problem and an equally structured intervention program. What is critical is that you learn how to approach and analyze both a person's needs and how he is attempting to meet them. It is on the basis of your perception of the problem that you will develop an individualized approach to problem reduction. For this to be possible, you need a body of relevant information about communication and a way of organizing it into a theoretical model. The model, which should never be considered either comprehensive or final, provides you with an organized way of thinking about why your client is experiencing communication difficulties and why certain intervention approaches might be most appropriate.

We will develop a theoretical model that provides a way of understanding what is involved in human communication. We will look at the role of experience and verbal language in the formulation of an idea and how that idea is encoded linguistically. Verbal language and articulation are intimately related; therefore, so are language and speech.

Communication Monitoring

Speech articulation is the method of patterning the acoustic signal that will carry the message information to the listener. To ensure that the signal we are producing is indeed what we intend it to be, it is necessary for the system to incorporate a vocal-articulatory self-monitoring component. Interference with the ability to self-monitor speech will result in deviation of speech patterns from the norm. These will go undetected by the speaker. Speech is monitored primarily through hearing. It is not surprising, therefore, that at some level of severity, hearing deficiency will prevent the normal acquisition of correct speech by very young children and will impair the maintenance of correct speech by adults. The monitoring component of the communication model is one that we must consider carefully. Our understanding of it will influence our analysis of speech errors made by persons with impaired hearing and the techniques we use in speech improvement education.

The importance of maintaining the fidelity of the acoustic signal has been stressed. I have pointed out already that environmental noise and reverberation often degrade the speech signal. Noise, in the sense of interference, may degrade the message in more than its acoustic form. Noise as *interference* is a valuable concept; in fact, that is how the term *noise* is used in information theory. We will consider all the interference factors, acoustic and nonacoustic, that may affect the communication process. We also will see how the human system has evolved to combat communication noise through use of the compensatory factor of *redundancy*, which exists in various forms at different stages of message processing. Redundancy, which derives from information in excess of that needed to permit comprehension, is one of our major resources in fostering more effective communication strategies in hearing-impaired persons. For this reason we will consider it in some detail both at the sending and receiving stages of communication.

It is important to avoid thinking of communication interaction as comprising the two mutually exclusive roles of speaker and listener. We always are playing both roles, though at any given moment we primarily will be talking or listening. Even as we listen we are sending messages back to the speaker who should be modifying what she is saying in the light of our responses. We will look later at the disturbance caused by hearing deficiency to the receptive-interpretive stage of communication. Before we do that, however, we will build our model to accommodate the various ways in which all sources of sensory information are received and integrated. We also will learn about this ongoing dynamic interactive relationship between the communication systems of speaker and listener.

Perception and Hearing Impairment

Every interaction between us and the world is based upon how we perceive things to be. Our perceptions govern our actions. Perceptions derive from the information we receive and, equally important, from how we process and evaluate that information. You probably already have a useful knowledge of perception gained from a psychology course. We will review the basic processes of perception for they include such important components as figure ground, attention, and memory. Most important we will see how perception is an active process, and how expectations influence how and what we perceive. This active stage of perception is responsive to training. Since hearing impairment changes the sensory information a person receives, it also changes perceptual processing behaviors. We will examine what these changes are likely to be, particularly in terms of how they influence the perception of the acoustic signal and the analysis of the information received in communication.

Of particular interest are the effects that hearing impairment has been shown to have on the development of language and speech in prelingually impaired children. These in turn affect a child's general learning abilities;

this fact will need to be borne in mind constantly when we plan strategies to enhance the child's learning capabilities.

Psychological Implications of Hearing Impairment

Distortion of the acoustic signal and possible related processing problems are the direct result of hearing deficiency. However these alone do not comprise the total effect of impairment of hearing. They constitute the disability; together they create varying degrees of handicap in different individuals and in differing situations. The degree and nature of the handicap demand considerable psychological adaptation on the part of the hearing-impaired child or adult. This is not always easily achieved; emotional reactions to being hearing impaired further complicate the problem (Sanders, 1980, 1988; Vernon & Ottinger, 1980). Furthermore, since the handicap is in communication, those who are close to the handicapped child or adult also will be affected both directly, by the increased difficulty in interpersonal interaction, and indirectly, by the feelings of sadness, inadequacy, frustration, and even guilt and anger that loved ones often experience (Williams & Darbyshire, 1982). The psychological ramifications of reduced ease of communication thus complicate the problem of being hearing impaired and must be addressed.

Everything we have outlined to this point pertains to the need for an understanding of how hearing impairment degrades the reception, analysis, and interpretation of information in spoken communication. We also have seen that language and speech encoding as well as speech monitoring may be affected, particularly in children with hearing deficiency. Knowledge and understanding of this factual information allow us to approach a hearing communication problem as multilayered. We will know that although the hearing deficiency is the root cause, it alone cannot describe the nature of the communication interference. It is hoped that the hearing deficiency will remain a fairly stable factor, but each of the other contributors to the process of communication will vary. Our task for each problem and for each situation is to determine at what stage or stages the system is inadequate. Intervention then can be targeted specifically for maximum results.

INTERVENTION

The particular intervention program you develop for any given child or adult will grow out of your understanding of communication and the ways in which impaired hearing causes it to break down. The knowledge you will acquire or review in the early part of this book will prepare you to examine practical assessment and management procedures. It is necessary to keep in mind during our exploration of intervention principles and approaches that although management and therapy overlap, they are not synonymous terms for the same process. Therapy usually encompasses procedures directed at habilitation or rehabilitation of the receptive or expressive components of communication, with the primary focus on spoken language. The word *therapy*, with its obvious medical derivation, is itself a limiting one, for the process involved bears little or no relationship to medical therapies. What we are involved in is a process of educating the child or adult, providing knowledge and tools and fostering the skills necessary for effective communication. This is what usually is understood by the term *speech, hearing, and language therapy*. Management encompasses this process but extends well beyond it. In management our concern is for all the factors that relate to and impact on the client's ability to meet effectively the communication and learning demands of his world. These might be thought of as the liabilities the person must meet communicatively and the resources available with which to meet them. We are, in fact, helping the person to recognize and understand the demands fully and to identify and capitalize on available resources. We will speak much of the various limiting factors related to communication and of how to minimize their impact. We also will examine possible resources and how to use them. The most important of all resources is residual hearing. However, to make that resource available, some form of amplification device must be used.

Amplification

To use amplification effectively as a resource, it will be necessary to understand what it can and cannot do. To help you with this, we will study those aspects of amplification necessary to ensure that no matter in what form you encounter a hearing aid or auditory assistive device, you will understand the basic principles it involves and how they relate to an individual's hearing deficit. We will look at some typical devices to see what features they share and how they differ in what they offer. Increasingly special amplification devices are used for hearing-impaired children in mainstream educational settings where they must become part of the teaching system (Ross, 1982). Classroom and specialist teachers, as well as speech-language therapists, encounter special amplification devices more and more often. So we will include in our discussion of amplification the special applications these have in education.

Intervention by Age Group

Although a problem-analysis problem-reduction approach underpins intervention procedures for children and adults, problems and needs are age-related in many ways. It is convenient to examine how management models and procedures need to be modified for various age groups. Hearing impairment in infancy and early childhood presents special problems that affect family-child interactions. The very fact that the child does not develop according to the parents' expectations causes anxiety. Not knowing what is wrong permits all sorts of fears to arise. Later, the diagnosis of hearing impairment, or even worse the labeling of the child as "deaf," will put the parents under considerable emotional stress. At this stage a counseling component must be primary in management. We will discuss counseling both from the standpoint of the parents' needs and from that of your feelings when called upon to provide support of this kind. After all, you probably have received little training or experience in counseling, yet you will be confronted by a need that ethically or humanistically cannot be ignored. The need for emotional support and guidance will be a component at every age level. The feelings of inadequacy, with which we all are familiar, are aggravated by functional limitations arising from a hearing impairment and exacerbated further by the feeling of being different. Such feelings will impede a positive and effective adaptation to the disability by increasing the handicap. Counseling support for this reason must be part of our management plan for children, adults, and families.

The overwhelming impact of hearing impairment in childhood is on learning. We will divide our discussion into the educational stages of infancy, preschool, and primary and secondary levels, examining how the changing needs demand different management approaches at each level. Hearing loss in adulthood presents different problems that arise from employment demands and social activities. Even during adult years, needs change, so our services must be adapted accordingly. Thus in addition to recognition of the very special set of circumstances to which each hearing-impaired person must learn to adapt, we recognize that some more general circumstances generate their own particular demands. For example, attendance at university, college, or trade school places the young person back in the educational environment but in a different milieu from high school. Similarly, retirement creates a changed set of demands for an adult than those experienced during working years, while a move of a retired person into a residence home, particularly into a nursing home, changes the demands yet again.

These changing needs emphasize the basic tenet of the management approach I advocate: it must be individualized, must address functional needs, must be creative, and must be based on a problem-solving partnership with the hearing-impaired person and his/her family or in the case of a child, with parents and teachers. If we can achieve this, we can anticipate having a significant impact in limiting the crippling effects that hearing impairment can have on the lives of children, adults, and their families.

2

The Acoustic Signal

The process of speech communication is based upon the acoustic signal that carries the speech code from speaker to listener. Since you already are familiar with at least the basics of speech production and acoustics, we will simply review those aspects pertinent to the communication model we are going to construct.

SOUND AS A REFERENT

Even before we reconsider the nature of sound in communication, it is important to remember the role it plays. Any living species that has evolved with an auditory mechanism depends upon sound for information about the environment. That information derives from the fact that movement in air causes acoustic vibrations. When these vibrations fall within the sensitivity range of an auditory receptor, in terms of both intensity and frequency, they activate the mechanism and sound reception takes place. When the pathway and neural centers above the level of the cochlea are intact, the sound will be detected. This is what occurs when we conduct pure tone tests of hearing. We generate a sound at a specific frequency and then determine at what intensity it evokes a response in a subject. Pure tones, however, are quite unlike either environmental or speech sounds since each is of a single frequency only. Both environmental and speech

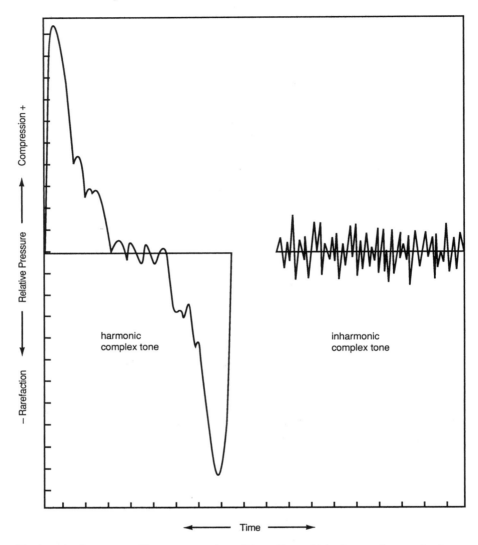

Figure 2.1 Spectrographic representation of the pattern of (a) a harmonic complex tone and (b) an inharmonic complex tone.

sounds are *complex*, that is, they are a mixture resulting from many simultaneous vibrations. This complexity is critical to the referential nature of sound because the frequency components can not only differ, but can also be arranged in different combinations. Each combination, if sustained briefly, produces a distinguishable pattern. We refer to patterned sound as *harmonic* (Figure 2.1a). The components of a harmonic sound can be analyzed electronically into the individual frequencies of which it is composed (Figure 2.2). The cochlear performs this same function.

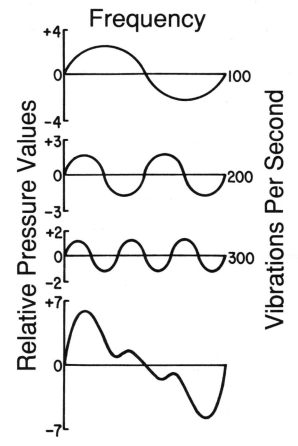

Figure 2.2 Depiction of a harmonic complex tone analysed into its component pure tones.

Complex sound is not always harmonic. When a vibrator oscillates in a random, nonrepetitive manner, it produces *inharmonic* sound (Figure 2.1b). Such vibrations lack pattern. The energy within them may be spread widely across the frequency range or may be concentrated within a narrow bandwidth. They also may vary in the frequency range they occupy. We refer to inharmonic sound as *acoustic noise*.

We know that the vibration of an object in air causes either harmonic or inharmonic complex sounds. When the frequencies contained in the complex sound are in the frequency and intensity range of the ear, the sound will be detected by an intact auditory system when the intensity is sufficient to gain attention. The brain quickly learns the connection between the detection of a sound and the fact that an event caused or is causing the sound. This in turn leads to a search for the source. The connection between the event and the sound establishes a *referential* role for sound. Sound now serves to refer to an event. In the same way we can link a speech sound pattern to an object, event, or an idea so that the speech sound becomes the *referent* to it.

Detecting a sound and then searching to find and identify the sound source is a time-consuming task. If we had to do this unceasingly for every perceptible sound occurring in our environment, we soon would become overwhelmed. We are spared such an impossible task by virtue of the complex nature of sound. Each vibrating body, whether it be a violin or the human vocal folds, vibrates differently. Each vibrator, therefore, sets up a pattern of vibration and a resultant acoustic pattern unique to itself. Thus sound patterns not only indicate an event, they also carry information specific to that event. Those patterns can be differentiated by the auditory system, allowing us to attribute specific meanings to individual environmental sounds and to different patterns of speech sounds. The acoustic signal thus comes to serve as a highly specific reference to either an actual event or to an internal value for such an event in the mind of the listener. This knowledge has significant relevance to the development of referential sound discrimination in children and to the impact that hearing impairment will have on this function in both children and adults.

We will have more to learn about the referential role of sound when we discuss communication and perception. What has been said to this point is sufficient to place a consideration of the physical characteristics of a sound into meaningful context. We have seen that a sound is generated when an object vibrates. The vibrating object sets the air molecules in motion in a manner that replicates its own vibrating motion, hence the referential potential of sound. A wave of patterned sound energy thus travels through the air medium. That energy wave can be described by its properties of *frequency, intensity*, and *duration*.

ENVIRONMENTAL SOUNDS

The sounds that occur around us are almost all inharmonic vibrations occurring in an unpatterned manner. Yet we can identify most environmental sounds because they do have discernible characteristics even though they lack pattern. The energy in these sounds is distributed differently by different vibrating sources. A tea kettle will concentrate its energy in the higher frequency ranges producing a whistle. In fact, as the steam pressure builds you can hear the energy band rise in pitch. Machinery vibrating at a slow rate will produce a low humming sound—the result of the energy being concentrated in the low range of frequencies. Some sounds have energy distributed across a wide frequency range, producing a rushing or roaring sound like a waterfall.

The intensity of sounds also helps to characterize them. We are startled by the thump of our heartbeat when it is amplified or when we stand in an anechoic room. We may have heard our heart beating, but never that loudly. We differentiate between the chimes of two clocks because they differ in loudness and pitch. Such differences perhaps seem insignificant to us because we receive such a wealth of information from our acoustic world, far more than we need to identify things. You will not find such luxury when working with a congenitally deaf child who must glean every available bit of information if she is to be able to build a referential picture from the little hearing that remains.

Clocks and kettles and cars and airplanes are not discriminated by pitch and loudness alone. Durational characteristics, including how a sound begins and ends, also carry important acoustic information (Levitt, 1981). For example, the tick of a watch and the tick-tock of a grandfather clock, in addition to having different frequency and intensity characteristics, differ in terms of the rate at which the tick event is repeated and in the duration of each tick. When the toilet cistern fails to shut off, we are alerted because we know how long it should run. It is the durational characteristic that we use to tell when the automatic choke is stuck on our car and is running the engine fast for a period longer than we expect.

The physical characteristics of environmental sounds differ in ways that permit them to be coded to their sources. Hearing impairment removes or distorts some of this information, sometimes to the point of making coding impossible. Part of the assessment of useful residual hearing in children with severe to profound losses includes determining how much potential remains and to what extent the child can be trained to use amplified environmental sound for functional purposes—that means to be able to detect and discriminate sounds in the environment sufficiently well as to know what is making a sound and to be able to respond appropriately (Boothroyd, 1982).

SPEECH SOUNDS

The use of voice to convey information is not confined to humans; it is widely practiced by birds and mammals. Humans, however, have developed this form of communication to a high degree of sophistication by developing a speech code to replace the cipher system used by animals.* Once

---

* Codes differ from ciphers because they allow a limited number of units to be combined and recombined to make an almost unlimited number of combinations. Ciphers contain units that are meaningful in themselves but cannot be broken down and recombined to make new units.

again, we need to consider only those aspects of speech production and acoustics that have bearing upon hearing impairment.

The Vocal Tone

Voice is not absolutely essential to speech communication; all that is necessary is a means of vibrating air passing through the oral cavity. This is evidenced by our ability to talk in a whisper and by individuals who must learn to use esophageal speech or to use an electrolarynx following laryngectomy. The glottis, however, is the most efficient means of vibrating the air medium with sufficient power to permit communication at a distance.

You will recall that the vibration of the glottis during vocal production produces a fundamental tone known as the *glottal tone*. The natural frequency of this tone is determined primarily by the anterior-posterior length of the vocal folds. The greater the length the lower will be the *fundamental frequency* of the glottal tone. The shorter the length of the vocal folds, that is, the smaller the larynx, the higher will be the pitch of the glottal tone. We perceive these differences in the different pitch levels of voices of men, women, and children, or in bass, tenor, alto, and soprano voices. "What," you ask, "has this to do with hearing deficiency?" Well, remember that the glottis produces the speech energy wave. That wave form is complex and for most sounds, harmonic. When the glottal tone is molded to impress articulated speech sounds upon it, all the patterning must occur as overtones of the fundamental. The fundamental frequency of the voice, therefore, determines the frequencies above which the speech pattern will be extended. The patterned information of the speech of men will be concentrated in the low to middle frequency ranges because it is all molded onto a low-pitch glottal tone, ranging from 124 Hz for /a/ to 141 Hz for /u/. The speech information of women, by contrast, is built on a glottal tone that ranges from 212 Hz for /a/ to 235 Hz for /i/, while young children code everything onto a glottal frequency ranging from 251 Hz for /æ/ to 276 Hz for /u/ (Levitt, 1978). The significance of these pitch differences for the purpose of our discussion lies in the effect they have on the relationship between sensorineural hearing deficiency patterns and where the coded information in a speech signal falls on the frequency scale. Two factors are important in this relationship:

- Most sensorineural hearing impairments show increasing deficit with increasing frequency, that is, greater impairment in the highs than in the lows.
- The higher frequency components of the complex speech wave are the weaker components.

So, as the pitch of the fundamental frequency of the voice rises from men's to women's and then even higher to that of children's voices, more and more information is pushed into the higher frequency ranges where hearing impairment is greater. The voice remains audible but the spoken message is perceived to be mumbled. Persons who come for hearing aid fitting often complain to me, "People don't speak clearly; they mumble, particularly women," and they tell me, "I simply can't hear what my young grandchildren say." Similar difficulties are encountered by hearing-impaired children in school. A child may hear a male teacher adequately but complain that a woman teacher fails to speak clearly.

Obviously we cannot insist on all male teachers for hearing-impaired children; they are rare creatures in the teaching world anyway. Nor can we advise hearing-impaired adults to confine their contacts to men. It is important, however, that we understand the relationship between the vocal pitch of the speaker and the discriminability of speech by the hearing-impaired listener. This will ensure that we take this factor into account in assisting the person's difficulties, in planning strategies to reduce the handicap, and in counseling.

I have spoken of molding the glottal tone to carry the speech pattern. We do this at two levels, generating the *suprasegmentals* and *segmentals* of speech.

Suprasegmentals

Suprasegmental characteristics produce the melodic intonational qualities of speech by varying frequency, intensity, rate, and duration. We perceive these pattern characteristics as pitch, loudness, rate, and duration, that is, the amount of time devoted to the production of a given unit of speech. We sometimes speak of suprasegmentals as *prosody*, or the *prosodic* aspects of speech. It was believed originally that the role of suprasegmentals was confined to the conveyance of emotive information or to the resolution of meaning. It has been suggested, however, that the basic function of suprasegmental patterns is to establish constraints that facilitate the identification of the coding patterns used at the level of syntax (Lefevre, 1973; Lieberman, 1967; Martin, 1972). The rhythm pattern of speech serves to identify highly encoded and, therefore, highly informative stressed syllables for early decoding.*

The suprasegmental information is heavily dependent on the patterning of the vocal tone. This suggests that an infant is capable of learning the basic rhythms of speech long before he or she has the capacity to process its segmental components. Evidence to this effect has in fact been provided by Condon and Sander (1973). These researchers demonstrated that even newborn (one-day-old) babies exhibit patterns of precise and sustained movements that are synchronized with the articulated structure of adult speech. The authors suggest that ". . . 'infant motor organization' entrained by these organized patterns for many months after birth may prepare operational formats for later speech" (1973, p. 101). If this assumption proves correct, the effects of hearing impairment on speech acquisition may indeed be maximal from birth. It certainly emphasizes the importance of suprasegmental components, both on the development of speech perception and on the ability to communicate within the normal melodic patterns of the language culture.

---

* For a discussion of this topic see Sanders, 1977, pp. 37–38, 136–139.

The role of early amplification in facilitating perception and production of normal suprasegmental patterning is obviously crucial. Our awareness of the probable importance of the lower frequencies of speech in the acquisition of spoken language is increased by such information. It may lead us, for example, to decide to emphasize frequencies below 1000 Hz for severely hearing-impaired children to provide listening and learning in favorable acoustic conditions.

Early babbling patterns and the subsequent development of jargon depend heavily on control of the vocal tone. Deliberate inflectional use of the voice precedes the ability to produce the specific sound of speech (Kaplan & Kaplan, 1971), the process we refer to as *speech articulation*.

Segmentals

We have seen that part of the molding of the glottal tone produces suprasegmental patterns that carry information. The greatest amount of information, however, is encoded into the glottal tone by the articulatory resonant system of the speech mechanism. You will be familiar with this system from other courses, so I will do no more than review it briefly.

The energy distribution of a complex sound wave can be rearranged by passing it through a resonant cavity. The nature of the pattern arrangement can be varied by changing the resonant sensitivity of the cavity. This is achieved by changing the shape and size of the cavity. The pattern arrangement changes because the resultant wave derives from the interaction of the frequency pattern of the energy entering the resonator and the sensitivity pattern of the resonator. To the extent that energy in a given frequency range in the sound wave matches the sensitivity of the resonator it will be enhanced, *resonated*. When no such coincidence occurs, the energy in those frequency ranges will be reduced, *damped*. A flexible resonator system, such as the coupling of the cavities of the pharynx, nasopharynx, nose, and mouth, permits the shape of the resonator to be changed to many different configurations. Each configuration arranges the complex energy wave of the glottal tone into a unique pattern leaving the fundamental frequency, or pitch, unchanged. Thus, each articulatory resonant pattern generates a correlated acoustic pattern. This relationship can be seen clearly in the production of the vowel sounds.

Vowels

In normal speech, vowels are produced with vocalization, the complex glottal tone energy being rearranged uniquely by each articulatory-resonant vowel production posture. The rearrangement of the total glottal energy, as it occurs in the production of the vowels /i/, /a/, and /u/, can be seen in Figure 2.3.

Consider what these spectra can tell us that is of importance to an understanding of auditory perception of vowels and the way in which hearing deficiency can impair this. Note that three amplitude concentrations occur for each vowel. They reflect the natural resonant frequencies of the

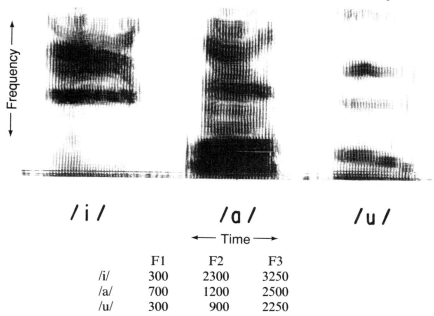

Frequency →

/ i /   / ɑ /   / u /

← Time →

	F1	F2	F3
/i/	300	2300	3250
/a/	700	1200	2500
/u/	300	900	2250

Figure 2.3 A spectrogram of the vowels /i/, /a/, /u/.

cavities while positioned to produce a given vowel. The position of these bands of energy, called *formants*, on the vertical frequency scale is different for each vowel; however, some of the formants of different vowels fall very close in frequency. The concentrations of energy weaken in intensity as they fall further along the frequency scale.

To identify a vowel in isolation on the basis of its acoustic structure alone, it is necessary to receive the first and second formant information. The F1 and F2 values for each of the vowels shown in Figure 2.3 are depicted. Look, for example, at the values for the vowel /a/. The first formant for this vowel peaks at 700 Hz, while the F2 value for /a/ is 1200 Hz. By contrast, F1 for /i/ is 300 Hz and F2 is 2300 Hz. It should be apparent from this information that a person with good residual hearing in the low frequencies but a deficit in the higher frequencies may well hear the F1 of both /a/ and /i/ quite clearly. However, because of high frequency deficit, the same person may hear the F2 for /a/ at 1200 Hz but not the F2 for /i/ at 2300 Hz. The likelihood of this occurring is increased when you realize that the total energy and duration of /a/ are considerably greater than those of /i/.

The values shown for the formants are for the natural vocal pitch of a male speaker. As we have seen already, vocal pitch changes with intonation and changes even more dramatically from male to female to child speaker. Vowel perception is dependent upon F1 and F2 information but not on the absolute frequency of each formant since this changes with the fundamental frequency of the glottal tone. An /a/ remains recognizable as an /a/ regardless of the pitch at which it is spoken, despite the different frequencies of F1 and F2 at each pitch. What remains constant is the difference frequency between F1 and F2 (F2 − F1). The increase in the frequency of the glottal tone from which these formants are derived naturally moves the formant values into the higher frequency ranges where hearing impairment is usually most severe. I need to point out, however, that the perception of vowels is not entirely dependent upon the reception of full formant information. As we will discuss later, the perception of speech is only partly dependent upon the signal received. Even in the acoustic signal itself, redundancy often permits the perception of something not actually received at the periphery. This is possible because of the influence of adjacent sounds on the production of a given speech sound in context. We will consider this influence after we have examined consonants.

Consonants

Vowels alone comprise just a small part of the sounds used in speech; few words consist entirely of vowels or dipthongs. The vowels carry the energy of speech but not very much information. It is the consonants that contribute most to the identification of words and phrases; we use more of them and they are more informative than vowels. Consider, for example, the word *multiplication*. You are more likely to fill in the gaps correctly when vowels are omitted, as in m-lt-pl-c-t--n than when consonants are omitted: -u--i--i-a-io-. Consonants may or may not contain vocalization and, therefore, may or may not have harmonic complex structure. A few consonants, notably /m/, /n/, /l/, and /r/, present harmonic wave forms very much like those of a vowel. Generally what differentiates a consonant from a vowel is that its production includes an articulatory movement that obstructs, or greatly restricts, the flow of air passing through the larynx to the articulatory resonant system. Consonants are described by the place and manner of their production. From the acoustic imprint of this information, it is possible for the brain to identify a sound on the basis of where and how it was articulated (Liberman, Shankweiler, & Studdert-Kennedy, 1967). Thus, information that a sound carries the evidence of a complete stopping of the air flow identifies it as being in the category of /p/, /b/, /t/, /d/, /k/, /g/ as does the subsequent release of air that identifies these sounds as plosives. Fricatives narrow the air passage but do not block it, producing the friction sound that characterizes /s/, /z/, /ʃ/, /tʃ/, /dʒ/, /f/, /v/. The point I wish to make is that articulation is creating a pattern of acoustic information characteristic of a given category of consonant sounds (e.g., fricatives, plosives, nasals). Within each category additional constraints, such as voicing and place of articulation, further delineate a given sound from other members of its category. No one piece of acoustic information can identify a consonant, for many share a particular characteristic (i.e., plosion). It is a unique combination of the various clues that unequivocally identifies a single consonant. The elimination or weakening of any of the informational constraints that contribute to the definitive identification of a consonant will cause it to be indistinguishable from other consonants in its category, may leave it audible but unclassifiable, or in extreme cases may cause it to be inaudible as an isolated sound. Fortunately neither consonants nor vowels are uttered in isolation. They are linked in the speech stream by the process of *coarticulation*, which results in acoustic *transitions*. These transitions provide a wealth of information that the hearing-impaired person draws upon for comprehension.

Transitions

We speak at a rate that precludes precise articulation of each speech sound. The exact articulatory postures by which, in phonetics, you learn to describe speech sounds, are *targets*. These targets always are approximated in connected speech, for that is essential to the identity of a speech sound, but rarely if ever are they fulfilled exactly. This fact necessitates, therefore, that our speech discrimination/recognition system has the capacity to tolerate the acoustic variations in a speech sound that derive from articulatory variability. This tolerance is achieved by processing speech at the syllabic level. A syllable contains the acoustic information arising from the smooth production of several sounds. Each of those sounds is melded, or fused, with its neighbors to constitute a unit. The fusing is made possible by the articulatory process you know as coarticulation. Coarticulation means that the articulation of a given speech sound in phonetic context is distinctly influenced by both the sound that precedes it and that which follows it. In fact, Daniloff (1973) has shown that though weakened as proximity is reduced, coarticulatory effects are evidenced backward and forward across as many as five phonemes. Consider the implications of this for speech discrimination and recognition. What this says is that at any instant in time, you are receiving not only acoustic information concerning the speech sound being articulated, but also *confirmatory* information of the two sounds that preceded it and *predictive* information about the two sounds that will follow. We use the term *parallel encoding* to identify this layering in, or sandwiching, of information in the acoustic signal that results from coarticulation. The parallel encoded information is to be found almost exclusively in the transitions between sounds.

Transitions arise from the movement of the articulators, primarily the tongue, toward and away from the target positions for adjacent speech sounds. Since there is no break in the vocal articulatory production, acoustic information is being generated between the targets. An example of transition information can be seen in the spectrum of a sentence shown in Figure 2.4. The articulatory movements between targets will vary depending upon the particular posture from which the articulators are moving away and the one they are aiming to assume. As a result, the transition between a given vowel and different consonants will vary but always will be constant for any given consonant-vowel combination in a given speaker. For example, the transition arising from /d/ to /i/ will be different from the transition from /d/ to /u/ (Figure 2.5a). Each transition, therefore, is characteristic of the adjacency of particular sounds. So each speech sound in context not only

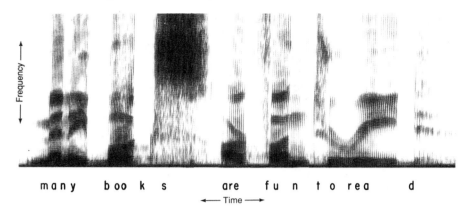

many   b oo k   s   are   fu   n   t   o   rea   d

← Time →

Figure 2.4   Sound spectrogram of the sentence "Many books are fun to read."

has its own acoustic structure, resulting from place and manner of production, but also embodies information about its neighbors. Your awareness of this information will be important in developing a rationale for intensive auditory training to increase perception by increasing confidence in using predictive information. Other constraint information arises from the intensity, frequency, and durational characteristics of speech sound production. We discussed how these characteristics help us to identify environmental sounds. They operate in a similar manner in contributing to the total pattern of information that characterizes any given speech sound.

Figure 2.5a   Sound spectrogram showing formant structure of vowels /i/, /a/, /u/ in transition from the consonant /d/.

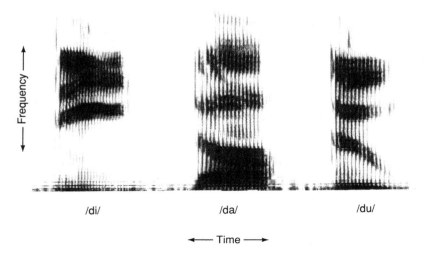

/di/   /da/   /du/

← Time →

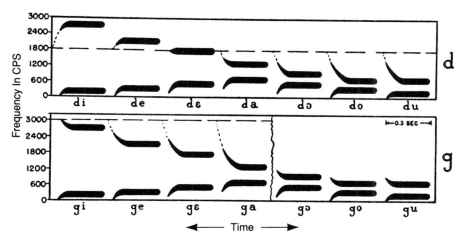

Figure 2.5b Transitions for the consonants /d/ and /g/ with various vowels. (Liberman 1957.)

Frequency Constraints

We have described the glottal tone as a complex sound wave whose energy is rearranged into formants by the articulatory resonant system. The pattern of formant distribution across the frequency range was seen always to characterize a specific articulatory resonant posture for a specific vowel or voiced consonant. The actual frequency bands that define the first and second formants rise and fall with the pitch of the glottal tone. The identifying information, therefore, cannot be the actual frequencies involved, for it has to be a measure that remains constant. That constant has been shown to be the difference-frequency between F1 and F2. This can be illustrated by simple number relationships. For example, the relationship between the following pairs (F2 minus F1) is constant even though the numbers change: $12 - 24, 25 - 50, 64 - 128$, as it is for $7 - 10, 14 - 17, 27 - 30$. Similarly the following $F1 - F2$ values for /a/ differ in absolute values but all have the same difference frequency: $680 - 1300, 715 - 1335, 766 - 1386$. This formant relationship can be seen clearly in Figure 2.5b. It explains why a vowel sound always is recognizable even though uttered at different vocal pitches. It also explains why, for many hearing deficit patterns, we cannot predict categorically whether a particular voiced sound can or cannot be discriminated. Our concern, therefore, must be to determine whether there are any pitch ranges, and any phonetic contexts, in which the sound is discriminable. This information is particularly important when attempting to improve a speaker's production of a given sound.

Formant frequency information is not generated in the production of unvoiced consonants. These, however, do have frequency characteristics that make them different. The energy in unvoiced consonants tends to concentrate in certain frequency ranges. For example, the /s/ sound at conversational speech intensity centers in a narrow band around 3600 Hz. The sh, /ʃ/, sound by comparison is broader in bandwidth and centers much lower on the frequency scale at around 1600 Hz. So, for a person with a high-frequency loss sloping sharply from 1500 Hz, /ʃ/ will be easily recognized but /s/ probably will be inaudible.

I wish to stress again that no one characteristic of speech is totally responsible for speech sound recognition even at the syllabic level. You should be thinking of each of these characteristics as contributing to a pool of clues to identification. What may seem a rather small amount of potential information available from one aspect of the speech signal may mean the difference between recognition and nonrecognition of a sound by a person with impaired hearing. It will be our task, later, to put all these potential resources together in our training model in a manner that maximizes the amount of information available to the hearing-impaired individual.

Intensity Constraints

The constraints imposed on the listener's decoding of the acoustic speech signal by intensity characteristics are less well defined, less precise than frequency clues. Hearing-impaired persons, however, often must manage on a very, very low information budget; every little *bit*, as information units are called, counts. Remember also that intensity and frequency are two measures of the same event, so if intensity in a given frequency range is reduced, the frequency cues may become inaudible. The symbiotic relationship between intensity and frequency explains why sounds, perfectly discriminable at some intensities, become blurred or inaudible when intensity decreases as it does, for example, with increasing distance. When we discuss amplification, you will see that tailoring the amplification pattern to meet various intensity needs at different frequencies can enhance discrimination better than amplifying the total speech signal equally.

The intensity of speech is determined by air pressure from the lungs and by the extent of vocal fold movement. The overall speech intensity varies from minimal loudness, around 30dB SPL (40dB HL*), to 80dB SPL (70dB HL) for loud conversational voice measured 3 feet from the speaker. Average conversational speech intensity is 50dB HL. These figures represent total sound pressure levels averaged over time. Speech intensity is different for different speech sounds and varies with intonation. Most of the energy, as we have seen already, is contributed by the vowels and is distributed at the low and midfrequency range of the speech spectrum. Consonants are weaker in intensity and have components in the higher frequency ranges. The different powers of speech sounds relative to the weakest sound /θ/ are shown in Table 2.1. As you can see, the relative differences are great. Even for persons with only moderate hearing deficits, the effect of an overall decrease in vocal intensity often reduces the intensity of the weaker sounds below audibility. It also is helpful to realize that the

---

* HL refers to *hearing level* reference OdB on the audiometer. *Sound pressure level* (SPL) is physical measure of all energy present reference .002 microbar.

TABLE 2.1 Relative phonetic powers of speech sounds as produced by an average speaker

ɔ	680	l	100	t	15
ɑ	600	ʃ	80	g	15
ʌ	510	ŋ	73	k	13
æ	490	m	52	v	12
ʊ	460	t®	42	ð	11
ɛ	350	n	36	b	7
u	310	ʤ	23	d	7
ı	260	ʒ	20	p	6
i	220	z	16	f	5
r	210	s	16	θ	1

Adapted from Fletcher (1953).

intensity values for the vowels, which here are represented for a constant phonetic consonant-vowel-consonant context, change as the consonants change. Even such minor details contribute to the sum total of contextual cues that the brain uses to identify speech patterns.

Durational Constraints

Speech occurs over time. Each component, sound, syllable, word, and phrase takes a certain amount of time to articulate. The amount of time varies sufficiently among sounds for the brain to use the information to further constrain the possible choices it must make in identifying a sound pattern. The sounds with the longest duration are the vowels, which range from 100–200 milliseconds in durations (Bode, 1975). Consonants are of much shorter duration, some as brief as 40 milliseconds. The shorter the duration of a sound, the more difficult it becomes for the listener to identify it (Gerber, 1974). Not only do these sounds provide the listener less decoding time, but because they are short, they tend to be less precisely articulated and thus carry less information.

By controlling the durational characteristics of speech, particularly at the syllabic level, suprasegmental information, that is to say, the melodic characteristics arising from variations in vocal pitch, duration, and intensity, is encoded. Duration is one of the characteristics of stressed syllables that results from a combination of intensity, frequency, and durational patterning. It serves the primary function of identifying the highly encoded syllables as well as adding emphasis to semantic content.

In processing speech, the absence of sound also may be informative. The brief silent interval that occurs before all stop consonants cues this category of sounds, while pauses of longer duration carry syntactic information. Each of these characteristics contributes to the speech patterns creating unique combinations to which linguistic values are ascribed. These sound qualities are informative. By contrast, other influences affect the acoustic signal negatively, weakening it, or adding or subtracting vibrations that, when blended into the original pattern, smear it. It is equally important that you be familiar with these negative influences and with the functional implications they can have for persons with impaired hearing. This will be our topic for the next chapter.

SUMMARY

In this chapter we considered the following important concepts:

- Sound serves as an equivalent of an event. Once we have made the connection between sound and its source, sound serves a referential function.
- Sound production produces complex waves. Those that are harmonic are patterned, those that are inharmonic are not.
- Acoustic patterns become learned so we are able to attribute meaning to them rapidly. They refer to internal values and memories.
- Speech consists mostly of harmonic patterns molded from the vocal tone. These patterns are both segmental and suprasegmental.
- The articulatory molding rearranges the energy in the glottal tone by varying the shape and size of the coupled resonator system. This produces concentrations of energy called formants. F1 and F2 are crucial for speech sound identification in isolation. It is the vowels that carry the energy.
- Articulation of consonants primarily involves the narrowing or stopping of the air stream. Consonants carry most of speech information.
- Consonant acoustic information is less intense, with higher frequency components than vowels. Discrimination of consonants thus is affected sooner by hearing impairment, particularly in the higher frequency ranges.
- The acoustic transitions that result from coarticulation meld sounds into larger patterns. Each sound thus contains confirmatory and predictive information about adjacent sounds; this is called parallel encoding.
- Frequency, intensity, and durational variations among speech sounds create patterns of informational cues that narrow the task of identifying the sound.
- The use of stress derived from intensity, frequency, and durational information identifies syllables rich in information, keys syntactic processing, and contributes to suprasegmental interpretive information.

Conclusion

From the topics we have discussed, we can conclude that the role of sound as a referent is crucial to our relationship with the auditory world. The referential function of sound is its communicative value both in terms of environmental sound and speech. The unique characteristics of acoustic events, most particularly of speech articulation events, enables us to attribute values to them that equate to our experience. In speech, acoustic patterns that relate directly to our language code are generated by the molding of the glottal tone by the articulatory resonant system. The continuous nature of the speech event results in a rich information-bearing pattern, each section of which bears new information as well as confirmatory and predictive information. The end result is to produce redundancy that actually reduces our dependence upon the processing of the fine details of the acoustic signal. This in part is necessary to help combat the negative influences exerted during the transmission of that signal.

3

Factors Limiting Acoustic Speech Processing

The problems resulting from impairment of hearing, as we will see, are many. However, at the base of them lies the inability of the cochlea to record accurately the pattern of acoustic information in the speech signal. That pattern provides the instructions essential for the easy reconstruction of the message being conveyed. If at any stage energy is added or subtracted, the pattern will be distorted with a resulting loss of information. The most obvious source of distortion is of course the defective cochlea. There are, however, a number of factors that may distort the signal before it reaches the ear. Given the loss of information resulting from the hearing impairment, these external factors often constitute critical negative influences on speech comprehension. A knowledge of these influences will be important when we discuss, for example, how the child with a hearing impairment hears in the classroom, how seating position affects auditory discrimination, how one aid may be better than two in noisy settings, and how amplification has been modified to combat acoustic distortion.

NOISE

We have described acoustic noise* as energy that is not informative to a listener; one might simply call it *unwanted* sound. This is a helpful definition because it takes into consideration whether the listener can use noise. We tend to think of acoustic noise in the general sense of sound generated by machinery, traffic, aircraft, lawn mowers, and so on. Yet you will agree that a neighbor's barbecue or pool party, to which you have not been invited, also constitutes noise, particularly when you can hear every word. The blaring stereo music also is unwanted, be it Beethoven or rock. Thus, noise has both acoustic and psychological correlates. In this section, we will consider only the acoustic factor; later we will discuss the impact of noise on attention, memory, and learning.

Acoustic Noise Levels

You know from personal experience that when you wish to pay attention to what someone is saying you want the room to be fairly quiet. A radio or TV playing, the dishwasher running, or other people talking makes it difficult to listen. This is because the energy in noise masks the speech signal. It blends with the speech signal, making it difficult to perceive the speech pattern in the total acoustic pattern. The greater the intensity of the noise, the greater will be the masking effect. In fact, if the intensity is great enough, as in some factories, conversational speech may be inaudible. Every environment contains acoustic noise; however, until it reaches 30dB HL, that is 30dB above audiometric zero, speech discrimination for normal-hearing persons will not be impaired. The frequencies in which noise will have its most serious effects lie, naturally, in the speech frequency range. Thus, tolerance for noise decreases as the energy extends into the middle and higher frequency ranges. This is because the speech energy in this range is weaker and also carries far more information. In Figure 3.1 you can see for classroom speech levels how the energy is distributed across frequencies from 125 to 8000 Hz, the average spectrum of speech over time, and the noise criterion. The noise criterion (NC-25) is the desirable limit of 30dBA that has been established for room noise originating from heating ventilation and air conditioning.* Unfortunately the noise criterion is seldom met, even in schools for the deaf because, in addition to the heating or air-conditioning noise, sound enters classrooms from the outside of the building, particularly in the warmer months when windows are open. It comes also from adjacent classrooms and from pupil activities. In a survey

---

* The term *noise* in this chapter refers to unwanted sound. In an information-processing context, the term refers to any influence that reduces information in the message during encoding, transmission, or decoding.
* Sound pressure levels can be expressed on an unweighted scale dBC in which the sound level meter is equally sensitive to all frequencies from 16–20,000 Hz or on a weighted scale dBA, which measures only the amount of energy to which the human ear is sensitive.

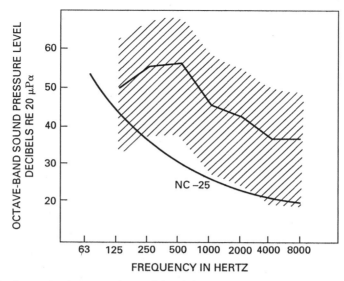

Figure 3.1 Approximate range of speech levels in a classroom (shaded region) and their relationship to NC–25 Noise Criterion Levels. The solid curve within the shaded region is the long-term average spectrum of speech. (From Bess, B. A. Freeman, B. A. & Sinclair, J. S. [Eds.]. *Amplification in Education*, p. 173) Washington DC: Alexander Graham Bell Assn. for the Deaf. 1981.)

of 47 classrooms in 15 schools (Sanders, 1965), I recorded average noise levels as high as 69dB in kindergarten classes with peak intensities to 75dB. The levels recorded in different types of classes are shown in Table 3.1. Later studies (Blair, 1977; Ross & Giolas, 1971) produced remarkably similar results.

Signal-to-Noise Ratio (S/N)

As you might expect, the human communication system has evolved a mechanism for combating the masking effects of acoustic noise; we call it the *Lombard effect*. This is the name given to the reflex that causes our vocal intensity to increase as environmental noise increases. It has been shown that our vocal intensity rises 6dB for each 10dB increase in background

TABLE 3.1 Mean values of ambient noise in occupied classrooms in four types of school environments. (Sanders 1965)

Type of School	Mean Value of Room Noise in dB Re: Sensation Level	Standard Deviation
Kindergarten	69	8.5
Primary school	59	6.2
High school	62	8.1
Special classes for the hearing-impaired child	52	4.7

TABLE 3.2 Teachers' speech levels in schools. (Cited in Pearsons, 1980, p. 167.)

CONDITION	*A LEVEL*
Background Noise Level	*50*
One meter from the teacher	71
Front of the classroom	64
Rear of the classroom	60

noise (Rupf, 1977). Pearsons, Bennett, and Fidell (1977) showed that in the classroom, the teacher uses a lecture voice level much higher than that of conversational speech, producing a decibel level of 71dBA measured at a one-meter distance from the speaker (Table 3.2). Up to a point, raising the voice increases intelligibility. However, for distances greater than six inches, the discrimination maximum drops sharply at intensities greater than 70dB due to distortion. Even more apparent is the limitation placed on maximum discrimination by distance from the speaker. This cannot be compensated for by talking louder; moving closer, however, results in dramatic improvement in intelligibility. This is a very important fact to communicate to the hearing-impaired person. Thus to some extent we can compensate for the masking effects of noise by involuntarily raising our voices, though moving closer is far more effective. When we do this, we aim to produce speech at an intensity level above the noise that maintains a constant favorable ratio of speech to noise; we call this the *signal-to-noise ratio*, abbreviated as S/N. Occasionally this will be referred to as the signal-to-competition ratio (S/C). When the speech signal is greater than the noise, the ratio is expressed in positive figures, indicating by how many dB the signal exceeds the noise, for example, signal = 50dB, noise = 30dB, S/N = +20dB. When noise exceeds the signal in intensity, the number will be negative, for example, signal = 30dB, noise = 50dB, S/N = −20dB. When signal and noise are equal, speech = 50dB, noise = 50dB, S/N = 0dB. When there is no noise in an environment in very low reverberant conditions, a person with normal hearing will obtain maximum discrimination. As the noise level increases, the ability to discriminate falls until a negative S/N ratio is reached at around S/N = −12dB, at which level speech ceases to be intelligible. The masking effect will be determined by the range of frequencies contained in the noise. The wider the noise bandwidth, the greater will be the masking effect. The greatest masking effect occurs when the competing noise is speech.

A number of researchers have investigated the relationship between S/N ratio and discrimination scores both for normal-hearing and hearing-impaired persons. At this point we are concerned only with those figures relative to normal hearing. The results indicate that noise alone reduces the word discrimination scores of hearing children from 95 percent in quiet to 80 percent at S/N = +6dB. A +6dB ratio represents the normal ratio of a teacher's voice to classroom noise in normal school classrooms. When S/N = 0dB, word discrimination drops to 60 percent (Finitzo-Hieber & Tillman, 1978). These figures, however, indicate *only* the effects of noise because they were made in a totally nonreverberant *anechoic* chamber. Reverberation itself reduces discrimination significantly as we will now see. Thus when noise and reverberation and distance are combined, the effects on speech discrimination, even by normal-hearing persons, can be devastating.

REVERBERATION

Reverberation is a phenomenon by which the *direct acoustic wave*, that is to say, the signal, bounces off reflective surfaces back into the acoustic space. The reflected *indirect acoustic wave* pattern then blends its out-of-date pattern containing old information with the direct wave carrying new information. The effect is to smear the speech pattern (Nabelek & Robinette, 1978). The bouncing of sound off walls, blackboards, windows, floor, ceiling, and other nonabsorbent surfaces in the room continues until the energy in the indirect wave is used up. We calculate the reverberation time, which is a function of the absorption characteristics of a room, by measuring the time it takes for the energy in a 1000 Hz tone to fall by 60dB once sound is terminated. Thus, a classroom with a 1.0-second reverberation time would have information one second old blended into the incoming direct speech wave pattern.

Speech discrimination scores in quiet have been shown to drop for normal-hearing listeners when reverberation times exceed 0.35 to 0.4 seconds (Bolt & MacDonald, 1949), though Crum and Tillman (1973) state a more liberal figure of 0.8 seconds. Table 3.3 shows the discrimination scores obtained by subjects listening in quiet in different reverberation times in three studies. It can be seen that a noticeable drop occurs between 0.5 and 1.2 seconds, but approximately 75 percent of the words remain intelligible. However, by the time 2 seconds is exceeded, the discrimination drops into the 65 percent range. Thus, rooms in which listening, and particularly learning, are to take place should have reverberation times of 0.6–0.8 seconds for large classrooms and 0.4 seconds for small rooms (Olsen, 1977; Ross, 1978). Unfortunately, normal school classrooms seldom even approach this goal. Thomas (1960) found reverberation times in classrooms to range between 1.3 and an amazing 3.4 seconds. Presumably in the latter case a child arriving a little late for school would miss nothing!

As you can imagine, when the two negative influences coexist, the resulting effect is serious and certainly exceeds the sum of each individual effect.

TABLE 3.3 Discrimination scores for normal-hearing subjects in quiet for various reverberation times

	REVERBERATION TIME IN SECONDS						
Study	*0*	*0.4*	*0.9*	*1.2*	*1.6*	*2.3*	*2.4*
Finitzo-Hieber & Tillman (1978)	95%	92%		76%			
Houtgast & Steeneken (1973)	99%			84%			66%
Moncur & Dirks (1967)	97%		80%		67%	60%	

INTERACTION OF NOISE AND REVERBERATION

The interactive effects of noise and reverberation have been demonstrated in a number of studies. The results obtained for normal-hearing persons in several of these are shown in Table 3.3. The discrimination scores in quiet listening conditions, as we have seen, deteriorate as a function of reverberation times that exceed 1 second. In a signal-to-noise ratio of +6dB, typical of regular classrooms, that decrease is severe at 1.2 seconds with discrimination for monosyllabic words dropping close to the 50 percent level. When long-term sound pressure averages for speech and noise are equal (S/N = 0dB), not an uncommon occurrence in noisy rooms, the score is reduced by a third even without reverberation. At approximately 1.5 seconds reverberation, two-thirds of the words become inaudible. Remember, these figures are for persons with normal hearing and language.

SPEAKER-LISTENER DISTANCE

The influence of room noise on speech intelligibility has been studied to determine at what intensity level interference occurs. Noise levels are calculated by averaging the energy at 500, 1K, 2K, and 4K. The *Speech Interference Level* (SIL) is then defined as the point at which communication becomes *just reliable*. The just reliable conversation level for normal-hearing adults corresponds to an effective speech-to-noise ratio of 0dB (Houtgast, 1980). Voice at normal conversational loudness at 1 meter is 65dBA; raised voice (i.e., lecture level) is 71dBA; very loud voice, 77dBA; and a shout, 83dBA. From Figure 3.2 you will see that in classroom noise of 60dBA, which is designated the speech interference level, a raised teaching voice (71dB) will cause conversation to fall to the level of just reliable at 7 feet and normal

Figure 3.2 Talker-to-listener distances for just reliable communication. This refers to free-field conditions. (From ANSI S3.14–1977.)

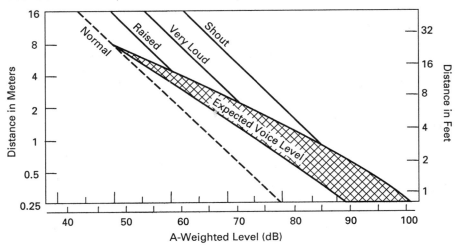

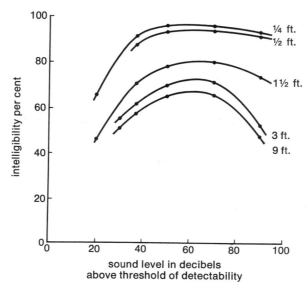

Figure 3.3 The effect of room acoustics on speech discrimination as a function of voice intensity and distance from the speaker. (John 1957)

voice level (65dB) at 4 feet. If the noise level rises to 70dB (S/N = 0), a teaching voice is just reliable at 4 feet while normal voice is barely understandable at 2 feet. It is well to remember that S/N = 0dB is an unfavorable ratio at which normal-hearing persons can *just* rely on their understanding of what is being said in normal conversation. Comfortable S/N ratios lie between +10 and +15dB for those of us with normal hearing and language. The more difficult the listening task, particularly if we are required to learn from a lecture, the better the S/N ratio we need to understand. Moving closer to the speaker does increase the S/N ratio and thus the tolerance for speech interference.

The effect of distance on speech intelligibility of normal-hearing listeners as a function of the intensity of the speech above threshold of detectability and the distance from the speaker was shown by John (1957). The speech was heard through a hearing aid. From Figure 3.3 it can be seen that speech at 60dB HL results in approximately 65 percent intelligibility at a 9-foot distance, a score not increased by increasing the voice intensity. At 1.5 feet the discrimination increases to 80 percent while at 6 inches the score approximates 100 percent. For distances above 1.5 feet, we observe a dramatic decrease in discrimination when the speech level is raised above 70dB HL.

CRITICAL DISTANCE

The distance of the listener from the speaker also impacts on the effects of reverberation. We discussed the problem of the listener's receiving the direct speech wave in competition with the reverberated indirect wave. At some point the intensity of the direct and indirect waves will be equal; this distance is called *critical distance* (Niemoeller, 1981); below it the direct speech wave will be dominant, while beyond it the indirect wave will dominate. The critical distance is inversely related to the absorption characteristics of the room. In classrooms with long reverberation times, the critical distance will be short, necessitating that a hearing-impaired child be moved as close to the teacher as possible. Seating distance from the teacher is thus a crucial consideration for the management of the hearing-impaired child both in terms of noise interference and reverberation effects.

DIRECTIVITY OF THE SPEAKER'S VOICE

Because a speaker's voice has a directional quality, its reception by the listener will be affected by the angle at which the speech signal reaches him. Different frequencies are affected by directivity to different degrees, with the high frequencies experiencing greater attenuation than the low ones. Figure 3.4 shows the relative sound pressure levels of the 500 Hz and 4000 Hz components of the human voice measured at different angles around the speaker's head. The 0 degree azimuth represents a position directly in line with the speaker's lips. The acoustic sound pressure decreases by 16dB at right angles to the lips (90° and 270°). We have seen that a teacher's voice averages 5dB above classroom noise. It is reasonable to assume therefore that a child who is just able to understand when spoken to face-to-face may lose comprehension completely when the teacher turns to address another

Figure 3.4 Directivity patterns for a typical human talker at 500 and 4000 Hz. Curves represent third-octave band data averaged over a group of three men and three women. (Niemoeller 1981.)

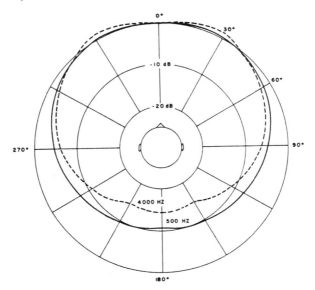

child. This situation becomes of great concern when a child or adult is wearing a single hearing aid, since speech originating on the unaided side will experience considerable attenuation by the time it reaches the other side of the head. The significance of this knowledge adds much weight to the argument for fitting two hearing aids whenever possible.

DIRECTIVITY OF THE LISTENER

Unfortunately one of the problems we still face when fitting hearing aids is ensuring that a person does obtain a binaural fitting except when contraindicated. One would not recommend two hearing aids, for example, when the hearing in one ear is within normal limits or when it has no usable residual hearing. Nor would two hearing aids be advised if the aided binaural discrimination proved poorer than the monaural results. With a few exceptions audiologists believe in the superiority of true binaural amplification. Unfortunately, we do not always practice what we believe. Sometimes the child or adult objects to two aids for psychological reasons, or even when acceptable two aids may not be an option financially. The acoustic advantage of two aids derives from a number of factors that we will discuss later. However, even considering just directivity emphasizes the binaural benefit.

Directivity of both listener and speaker "effectively increases or decreases the direct-to-reverberant sound ratio at the eardrum depending on the orientation of the listener's head" (Niemoeller, 1981, p. 173). Figure 3.4 indicates the variations in directional sensitivity of the human ear as measured on the KEMAR manikin designed by Knowles Electronics, Inc., for acoustic research and measurements. The greatest sensitivity of each ear occurs between 60 and 90 degree angles from directly ahead of the listener. It is obvious that two ears are essential for all around pick-up of sound and that a binaurally hearing-impaired person will have increased difficulty in hearing what is said on the unaided side if only one aid is worn.

SUMMARY

- Factors that limit the reception of the acoustic signal are highly detrimental because they further reduce information already diminished by impaired hearing.
- Acoustic noise is defined as unwanted sound.
- Noise is most detrimental when it falls in the frequency range of speech, most particularly in the 500–4000 Hz range.
- Noise is less important if the signal intensity is raised well above that of the noise resulting in a high ($+$) signal-to-noise (S/N) or signal-to-competition (S/C) ratio.
- An S/N of $+6$dB is representative of a teacher's speech in a school classroom.
- Reverberation refers to the decay of a sound in a room. Decaying sound (echo) distorts current sound patterns and reduces information.
- Classroom reverberation times in the 1.3–3.4 second range far exceed the recommended range of 0.4–0.8 seconds.
- Noise and reverberation interact to result in serious sound pattern distortion with a resultant drop in auditory discrimination.
- Distance from the source further reduces information by decreasing signal intensity.

Just reliable conversational distance is a factor of the level of speech and the noise interference level. In 63dB of noise, conversation drops to just reliable at 3 feet.
- Critical distance refers to the distance at which reverberation seriously diminishes speech intelligibility. It is inversely related to the absorption characteristics of the room.
- Directivity is the measure of the angle of a sound source to an ear—a factor that significantly affects discrimination in poor acoustic environments. The ear is most sensitive at an angle from 60–90 degrees from directly ahead.
- Directivity makes binaural hearing very important in most communication situations.

Conclusion

We can conclude, therefore, that our concern must be directed as much to the acoustic signal in the transmission stage between speaker and listener as to the compensation for predicted distortion of that signal at the cochlear. The primary influences to be combatted are noise and reverberation, since in combination these result in significant decreases in speech discrimination by hearing persons. Maximizing the signal-to-noise ratio is the primary goal. We endeavor to achieve this by ensuring that the listener is within the critical distance and that both speaker and listener directivity is optimal. We also look to technology to help us overcome the negative effects of long reverberation time.

4

The Visual Signal

Asked whether vision plays an important role in speech communication, most people probably would say no. After all, blind people seem to understand speech without difficulty, we have no problem listening to the radio, and we talk on the telephone all without the aid of vision. It appears that under favorable conditions there is more than enough information in the acoustic signal for it alone to convey the information necessary for the listener to comprehend the spoken message. We have already seen that coarticulation encodes extra information into speech patterns, and later we will see that because of language familiarity, under normal circumstances we depend on only half the acoustic information to reconstruct meaning. Even so you probably prefer to watch news on TV rather than to listen to it on the radio, you choose to sit in the front of a lecture hall or church in order to see the speaker clearly, and you are willing to pay more for orchestra seats when attending a play or even a concert, particularly if there is a soloist. What does this suggest? It implies that those of us with normal hearing appreciate seeing what is occurring even when the visual signal includes no more than a view of the person speaking. Obviously we derive information from the visual signal that enriches that available in the auditory signal. In so doing *visual information decreases our dependency upon listening,* reducing the need to process the details of the acoustic pattern. This, in turn, allows us to devote more of our attention to the linguistic pattern, to note the choice of words and the manner in which the message is phrased. We have more time as the speaker is talking to consider the meaning of what is being said. Sometimes, when listening to a nonnative English speaker, the language and articulation deviate so much from the norms for English that by the time we have realized what has been said we have lost track of the message.

Hearing impairment, by reducing acoustic information, puts a heavy stress on the speech perceptual processing system. It slows down the rate at which the signal can be decoded, making it difficult to follow the meaning of what is being said. Thus we must look to every potential source of supplementary information. Vision is such a source, so it is of importance to examine the nature of visual constraints in communication so that we can build visual communication training into our intervention model. First we will examine the sources of visual information that contribute to the reception, comprehension, and interpretation of spoken language; then we will consider some of the significant characteristics of visual cues received.

RELEVANT VISUAL INFORMATION

Speech communication is part of a larger communicative act. We participate in a continuous stream of communication events, each occurring in a particular setting, each involving different participants playing different roles. We wear different costumes in different roles, vary the manner in which we communicate to fit each role, and use different props to support our part. Goffman (1967) describes face-to-face interaction in natural settings as comprising "glances, gestures, positionings, and verbal statements that people continuously feed into the situation, whether intended or not." This is the resource of information that we try to enable the hearing-impaired person, child or adult, to use more efficiently. Just as Sherlock Holmes at the scene of a crime observes clues that dear Dr. Watson had not noticed, so can hearing-impaired people learn heightened awareness of extra information available to the visual system. Information, however, as I already pointed out, is not in itself meaningful. To be referential it must be fitted together to make a pattern. Visual communication enhancement requires that training activities heighten a person's awareness of the speech communication act *in context*. We try to increase the person's ability to select visual information relevant to the verbal communication, thus decreasing dependency on the auditory channel that cannot receive its full quota. Ultimately, as we will discuss in some detail later, our aim is to increase the accuracy with which the person can *predict* the general topic and the probable evolution of the linguistic message.

Since this is the conceptual basis for visual communication training, you need to be familiar with the components that contribute to the visual information. Consider first the "settings" in which communication takes place, that is, the environmental constraints.

ENVIRONMENTAL CONSTRAINTS

What we say to each other is not determined by the environment, but much of our conversation tends to arise from and be influenced by the setting we are in and the activities we pursue in that setting. It is quite possible to discuss a weekend ski trip in the setting depicted in Figure 4.1a, but it is far more likely that your discussion would center around dental problems. Similarly the second scene (Figure 4.1b) is less likely to give rise to a conversation about the value of dental floss than to a discussion of the chances of the university's team winning the big homecoming game.

The setting also includes the people present. We have definite expectations that people will conform to an image that fits into the setting in which we encounter them. This image is influenced by the person's dress code and the tools and instruments of his/her trade or profession. A burly football player in full gear would appear as incongruous in Figure 4.1a as would a dentist in a white coat in Figure 4.1b. A long time ago, Reusch and Kees explained that "The interpretation of mutual roles serves the purpose of clarifying the verbal, gestural and action messages that people consciously convey to each other. . . . Those who are quick to recognize roles are at an advantage in dealing with social situations" (1956, p. 72). Even before that, Nitchie (1912), who became severely hearing impaired and developed an integrative method of teaching lip-reading, advocated that we attempt to develop in the hearing-impaired person what he called "intuitiveness." Intuitiveness is the ability to make accurate predictions on the basis of minimal patterns of nonverbal and verbal cues. Reusch and Kees also emphasize this ability:

> In the practice of communication we are continually assessing our material surroundings, making attempts at identifying others and their roles, their status, and their group membership in order to arrive at a kind of diagnosis

Figure 4.1(a)(b)

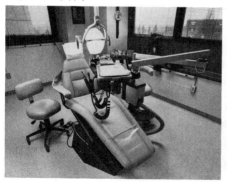
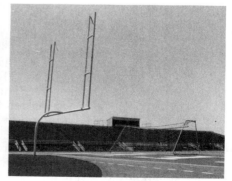

that will combine all these features into an integral pattern: the social situation. In the truest sense it is the social situation that determines the context and nature of any communicative exchange. (1956, p. 37)

Or, to quote Peters:

We know what the person will do when he begins to walk towards the pulpit in the middle of the penultimate hymn or what the traveler will do when he enters the doors of the hotel, because we know the conventions regulating church services and staying at hotels. (1958, p. 7)

Our goal is to increase hearing-impaired persons' intuitiveness—to heighten their awareness of situational constraints so they can make better predictions about what may be said. Ease of communication, for all of us, depends upon our ability to think ahead of the actual words and to need the acoustic signal primarily to confirm our predictions. Hearing loss places a premium on this ability.

This knowledge of communication behavior, particularly in relation to the perception and use of spoken language, is the basis of *pragmatics*. We will consider the nature of pragmatics and its role in communication assessment and intervention in some detail later in our discussions.

CONSTRAINTS OF IMPLEMENTAL ACTIVITIES

When I teach students about visual communication, I often ask them out of context and without voice, "Does anyone have change for a $20.00 bill?" Rarely does anyone have any idea what I have said even when I repeat it. I then take my wallet from my pocket, remove a $20.00 bill and hold it out looking enquiringly at different students as I ask again without voice, "Does anyone have change for a $20.00 bill?" Everyone understands, though no student ever has $20.00! This situation evidences the role of the constraints generated by our actions. A motorist who stops a car, winds down the window, and asks a question is likely to require directions, as is a pedestrian holding a street map in her hand. To these implemental activities are added postures and expressive movements that convey an emotional state. These are primarily of an involuntary nature, but they are informative. We may find it difficult to say exactly which muscle actions are involved in a look of surprise, but we recognize and know how to assume such an expression. Several investigators have shown that we can recognize emotional states when illustrated by photographs. This is so both for actors posing (Coleman, 1949; Fry & Whetnall, 1962) and for authentically elicited emotions (Dolanski, 1930). We expect certain facial expressions to relate to certain situations that in turn limit the possible verbal messages we would consider appropriate (Figure 4.2).

Nonverbal information also is transmitted through posture and movement. People's moods can be predicted by the way they walk, stand, sit. Depression tends to weigh our body down; we slump in a chair, round our shoulders, slow our movements, drag our feet. Excitement, by contrast, agitates us, expands movements, quickens pace. Guilt is often "written all over our face." "OK," mother says, "what did you do?" Anger contorts the

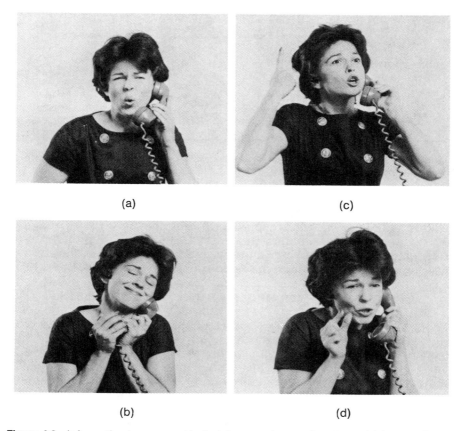

(a)

(c)

(b)

(d)

Figure 4.2 Information is conveyed in facial expressions and gestures: (a) learn estimate for fixing the fender; (b) learn husband still loves you in spite of fender; (c) get out the vote; (d) tell the store to send those *teeny-weeny* tomatoes for the party. (Photographs courtesy of Ormond Gigli, Inc.)

face differently from pain; sorrow slackens facial muscles and elongates the face. Fear furrows the brow, widens the eyes, and tenses facial muscles, whereas surprise lifts the brow and opens eyes and mouth. These are for the most part involuntary movements, unlike gesture that constitutes a more culturally bound nonverbal language system.

GESTURAL CONSTRAINTS

We gesture with our head, face, tongue and lips, shoulders, arms, and hands. We all recognize the significance of the nod of approval or agreement, the head shake that signifies denial, the protruded tongue, the blown kiss, the shrug of the shoulders, or the extended hand in the classroom. We come when beckoned, stop when a hand is extended toward us at 45 degrees

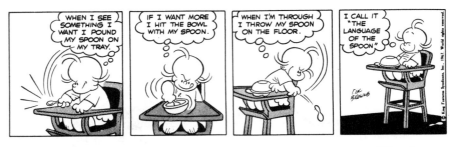

Figure 4.3 Gestures can often prove very meaningful. (Cartoon courtesy of King Features Syndicate, Inc.)

with the palm open, shake the same hand when held extended at waist height, smile knowingly in response to a wink. We know the language of gesture that so often accompanies words: "Gestures are used to illustrate, to emphasize, to point, to explain, or to interrupt; therefore, they cannot be isolated from the verbal components of speech" (Reusch & Kees, 1956, p. 37).

In normal conversation gestures are used as signs, that is, the meaning of the gesture is related closely to the act itself (Figure 4.3). Gestures serve the secondary function of augmenting or modifying the spoken message in some way. It is possible, however, for gestures to be given symbolic value. When this occurs the meaning is arbitrarily assigned a gesture that now *stands for* the object, event, or idea rather than being an extension of it. Many such gestures derive from the concept but others, such as a thumbs-up sign to indicate approval or a circle made with thumb and first finger to indicate perfection or success, are totally arbitrary in construction. In such cases, it is impossible to interpret the gesture unless you are taught the meaning, as in sign language.

CUES ARISING DIRECTLY FROM THE SPOKEN MESSAGE

Finally, we must consider the contribution made to speech intelligibility by the visible characteristics of the spoken message itself.

The organs of articulation that contribute most to the visible aspects of speech are

1. *The lips.* Cues to recognition may be derived from various degrees of lip rounding or spreading, ranging from the marked rounding that characterizes the production of the vowel /u/ as in *boot* and the /w/ in *wind*, to the spread lips for the vowel /i/ in *meek*. Protrusion and lip rounding together help in recognition of the /tʃ/ in *church* and /ʃ/ in *ship*.

    Cues to the bilabial plosives /p/ and /b/ and the bilabial nasal /m/ are obtained from observing the lips being brought together. The contact of the lower lip and the upper teeth facilitates the recognition of the labial dental fricatives /f/ and /v/.

2. *The tongue.* Observation of the tongue position contributes valuable information to the recognition of such sounds as the lingual dental $/\theta/$ and $/\delta/$ in *think* and *these*, the $/l/$ in *letter*, the lingual alveolar plosives $/t/$ and $/d/$, and the lingual nasal $/n/$.

3. *The jaw.* From observation of the degree of opening of the jaw, together with information about other articulators, we obtain cues important in the differentiation between vowels—for example, between $/a/$ as in *a*rm and $/i/$ as in h*i*m.

To the information obtained from these articulators, we must add that contributed by the secondary movements of facial muscles associated with the articulation of certain phonemes. For example the lip-rounding and lip-spreading characteristics of $/\int/$ and $/s/$ provide clearly differentiated visual speech patterns, though they are not essential to the acoustic production of these sounds.

An observation made by Woodward (1957) and supported by Brannon and Kodman (1959) was that the visibility of movements was related to their place of articulation. Mirror observation of your own speech will illustrate this relationship. You will notice, for example, that the bilabial clusters $/p/$, $/b/$, and $/m/$ and the lingual dental clusters $/f/$ and $/v/$ are far easier to recognize than the lingual alveolar clusters $/t/$, $/d/$, $/n/$, and $/l/$ or the lingual velar sounds $/k/$, $/g/$, and $/\eta/$. It is, however, not true and the relationship between visibility and place of articulation is on a one-to-one basis. Because the formative movements of the lingual alveolar fricative sounds $/s/$ and $/z/$ and the alveolar fricatives $/\theta/$ and $/\delta/$ occur at the same place of articulation as the $/t/$, $/d/$, $/n/$, and $/l/$ cluster, they should be equally hard to recognize. In fact they possess high visibility bestowed upon them by the secondary revealing movements of the lips.

In an attempt to obtain more information about what can be derived from the visible aspects of speech in the absence of sound, I conducted a small project involving 20 college students with normal hearing. I found that when I asked them to recognize phonetically balanced monosyllabic words from visual cues alone, the mean score based upon 100 words was 7.0 words correctly identified. In other words, when visual perception of the spoken word provided the only source of information about the message, only 7 percent of the material was correctly identified.

Utley (1946) administered her film test "How Well Can You Read Lips?" to 761 deaf and hard-of-hearing subjects. The mean score obtained on the word-recognition part of the test was 6.9 words (19 percent) of a possible total of 36. The words in this test were, however, not monosyllabic but were selected from a test of the first 1000 most frequently used words. They included a number of bi- and trisyllabic words, which increased redundancy, and a score of correct was given on the basis of recognition either of the test word or of any of its homophenes. Even so, less than one-fifth of the words were recognized by experienced lip-readers.

If we view these results in the light of our understanding of the factors that limit the visual reception of speech, the low scores obtained through vision alone will not be surprising. The little information one is able to obtain from the visible aspects of the spoken message signal itself is derived from the revealing movements of the articulators.

How much visual information is available to the viewer in normal conversational speech is extremely difficult to determine because conversation is rich in all the other visual constraints we have discussed. Furthermore, conversation involves language, so it is hard to know how much of a viewer's comprehension derives from visual constraints and how much from her ability to generate linguistic predictions. Estimates of the percentage of the phonemes of English that are visibly distinguishable vary from 11–57 percent (Berger, 1972). More often a phoneme can be categorized as one of a particular group but is not discriminable from others in the same group. Such groups are called *visemes*. The number of viseme groups has not been categorically determined. Woodward and Barber (1960) and Fisher (1968) identified four and five viseme groups respectively for consonants while Binnie, Jackson, and Montgomery (1976) identified as many as 10.

After a period of training the number of consonant visemes which subjects differentiate with 75 percent consistency in an experimental task varies from six (Walden, Erdman, Montgomery, Swartz and Prosek 1981) to nine (Walden, Prosek, Montgomery, Scherr and Jones 1977). As we have seen, a number of factors other than the actual articulatory movement influence the visibility and distinguishability of a particular phoneme. Moreover, in conversation the identification of individual speech sounds seldom occurs since we process holistically to determine meaning not structure. As Boothroyd states:

> Speechreading is inherently a linguistic activity. The message to be perceived does not consist of speech patterns but of the linguistic structures those patterns represent (Boothroyd 1988, p. 77).

The significance of these findings lies in the implications they have for how we view vision as a supplementary source of speech information, and particularly how we plan to use it in teaching our client to improve communication effectiveness. It is apparent that visual lip-reading of speech sounds alone cannot provide adequate information for comprehension to occur.

CENTRAL NERVOUS SYSTEM EFFECTS

As in the case of auditory perception of speech, visual perception depends not only on reception but on the efficiency with which the signal information is processed by the central pathways, neural centers, and the cortex, in the case of visual stimuli, and by the occipital lobes of the cortex. Two studies (Shepherd, 1982; Shepherd, DeLavergne, Frueh, & Clobridge, 1977) assessed the relationship between the neural firing time (latency) of the visual system and scores obtained on the Utley Test of Lipreading (1946). In both studies, electroencephalography, a measure of changes in the electrical activity of the brain, was used to determine the neural firing time in response to low-rate random visual flashes. The scores obtained on the word and sentence parts of the test were then correlated with the firing times. It was found that a significant direct relationship exists: the shorter the latency period (i.e., the neural response), the higher the speech-reading score.

In a subsequent study, Lesner and Sandridge (1984) investigated the effects of age on speech-reading performance and its correlation with visual neural latency times. They showed that in the older group of subjects with normal hearing, latencies were significantly longer than those of the younger group, as were the scores on the CID Everyday Sentence Test presented visually only on videotape. They noted, however, that the test scores obtained by a hearing-impaired older group were superior to those of the older group with normal hearing. This indicates that in some manner adaptation to hearing impairment permits a person to develop speech-reading skills despite reduced visual neural efficiency.

The value of the visible signal of speech lies in the possibility of using visible speech patterns to identify meaningful units of speech, words, and phrases. As I will discuss later, such recognition is as much an active perceptual process as a passive receptive one. Thus the contribution of the visual signal, in all its forms, is to add information to a pool that is contributed to by two or more sensory systems and, equally important, by the ability of the perceptual system to generate rational expectations.

We can be certain, therefore, that speech and its visible manifestations are inseparable in communication from language and cognition. We can be sure also that, like the acoustic signal, the visible speech signal is subject to limitations. These we will consider in the next chapter.

SUMMARY

- Visual information decreases dependency on acoustic information and thus is a resource for hearing-impaired persons.
- The greater the information contributing to the overall pattern, the less we need to process fine details.
- Speech communication occurs as part of a holistic communicative event related and constrained to various degrees by the environment, the persons involved, dress codes, and voluntary and involuntary behaviors including gestures and facial expressions.
- The act of speech articulation generates correlated visible speech constraints. The amount of visual information extracted at the word level is, however, low even for experienced lip-readers, less than 25 percent, suggesting we need larger chunks of the spoken message in order to make maximum use of visible speech constraints.
- Visual perception is affected by central processes as well as by peripheral reception.
- It has been shown that a positive correlation exists between the efficiency of the neural firings of the visual pathway and the ability to speech-read.
- The normal aging process decreases the rate of neural transmission.
- Older individuals with hearing impairment nevertheless can acquire compensatory visual-processing skills to raise performance above that of their hearing peers.

Conclusion

Hearing impairment, by reducing auditory information, places a greater premium on the visual information relevant to communication. Visual information increases the number of constraints within which predictions are made, thus facilitating rapid processing. It also influences how we interpret acoustic cues in the presence of intersensory (auditory-visual) cross verification of predictions. By narrowing the constraints thus, we need to process less of the signal to identify it. Relevant visual information must be seen as integrating cues derived primarily from the act of communication but with the support of situational cues.

Like auditory perception, we process visual information in as large a chunk as possible. Thus we watch for meaning rather than for individual articulatory movements when processing visible speech. The ability to do this well is influenced by the efficiency of the neural coding, an ability that decreases with age. However, studies show that compensatory learning can surmount many of the negative effects of aging on speech-reading competence.

5

Factors Limiting Visible Speech Processing

FACTORS WITHIN THE LISTENER

Opthalmological Factors

In view of the importance that visual information has in compensating for the reduced auditory information arising from impairment of hearing, you would think that optimal visual function would be our first concern. It is not. To make matters worse, the two periods when visual problems are most likely to be detected, that is, during early school years and during middle age, are the same periods when hearing deficiency is often first noticed. It has been convincingly documented that the incidence of visual difficulties is higher among deaf children than among their normal-hearing peers (Green, 1978).

Greene's (1978) in-depth screening of the vision of 156 deaf school-age children demonstrated a significantly higher incidence of visual anomalies than is present among hearing children of the same age. The increased incidence shown for hyperopia was 4 times greater, strabismus 2.5 times greater, amblyopia 8.5 times greater, and other binocularity disorders 3 times greater. Pathology among the deaf children was shown to have an incidence 12 times greater than among normal-hearing children. In an earlier study Pollard and Neumaier (1974) reported the incidence of ocular defects among deaf children to be between 20 and 60 percent. These findings emphasize the paramount importance of thorough in-depth visual testing of hearing-impaired children.

A notable cause of congenital auditory and visual problems is maternal rubella, which affects the infant, particularly if the mother contracted the disease during the first three months of pregnancy. Increasing age, which produces a deterioration of both visual function (presbyosis) and auditory function (presbycusis), is a condition we can all expect to face. Although many adults become aware that they are experiencing difficulty with visual acuity, the amount of deterioration is often fairly marked before it draws attention to itself. Up to that point, many people unconsciously compensate for the problems they are experiencing. It is possible that some people, to a certain extent, psychologically may reject the idea that they might need glasses. People who already wear glasses might not want to go to the expense of reexamination and possible replacement of their current pair. The visual difficulty may, therefore, only evidence itself in the hard-of-hearing adults as part of the total deterioration in their ability to communicate as a result of the less-than-normal visual acuity. Such people are unable to compensate to any marked degree for the loss of hearing by greater dependence upon visible cues to speech. In a visual-communication training activity, they may suggest many different reasons why they have been unable to develop this skill. It may not occur to them that they may be calling upon their eyes to perform a task that is too fine for their visual acuity to handle. Because vision constitutes such an important component in the total information-processing system that we utilize in training or retraining people with impaired hearing, we now need to consider some of the most important factors that influence the effectiveness of visual processing of information.

Visual Acuity

Despite the obvious importance of vision in the processing of visual speech information, not until 1970 was the report of a systematic investigation that related the performance of the peripheral visual mechanism to lip-reading performance published. Sixteen college students with normal hearing participated in the study by Hardick, Oyer, and Irion (1970). The subjects were drawn from a pool of 52 students who had taken a filmed lip-reading test (Utley, 1946). The two equal groups of subjects chosen had obtained the eight highest and eight lowest scores on the test. The original pool of students represented a random sample with respect to skills in visual speech processing. The main purpose of the investigation was to determine whether, on the basis of optometric findings, normal-hearing subjects who demonstrated an ability to process a relatively large amount of visible speech information could be discriminated from those who performed poorly. The measures of visual function included visual acuity, refraction, astigmatism, and ability of the eye to discern form movement and color. Accommodation, peripheral vision, eye-blink rate, stereopsis, and phoria—that is, the tendency of the visual axis of one eye to deviate when the other eye is covered and fusion is prevented—were also assessed. The result of this examination revealed that visual performance varied along only two of the parameters tested, visual acuity and eye-blink rate. Subjects were thus given an optometric rating mainly on the basis of binocular acuity.

The lip-reading scores obtained by subjects with high visual acuity rating and the scores of subjects with visual deficiencies were compared. The results indicated that the subjects in the normal group obtained significantly higher lip-reading scores on the sentence subtest and on the overall test score, but not on single-word identification or the story comprehension.

The authors of the study concluded that their results indicated that even a relatively minor deficiency of acuity will significantly lower scores on a lip-reading test. This is a conclusion strongly concurred with by Parasnis and Samar (1982) and by Johnson and Snell (1986). They questioned the validity of previous research into visual communication skills because rarely, if ever, were the test subjects controlled for visual acuity.

Visual Defects

A variety of visual defects occur in children and adults. Some are peculiar to our later years and often significantly affect our ability to see the visual cues to speech, to see visual aids to teaching, and to see printed material clearly (Karp 1988). These defects are summarized in Appendix 5.A. Visual problems are likely to remain undetected until well advanced unless the eyes are tested. Children with visual defects may be quite unaware that the world should appear differently from the way they see it. Furthermore, in the early years most children tend to be farsighted. Thus, the gradual onset of myopia, most commonly occurring during the first years of school, may escape detection. It is not until the visual deterioration evidences itself in the child's failure to make progress in school that visual acuity is questioned. The hard-of-hearing child stands in double jeopardy in this respect. We are only too likely to attribute educational retardation entirely to the hearing impairment and thus completely overlook the role of vision. Similarly, vision requires special attention in the older person since the aging process makes older people particularly vulnerable to visual difficulties.

The importance of evaluation of peripheral visual function in any child or adult with a hearing impairment cannot be emphasized too strongly. Optimally, corrected vision should be a prerequisite to a person's enrollment in a rehabilitation management program. This is important because such intervention procedures almost of necessity will include training designed to develop supplemental skills in the visual processing of speech to compensate for information lost as a result of impaired hearing. Thus, in keeping with our concern for the total process of communication, it is essential that we make particularly certain that in addition to providing the hearing-impaired person with all possible help in receiving and interpreting the auditory signal, we also ensure that the visual pathway is operating at its optimum level. This requires that each person with a hearing impairment receives a thorough examination of visual function by an ophthalmologist or optometrist. Reexamination should be made every two years.

FACTORS IN THE ENVIRONMENT

Lighting Conditions

The efficiency of the human eye is markedly reduced when the light intensity is strongly increased or reduced suddenly. Consider, for example, the effect of extinguishing the lights in a bright room. The initial reaction is that you are in total darkness. However, you gradually become able to distinguish the shapes of objects that were previously not visible. This phenomenon is known as *dark adaptation*. Similarly, sudden exposure to bright light after a period in a relatively darkened room results in a sensation of glare until your eyes adapt to the new light conditions. Light adaptation is very important to hard-of-hearing subjects in communication, because they are dependent upon the visible aspects of speech as an aid to comprehension. If they move from brightness to a dimly lighted environment, they experience a temporary decrease in visual sensitivity because of the low level of illumination. They experience similar difficulty in bright light.

Visual acuity can be defined as the ability of the eye to distinguish fine details. Perhaps the most important factor affecting visual acuity is the light intensity. The amount of light that needs to be present in the environment to permit the clearest vision varies depending upon the nature of the visual task. Generally speaking, the finer the nature of the work the eyes are required to do, the more illumination is required. For example, you may be able to peel an apple, count coins, or arrange flowers in relatively poor light. However, threading a needle, removing a splinter from a finger, or reading small print on a label all necessitate a much greater amount of illumination. Up to a point, performance on even larger tasks may be improved by the provision of extra light; however, too much intensity will produce glare, which reduces acuity. The light must be directed on the activity or object being observed; if the light is directed toward the viewer, it will tend to decrease that person's ability to perform the task accurately.

The visual task confronting the listener in a communication situation is to see and utilize the constraint cues arising from facial expressions and, more specifically, from the visible characteristics of speech articulation. The influence that various levels of constant illumination have upon the ability of hearing-impaired persons to speech-read has not been subject to extensive study. Thomas (1962) appears to have been the first to investigate the effect of several constant light levels on the visual recognition of messages with highly familiar content. Thomas found that speech-reading performance of trained subjects was not significantly different under excellent or adverse conditions. At a distance of ten feet from a speaker, Thomas's subjects showed no deterioration in their ability to identify test items correctly until the level of lighting was reduced to approximately one-half foot candle power, which is the minimal amount of light necessary to be able to just see the speaker's face.

Erber (1974) studied the effects of facial and background illumination on the ability of profoundly deaf children to recognize words by visual cues alone. He compared the mean word-recognition scores obtained when the speaker was seated in front of a highly reflective surface with those obtained when a low reflective, black background was used. Erber's results revealed little difference in the scores obtained by the deaf children when lip-reading under these two conditions of reflected light. He concluded that the intensity of a light source at the level of the mouth, which illuminates both mouth and face, affects visual recognition of the spoken word only minimally. Thus, background reflection of light does not appear to be a significant factor in visual-communication performance. Further study by Erber concerned the influence of a highly illuminated background (300 footlamberts) on the ability of the children to visually recognize words presented under varying levels of illumination of the speaker's face. This part of the investigation demonstrated a highly statistically significant effect. The mean difference between the word-recognition scores for low (3 footlamberts) and high (30 footlamberts) facial illumination against the background glare (300 footlamberts) was 49 percent.

The conclusion drawn from these studies is that contrary to conventional wisdom, once appropriate light adaptation has occurred, speech-reading can be performed equally well in high- or low-intensity light levels. However, contrast between the level of illumination of the speaker's face and the background exerts a highly significant effect on speech-reading performance, at least among the deaf children studied by Erber. Erber concluded from this research that the level of contrast between facial and background illumination is the critical factor. Thus, when facial illumination is high, the effect of a bright background on a listener's ability to use visible speech cues will be negligible. However, the reverse is true when, for example, the listener stands with his or her back to a sunlit window with no other light source to equally illuminate the face. Erber makes the important point that persons with normal language abilities do not depend upon the perception of every speech element for speech recognition, even under adverse listening conditions. Young children with impaired hearing, on the other hand, require every available external cue to compensate for their low linguistic redundancy. Thus, concern for adequate contrastive lighting conditions in educational settings is justified.

Another important factor in determining the fineness of details observed by the eye concerns the angle at which the light strikes the retina. When a person focuses on an object, the light reflected from that object is directed on the fovea of the retina. The ability to see an object 20 degrees to one side of the center of focus is reduced to a visual-acuity level approximately one-tenth of the foveal vision, because the light rays at this position will not be as sharply focused (Kendler, 1963). Thus, to teach deaf children the names of objects or to point out a particular picture, try to bring the object close to your face so that it is in clear focus.

Viewing Distance and Angle

Visual acuity is also affected by the angle and distance between the eye and the object observed. The greater the separation, the poorer visual acuity becomes. Neely (1956) attempted to quantify the effects of distance and the angle from which the listener observes the speaker. Using a trained speaker and 35 male listeners with normal hearing and vision, Neely compared the scores obtained by the subjects on a multiple-choice intelligibility test at 9 different seating positions. These positions were 3, 6, and 9 feet and 0, 45, and 90 degrees from the speaker. Distance, within the limits tested, did not affect intelligibility, though the scores obtained by subjects directly facing the speaker were higher than those obtained for subjects at 45- and 90-degree angles. Berger, DePompei, and Droder (1970) extended the viewing-distance factor. These researchers assessed the effect of distance upon the ability of normal-hearing adults to distinguish between vowels in monosyllabic words using only visual speech cues. Their results confirmed those obtained by Neely (1956) but extended to 24 feet the range within which visual speech discrimination is not affected by distance. Using two speakers, Erber (1971) also examined the effect of distance on the lip-reading performance of profoundly deaf children. The speakers' faces were lit directly at mouth level. The test items were monosyllabic words, two-syllable words with the stress on the first syllable (trochaic), and two-syllable words with equal stress on each syllable (spondaic). The study revealed that word-recognition scores for the subjects increased as the distance decreased from approximately 11 percent at 100 feet to approximately 75 percent at 5 feet. In a later study, Erber (1974) reported that the scores obtained by his subjects, viewing from angles of 0 and 45 degrees, decreased in a linear manner as a function of increasing distance. However, when the speaker was viewed from the side (90-degree angle), the mean scores were not further enhanced by decreasing the speaker-child distance below 12 feet.

Erber also investigated the effect of the angle of viewing on visual reception scores obtained by the profoundly deaf children tested. He found the best visual reception of speech to occur for either the 0- or 45-degree viewing angle. Erber notes that these findings do not exactly concur with those obtained by other researchers. Neely (1956), for example, found that the 0-degree horizontal viewing angle produced slightly higher scores than the 45-degree angle, whereas Larr (1959) and Nakano (1966) both reported that the 45-degree angle was superior to the 0-degree viewing angle.

In a different approach, Berger, Garner, and Sudman (1971) compared the effect on visual speech discrimination of viewing the subject from below the level of the face (-35-degree angle), which is equivalent to how a child sees an adult, with face-level viewing (0-degree angle). The adult subjects had normal hearing. No significant difference was found in the scores obtained for the two viewing angles.

Thus, for children and adults, the optimal viewing position for visual perception of speech appears to be a horizontal angle of 0 to 45 degrees at a distance of no greater than 6–10 feet (Caccamise, Meath-Lang and Johnson, 1981). A 90-degree viewing angle appears to be disadvantageous to optimal visual recognition of speech, reducing performance by 11 to 22 percent.

VISIBLE ASPECTS OF SPEECH PRODUCTION

The production of various speech sounds is made possible by the modification of air flow from the lungs brought about by the changes in the shape and size of the supralaryngeal resonators. These changes involve the movement and positioning of the jaw, lips, tongue, and soft palate. Each speech sound involves a distinctive articulatory movement. Under favorable viewing conditions, part, but seldom all, of this movement will be visible to an observer. A movement may be considered as having a *formative aspect* and a *revealing aspect*. The formative aspect includes the movement of all articulators essential to the production of a particular sound; the revealing aspect involves only those visible movements of articulators that may be involved in or associated with its production. For example, the formative aspect of the speech sound *sh* /ʃ/ involves elevation of the soft palate, the grooving of the tongue, and the elevation of the sides of the tongue to make contact with the upper teeth. None of these movements is easily visible. The revealing movement associated with /ʃ/ is the puckering and protrusion of the lips, a movement associated with, but not essential to, the acoustic production of the sound.

In a number of phonemes, some of the formative movements may also be revealing, as are the lip movements in the production of the bilabial plosives /p/ and /b/, or the tongue movement in the production of the voiced and unvoiced lingual dental fricatives /θ/ and /ð/.

Since these visible stimuli arise directly from the production of a specific phoneme, they provide a valuable source of additional information concerning the spoken word. If it were possible for the eyes to receive and identify each phoneme or word spoken purely on the basis of its visible characteristics, and if the conditions for viewing the speaker were always optimal, then the hard-of-hearing subject would not be handicapped by the inability to receive the auditory signal correctly. Rehabilitation of the hearing-impaired person would simply involve training the person to replace the use of ears by eyes in the reception of the message signal. Unfortunately this is not the case. The visible aspects of speech are subject to a number of important limitations that exist within the visual message signal itself, within the environment through which it travels, and within the person who is acting as the receiver. At this time, we are concerned only with the factors that pertain to the message signal and the environment.

Four major factors influence the usefulness of the visual signal as a conveyor of information:

1. The degree of visibility of the movement
2. The rapidity of articulatory movements
3. The similarity of the visual characteristics of the articulatory movements involved in the production of different speech sounds
4. Intersubject variations in the visible aspects of articulatory movements involved in the production of any given sound

Degree of Visibility. The visual recognition of the speech sound is dependent upon the revealing aspects involved in its production. These vary considerably for each phoneme. The only phoneme that can truly be said to possess no revealing visible characteristic in its production is the aspirate /h/; however, for a considerable number of phonemes, the revealing characteristics are relatively obscure, and accuracy of recognition cannot be absolutely guaranteed even for a trained observer.

The range of visibility of normal conversational sentences varies from a minimum of 47 percent to a maximum of 83 percent, with the average falling between 65 and 70 percent. (USWAPA 1939)

Rapidity of Articulatory Movements. Nitchie (1912) pointed out that in ordinary conversational speech, a speaker averages approximately 13 articulatory movements per second. The eye, on the other hand, is capable of consciously recording eight or nine movements per second. According to these figures, the eye therefore misses approximately a quarter of all sounds produced, though it must be remembered that not all the sounds are clearly visible to the observer in the first place. Nitchie draws attention to the fact that although the average duration of the articulatory movement is one-thirteenth of a second, speech sounds are produced that are both shorter and longer in duration. Using a motion-picture camera, filming at 16 frames per second, Nitchie found that many of the speech sounds were too rapid to be recorded by the camera, indicating a duration of less than one-sixteenth of a second. The consonants were found to be of shorter duration than the long vowels, which had a duration of two-sixteenths to three-sixteenths per second, although some short vowels were articulated as quickly as many of the consonants.

The importance of the rate of articulation is supported by the findings of Mulligan (1954), who investigated the effect that speed of projection of a movie film had on the viewers' scores on a test of lip-reading. Mulligan showed the film at two speeds—slow (16 frames per second) and normal (24 frames per second)—and found that the slower speed resulted in higher scores on the test.

On the other hand, a later study conducted by Byers and Lieberman (1959) produced contrary evidence. These researchers subjected four groups of experienced lip-readers from a school for the deaf to a sentence lip-reading test adapted from the Utley test (1946). By modifying the speed in filming and the speed of projection, they were able to produce controlled variations in the speaker's rate of utterance. Using four rates, normal (120 words per minute), and two-thirds, one-half, and one-third slower than normal rate, they studied the subjects' performance on the test under each condition. The results indicated no significant differences between the four rates of presentation. The authors concluded that within the range studied, variation in rate did not affect the degree of correct recognition of the visible aspects of the spoken word. This was found even though one of the rates was one-third of normal, and despite complaints from the viewers that the films were being shown at too slow a speed. They were of the impression that lip-reading skill is adaptable to quite an extensive range of articulatory rates.

The reason for the discrepancy between the results in these two studies may rest within the subjects used. Mulligan's findings are based on the performance of college students with normal hearing, while those of Byers and Lieberman were obtained from a group of deaf subjects, all of whom had had at least two years of formal lip-reading training. It may well be that we are not justified in generalizing data collected on subjects with normal hearing to the performance of subjects with hearing impairment. It has been demonstrated by Sumby and Pollack (1956), Neely (1956), and Sanders and Goodrich (1971) that for subjects with normal hearing, increased distortion of the auditory aspects of speech results in an increased dependence upon the use of visual cues. It may reasonably be presumed that a subject with a marked congenital auditory impairment will have come to depend heavily upon the contribution that vision is capable of making to speech intelligibility. This dependence will undoubtedly have resulted in a degree of skill—which the subject with normal hearing has not been called upon to develop—in making use of this information. When each of these two groups, the normal and the hard-of-hearing, are presented with a task involving the ability to obtain information through the recognition of visible speech characteristics, the hard-of-hearing subject is at an advantage. As a sophisticated user of information, a hearing-impaired person's tolerance for changes in speech rate is much greater than that of the person with normal hearing, who finds that he or she performs best when the material is presented at a slower speed.

If this is in fact so, then it has important implications for the training of beginning lip-readers. Factors that may not be important for the sophisticated lip-reader may well be crucial in the early learning stages. The role of rapidity of articulatory movements in the learning and maintenance of visual communication requires more investigation before we can confidently say that rate is not important.

Similarity of Visible Articulatory Movements. As was explained in our discussion of the acoustics of speech, each phoneme in the English language has a unique acoustic structure. The phonetic alphabet recognizes this in that, unlike the alphabet of written English, there exists a discrete symbol for each sound. The uniqueness in acoustic structure is that no two sounds are articulated in exactly the same way. In other words, for a given sound the formative movements that constitute the total articulatory movements are different from the formative movements of all other sounds. This is not, however, true for the revealing movements, which are confined only to the articulatory movements that are visible. Many speech sounds are revealed by identical visible movements. Such sounds are known as homophenes.* Homophenous consonants comprise the viseme categories we discussed in the last chapter. The adjective *homophenous* may be applied both to individual phonemes such as /p/, /b/, /m/, which are identical in revealing movements; to groups of phonemes such as /nt/ and /nd/; or to words, such

---

* The term *homophenes*, which refers to phonemes that are identical in the visible aspects of their articulation, should not be confused with the similar term *homophones*, which refers to letters or symbols that have the same sound as others. These are synonymous with visemes.

TABLE 5.1 Homophenous clusters of initial English consonants (after Woodward, 1957)

(a)	p	b	m					
		f	v					
		w	r					
(b)	tʃ	ʤ	ʃ	ʒ	j			
	t	d	n	l	s	z	θ	ð
	k	g	h					

as *bad, mat, pan*. In normal conversational speech, it is quite impossible to distinguish between homophenous items. A study of the vowels and consonants of English indicates that the vowels do not exhibit any strictly homophenous formation, though some of the vowel sounds do present difficulty and only appear different to a trained observer. A list of homophenous groupings of consonants is given in Table 5.1. The homophenous groupings of consonants indicated in this table were established by Woodward (1957). Woodward made a linguistic analysis of the phonological, grammatical, and lexical aspects of lip-reading stimulus materials and hypothesized that the absolute visibility of a given speech item was dependent upon the area of articulatory placement involved. She presented a filmed series of paired syllables to a group of subjects with normal hearing and asked them to judge the two items as same or different. From an analysis of the results, Woodward established the consonant classifications already indicated. She concluded that although in context it is possible to distinguish between many of the phonemes within a set, differentiation cannot be based upon visual comparison alone.

In a more recent study Kricos and Lesner (1982) showed that viseme groupings vary with the ease with which a person can be speechread. However, across studies which have reported viseme, or homophenous, groupings since the Woodward (1957) study, general agreement has emerged concerning the consistency of four consonant viseme categories. The consonants within the groupings /p,b,m/, /fv/, /θ,ð/ and /w,r/ are identified with a high level of consistency as homophenous. Other groups vary somewhat from study to study. It is of note that training has resulted in some subjects learning to differentiate /s,z/ from /ʃ,ʒ/ (Walden, Prosek, Montgomery, Scherr and Jones, 1977), leaving /t,d,s,z,l,n,k,g,h,j/ as the most variable consonants in terms of differentiation. In reviewing the research Jackson (1988) states:

> This discussion once again points out that there is no one viseme system that accurately describes the visual characteristics of all phonemes for all talkers (p. 103–104).

It must be concluded, therefore, that the visual similarity of homophenes compels the observer to rely on the linguistic redundancy of the material to provide the information necessary to differentiate between them.

On the basis of tests conducted with different passages representing colloquial English, Nitchie (1912) estimated that almost every word contains one or more homophenous sounds, that more than 40 percent of the total number of sounds in the test sample have one or more sounds homophenous to them, and furthermore, that approximately 50 percent of the words in the sample constitute homophenes of one or more other words.

Intra- and Intersubject Variation of Articulatory Movements. Careful analysis of the speech of a given individual reveals that the manner of articulation of a given speech sound varies at each production. It has been demonstrated experimentally that exact duplication of the manner of production is not possible, even when a subject makes a special effort to achieve this. The variation, which always exists to some degree, is frequently found to be quite considerable. Although these deviations are observed in the production of all speech sounds, they are especially noticeable in the production of vowels. In spite of these variations, there exists for each phoneme a fundamental movement pattern, which remains essentially the same. Kantner and West (1941, p. 29) use the analogy of movements involved in writing to illustrate this point. They explain that even though letters of the alphabet may be produced in a variety of different ways, the movements tend to become stereotyped within an individual, making it possible to identify a person by his or her handwriting. An expert is able to recognize these stereotypes even when an attempt has been made to disguise them.

In the production of speech sounds within the individual, this stereotyping occurs as a result of the necessity to ensure that the acoustic characteristics remain within the limits of a phoneme so that the meaning of a group of phonemes (a word) is not interfered with. A second factor is the influence of a physiological tendency to stereotype movements.

When we extend our interest in the variability in speech-sound production to the changes occurring in the way in which different people produce a given speech sound, we find that the differences are frequently quite marked. It has been suggested that these interpersonal variations can be attributed to three causes: (1) variations in anatomical structure of the speech mechanism; (2) interpersonal differences in auditory perception of speech sounds; and (3) regional or social variations occurring where speech sounds have developed in a different manner from those of people in other areas or social milieux.

Obviously, the stereotyping of sound production between individuals is dependent upon the acoustic factor. Auditory feedback ensures that the output—that is, the acoustic pattern of the speech sound—stays within the person's perceptual limits for that particular phoneme. It is these limits, rather than the specific articulatory movements, that different speakers have in common. Because it is possible to produce a sound in a variety of ways within the phonemic limits, it is understandable that the visible, or revealing, characteristics may vary somewhat from person to person.

As we have already noted, a careful comparison of the visible characteristics of English phonemes indicates that for some, the movements essential to the normal production of the sound—that is, those upon which the phonemic value of the sound is dependent—are quite visible to an observer. In these instances, the sound may be considered to be formed and revealed by the same movement. For other sounds, the formative movement is concealed from the observer. However, it has been demonstrated that the articulation of certain phonemes commonly involves movements of groups of facial muscles that are quite unnecessary for the normal production of the acoustic properties of the sound (Lightoller, 1925). These movements constitute associated, but under normal conditions of oral communication, unessential, accompaniments to the formative movements.

It would seem rather odd that an organism should preserve such apparently useless movements. The answer rests, perhaps, in the underlying philosophy of this text—namely, the totality of the act of communication. We may thus presume that these seemingly unimportant movements do, in fact, have a role to play. Although they do not contribute to the recognition of the acoustic aspects of the sound, they are directly associated with it. They constitute, therefore, part of the total identity of the sound. Under normal listening conditions, we do not need to make use of these visible characteristics; however, under conditions of auditory distortion, recognition of the sound may be dependent upon the ability of the listener to utilize this built-in visual redundancy. For example, for many hearing-impaired subjects, the recognition of such sounds as /sh/ and /s/ is dependent upon the associated secondary lip-rounding and lip-spreading, since the formative movement, which is lingual alveolar, is practically invisible.

It is the secondary movements that are most subject to variation. The visible aspects of a sound that are revealed by its associated rather than by its formative movements may vary sufficiently from one speaker to another to present a problem of identification. As will be explained in the following chapter, the recognition of vowel phonemes is a function of auditory judgment rather than the exact nature or extent of the movement. The pitch, resonant qualities, and duration are all important contributing factors. The actual articulatory movements of vowel production vary considerably, making it difficult to differentiate between them on the basis of their visible appearance. Consonants, on the other hand, require more exact positioning of the articulators and tend, therefore, to exhibit somewhat less variability of revealing characteristics. When we examine the visual nature of the articulatory movements in consonant production, we find that a number are revealed by their secondary characteristics alone. Those that are considered visible are /r/, /s/, /z/, /t/, /ʃ/, /ʒ/, /j/. It is these consonants that are particularly subject to interspeaker variability.

We have discussed the four major factors that influence the usefulness of speech as a form of visual communication. We have also considered the effect on speech-reading of some of the conditions that are known to affect the efficiency of the human eye. These included the phenomenon of dark adaptation, variations in light intensity, the position of the object in the visual field of the observer, and the distance between the eye and the object viewed. In addition to these, we also discussed the effect of certain defects of vision. Unfortunately, when we look to the literature to provide us with data concerning the interrelationship between these various conditions and the communicative value of the visible aspects of speech, we find little available. This remains an area that requires further systematic investigation.

We may conclude that the value of the visual message signal in communication will be influenced by environmental conditions. Until we have definite evidence to indicate the contrary, we must take these factors into consideration when planning rehabilitational training in the area of visual communication.

SUMMARY

- Vision is a valuable system for the intake of information relevant to speech communication; yet, the optimal functioning of the vision of hearing-impaired persons is generally neglected.
- The incidence of visual problems among hearing-impaired school-age children has been shown to be considerably higher than among their hearing peers. Visual problems, like hearing problems, have a high prevalence in the elderly population.
- Research has indicated that even a mild visual problem reduces a subject's performance on speech-reading tasks. Visual acuity was shown to be the most important visual attribute for speech-reading.
- Myopia (poor distance vision), hyperopia (poor close-up vision), and astigmatism (visual distortion) are common visual defects that affect usefulness of potential visual cues.
- Glaucoma and cataracts threaten the visual function of adults over 40 years of age.
- Appropriate lighting for speech-reading requires maximum contrast between high facial illumination of speaker with low background light levels.
- Dark adaptation must occur before maximum speech-reading potential is restored when moving from well-lit to poorly lit environments.
- Level of lighting does not appear to be critical once dark adaptation has occurred.
- Optimal distance for speech-reading has been shown to be 5 feet. Optimal viewing angle is 0–45 degrees. No significant difference was found between speech-reading scores obtained for face-to-face (0 degree angle) and a lower (-35 degree) viewing position.
- Visible speech cues are reduced by the low visibility of revealing articulatory movements for approximately half of the consonants and one-third of the vowels.
- Rapidity of articulation of normal speech exceeds the capacity of the eye to record information by about one-third.
- Similarity of revealing articulatory movements (homopheneity) reduces visual recognition of phonemes by approximately 60 percent. Approximately one-half of all words in conversational speech have homophenous counterparts.
- Intraspeaker variability of articulation arising from coarticulation and interspeaker articulation differences contribute to a reduction of the information that can be extracted from the visible speech signal.

Conclusion

Vision provides the primary support system to audition in speech communication. Thus, even a mild impairment in the visual system will reduce the compensatory resources available when hearing impairment reduces auditory information. Visual deficiencies are among the two sections of population most subject to hearing impairment, namely, the young and the elderly. This requires that a current professional visual examination be available on all hearing-impaired persons and that corrective lenses, when prescribed, be used. Environmental control can optimize speech-reading up to the limits of a person's visual capabilities. Maximizing illumination on the speaker's face, reducing speaker-listener distance, and staying within a 0–45 degree viewing angle are practical steps to maximize use of visual cues. It is important, however, to recognize the limitations placed upon visible speech as a source of information. The detraction factors are low visibility, similarity, and rapidity of articulation and intra- and interspeaker variability.

Appendix 5.A
SUMMARY OF MAJOR VISUAL DEFECTS

Myopia

Cause: Abnormal elongation of eyeball
Result: Blurring of distant objects
Unimpaired near vision
Effect: Difficulty in observing facial expressions and visible speech movements at 15–20 feet
Difficulty in seeing visual aids at a distance

Hyperopia

Cause: Shortened distance between cornea and the retina.*
Result: Normal distance vision but blurred images at close distances
Effect: Early compensation by *accommodation*, that is, strong contraction of ciliary muscles to control shape and thickness of lens; may result in periodic blurring of image, short visual attention span, headaches, difficulty in speechreading at conversational distances, poor reading ability

Astigmatism

Cause: Irregularity in curve of cornea
Result: Uneven focus of light waves from the same source
Effect: Objects appear fuzzy, elongated, or flattened; parts of a speaker's face will be out of focus

Glaucoma

Cause: Increased pressure of fluid in the eyeball
Result: Pressure on optic nerve and its blood supply
Effect: Slow incidious development; detected early only by special pressure test, later symptoms may include mild headaches, aching eyes, transitory visual blurring, poor dark vision, halos around lights, partial loss of side vision

Cataract

Cause: An opaque covering of the lens of the eye
Result: A cloudiness of the lens
Effect: Blurring of near or distant vision, black spots in visual field, or perception that object parts are missing

Macular Degeneration

Cause: Degeneration of the retina in the macular region, that very small area responsible for sharp focal vision, results usually from prolific growth of blood

---

* Cornea: transparent covering of the eyeball, pupil, and iris. Retina: sensory cells located on the innermost part of the eyeball that code visual patterns into nerve impulse patterns

vessels in the retina, may be inherited, occurring before age of 20, or may occur with aging.

Result: Loss of vision in central focal field about one-quarter of an inch in diameter, may be treatable surgically in early stages

Effect: Speech articulation movements may be in field of lost vision, use of peripheral vision to compensate results in poorer focus of image.

For every disorder, a large majority of persons may be helped by professional intervention.

6

Relevant Principles of Perception

In our discussion of the auditory and visual speech signals, we have mentioned in passing that the role of the stimulus, be it speech or nonspeech, is to *evoke* in the listener a value *equivalent to* the value at the source. This view of communication makes the listener a very active participant in the receptive stage of communication. He interacts with the environment and with the people in it. Listening, even merely hearing, is an interactive rather than a passive process. Thus the perceptual system not only is involved in how we interpret what we hear, it also determines what we expect to hear, what we pay attention to, and how we process the patterns we select. In a fascinating book called *Ways of Seeing*, John Berger says:

> It is seeing which established our place in the surrounding world; we explain that world with words, but words can never undo the fact that we are surrounded by it. The relation between what we see and what we know is never settled. (Berger, 1986, p. 7)

The same statement can be made for hearing. The reason for the flux in the relationship between the environment and the "knowing of it" is that our perceptual system is dynamic, and our experience and our repertoire of values are growing and changing constantly. The child who is born severely or profoundly hard-of-hearing literally lives in a different world from a hearing child. The absence, or near absence, of audible sound represents more than a deprivation of acoustic information; it results in a devel-

opment of ways of perceiving, of "knowing" the world, ap
world of relative silence rather than to a world bustling wi'
deaf child's world is just as valid to her as our world is to us, b
ship between the environment and what she knows will be di̶ᵢ.
standing the rationale for the child's behavior, understanding her neeas,
requires that we review even the most basic roles of the senses.

THE ROLE OF THE SENSES

Though we particularly are concerned with the role of hearing in speech,
we must not forget that hearing, together with the other senses, has a more
fundamental purpose. The major function of sensory processing is to provide information. This information reaches us through both our peripheral
and our internal sense organs, which provide a continual flow of data concerning changes in our bodies and in the environment. We are able to
initiate appropriate behavioral responses based on the analysis of information received.

Awareness

At its most primitive level, perception constitutes a preconscious awareness
of our relationship with the environment. An ongoing monitoring of this
relationship, together with the resultant adaptive behavior, accounts for the
comfortable feeling of being a participant in the world around us. If this
coupling is disrupted—for example, if we are suddenly plunged into darkness or if we enter a sound-isolated chamber—a feeling of anxiety, sometimes acute, is almost certain to occur.

Ramsdell (1970) stresses that the most serious effect of acquired hearing impairment is a loss of this "feeling of relationship with the world." It
is our ongoing monitoring of the activities of daily living that makes us feel
like participants in the events occurring around us and enables us to react
to them:

> The constant reaction establishes in us states of feeling that are the foundation
> of our conscious experiences, a foundation which gives us the conviction that
> the world in which we live is also alive and moving. (Ramsdell, 1970, p. 438)

The auditory system is particularly important to this background monitoring because the information it receives arrives from all around us.
Sound is not easily blocked out by physical objects, as visual information is,
nor does the monitoring cease when we sleep.

The child in whom this preconscious auditory monitoring capability
is either congenitally absent or deficient as a result of impaired hearing may
be expected to feel less confident in dealing with the environment than do
his hearing peers. It is essential that we remember this aspect of the role
of hearing when we consider providing early amplification for hearing-
impaired children. With young children our first concern must be to establish this auditory coupling with the environment at as early an age as possible to ensure increased stability in the child's perceptions of his or her

relationship to the physical world of people, things, and events. Thus, the fitting of a hearing aid may be justified even when the only benefit it provides is to facilitate environmental awareness. This is so because the way in which the perceptual system and, thus, adaptive behavior will evolve depends upon the sensory experiences to which the child is exposed during the early formative years.

Deterioration of hearing in children and adults who have had normal hearing reduces the efficiency of the monitoring process. The effects will be most dramatic in cases of rapid loss of hearing, which sometimes produces a state of depression necessitating psychological guidance. In the more common event of a gradual reduction in hearing, the effect tends to be insidious. Unfortunately, feelings of progressive detachment and isolation, which lead to loneliness and insecurity, frequently are misinterpreted both by the person with this problem and by those around him or her (Ramsdell, 1970; Sanders, 1980, 1988b).

In addition to general awareness of the world, our sensory systems provide us with information about specific changes. Any one of these may constitute a potential threat necessitating immediate action or may require less dramatic behavioral adjustment. In either case, awareness leads to attention and a suitable level of information processing. Without awareness neither attention nor appropriate adaptation would be possible. Awareness, therefore, serves as the basis for protection, orientation, and communication.

Protection

The most important information we receive is that which provides warning of a threat to our safety. The ability to perceive and react appropriately is essential to the preservation of the individual. Warnings from our internal sense organs alert us to possible sickness or disease, while those received through our peripheral sensory receptors indicate potential external danger. The startle (moro reflex) and eye-blink (auropalpebral reflex), which occur as reactions to a loud sound, are examples of the most primitive of the auditory defense processes. Children with severe congenital hearing deficits will be unaware of the significance of intense or unusual sounds, since they are inaudible to them and play no part in their perception of the environment. If by use of amplification we are able to bring these sounds within their hearing sensitivity, it will be necessary to train the children to recognize and adapt appropriately. Thus gross sound-discrimination training must be an important component of the auditory training of young children. It creates environmental awareness and teaches children to make use of sound to predict what is happening around them. A hearing-impaired child who has received amplification and training in environmental sound awareness and recognition will be safer than a child for whom this aspect of training has been neglected.

Orientation

In addition to awareness and protection, sensory information contributes to spatial orientation, which is dependent upon the integration of data received from internal and external sensory mechanisms. From these sources we obtain not only information relevant to posture and balance, but also information concerning the position of our body relative to objects around us. The role of hearing in spatial orientation is, perhaps, underestimated. You are probably unaware of the number of times you safely cross a road without looking, depending on your ears to tell you that no cars are coming. Your ability to walk confidently down a familiar staircase in the dark without falling is partly due to the auditory feedback you receive from your footsteps, which tell where you are in relation to the bottom. In a strange house, you literally may need to feel your way down the stairs. This use of the auditory aspects of spatial perception is most clearly illustrated in the blind subject. Several experimenters (Cotzin & Dallenbach, 1944; Dolanski, 1930; Kohler, 1944; von Senden, 1960; Supa, Cotzin & Dallenbach, 1944), working under controlled laboratory conditions, have demonstrated that both blind subjects and sighted subjects temporarily deprived of vision are able to detect the presence or absence of target objects placed before them purely on the basis of echo reflection from the objects. The sound made by a person's body movements and footsteps as he or she approaches an object is sufficient for detection and avoidance (Cotzin & Dallenbach, 1944; Kohler, 1944). There is even evidence that it is possible to discriminate with a high degree of accuracy between various shaped objects and to a lesser extent between materials of different qualities (Rice, 1967).

Orientation of our systems to sound sources also enables us to adjust rapidly to demands expected from relevant stimuli. In speech communication, awareness that someone has spoken, which can be determined merely by identification of the vocal tone, is followed by orientation to the speaker. We look up when spoken to, we turn toward the speaker. We expect this same behavior when we address someone. Absence of this response, which often is evident in the communication behavior of a blind person or of someone who deliberately ignores us, is disconcerting. As listeners we usually feel more comfortable when we watch a speaker. For a person with reduced hearing sensitivity, rapid visual orientation is even more important, because visual cues may greatly facilitate comprehension of a remark that might not be understood by hearing alone; it also maximizes the benefits of directivity.

Preconscious monitoring, which contributes to basic awareness and orientation, is thus important to the overall level of adjustment. If an ability can be shown to contribute in some way to normal adaptive behavior, impairment of that ability will modify certain aspects of the person's perceptual function. Awareness of these subtle changes may help us to understand the problems we seek to solve. Certainly the studies referred to previously emphasize the importance of recognizing that sense modalities do not function as independent mechanisms. To consider hearing only in relation to its role in speech perception is to fail to understand the complexity of the problem of hearing impairment.

THE PERCEPTUAL PROCESS

We have discussed how the ability to discriminate among various stimulus patterns allows us to assign appropriate meaning and to respond accordingly. When we respond in a discriminating manner, we show that we have perceived a particular group of stimuli, a "stimulus complex," as different from all other stimulus complexes. This permits us to attribute a particular meaning to it. It may help you to understand this process of perception if you look up from this text for a moment and glance around you. Now ask yourself what you see and hear. Your answer almost certainly will include a list of people, things, and activities that you have observed, together with the sounds associated with them. Depending upon where you are, you may perceive your roommate sitting in a chair studying, a clock ticking on a bed table, a news program on television, or the siren of a fire engine or ambulance in the distance. The first thing to note is that the stimuli reaching you are all complex in nature and that you are aware not of the individual stimuli, but of the objects and activities that give rise to them. You see people, not rays of light, hear voices, not component sound vibrations. Your reaction is to *patterns* of stimuli; you are not usually aware of the component parts. You may look at each of the pieces of this perceptual jigsaw in isolation, but when you put them together they constitute a picture that only then are you able to recognize. As Hilgard says, "The total impression from organized stimuli has properties not predictable from the parts in isolation" (1957, p. 363). We should bear this in mind when we discuss the analytic and synthetic approaches to the teaching of auditory and visual communication skills.

The second thing that you may note about your observation of your environment is that you are familiar with almost all of the things you see and hear in it. You have encountered them on previous occasions and in other settings. Nevertheless, your orientation toward them on this occasion may be somewhat different from what it was before. This is because your perception of the object or activity is determined not only by its immediate setting but also by your past experience of the same or similar object, event, or idea. Note how, on separate occasions, you often respond differently to the same stimulus complex, and how different reports of the same event may be received from a number of observers.

We note, then, that we react to groups of stimuli as an integrated whole, a *gestalt*. This gestalt is the result of the interaction of all the component stimuli; the identity of the individual components may not be perceived consciously. Indeed, in the early stages of learning, it may not be possible to isolate and identify them consciously. We respond to the "catness" of a cat, rather than to the individual attributes of a cat, a phenomenon referred to as *physiognomic perception* (Coleman, 1949). We also notice that we are influenced in what we perceive by our previous experiences. How do we organize these multitudinous stimuli in order to make possible the designation of meaning? In communication two phenomena are particularly important in this process: figure-ground perception and closure.

Figure-Ground Perception

The general constancy of most of our perceptions implies the existence of an underlying organizational pattern. The first of these is the phenomenon of *figure-ground.* This may be defined as the perceptual process by which a particular object or object quality is seen to stand out against a background constituted by the remaining objects or object qualities.

It is clear that some filtering system is functioning in the newborn infant to protect him from the bombardment of stimuli which impinge upon his sensory system. Broadbent (1958) and Spitz (1965) have referred to a "sensory barrier" which prevents the child from being overwhelmed by the quantity of peripheral information. The barrier probably derives from an as yet rather unsophisticated neural system combined with an inherent or early developed capacity to favor certain stimulus patterns while suppressing the processing of others. For selection of stimuli to be possible some sounds must already have been differentiated and identified with their appropriate stimulus. We know that infants respond to sounds even in utero, evidencing heart-rate deceleration (Johansson, Wedenberg and Westin, 1964), and at birth evidence greater response to the mother's voice than to a stranger's voice (DeCasper and Fifer 1980). Thus it would seem that a congenital predisposition or an ability acquired prior to or very soon after birth ensures that significant sounds are processed as figures while nonsignificant sounds are screened for blocking or attenuation, unless of a sufficiently high intensity to evoke reflexive, or later, investigative response. We will see clear evidence in this differential response to meaningful and non-meaningful sounds when we discuss development of the very young child in Chapter 14. We will observe that thresholds for response to various sounds improve markedly during the first years of life, with speech response threshold showing the greatest and most rapid change.

For a child to learn to pay differential attention to various sounds it is necessary for his brain to separate stimuli, that is to say, to weigh them at each instant in time. This makes certain stimuli stand out more distinctly than the rest. A number of factors within the child and within the stimuli will determine which are most attention-getting. The group of stimuli that at a given instance in time command the child's attention become the figure; the remainder constitute the (back)ground. This phenomenon of figure-ground perception appears to occur even when practice has been denied. The research findings of von Senden (1960) on the experience of congenitally blind adults following surgical removal of cataracts showed that after an initial period of recovery, patients evidenced figure-ground perception ability. Without previous visual-perceptual experience, they were able to organize the stimuli into a figure-ground relationship. Lawson has explained this function:

The code interpretation of how an infant learns to differentiate a primitive figure-ground unity to perceive an object as a whole is based on five related assumptions. The first of these is that every perception involves an etiology and a prognosis, i.e., any perception is based on past experience and contains a predictive element. . . .

The second assumption is that every visual perception includes a figure-ground unity. The third assumption is that every perception results in some behavior. The fourth assumption is that following perception of a unity there results an automatic shift of focus to some part or subfigure within the whole. The fifth assumption is that through eye movement (behavior) other parts or subfigures of the whole are sought and the perceived parts are then related and recorded in the memory code.

If we accept all these assumptions, we may say a human infant begins by perceiving a figure-ground unity. He then changes his focus from the figure as a whole to some part of the whole. If he can differentiate lines and angles and can follow the contours of the figure by eye movement, he can differentiate parts of the whole and relate them. If we assume that each movement of the eye is recorded and that the parts of the figure also are recorded, then after the record is complete, perception of any part of a figure would activate the record, firing the entire sequence and producing perception of the whole. (1967, p. 17)

Figure-ground perception is not confined to vision; it also occurs in hearing. It makes it possible for you to attend to a particular sound source against a background of other environmental noises and to shift your attention from one sound source to another. It accounts for the fact that you are able to listen to what one person is saying at a cocktail party, even though everyone is talking, and that you can recognize the melody of a piece of music against the background of accompaniment. It is important to recognize that perception of figure-ground does not constitute the ability to attribute meaning to a stimulus. A person exposed to sound for the first time is able to hear something against a background but will not at first have any knowledge concerning what this something may be. Subjects studied by von Senden were unable to make even the simplest visual discrimination between shapes until they had been given extensive training.

We can find equivalents to the visual code interpretation, described by Lawson, in theories of auditory code interpretation of speech. The infant begins by perceiving figure-ground unity, identifying human speech as an entity. The child responds initially to the emotive content of what Mother says rather than to the language structure itself. The child learns to interpret Mother's mood from the intonation patterns of her speech. Freelander (1970), for example, demonstrated that infants aged 9 to 18 months clearly prefer certain types of speech stimuli. They prefer melodic to monotonic speech, they are more responsive to familiar voices than to unfamiliar ones, and they prefer varied content to repeated content (Mehler, Bertonicini, Barriere et al, 1978). As children's exposure to speech increases, they begin to associate word patterns to intonational patterns. They change their focus to include the key elements of the segmental structure. We saw that the differentiation of the parts of visual patterns is enhanced by the development of the ability to distinguish component lines and angles. Similarly, in auditory perception, the recognition of the underlying phrase markers, cued by intonational patterning, enhances the recognition of syntactic structures.

Cognizant of the role that figure-ground plays in auditory pattern interpretation, we recognize the need for such basic perceptual training in auditory discrimination as part of our program of aural rehabilitation for those with impairments of hearing sensitivity. A distinct difference exists in the manner of processing speech and nonspeech. The author concurs with Ling (1976) that the auditory discrimination of nonverbal sounds and speech sounds is not, therefore, part of the same developmental process. However, commitment to a program of intervention directed at facilitating maximum adaptation to the environment, rather than concentrating exclusively on speech discrimination, means that we should provide training in environmental sound discrimination as well as in the recognition of meaning in the speech signal. We may also train the child to make speech and nonspeech discrimination decisions. Rhythm training of nonspeech and speech patterns appears justified because rhythm, both of speech and nonspeech, is perceived in the nondominant hemisphere of the brain, while speech is perceived in the dominant hemisphere. The relationship between speech and nonspeech perception is not, therefore, exclusive.

Closure

The second important factor to consider in perceptual organization is *closure*. This term refers to the tendency we have to perceive an incomplete figure as being complete. It accounts, in part, for the ability of a person to recognize a spoken word or a sentence on the basis of limited visual cues, or for a person with a marked hearing loss to perceive correctly certain sounds that are inaudible to him or her. Closure obviously is dependent upon prior experience with the whole figure at either the acoustic or linguistic level. It is important to complete correctly a figure with which one is unfamiliar. Given parts of a relatively unfamiliar sentence, you may be unable to complete closure:

_____ has a _____ suffered _____ _____ tragedy.*

However, the task is relatively easy if you are familiar with the whole:

Don't _____ all _____ eggs _____ _____ basket.†

When you encounter an unfamiliar situation, you attempt to understand it by analyzing its components. In so doing, you are able to establish the relationship that exists between the whole and its parts. On future occasions it may not be necessary actually to receive the total stimulus complex in order to recognize it. As has been discussed already, perception of part of the stimulus will frequently be sufficient to call forth a memory of previous perceptions of the same or related experiences. Every stimulus complex

---

* Never has a man suffered such great tragedy.
† Don't put all your eggs in one basket.

has, for each of us, a minimal number of component stimuli necessary for its accurate perception (recognition). This minimum constitutes the *minimal perceptual invariant*. The minimal perceptual invariant need not be a consistent pattern of stimuli. It may be different on different occasions, but whichever combination of stimuli is utilized, it provides the essential elements for recognition.

THE NEED FOR A PERCEPTUAL MODEL

When we work with the hearing-impaired child or adult, our primary goal will be to improve comprehension in various communication and learning situations. We aim to increase the person's ability to recognize the acoustic and visual patterns of spoken language. We need to recognize, however, that in most cases, even with optimal amplification, the amount of acoustic pattern detail will remain limited by the capacity of the damaged cochlea to respond to all frequencies. We can raise sound intensity to a level that stimulates residual auditory nerve fibers not activated by normal conversational speech intensities. Unfortunately, the auditory fibers at this level of intensity are not able to replace the finer sensitivities of those normally activated by conversational speech. Thus even with the added information, the pattern remains distorted. Remember, amplification does not replace deficient auditory capability; it only makes residual potential available.

Our intervention, therefore, has to aim at improving perceptual processing to compensate for the information deficiency that remains even after optimal signal enhancement. This involves increasing the internal ability to predict the probable pattern, that is, to increase expectancy and, therefore, to facilitate closure of a pattern through familiarity with that pattern in context. We seek to help children build the best possible internal representation of the pattern and to teach them to link it to as many related situational, contextual, and linguistic predicters as possible. For adults with acquired hearing deficit, we must strengthen those related cues.

What I am trying to emphasize is that you are not going to be training ears, you are educating or reorganizing perceptual processes. These include more than just auditory perception; they extend to all systems of perceptual processing through which communication information can flow. These are needs and circumstances best addressed by a single-sense analytical approach, but for the most part we analyze cautiously, always aiming to enhance the ability of the person to synthesize the total pattern. For this reason an understanding of perception in communication will guide us in developing our intervention plan.

SUMMARY

- Perceptions are evoked by information received and the manner in which it is processed.
- Perception is an active process involving the organization of the sensory systems to favor processing of predicted patterns.

- Congenital or early acquired hearing impairment changes the child's perceptual organization.
- The fundamental roles of hearing serve awareness, protection, and orientation.
- Awareness is both conscious and preconscious. The latter is a continuous monitoring of the auditory environment from which we derive our perception of ourself relative to our auditory world.
- Acquired hearing impairment reduces auditory monitoring efficiency, eroding a person's sense of well-being.
- Auditory monitoring contributes even more than vision to protection because it is an all-around sense unimpaired by obstructions, unhindered by darkness. An individual's safety thus is reduced by hearing impairment.
- Orientation to sound facilitates rapid response to environmental stimuli and contributes to safety. Orientation identifies objects in spacial relationship to an individual.
- Perceptual organization establishes a hierarchy of stimulus values. The assigned priorities change constantly.
- In concert with orientation, established stimulus priorities permit figure-ground perception essential to stimulus processing.
- Rapid perceptual processing is possible because of the phenomenon of closure.
- Closure is the ability to predict the whole from landmark components, obviating the need to process each detail.

Conclusion

Perception is a result of our immediate relationship with our environment, which we know primarily through our senses. Hearing impairment changes our relationship to the world. More basic than the impediment it presents to speech communication is its effect on critical perceptual processes. These include the preconscious monitoring of our environment, with its resultant sense of well-being, the role hearing plays in protection, and its contribution to our awareness of and orientation to events occurring around us.

It is important, however, to realize that perception is far more complex than sensation. We perceive people, things, and events holistically, with relatively little awareness of their component stimuli. This results from the constancy of perceptions, which, in turn, derives from an underlying organizational pattern included among the processes. Contributing to that organization is figure-ground perception. This prevents the chaos that would result from all stimuli being equally competitive and permits us to determine what we react to. A second process important to our discussion is closure, which obviates detailed processing. Familiarity with a pattern permits recognition once a given amount of information has been deduced.

7

A Perceptual Model

Many models of perception exist in the psychology literature, each representing a particular theory. In seeking a perceptual model to help us understand how we perceive spoken language, I required one that was relatively simple. It also had to offer a practical way of analyzing the interference with perceptual processes that results from hearing impairment.

The model of perceptual processing proposed by Solley and Murphy in their book *Development of the Perceptual World* (1960) meets these requirements. They state that perception is a process that "is extended in time and . . . consists of a series of interdependent subprocesses, or stages which can be partially ordered in their succession" (p. 18). Their schematic model (Figure 7.1) involves five stages: (1) perceptual expectancy; (2) attending; (3) reception; (4) trial and check; and (5) final perceptual organization. Unfortunately, whenever you try to depict a process, its dynamics are lost, leaving a static compartmentalized model. As Solley and Murphy point out, the ordering of the stages is only partial and the subprocesses are interdependent. To target your remedial or educational efforts for maximal communication effectiveness, you need to determine at what stage or stages the problem is occurring and how difficulty at a given stage impacts upon other stages. With this in mind, we now can consider the Solley and Murphy stages in detail.

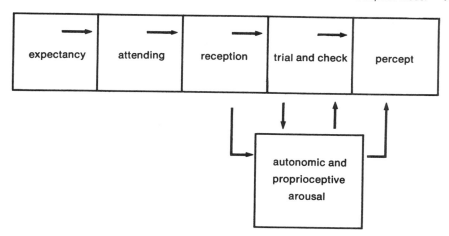

Figure 7.1 A model of the perceptual process. (After Solley & Murphy, 1960.)

EXPECTANCY

I have stressed repeatedly that perception is a process involving the verification of our expectations. I have emphasized the active nature of the perceptual process. We build from birth an ever-expanding knowledge map of our world. We represent internally in memory the concrete world and our experiences with it. We relate and correlate experiences so that we have webs of experiential memories. This ensures that rarely do we ever encounter a totally novel situation, one that has no relationship to any one of our past experiences. Thus we develop expectations.

Expectancy consists of the ability to predict, with some measure of reliability, the probability of a given pattern of stimuli and the likely evolution of an event. Solley and Murphy explain:

> We know from countless acts of commerce with our environment that we can expect such and such a stimulus to follow or occur with another set of stimuli. The ebb and flow of experience is such that we are constantly being bombarded by stimuli, and it is only by developing expectancies and schemata that we are able to deal with this array of stimulation. (1960, p. 156)

In other words, we prepare our perceptual system to facilitate the detection, reception, and analysis of what we expect to receive. Stevens and Halle (1967) describe this as *analysis by synthesis*. We identify patterns based upon the constraints we perceive. We use the constraint rules stored in our system to synthesize internally an expected pattern, a computed probability, an *expectancy*. Analysis consists of comparing this expected pattern with what actually is received. The process is accommodated by the trial-and-check stage of our model.

Expectancy directs us to search for a given stimulus or patterns of stimuli and so increases the probability of our becoming aware of them. An examination of the auditory system as a pattern processor (Sanders, 1977) reveals considerable evidence to support the theory that expectancies result in the tuning or *gating* of the neural pathways. Gating is rather like setting up a flow chart to ensure the rapid transmission of a commodity to where it is expected to be needed most at a given time. As the anticipated needs change, the switches are reset to redirect the commodity flow to appropriate centers. In neural gating it is believed that the thresholds of those neuron combinations not expected to be relevant to the processing of the next segment(s) of the message are raised by means of neurochemical action. At the same time the thresholds of neurons that are predicted to be relevant are lowered, increasing their sensitivity to anticipated message components. In this way processing is accelerated by eliminating the need for all possible combinations of neurons being tried until the appropriate one is identified. The auditory system thus may be set up as a flow chart appropriate to expectancies, providing preferential treatment of relevant components of the message signal. Expectancy and the resultant level of neural gating influence how the signal is processed. When we are unable to predict the message evolution, we are forced to analyze the acoustic signal at the phonetic level until morphologic and syntactic units are reconstructed. This analytical process commonly is referred to as *bottom-up processing*. It occurs when the message is unfamiliar, complex, or distorted; it is slow and laborious. When the constraints are high, when we can predict the evolution of the message, we quickly shift to the processing of much larger units, barely checking the signal to verify our morphologic, syntactic, and semantic predictions. This rapid synthetic procedure is referred to as *top-down processing*.

We will discuss later how a knowledge of language rules allows us to develop linguistic expectancies for speech sound, words, sentence patterns, and semantic values. In this respect expectancy reduces dependency upon the details of the acoustic signal, thus allowing high rates of information flow. Linguistic expectancy also helps to combat the noise in the system. Hearing impairment, which filters out acoustic information, increases our dependency on the remaining acoustic cues. Persons with hearing difficulty are forced to process the details that those of us with normal hearing do not need. This slows processing. Unless normal communication rate is slowed and the linguistic information enriched, the system becomes overloaded and comprehension breaks down. Expectancy of both nonverbal and verbal speech cues is, therefore, particularly important to a person with impaired hearing. The value of expectancy increases considerably when message signals are received under adverse acoustic conditions, such as those imposed by hearing deficiency. By giving priority to expected patterns embedded in the multiple stimuli impinging on our sensory systems, we make attention possible.

ATTENTION

Solley and Murphy consider the process of attending to be biological: "Some sort of competition among the various perceptual tendencies must be resolved by a priority system within the living structure itself" (1960, p. 178).

This involves the selective adjustment of the sense organs, an assumption supported by a growing amount of neurological data.

It has been demonstrated that two sets of nerve fibers are found in the auditory pathway, afferent and efferent. Afferent fiber carry neural impulse patterns away from the cochlear. They ascend the auditory pathways by both the direct and indirect route, passing through the neural centers and terminating in the auditory cortex. Parallel to, but flowing away from the cortex, connecting to the various nerve centers of the auditory system is another set of fibers known as the efferent system. These run from cortex to cochlea. During selective attention it appears that these efferent fibers exert an inhibitory influence on the nerve cells around the focus of excitation, thus sharpening its activity—a type of neural figure-ground function:

> There is strong evidence that this descending inhibitory influence may play a role in "editing" the flow of information by acting to suppress some of the input from the periphery of the receptive field and thereby producing an effective inhibitory surround to the main focus. (Brazier, 1964, p. 1427)

Furthermore, it has been suggested (Neisser, 1967) that we process the patterns to which we attend in a much more sophisticated manner than information from other less important sources.

It is apparent that figure-ground expectancies and selective attention are interdependent processes that serve to rank order environmental stimulus patterns according to our changing needs. The ordering of stimulus patterns is accommodated by two types of attention that relate particularly to our understanding of the process by which learning and relearning of communication patterns occur when a hearing impairment is present. Lawson explains the difference between nonspecific and specific attention thus:

> First, there is the awareness essential for carrying out a learned behavior pattern. A person who has driven an automobile for years performs the manipulations of driving automatically, without paying attention to the details of steering, accelerating, shifting, or braking, as long as the pattern unfolds as expected. However, should the accelerator get stuck, or brakes fail, or any other event occur that is contrary to the normal behavior pattern, then the second kind of awareness of attention would go into operation. Specific attention is now directed to the cause of the disruption and the person is alert to new sensory input, unexpected in terms of normal driving behavior, but expected in view of the disturbance. (1967, p. 98)

These quotes relate well to the processing of language patterns and have implications for auditory training procedures. We need to remember constantly that the successive acts of attending, in close contiguity with one another, are a prerequisite to the integration of the separate bits of sensory information into a meaningful pattern. Children with impaired hearing must be taught listening habits. The fact that amplification brings acoustic information within their reach does not ensure that they naturally will acquire optimal use of it. It is our role to motivate the children to pay attention while we ensure the repeated sound-pattern presentations they need to fuse the parts into a meaningful whole.

Lawson's reference to two types of attention should remind us that the patterns we present can be processed sequentially or in parallel. It has been suggested by Neisser (1963) that in responding to new patterns of stimulation, we use a step-by-step serial procedure to examine the individual features in order. This is a rather slow process, prone to compounding of any error occurring in the early stages of processing. Furthermore, if there are a large number of components, heavy demands are made on short-term memory—something we will discuss later. Nevertheless, it seems we pay attention to detail until we are familiar with the landmark cues and are able to sense the overall pattern emerging. Once this occurs we shift to the parallel processing of information, making it possible to pay no more than scant attention to familiar patterns. In parallel processing we examine the components simultaneously so that the pattern emerges immediately with little need for storage. Familiarity with the pattern means that we can predict it on the basis of little information; thus, tolerance for distortion arises from the inherent redundancy.

Much work with children who are hearing handicapped involves teaching them to become familiar with new auditory-visual speech patterns, and with new linguistic patterns. We need to be aware of the shift in the type of processing that occurs when sensory perceptions become integrated into a meaningful whole with the resulting change in the type of attention. Although we must ensure the availability of the complete pattern of information, we also need to have insight into the possibility that the child is processing the pattern serially while we are dealing with the whole in parallel. Attention is thus the intense focus of the expected figure, a process that holds the perceptual system in an optimal state for reception of relevant stimulus patterns.

RECEPTION

We have examined the acoustic and visual signals that carry information about things, people, and events occurring in the environment. The event of greatest importance to us is of course speech, which generates both auditory and visual patterns. Reception of the speech signal is the function of the peripheral organs of hearing and vision. We have discussed the physical nature of both signals and the factors that limit the fidelity of transmission. We also considered the visual deficiencies that may reduce signal reception. Later we will examine in some detail the effects of hearing impairment on auditory reception.

At this point it is sufficient to iterate that reception of the auditory signal depends first upon the integrity of the conductive mechanism, which reacts and replicates mechanically the acoustic energy wave. The tympanic membrane and the ossicular chain must pass the intensity and frequency information of the energy pattern to the cochlea. The cochlea in turn must have the full range of sensitivity to record and convert faithfully into neural impulse patterns a replica of the mechanical pattern. The crucial requirement is that the pattern set up in the auditory nerve be an accurate replica of the pattern generated by the source, particularly when that source is the vocal articulatory system of a speaker. Bear in mind that although the acoustic speech signal contains all the information necessary to reconstruct the speech event, the listener's auditory system does not receive the acoustic signal. It receives a *copy* of the sound wave pattern *as it was recoded* into neural energy at the cochlea. Thus the receptive stage is all-important in determining whether the listener receives all the intensity, frequency, and durational information that constitutes the true pattern. Any loss or distortion of components of the pattern changes perceptual processing in a manner we will explore when we discuss the effects of hearing impairment.

We tend to think of the function of the cochlea as purely that of a transducer of the energy pattern flowing through the endolymphatic fluid and replicated by the mechanical movement of the basilar membrane and its structures. It is, however, also an analyzer since it breaks down the complex wave into its frequency and intensity parameters. These then are displayed in the ventral and dorsal cochlear nuclei in a manner we refer to as *tonotopic organization*, that is, in a frequency distribution from low to high. What happens from here upward to the brain remains in the realm of hypotheses. I find a combination of two theories helpful in understanding what might happen. The theories, *feature detection theory* and *analysis-by-synthesis*, help clarify the trial-and-check box in the model.

TRIAL AND CHECK (ANALYSIS-BY-SYNTHESIS)

Before the stimulus is finally structured as a percept, the model depicts a stage in which a hypothesis is made about what the signal pattern will be. An internal model of an expected pattern is synthesized from knowledge of prior components of the stimulus and from more general situational and contextual constraint factors. This ongoing pattern prediction, created from information fed forward from earlier segments, is then compared to the actual signal received. The comparison, thus, is between expected and actual input. Solley and Murphy have borrowed the term *trial and check* from Woodworth (1947).

The purpose of this stage, then, is to compare the expected perceptual pattern with what has actually been received. If the predicted event concurs with the perceived event, it is possible to attribute meaning to it. If a discrepancy is revealed, then the organism is directed both to obtain more information through reobservation and to recheck the files of associated memories in an attempt to identify the incoming stimulus complex. Within-channel trial and check might occur, for example, when a friend introduces you to her fiancé. From your friend's previous description of her fiancé, you will have built up an expected perceptual pattern. When you meet him, you may find that he is quite different from what you had envisaged; your predicted image does not concur with what you now perceive: "He's not a bit like I had imagined him." You then seek to eliminate the discrepancy between what you had previously anticipated and what you now observe in order to ensure future recognition. Future recognition thus necessitates your restructuring your image.

The same trial-and-check process has been offered in several mediated theories of speech perception. Each theory postulates that the perception of spoken language involves the active generation by the perceptual system of an internal model against which the incoming speech-pattern information can be compared for verification. The internal model can be synthesized at any level from articulatory to syntactic. The actual level at which we conduct this "analysis by synthesis" depends upon the ease with which we are able to develop accurate predictions at any moment in the process. The poorer our internal prediction function, the more dependent we are on information derived from the acoustic signal. Moving to more detailed analysis slows down and generally impedes communication interaction. Thus the person with impaired hearing is forced to ask for clarification or repetition of what has been said. As a result, communication may be reduced to an unsatisfying level of interaction.

In attempting to understand the trial-and-check (or analysis-by-synthesis) component, remember that it is not confined to any one sensory channel. We recognize that a given object or event simultaneously emits stimuli of various types. We may see, hear, and touch a particular object. In doing so, we initiate a trial-and-check procedure for each channel. We know that in the brain interconnecting fibers travel between various subcortical centers strongly suggesting the existence of a complex system involving reception, integration, analysis, association, and interpretation of data from all sensory end organs. The trial-and-check process occurs, therefore, not simply *within* a sensory channel, but also *between* sensory channels. When we perceive and attribute meaning to something, we do so because there is harmony between the perceptual structures in each channel. If, for example, you were to see what you thought to be a vase of freshly cut roses, but on touching them felt the texture of silk and noted the absence of any scent, you would reject the visual percept that you had already satisfied with the trial-and-check process for that sensory channel.

Between-channel trial and check would be important in a communication situation in which a speaker might perceive a person to say, "Did you hear that John Smith lost his life in a car accident?" This sentence would make sense in context and would pass an auditory trial-and-check stage. If, however, the observer noted that the word heard as "life" showed lip rounding of the initial sound, he or she would not achieve auditory-visual, interchannel trial-and-check agreement. If the word has lip rounding for the initial sound, it cannot be "life"—it must be "wife." The observer will therefore reject the initial perception and replace it by, "Did you hear that John Smith lost his wife in a car accident?"

The amount of trial and check necessary is a function of the predictability of the event. When redundancy is high, as in favorable listening or viewing conditions, it is not necessary to carry out extensive trial and check. However, when high noise levels in one sensory channel reduce redundancy, then trial and check both within and between sensory channels becomes vital to comprehension. Our justification for training the hard-of-hearing person in visual communication skills is based upon this awareness of the part that intersensory-channel trial and check contributes to the correct decoding of the message signal.

Trial and check depends, therefore, upon our familiarity with the evolving message and with the language within which it has been encoded. As that predictability drops, we must process the incoming patterns in greater detail. When we need more information, we probably extract it from the neural equivalent of the acoustic signal by the process of feature detection.

According to this theory, the neural system has an array of neuron feature-detector units, each sensitive to a specific acoustic feature. By feeding neural representations of the acoustic features through this system, the presence or absence of every feature can be determined. A unit will fire only when all the criteria for its particular feature are present. Patterns of neuron firings thus come to represent phonologic values. The model developed by Hemdal and Hughes (1967) illustrates this process (Figure 7.2). In this model the incoming acoustic signal is subject to a series of questions, the answers to which determine the nature of further analysis

Figure 7.2 Independent time segmentation classification. (Hemdal & Hughes 1967, p. 448.)

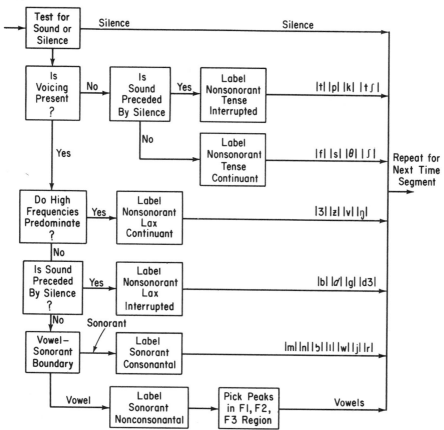

until the category of sound has been identified. For example, the presence of voicing excludes all non-voiced sounds from the probabilities, while the presence of high-frequency energy and a preceding interval of silence eliminates all but the /b/ /d/ /g/ /d/ phonemes. It is important to note that the input data will not be perceived in terms of the external stimulus, *but in terms of how the system has processed it.* The peripheral data undergo numerous transformations:

> By the time the temporal spacial patterns reach cortical circuits, the code may bear little relation to the original stimulus pattern. Indeed, perception may be so altered by the reticular system that it represents a distortion of the actual nature of the stimulating world. (Berry, 1969, p. 101)

In Kohler's words:

> What the subject sees then is not constructed from bricks; rather what the subject sees represents the results of encoding routines or cognitive operations that work on whatever materials are available. (1967, p. 224)

These statements emphasize that the impact of a hearing impairment will depend upon the degree to which the internal encoding routines are intact. As Kohler explains, these "cognitive operations . . . work on whatever materials are available." When language and speech learning have been well established, the degree to which a reduction of acoustic information can be compensated for by cognitive processing routines is remarkable. I often wonder how someone with a significant hearing loss has managed to cope so well for so long without amplification. However, these internal resources are not present in the child with a congenital hearing deficiency. Hearing impairment for these children is as much a cognitive-linguistic problem as it is a receptive one. It is difficult to generate *trial* expectations against which to *check* the incoming pattern when the internal repertoire of cognitive linguistic knowledge is so impoverished. Linguistic closure is seldom a viable option for young congenitally hearing-impaired children. They simply have not acquired the experience necessary to make a tentative hypothesis to perform the two-stage trial and check described by Woodworth:

> When a new percept is in the making—when an obscure stimulus-complex is being deciphered, or when the meaning of a cue or sign is being discovered—an elementary two-phase process is observable. It is a trial-and-check, trial-and-check process. The trial phase is a tentative reading of the sign, a tentative decipherment of the puzzle, a tentative characterization of the object; and the check phase is an acceptance or rejection, a positive or negative reinforcement of the tentative perception. (1947, pp. 123–124)

This processing of the incoming signal appears to fluctuate between detailed analysis when predictions are low and a rapid scanning of the signal simply to check it against our trial, when we are fairly confident we are understanding correctly. The demands placed upon attention will vary accordingly. We will notice shifts in the amount of attention we pay to the acoustic signal as familiarity with the topic, the vocabulary and language structure, and our interest in the topic vary. These concepts should play an important role in our understanding of the complexity of the communication problems that derive from impairment of hearing. They also should influence both our concept of the needs that are created and the most appropriate approaches for meeting those needs through cognitive, linguistic, and perceptual enhancement of listening behaviors. These strategies will, however, need to go beyond improving reception attention and trial and check, for unless a library of experiences is developed there will be no resource of internal redundancy upon which to draw. That resource is stored in memory, which plays a critical role in auditory perception.

MEMORY PROCESSING

Because the acoustic speech stimulus is continuous and unsegmented, the listener at no time has available more than the minutest part of a meaningful segment. Therefore, it is necessary for the brain to record the acoustic information. It must be allowed to accumulate until enough of the pattern emerges for probabilities to be computed and predictions generated. Storage is believed to occur in three stages, each of which is different in nature. The stages or types of memory are

1. *Echoic* memory
2. *Short-term* memory
3. *Long-term* memory

Echoic Memory

Echoic memory consists of an echo of the actual neural equivalent of the acoustic pattern. The amount that can be stored is small, only 2 to 3 seconds in duration (Bjork & Healy, 1970; Crowder & Morton, 1960; Estes, 1970). Echoic memory storage allows sufficient pattern image to be pictured for the extraction of distinctive features and essential suprasegmental information. It can be envisaged as an oscilloscope screen on which the most recent pattern information continuously enters at the left and moves rapidly across to the opposite side fading as it travels. The screen can depict only a 2–3 second section of the continuous pattern flowing across it. What appears in echoic memory depends upon how faithfully the acoustic signal is replicated neurally by the cochlea. All processing above this level will reflect any deficits at this stage. Deficits must be compensated for by closure strategies based upon the ability of the brain to predict the missing information. The characteristics of echoic memory are

- It is an analog or replica of the pattern at the cochlea.
- It is short in duration.
- The information is fast fading with no recall potential.
- It is nonsegmental.

Information is restructured out of echoic memory into short-term memory.

Short-Term Memory

Short-term memory differs totally from echoic memory because the information has been changed from raw data into segmented linguistic form organized according to the rules of the language. It is at this level of processing that we first are able to exert conscious control over memory content. For example, we are able to renew the linguistic pattern by rehearsing what we heard, either overtly or covertly, or we may recode it into a mnemonic key to aid future recall. Short-term memory is, however, also limited in capacity. Miller (1956) has explained that the number of stimulus units that we can hold in conscious memory is limited to between five and nine. This holds true whether we are trying to remember numbers, words, or any other kind of unit. To surmount this limitation, we must combine smaller units into larger chunks. Although these are subject to what Miller refers to as the limitation of the "magical number seven plus or minus two," each unit represents a relatively large amount of information. In processing spoken language, chunking into more and more complex units results from progressively restructuring the information up through the linguistic hierarchy from phoneme through morpheme to syntax. In this way we can remember several sentences just as they were spoken, but we cannot retain an equally long string of unrelated words.

Short-term memory is characterized by the fact that it is

- Segmental
- Linguistically based
- Available for rehearsal, which prolongs the pattern
- Expandable through chunking

It is a memory that has linguistic *structure* as its primary responsibility, though comprehension for short duration also is a secondary function. For conceptual processing and recall and thus for the process of learning, we must depend upon long-term memory.

Long-Term Memory

Long-term memory is concerned with concepts, ideas, facts. Here the emphasis is on the *meaning* or *content*, not the structure of the message. The original language pattern fades while the semantic value and the webs of meaning linking the information to other relevant information are retained.

Access to that information necessitates that it be restructured back into an equivalent linguistic pattern. It is important to recognize that because the original language structure was not stored, the accuracy of recall of a topic will depend upon the ability of the person to use knowledge of language rules to restructure an equivalent message. Memory for spoken language content, therefore, is influenced by the ability to construct a linguistic message from an acoustic pattern, and later by the ability to reconstruct an equivalent language pattern when the information needs to be retrieved. Long-term memory thus is storage of *meaning*, which involves correlation of new information with relevant existing information. Access to long-term memory requires the ability to restructure the memories into linguistic forms.

Each of the stages in perceptual processing requires very complex activities. It is not surprising, therefore, to find evidence that suggests that through learning a part of the process becomes relegated to an internal monitoring system. This system exerts an active influence not only on how stimuli are processed, but also on the sensitivity of the system to different stimulus patterns. This role has been attributed to the autonomic and proprioceptive arousal system.

AUTONOMIC AND PROPRIOCEPTIVE AROUSAL SYSTEM

In recent years there has been a considerable growth of interest in the role of the feedback mechanism by which the sensory perceptual system monitors its own behavior. We have mentioned already the efferent fibers that run from cortex to periphery, tuning the sensory systems in preparation for the expected pattern.

Clear evidence is available, therefore, of the existence of a servomechanism within the auditory perceptual system. This afferent-efferent loop changes a passive sensory system into a dynamic tunable one under the control of higher processing levels. The capability exists for the processing of the input signal, indeed for its very reception, to be preset by higher-order neurons on the basis of computed expectancies. Rather than "feedback" we would envisage a "feedback-feedforward" process preparing the system to respond in a weighted manner to any components of the total stimulus array that are predicted as relevant, while rejecting the upward flow of other stimuli. Thus stimuli either are processed upward to conscious levels of awareness, or processed no further than a preattentive level.

According to Solley and Murphy, the organisms' constant sensory scanning activities constitute the heart of perception. These result from homeostatic factors, from specific needs or sets. Initially random in character, this scanning for exteroceptor cues becomes more patterned. It is not unreasonable to assume that scanning becomes more selective, more appropriate, as the neural system becomes tuned in accord with expectancies. As early parts of the incoming signal confirm crude expectancies, more accurate tuning of the perceptual system is possible, resulting in more effective scanning procedures. French (1957) is of the opinion that the internal scanning process probably constitutes part of the function of the reticular formation, which, he suggests, develops differential sensitivity to stimuli. This view is certainly in accord with neurological theories of speech perception (Abbs & Sussman, 1971; Uttley, 1954, 1959, 1966) and with what is known about the efferent system. French proposes that the attention pattern results from the action of both the arousal system and a cortical probability calculation. Solley and Murphy also suggest that we scan for internal memory cues to identify a match between the incoming stimuli and memory traces left from previous stimuli. Active mediative theories of speech perception view the process as more generative (Lieberman, Cooper, Shankweiler, & Studdert-Kennedy, 1967; Stevens & Halle, 1967). According to these theorists the system actually generates a pattern based upon probability computations. It is against this pattern that the incoming signal is compared for verification of predictions. Neisser (1967) proposes that "this constructive process is itself the mechanism of auditory perception." Thus those components that do not match constitute the ground, as discussed earlier. "Scanning moves to that which is congruent with established set and excludes that which is noncongruent" (Solley & Murphy, 1960, p. 253). It seems justified, therefore, to modify the model in Figure 7.1 to show the arrows running in both directions between each stage to represent the tuning in the system we have discussed.

We have talked repeatedly about the need to enrich total perception for the hearing-impaired person in all available ways. The question arises whether it is feasible to sensitize the student to such internal cues. If this is possible, we may be able to evoke what Solley and Murphy refer to as a new "search set." The authors are reassuring; they refer to an experiment by Seward (1931) in which it was shown that on a repeated visual-perceptual task in which no results were given to the subject between trials, the number of correct responses increased progressively. This indicates that repeated exposure to the sensory data arising from a perceptual act, even in the absence of external feedback, may lead to the modification of the response to more closely approximate reality. Evidence that this may be true for the perceptual act of interpreting visual speech cues can be derived from the present author's work with Goodrich (Sanders & Goodrich, 1971). Examination of the mean scores obtained by normal-hearing subjects on four successive visual-discrimination tests of monosyllabic words with no feedback given revealed that the mean items correctly identified rose from 6.60 on the first presentation to 8.00 on the fourth. This tendency encourages us to persevere with many aspects of auditory and visual communication training, even though to date we lack experimental proof of value. In the words of Solley and Murphy (1960): "To the extent an individual can learn to discriminate and recognize these cues he can gain greater control over his perceptual system and, hence, become more viridical in his perceptions" (p. 260).

THE PERCEPT

The ultimate result of these progressive stages is the *percept*. This final structuring of the perception permits meaning to be attributed to the stimulus complex. The stimulus is interpreted in a particular way on the basis of previous experience. The phenomena of figure-ground and closure play an important role in determining the final percept. We have seen that the determinants of the figure-ground relationship lie both within the stimulus and within the individual. It is a dangerous oversimplification to consider the environment and the individual as independent entities. They are, in fact, so interrelated as to constitute one system. It is rather like stirring chocolate cake batter into a white cake mixture to make a marble cake. In places, the cake is clearly all white or all brown, yet in general, the colors run together so as to be inseparable.

The process by which we finally attribute meaning is highly complex but clearly involves the fusion of selected external stimuli with the memory of past experiences. This brings about an interpretation that most reasonably fits in with the information that has satisfactorily passed the within-channel and between-channel trial-and-check stage. This process is never completed; our perceptions can never be reality, because absolute reality is really nonexistent. We are not attempting to specify a "something" out there, but rather to specify the significance of the result of our interaction with that "something." That is, we perceive in terms of how we process stimuli. So the trial-and-check process constitutes a continuous servo-mechanism, causing us to reevaluate constantly our perceptions in light of the never-ceasing intake of additional sensory data. The amount of perceptual change must be a function of the ability of the individual to use the additional stimulus input; such ability is determined by motivation, awareness, and a library of perceptual experiences. Through a systematic program of aural rehabilitation, we aim to provide the hard-of-hearing person with an enhanced ability to do this.

We have now set the stage for a consideration of the perception of the auditory and visual speech signal.

Each of the perceptual processes we have considered contributes to the highly complex act of human communication. We probably never will know exactly how we enable another person to understand what we are thinking, or how that person can effect that in us. Yet to enhance that process is the charge we accept when we work with communicatively handicapped persons. To even begin to plan what we can do, we need a way of representing the problem. It is to assist us in this task that various communication models have been developed.

SUMMARY

- Perceptual models must accommodate the fact that perception involves a complex of somewhat linear interdependent subprocesses and stages that function overtime to produce a percept.
- The subprocesses in the Solley and Murphy model considered here are (1) expectancy, (2) attention, (3) reception, (4) trial and check, and (5) perceptual organization.
    1. *Expectancy* derives from probabilities. These lead to predictions concerning how a message likely will evolve at each level of linguistic structure.
    2. *Attention* is the result of selective processing. The neural system is tuned to favor expected patterns over unexpected patterns and to prioritize the processing of available stimuli.

        Selective processing is thought to be effected by the efferent system.

        Two types of attention have been postulated: preconscious nonspecific attention, which is a monitoring of well-learned behavior; and specific attention involved in learning and problem solving.
    3. *Reception* refers to the process of detecting and representing sensory stimuli by neural patterns.

4. *Trial and check* is the process of testing a hypothesis regarding a pattern evolution by comparing predicted patterns to actual patterns. This occurs by sampling major features rather than by careful analysis.

- *Internal monitoring* through *feedback* maintains the effectiveness of the system.
- Three stages of *memory* are involved in perception: *echoic memory* retains an image of the sensation pattern just long enough to extract its features; *short-term memory* stores linguistic patterns derived from the raw data; *long-term memory* stores meanings, ideas, concepts.
- The autonomic and proprioceptive arousal system provides an ongoing feedback-feedforward function by means of an afferent-efferent loop. The autonomic arousal system constantly and progressively tunes perceptual processing to accommodate expected patterns.

5. The percept is the product of analysis and interpretation of related sensory patterns from the relevant modalities. The percept is shaped by memory associations and comprises an internal experience.

Conclusion

Perception is a highly complex process that results from the interaction of sensory stimuli with the sensorineural system. The process is active and is affected by the tuning of the system by the action of the efferent fibers. Tuning is used to facilitate the rapid analysis of predicted pattern components and to dampen sensitivity to those components predicted to be less relevant. It prioritizes processing, a function we call *attention*. The nature of attention itself is adapted to accommodate detailed processing (specific attention) of unfamiliar tasks and the preconscious or barely conscious processing (nonspecific attention) of familiar information or activities. To facilitate rapid processing, stimulus patterns in echoic memory are checked against predictions. This trial and check is repeated at each linguistic level in speech processing, which involves short- and long-term memory. The end product is the percept, which is an internal representation derived from sensory information, the process of analysis, and memory of related experience.

8

A Model of Communication

THE NATURE OF MODELS

Having identified the prerequisites to communication, we now must try to envisage a way in which the human communication system processes the information we receive from and send to each other. To do this we use a model. There are many models of communication, each attempting to identify the components of the process, how they relate to each other, and how they function. Subdividing the components and stages, as we do when we develop models, exposes us to the risk of a simplistic view of the problem and how to deal with it. Yet a degree of analysis is essential to problem solving. It enables us to differentiate among breakdowns occurring at different stages of processing, even though the presenting behaviors may be the same. Models do not represent *how* communication processes work. They are simply representations of how we envisage those processes *might* function given what we know about the system. Models are important for a number of reasons:

- They provide us with a way of envisaging the processes in a logical manner.
- They integrate what we know about communication based upon research and observation.

91

- They permit us to develop rational hypotheses concerning what we do not know.
- They provide a rationale for the development of hypotheses regarding how we might intervene to reduce problems.

We remain far from a comprehensive knowledge of the intricate processes of human communication; indeed, we may never fully understand them. However, we know enough to be able to construct theoretical models based upon research, empirical data, and reasoning. The purpose of such models, of which there are many types, is not to explain communication. A model serves rather to integrate what we know from a variety of fields of study into a holistic picture. We then can use a given model to examine the component units to see how they relate and to test the model's integrity and usefulness in understanding the communication process.

The advantage of a model is that it provides us with the basis for understanding the communication problems associated with impaired hearing and it affords a rationale for the intervention procedures we develop. However, you must keep in mind, always, that models still remain largely hypothetical, should be reconsidered constantly in light of new factual information, and are of value only to the extent that you can use them practically. We now will examine each of the prerequisites essential to communication beginning with equivalence of experience.

PREREQUISITES TO COMMUNICATION

Consider seriously the act of communication. You cannot help but be amazed that a process so complex that we can do little more than speculate as to its true nature occurs unconsciously, effortlessly, and with few flaws most of the time. Those of us with normal hearing rarely pay attention to the sounds of speech; we perceive instead meaningful messages. Similarly it is seldom that we trip over our tongues, or say something that surprises us as much as our listener. It is important to keep this automaticity of spoken language comprehension and production in mind in our study of communication breakdown. Ultimately our efforts must lead to maximal communication effectiveness with minimal attention to the process itself. We must aim to make habitual in the child or adult the procedures we use in our intervention strategies.

The problems of the person with impaired hearing arise from difficulty in understanding what others are saying about an unlimited number of possible topics in a wide variety of situations. When the impairment is congenital or occurs early in life, the child's ability to learn optimally through audition, the manner by which so much of our knowledge normally is acquired, will be affected. The acquisition of verbal language skills particularly will be involved. For a person with a hearing problem, therefore, the overriding difficulty is to define and share experience.

Satisfactory communication is dependent upon two or more people's sharing of a common means of interaction. This necessitates the development of a communication system in which the participants have compatibility. The person with impaired hearing will experience a communication handicap in proportion to the degree to which his or her handicap reduces this compatibility. It is the aim of habilitation/rehabilitation procedures to develop compensatory strategies to reduce the impedance between the individual and the larger communication matrix into which that person must fit.

THE STORE OF EQUIVALENT EXPERIENCES

When communication occurs successfully between two people, it means that Subject A has managed to cause Subject B to experience thoughts that represent the ideas Subject A wished to communicate. The important point is that the thoughts the listener experiences are her own. They are *equivalent to* those of Subject A and are *evoked* by Subject A, but they were neither sent nor received.

The first requirement for successful communication is, therefore, that each participant possesses a store of experiences to which others may relate. Similarity of stored experience is a prerequisite. When experiences between people are noticeably different—as occurs, for example, between racial or cultural groups—communication becomes difficult even when the parties are able to use a common language code. This is relevant to our understanding of the problems arising from hearing impairment.

When we encounter a young, congenitally severely hearing-impaired child, we are acutely aware of that child's difficulties in using language to express ideas. It is easy for the problems of linguistic proficiency to conceal the fact that the child's communication handicap goes much deeper than the use of structural language. So much of what we know is acquired through use of verbal language. Even our perceptions of direct experience are modified by the manner in which we encode them linguistically. Because of language deficiency, the young hearing-impaired child's experience of the world will be less sophisticated than that of his hearing peers. Unless special help is provided, the child will not be able to participate equally in shared experiences as his peers do through their use of language. Thus we must not overlook the fact that although difficulty in the use of the language code appears to be the problem, the situation is complicated even further by the limits placed upon the acquisition and storage of experience. The reduced compatibility between the store of experiences of the hearing-handicapped child and hearing peers places the roots of the problem even deeper than the coding and transmission processes.

This becomes an increasingly influential factor as the growing child with normal hearing adds more and more abstract experiences to knowledge of the concrete relationships of the physical world of people and things. In order to perceive, store, and communicate at an abstract level, use of an increasingly sophisticated language code is essential. The child with a congenital or early acquired hearing deficit will almost certainly be unable to add to his store of experience at the same rate as hearing peers. This is not to say that the hearing-impaired child is less intelligent or less capable than his hearing counterparts. The problem lies in the impairment of auditory processing of information resulting from the hearing deficit. The ultimate impact of the impairment on the child's learning rate will depend on many factors. The child's innate intellectual potential, personality, parental and environmental influences, and the age at which intervention is begun are among the most important. However, the amount of useable residual hearing, together with the age at which amplification is provided and the success with which it is used, will exert a highly significant influence on the successful acquisition of knowledge.

Most of what a child comes to know about the world is self-deduced through exposure to events in context. We learn mostly by a process of absorption, similar to osmosis, rather than by direct instruction. Yet for experience itself to influence behavior requires refinement, clarification, correlation, and storage. This is particularly true if experience is to serve to permit a person to predict ahead. We use linguistically stored information about past experience to define what appear initially to be novel situations or problems. The processes necessitate the development of some form of symbolic language, though it need not be spoken language. Without the language tool, the experiences of the child with impaired hearing will be different from those of hearing peers. These experiences also will be impoverished, compared to those of his hearing peers, and their rate of acquisition reduced. This is so because poor language-coding abilities limit the manner in which the hearing-impaired child can deal with direct experience. The hearing-impaired child will have difficulty in defining an event, in storing information about the event, and in correlating the event with memories of past experiences. The discrepancy will rapidly accelerate as children with normal hearing move from the period of concrete thinking to more sophisticated processes of abstraction. Abstraction involves the ability to deal with things, people, events, and feelings that are not currently occurring. Abstraction allows us to deal instead with the symbolic referents into which those experiences have been encoded. We can thus overcome the limitations imposed by time and space, to deal with what one student aptly referred to as the "not here—not now."

The problems arising from congenital or early acquired hearing impairment thus affect the store of experiences that dominate the compatibility between the hearing-impaired child and those with whom that child must communicate. The degree of impedance, at this most basic level, will depend on the compatibility between the experiences of the communicators. This is why hearing impairment occurring very early in life exerts such a profound influence on normal cognitive and linguistic development. It explains why children who have had hearing for only one or two years, or even for no more than a few months before it is lost, evidence so much more natural auditory responsiveness when amplification is provided than a child with a true congenital hearing deficit. It also explains the concern of audiologists, teachers, and speech-language pathologists for early diagnosis and intervention.

The effect of hearing impairment on the development of a store of common experiences decreases as the age at which the hearing impairment occurs increases. The effect is related closely to the language level at the age of onset, but its influence is felt even in the older school-age years. At that time, the filtering out of auditory information affects the acquisition and understanding of the more sophisticated forms of language play, such as humor, sarcasm, double-entendre, or punning. These more subtle limitations may not be evident in standard test results, but they often show up in anecdotal accounts of difficulties experienced.

The separation of experience and language is thus an artificial dichotomy; they can be considered separate only in the early years when experience precedes language. As language develops, exposure to new verbal expressions or new vocabulary often initiates a search for an experience or meaning to relate to the language.

Hearing impairment also must be understood in terms of its impact on the learning process. Test results that indicate that a child has adequate language skills do not reflect the difficulty the child is almost certain to have in using those skills under adverse listening conditions. To be able to use linguistic skills successfully, the child must receive the spoken message with a clarity adequate to permit language decoding. The test environment usually provides optimum listening conditions. School classrooms, as we discussed in Chapter 3, constitute notoriously poor listening environments. Under the conditions of noise and reverberation that the student is likely to encounter in school, even a mild hearing impairment can impair speech comprehension. Difficulty is frequently experienced in following directions and in feeling confident to act even upon what has been heard. The effect of such reduction in the clarity of the speech signal has a still greater impact on the student's ability to learn from orally presented information, which may be difficult to understand even when heard clearly.

A COMMON LINGUISTIC CODE

In discussing the importance of a common store of equivalent experience, consideration of the influence of language is unavoidable. It is apparent that language and experience are related intimately. Language not only molds experience, it also serves as a valuable tool that facilitates the acquisition of new experience. We use our language system to code experience for storage and easy retrieval. In this way we are able to deal with the world abstractly, which infinitely affects the manner in which we can interact with others. Instead of confining our discussions to things present or to events as they occur, we are able to override the constraints of time and space by tapping into the abstractions of those occurrences now stored in the referential language system. Symbolic coding permits us to transform concrete experiences into abstract ones. When we function linguistically, we do so by manipulating the code to formulate the referential patterns equivalent to the experiences we wish to consider. Communication occurs when two or more people use a language code to cause each other to formulate equivalent coexperiential abstracts. The ability to do this successfully necessitates not only that participants each have a store of equivalent experiences, but also that they share a common language code.

When we think of a language code, we automatically think of spoken language because in all cultures, in all societies, spoken language is the common basis for communication. Languages differ in the actual symbols that have evolved, and this presents a communication barrier between people from different language cultures. In addition, different languages result in individuals' experiencing the world differently from one another. Nevertheless, all languages are based upon the ability of human beings to restructure experience into a symbolic code.

The potential to do this is almost certainly part of our genetic endowment. The newborn child with normal sensorimotor capacities, capable of learning *a* language, is, therefore, capable of learning *all* languages equally well. As the child begins to develop a particular language, the ability to acquire fluency in others decreases as the years pass. Even so, a child who has a need to learn several languages will retain far more of the facility that permitted the first language to be learned than will the monolingual person. This decreasing capacity to learn other languages as we grow older does not represent a particular handicap to most of us. Recognition of this phenomenon, however, should have great impact upon our appreciation of the problems of the prelinguistically deaf child. For such a child, the task is not second-language learning, but the acquisition of a native tongue. The longer we wait to take intervention steps to stimulate language learning, the harder this task will be and the more limited the child's potential for optimal achievement.

Linguistic Coding

The language coding process entails

- A set of internalized values or experience memories
- A set of symbols keyed to those values
- A set of rules that govern the manner in which the symbols may be combined to form complex patterns to facilitate rapid communication about an unlimited number of values or experiences

Values

Values refer to memories and experiences. We become aware of them only when they are called to consciousness. This may occur when a sensory experience evokes associated memories or most commonly when language taps into memory. At this level of processing, we stand at the boundary, or *interface*, between raw experience and the details of experience encoded into linguistic structures or patterns. Communication begins and ends at this interface, where language evokes perception of experience, or, in expressive communication, where the experience is encoded into the language form. In a way, the concept of a true boundary is misleading, for there is, as we have discussed, a considerable overlap between language and experience. The meaning of experience must mesh with the symbolic level of processing if communication is to occur. Semantic perception involves the evoking of units of speech as large as a phrase or several phrases. At this level the patterns are treated holistically with little or no awareness of the individual components. This is the level of identification of *meaning*, the level of *understanding*. However, holistic pattern processing first requires that a sufficient number of individual components at lower linguistic levels—that is, phonemes, words—be identified in order to predict without ambiguity the future pattern development and to identify the associated meaning. These tokens exist in a layered or *hierarchical structure* and may be identified from the information generated by the speaker and broadcast into several media.

Tokens

Tokens are elements of the language structure that may be identified and reconstructed by the "listener" from the pattern of information received by his or her sensory system. It is again necessary to stress that tokens are learned, that they *exist within the speaker and receiver*, but not in the physical stimulus. The pattern contains only the information necessary to identify the token. This requires that the receiver be sensitive to enough of the physical stimulus to identify the pattern unambiguously. The receiver also must be experienced in transforming the physical pattern of information to the abstract linguistic token. The child with a congenital hearing impairment experiences difficulties with both of these stages, whereas a person with a postlinguistically acquired hearing deficit has trouble with pattern reception only.

Linguistic tokens are the building blocks of linguistic communication. They may be encoded by articulation (speech), broadcast acoustically (sound waves), and received auditorily (hearing and auditory perception). Similarly they may be encoded physically by the hands (signing, fingerspelling), broadcast visually (light waves), and received visually (seeing and visual perception). Visual encoding of token information has also been successful using colored plastic chips to represent different linguistic values (Carrier, 1976; Premack & Premack, 1974). The vibrotactile channel, another avenue for the encoding of linguistic patterns, has relevance in teaching children with minimal residual hearing (Englemann & Rosov, 1975; Erber & Cramer, 1974).

Rules

I mentioned earlier that tokens exist in a hierarchical structure. At each level, a set of rules peculiar to a particular language culture governs the ways in which tokens may be combined. In effective communication both the speaker and listener are familiar with these linguistic rules, which exist at each level of processing of the verbal message and are used both in encoding and decoding. The shared knowledge of these rules permits the tokens to be restructured into patterns of increasing complexity. Thus, the pattern at each level derives from the application of a rule to the tokens at a lower or *deeper* level, changing the form but not the value of the message. The human mind learns to recognize rapidly the implied value of a pattern at a given level. It is not necessary to decode a particular pattern to its essential ingredients because its meaning can be predicted from a knowledge of the rules governing restructuring of tokens.

The size of the tokens varies from phonemes to sentences. There has been much debate over the question of the size of the perceptual unit used in speech perception. It is assumed that the *minimal* elements of speech perception are located below the level of the phoneme (Lehiste, 1972). It is likely, however, that in normal communication we process a chunk of the signal no smaller than is necessary to identify a token at the highest level. Only in phonetic transcription or in spelling are we interested in processing individual sounds. Usually, we do not even have to pay attention to individual words, but listen instead for the meaning.

We will discuss this further when we consider speech perception. It helps to remember, however, that the child with impaired hearing has reduced familiarity with the rules for identifying or generating syntactic patterns. Thus, the ability to process the surface level of the larger pattern is reduced, forcing the child to depend more heavily on the processing of smaller units. A hearing-impaired child, therefore, has much greater need of the extrinsic information contained in the acoustic signal of which, paradoxically, such a child receives less than a person with normal hearing.

INFORMATION PROCESSING

Before we leave our discussion of the role the cognitive-linguistic system plays in communication, it is necessary to examine how the constraints of language structure operate. We need to understand how abstract language patterns in one person's mind can effect the construction of equivalent patterns in the mind of another. This is achieved by the transmission and processing of *information*. Note that the meaning of the term *information* here derives from statistical theory having to do with probability. Its use, however, is highly appropriate in the context of our discussion because our model of communication is built upon predictions made by the listener on the basis of his or her ability to compute probabilities.

Information was described by Shannon and Weaver (1967), who evolved a mathematical model of information transmission, as "the informativeness of the symbols in a message relative to one's expectation of those symbols." In other words, the components of the pattern at all levels of processing are informative to the extent that they are needed and used to constrain choice.

Phonemic Constraints

That which we expect, whether it be individual speech sounds, a sentence, or a whole phrase, does not convey very much constraint value—that is, information. The unexpected is, by contrast, highly informative. Thus, the role of information is to limit choice on the basis of expectancies computed from a knowledge of probabilities. Carroll (1964, p. 55) illustrates this with three strings of ten-letter messages with the tenth letter missing:

P	R	R	N	W	B	I	T	K	—
A	A	A	A	A	A	A	A	A	—
G	E	N	E	R	A	T	I	O	—

Carroll points out that the informativeness of the missing symbol is great in the first example because the symbols are in random sequence. The probability of a given letter occurring in the tenth position is uninfluenced by those preceding it and is, therefore, low. In the second example, if the selection of the letter A for the missing symbol proves correct, it will convey little information because one would have had little difficulty predicting it. If, on the other hand, it proves not to be A, the missing letter would be highly informative. The missing N in the third string of letters may be predicted with a high degree of success because the choice of the letters is severely restricted by all of the preceding letters and is further constrained by the imposition of morphological constraints and the semantic criterion—that is, for the result to be a meaningful English word, an N is required for completion.

Structural Constraints

At each level of linguistic processing, a different set of probabilities operates. For a person familiar with the linguistic rules the speaker is using, the linguistic constraints operating at the phonemic level begin to generate probabilities as soon as the first phoneme is identified. This is so because the listener's mind has subconsciously learned the rules that determine the relative statistical probability of occurrence of a given phoneme immediately following or preceding any other given phoneme. As the number of phonemes decoded increases, the probabilities for succeeding phonemes continue to narrow with each additional phoneme until only one is possible. To understand how we narrow the choices to one phoneme, it is necessary to recognize that as phonemic pattern builds, we begin to derive enough information at that level to allow us to shift gears and to begin to process according to the higher constraints of the morphological level. At this level we are concerned with the requirement that phonemes be grouped into meaningful forms such as *ing, ly, ness,* or into whole words. These forms comprise the basic elements of grammatical structure and are slotted into the syntactical constraint patterns until syntactic predictions begin to be possible. As soon as this occurs, perceptual processing begins to operate on probabilities computed at the syntactic level of pattern reconstruction. This obviates the need for time-consuming processing of individual units, shifting the reconstruction process to the generating of much larger patterns on the basis of syntactic constraints.

Contextual Constraints

Even familiarity with the structural rules of a language frequently proves insufficient to permit a message to be understood under conditions of distortion. If, however, the topic of conversation is made known, the distorted signal may be interpreted because it is in context. The effect of contextual and/or semantic constraints is to limit the choice of words and phrases that may be used to convey a particular meaning. A conversation on the topic of baseball eliminates the use of most vocabulary that might be appropriate to a discussion of, for example, music. It is in this way that we often reject a particular interpretation of a distorted message because it appears to be unrelated to its context. Certainly a relationship exists between the semantic and syntactical constraints. We are aided in our interpretation of the signal by the knowledge that nouns are naming words, that verbs designate activities, and that adjectives describe properties or characteristics. Yet, as Cherry (1957, p. 119) points out, meaning may be conveyed by a chain of nouns—for example, woman, street, crowd, traffic, noise, haste, thief, bag, lost, scream, police.

The reader, by virtue of a knowledge of syntax, can predict the missing elements, but it is also likely that the reader has experience with the types of contexts in which these words may occur, particularly when they occur in this order.

Situational Constraints

In addition to the effect that context has on the choice of vocabulary, the speaker is limited further in the choice of mode of expression by the actual situation in which he or she is to communicate a message. The same message may be expressed in a variety of different ways, and different words and phrases can be used according to the speaker's evaluation of the nature of the audience. A message may be communicated to a roommate in a form that may be totally inappropriate to convey the same information to one's parents. Situational constraints may be considered to be a function of the people present, the relationship of the speaker to these people, and the social structure of the particular environment. The form of expression of a message that passes between a professor and a student may be predicted as being different from the same message passing from the student to another student. This will be influenced by the relationship that exists between these two people. Between individuals who have had little or no previous contact, the message will be influenced primarily by the speaker's evaluation of the role and social standing of the listeners.

The influence of environmental factors upon a topic of discussion and upon the manner in which the information is conveyed will be appreciated by the listener if that person imagines herself in each of the following situations: in the main aisle of a large cathedral just before morning service, at an informal student party, in a seminar group, at the question period in a large lecture meeting, or on a first date in a small cocktail bar.

Redundancy

The result of these various constraints is to produce what is known as *redundancy*. This may be defined as that part of a message that can be eliminated without a significant loss of information. Carroll (1964, p. 56) explains it as "the property of texts (language contexts) that allows us to predict missing symbols from the context." It must not be confused with simple repetition of all or part of the message signal, though repetition may affect redundancy. The idea of redundancy is perhaps more easily understood if it is considered as the result of the interaction of certain factors within the speaker (and therefore the message signal), the environment, and the listener. It is not possible to state a redundancy figure for a given message signal without considering these three variables. What may prove to be redundant for one listener may not be so for another. A message signal in one set of environmental conditions may have high redundancy, whereas in a different environment the redundancy of the same message signal may be reduced severely. Similarly, a message spoken by a person whose native tongue is English may become extremely difficult to understand when spoken by a foreigner whose English is characterized by a heavy dialect. The most important factors influencing redundancy are shown in Table 8.1.

Shannon and Weaver, 1967, showed that for the average adult reader, the redundancy of written English over any series of no greater than eight letters is approximately 50 percent. Thus, when we are operating under the constraints of written English, half of what we write is freely chosen, whereas the other half is determined by the structure of the language. In normal conversational speech, under favorable conditions, the level of redundancy is higher. Most of us can recall instances in which we have been able to maintain a conversation with one person while listening to the conversation of two people standing close to us.

TABLE 8.1 Factors influencing redundancy

Factors within the Speaker
    Compliance of the speaker to the rules of the language
    Compliance to the patterns of articulation, stress, intonation
    Size of vocabulary from which the message is composed
    Appropriate choice of words to convey the message

Factors within the Message Signal
    Number of syllables within the word
    Number of words within a sentence
    Number of different words (type-token ratio†)
    Amount of context
    Amount of repetition
    Frequency bandwidth of acoustic signal
    Intensity of acoustic signal

Factors within the Environment
    Amount of acoustic noise
    Amount of reverberation
    Amount and intensity of other environmental stimuli
    Number of potential clues related to the message

Factors within the Listener
    Familiarity with the language rules
    Familiarity with the speech patterns of the speaker
    Familiarity with the vocabulary used by the speaker
    Familiarity with the topic of conversation
    Fidelity of reception of the acoustic message signal
    Awareness of and ability to interpret related stimuli

---

† Type-token ratio: $\dfrac{\text{number of different words}}{\text{(total number of words)}}$

TABLE 8.2 Sources of noise

Within the Speaker
  Inadequate vocabulary
  Poor syntax
  Semantic ambiguity
  Imprecise or deviant articulation of speech
  Poor vocal production
  Improper stress and inflection

Within the Environment
  Acoustic signal
    Acoustic noise resulting in masking of the message signal
    Distortion of the frequency pattern of the message signal
    Reverberation
  Visual signal
    Poor lighting
    Visual field limited
    Competing visual stimuli

Within the Listener
  Unfamiliarity with the vocabulary of rules of the language
  Failure to identify correctly the topic of the message
  Incorrect recognition of auditory and/or visual signals because of similarity between sounds
    or between the visible characteristics of some articulation patterns
  Distracting stimuli
  Psychological factors, such as poor intellectual ability, poor motivation, poor attention span,
    high distractibility, preoccupation with something else, prejudice against the speaker or
    topic of conversation, and so on.

Noise and Redundancy

Closely related to the concept of information is the concept of *noise*. In communication terminology, this term is far more inclusive than the concept of audible noise. Noise may be considered the effect of any factor that adds confusion and so reduces the amount of information conveyed. In any communication situation, the listener is faced with varying amounts of noise in the system. This may be inherent within the message signal itself, it may be a function of limitations in the listener's ability to receive and decode the message signal accurately, or it may exist in the channel through which the message signal travels.* Table 8.2 indicates the major sources of noise in oral communication.

The importance of redundancy lies in the role it plays in helping to combat these noise factors. If the redundancy of a particular message is relatively high, then its resistance to noise or distortion is also great, permitting the receiver to obtain enough information to enable him or her to predict the missing elements of the message. The amount of redundancy in any given speech sample is, therefore, a function of the interaction between the speaker, the listener, and the message signal. It must be stressed

---

* The term *channel* refers to the pathway through which the message signal travels. This includes both the neurological and the environmental pathways—for example, auditory channel: hearing and sound waves; visual channel: vision and light waves; tactile channel: touch and low-frequency vibrations.

that the value of redundancy is limited by the extent to which the receiver is able to utilize it. Unfamiliarity with the linguistic structure or ignorance concerning the context of the message will affect seriously the benefit that the listener can derive from redundancy of speech material.

An understanding of the role of noise and redundancy in communication helps us to appreciate how it is that a person with what appears to be quite a severe auditory handicap often can function adequately in a communication situation. At the same time, it emphasizes the need for developing in the individual an awareness of an ability to capitalize on other factors that contribute to redundancy.

The concept that human communication is a process based upon the ability to predict the next "bit" of information has been summarized succinctly by Peter Laurie in an article entitled "The Explorers" in the British *Sunday Times Supplement*. Laurie writes:

The idea of the mind computing the probabilities of what's coming next has proved an essential key in the fast-growing new branch of psycholinguistics. One of the problems here is to elucidate the processes of hearing speech and decoding it into ideas. A good deal of experimenting has been done on this now, starting with the work of Professor Colin Cherry at Imperial College, London, at the beginning of the 1950s. It appears that hearing and understanding a spoken message involves several layers of computation. At the first level we can pick out from the noise around us—a cocktail party, say—one voice. We can tell the rate it's speaking and the direction it's coming from. Even something as apparently simple as this is in fact very sophisticated. It involves, to keep track of the tone of voice, making a statistical analysis of the characteristic sounds of that voice, storing this and comparing all the incoming sounds with this to pick out the ones we want. Then to find its direction we have to store the last second or so of this voice's input into each ear and shuffle the two records until they match to find the time delay between the two ears.

The sounds from the selected voice are stored for less than a second and passed on to the next level where they are translated into the equivalent sounds one could make oneself, and stored again—this is how one can make a stab at the last few syllables of something in a foreign language. This transfers again into a store where the sounds are identified with meaningful words—the short term memory we use to hold a telephone number between directory and dial. Unless the number is consciously repeated and reinserted, it fades after six seconds or so. Then the words are recorded again as ideas and transferred into long term memory. Interest focuses at the moment on this transfer from short term into long term store and back again. It is suggested that as one listens to a speaker, one runs ahead, using the statistical structure of the language to throw up the probable next words out of the long term store and matching them in one's head against those in the short term store. What we remember, or understand, is not the *sound* of the word we hear, but the *idea* stored in our heads that would generate the sound nearest to it. It's as if we were using a dictionary, flipping through it until we find a word that seems to match the word we hear and reading off the meaning. The fact that there's only one central dictionary is shown by the impossibility of speaking effectively while reading, writing, or listening.

This dictionary is not, however, arranged alphabetically, but by a continuously shifting scale of probabilities, and these are influenced by who is speaking, the situation we are both in, and particularly by what has just been said. So when one goes to answer the phone, one's dictionary already has some likely phrases ready to hear, like "Hold on, I have a call," and when you've got that far you hear "for you" automatically. But if the operator said, "Hold on, I have a call for umbilical hippopotamus," the last two words—having a low assigned probability—would not be found until it was too late, and so wouldn't be heard. That the brain works somehow like this was shown by an English psychologist, David Bruce, who made a record of a voice speaking against a background so noisy that nothing could be understood. He played this to a group of listeners who were told it was a talk about football. Then he played them one about hire purchase, and another about politics. Each time, given a cue, they could follow the sense; they were astonished to be told afterwards he'd played the same record each time. (March 19, 1967)

Summary of Information Processing

To summarize information processing, we can say that information refers to the contribution any element of a pattern makes to the identification of the speaker's intent. A message component is said to be highly informative when it is not predictable. Each bit of information contributes to the identification of a meaningful unit of the language. The rules of a language operate at the level of phonemes, morphemes, syntax, and semantics. We process the incoming bits of information at each level only until we identify enough constraints to permit us to move up to the larger, more meaningful units at the next level. The more of the pattern that is apparent, the easier prediction of meaning becomes. The prediction of meaning from phonemic and structural constraints is enhanced by the effect of context, which relates to the rules of semantics. Finally, the constraints generated by the situation in which the communication arises further contribute to the probability of what is said. A given number of constraints are necessary to permit comprehension of a particular message by a particular person in a given place and time.

Constraints in excess of the required minimum constitute redundancy. They reduce the pressure on the listener, who does not have to pay attention to each bit of information. Factors within the speaker, listener, or environment that hinder the encoding, transmission, reception, or decoding of the message are known as *noise*. When noise occurs, the task of comprehending becomes more difficult. The listener is forced to draw upon redundant information to compensate for the increased difficulty. If insufficient redundancy exists to compensate for the effects of noise, the message will be distorted and misunderstood.

We now can consider the components of a model of communication.

COMPONENTS OF THE MODEL

Before we develop a model, we need to think about what we wish it to accommodate. Human communication in general, and speech communication in particular, is multifaceted, but it can be viewed conveniently in terms of the components shown in Figure 8.1. Follow each of these stages through the model. The numbers are keyed to those in the figure.

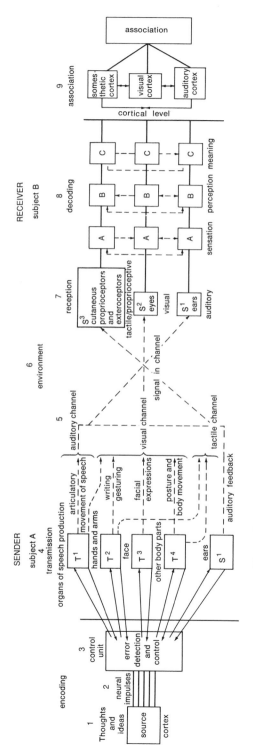

Figure 8.1 The components and stages of a human communication model.

THE SENDER

1. Thoughts and ideas originate in the cortex where they are coded into language.
2. The language pattern is recoded into neural impulses to the organs that will transmit the message.
3. On route to the transmitting organs, the message passes through a control unit whose function is to monitor and maintain the correctness of execution of the message signal.
4. The message signal reaches the transmitters. These are the organs of speech; the facial muscles of expression; the hands and arms used to gesture, sign, or write; and the whole body, conveying information by posture and movement.

THE ENVIRONMENT

5. Each transmitter broadcasts into at least one of three channels: auditory visual, or tactile. The speech organs broadcast into both auditory and visual channels.
6. The signal passes into and is subject to the influences of the environment; it will experience various degrees of distortion as a result of any competing stimuli.

THE RECEIVER

7. To be sensitive to the signal, the sensory organs of hearing, vision, and touch must be capable of detecting, at an adequate level of intensity, the full range of components of the signal that comprise the message information.
8. The signal is detected, recorded, analyzed, and recoded into meaningful linguistic patterns. Information in the different channels is cross-checked for compatibility.
9. Meaning is assigned, associations are made with past similar experiences, and the message is interpreted.

During communication at any one movement, our role is predominantly either that of sender or receiver. However, even while in one role we continue to function in the other, albeit to a lesser degree. That is to say, as I speak to you, I am also the listener. I note your vocal reinforcers, your head nods or shakes, your smiles or grimaces. I transmit similar cues to you while you are speaking to me. We influence each other in our communication interaction throughout our conversations through the simultaneous sending and receiving of verbal and nonverbal message codes.

The components we will consider therefore are

THE COMMUNICATOR/SPEAKER

- The concept or idea
- The linguistically coded message
- The articulatory encoded message

THE ENVIRONMENT

- The medium
- Airwaves
- Light waves
- Tactile vibratory waves
- Interference (i.e., "noise")

THE RECEIVER/LISTENER
- Reception/pattern replication
- Pattern analysis
- Linguistic reconstruction
- Semantic evaluation
- Conceptualization/interpretation

Even before we discuss and expand upon these components, it is possible to see that lack of comprehension of what a person says may result from a problem at any one or at several of these stages. It is not necessary to be hearing impaired for comprehension difficulty to occur. If a speaker has only a limited knowledge of English vocabulary and structure, we can expect difficulty in understanding him. Our difficulty with this person will be exacerbated further if he also has poor English pronunciation or uses inappropriate stress patterns. Providing auditory training, or even a special amplification system to a hearing-impaired college student faced with a foreign instructor will do nothing to alleviate this problem. On the other hand, if it can be shown that the difficulty in comprehending course content derives from poor room acoustics rather than from the deviant speech/language patterns of the instructor, we will know what intervention options are available. Thus, each person's difficulties in comprehension must be subject to diagnosis to determine at which stage of the communication process the problems occur. Then, within each stage, we must decide at what level or levels the problem lies. The course of action we prescribe must be determined by such a situation-by-situation analysis.

STAGES OF PROCESSING

Consider now each of the stages involved in the act of communication.

Encoding

Need: The Communicator. Communication begins with a *need*. We must be motivated to communicate. The number of different needs is infinite. We may speak to identify physical states, "I'm hungry"; or feelings, "I'm worried"; to obtain information, "Is dinner nearly ready?," "Do you think she'll be all right?"; to effect action, "Please pass the bread," "Call and see if she arrived safely"; to provide information, "This casserole is delicious," "She said the driving wasn't bad at all"; and so on. Even communication at the most sophisticated level derives from need: a need to teach, for example, "Piaget maintains that initially the child is incapable of making any distinction between himself and what is not himself"; or perhaps a need to negotiate, "We propose to match your offer of $37 per share if we are allowed to purchase a controlling interest."

The relevance of need lies in the obligation we have to focus our intervention procedures on the specific needs that our clients, children or adults, will experience. The academic and social needs of a third-grade child will be different from those of a student in tenth grade. The needs of a young unmarried hospital nurse will differ, both in terms of occupation and social life, from those of a married bank manager with two teenage children. It is helpful in analyzing communication problems to go back one step further, since needs arise from demands. When we understand the demands placed upon the tenth-grade student by teachers and by peers, when we have insight into demands the bank manager faces daily at home and during the week at work, we can anticipate and seek to provide appropriately for needs.

Need: The Listener. Need gives rise to motivation. The fact that need motivates speech is fairly obvious. It is less obvious that there must be need in order for us to listen. By listen I mean to process and evaluate the message signal, rather than simply to receive or hear the signal. Your attention to what I am explaining now will be enhanced greatly if an approaching exam requires you to understand and remember the points I make. Most of the time we process the spoken message, we receive in a fairly cursory manner. We can do this because of our sophisticated cognitive-linguistic expectancies. We need only half the acoustic signal to confirm our predictions. As hearing impairment erodes the acoustic information, the task of paying auditory attention becomes increasingly difficult and frustrating. For the child in school the impact is more serious. The school-age child has little familiarity with the content of academic subjects nor, to a considerable degree, with the vocabulary and language of new content. Frustrated by the adverse acoustic conditions of the classroom, the child loses the motivation and, therefore, the need to listen. Thus, in the case of both child and adult, need is redefined to accommodate the reality of a world filtered through hearing impairment. A reduced interest and motivation for communication is forced upon them.

The impact on need of hearing impairment of moderate to profound severity is extremely serious when it occurs prelingually. So long as a child remains functionally deaf, there will be an absence of the need to communicate orally regardless of the audiometric classification. The child will need neither to listen nor communicate by auditory or oral means. In these children, deprivation of the ability to hear spoken language results in the stabilization of a biologic-perceptual system that excludes spoken language (Furth, 1974). You must recognize this dramatic effect of hearing deficiency on the need and motivation to talk experienced by the prelingually hearing-impaired child in order to plan a realistic approach to communication training. Your understanding of the role of need and motivation in the communication process must translate into management and counseling strategies. These must be designed to address this basal level of breakdown with the intent of creating need where it does not exist.

The need to communicate results in the evoking of a concept or idea based upon experiences relevant to the need. In other words, we conceive of the need within the framework of experience.

Experience-Related Concepts

As we discuss each of these stages, I wish to remind you once again that we are discussing what in fact is a totally integrated process. In reality all stages are one; the process is circular and operates forward and backward simultaneously in a quality-monitoring manner, occurring with the rapidity of neurological processes. Thus, experience, concepts, and language do not exist independently. It is only for the purpose of trying to envisage what is happening that we can afford to treat components as though each had an independent identity.

The felt need translates into thought, into concepts. These concepts derive from the memories we have of past experiences related to the need. This is why a need in one person may evoke positive feelings and action, while in another the associations linked to that need cause the concepts evoked to be negative. The significance of this stage for us is that a large part of our work with children, and to a lesser extent with adults, will be directed at building new or different experiences related to concepts. The concepts of small children initially are very simple and do not relate to other concepts with the richness that characterizes adult thought. As children grow they gain experience in a direct manner, but increasingly they add to experience vicariously. Vicarious experience is dependent primarily upon language. Even visually perceived events, both those that are real and those seen on television or in picture books, are molded by verbalization. Since verbal language is primarily auditory, functionally deaf and even hard-of-hearing children are handicapped in experiencing the world. The essential point is that a *word is not an experience, but it serves to evoke an experience* and has the power to mold experience. The complexity of what it evokes will depend upon the richness of the concept that embodies that experience. Communication is diminished in effectiveness, or even may break down, when there is a significant difference in the experiences of the speaker and listener. This is because the listener is perceiving the concepts that the speaker *evokes* in him by her words, not the concepts that gave rise to those words. In working with hearing-impaired children, analysis of communication effectiveness must include the question, "Does this child have an appropriate concept for this word and if so what is the extent of that concept?"

When analyzing difficult communication situations encountered by the young student or the adult, you must ask whether there may be difficulty in conceptualizing what is being discussed rather than, or in addition to, difficulty in hearing the presentation. Problems at different stages require different intervention strategies. Conceptualization is heavily influenced by linguistic knowledge that permits the storage and reconstruction of information related to experience. Thus, once again it is artificial to separate the two, but we will do so for our convenience.

NEUROLINGUISTIC CODING

The idea or concept is actualized for most individuals by linguistic coding, that is to say, we think in a language. It is not essential that the language be verbal; deaf persons think equally well in sign language, while scientists conceptualize problems using mathematical or chemical language codes. Our interest, however, is in verbal language communication, which depends upon the correlation between what we think and the acoustic speech pattern or sign pattern we generate. The concepts or ideas we wish to communicate first must be encoded into linguistic symbols that relate to or denote the person, object, event, feeling, and so on to which we wish to refer. Simply put, ideas must be encoded into meaningful language units (Figure 8.2). The first of these units is the semantic level.

Semantics

NARROW: BEACH: STEEP: PATH: DESCENT:

You may have experienced directly or vicariously the conceptual values to which these words refer, but without the appropriate words both those given and those that will link, augment, and clarify them, you will be unable to formulate the experience linguistically. You may know a person who hoards every penny he acquires, lives in apparent poverty despite substantial wealth, and never lends money to help a person in need, but you cannot communicate this experience without such words as stingy, parsimonious, Scrooge-like. The experience and the semantics in a hearing world are interwoven. We learn the semantic values and the contextual influence of words on meanings as we experience; we hear people commenting about events. The functionally deaf child lacks the luxury of learning by osmosis. For her, experiences must be labeled deliberately and repeatedly. The experience itself must be recreated many times to allow the semantic equivalents to be taught first in a given context and later in other contexts. Inability to communicate a given experience may originate at this basic entrance level to the language code. Teaching techniques for that particular breakdown must be targeted appropriately.

The concepts identified by

NARROW: BEACH: STEEP: PATH: DESCENT:

become much clearer when recoded into semantic units that comprise the *deep structure* underlying what we say:

The path descends.   The path is steep.   The beach is narrow.

Further clarification arises from grammatical and syntactic restructuring.

Syntax and Grammar

The three semantic units just stated must be recoded into a complex surface structure that represents the way we speak. This requires a knowledge of the rules that govern the patterns of word types acceptable in a particular

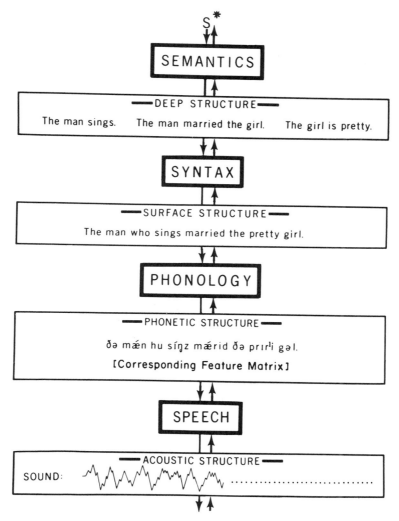

Figure 8.2 An illustration of the assumption that the sounds of speech are a separate level of language, connected to the phonetic structure by a grammatical recoding similar to syntax and phonology. (Liberman, 1970, p. 302.)

language. In English we would not say as we would in German, "It is today very fine," or as in Norwegian we would inquire, "How stands it to with you today?" The syntactic patterns enhance the semantic clarity and allow for rapid encoding and decoding of information. Grammatical rules further speed up comprehension by providing information concerning time, number, ownership, relationship, and so on.

"The steep path descends to a narrow beach" tells us something subtly different from "The beach led to a steep descending narrow path," yet the words are almost identical.

Communication breakdown may occur either in the expressive or receptive stages if the complexity of syntax required to encode or decode the deep structure exceeds the speaker/listener's capability. We must be alert to the communication difficulties that hearing-impaired children experience as a result of poor development of syntactic knowledge. The structure of the language used in learning grows more complex as the child progresses through the school years. Ideas and experiences embedded in surface sentence structure too complex for the child to decode into deep structure will not be accessible even when content is familiar. Even for a hearing-impaired adult, the complex syntactic structure of a message may overload a system that must devote much of its attention to the more basic process of making linguistic and conceptual closure from limited information.

Phonology

The phonology of our language comprises the boundary between our world of thought and the physical world that separates us from our listener. At this level linguistic patterns must be converted into acoustic patterns. Oral communication can occur only to the extent that we can produce and receive the acoustic patterns coded to phonology. The sound patterns that we combine to make word units are just as culturally rule bound as at every other level of language structuring. "Przyszlosci" is a perfectly acceptable phonologic pattern in Polish but utterly irregular in English. Phonology encompasses both phonemics, that is, the units of sound that have the potential to change meaning (e.g., M*u*te/m*oo*t), and phonetics [mjut/mut], the acoustic pattern itself. Phonetics and articulation are totally intertwined since we produce the speech sound by speech articulation. Because the hearing impairment distorts or eliminates the reception of accurate acoustic models of speech, breakdowns in communication are common at the level of articulatory encoding/decoding.

ARTICULATORY CODING

The phonologic values must be encoded into patterns of articulation that in turn pattern an acoustic wave. It is necessary, therefore, that the neuro-linguistic patterns be restructured into equivalent patterns of neuromotor commands to the breathing mechanism, vocal folds, and the articulatory resonant system of speech. It is to be expected that a process that involves so many transformations will require careful monitoring and a system of self-adjustment to maintain the desired accuracy of output. This quality control is achieved through a feedback system. Articulatory problems arise when the child's internal model, which represents how he hears us say the sound through the distortion of the cochlea, is incorrect. He will produce the distorted sound that matches the distorted internal model and thus is reinforced.

QUALITY CONTROL

To assure that a production unit maintains a particular standard of operation, it must incorporate an ongoing system of assessment and control of the quality of the product *as it is in the process of being produced*. This is as necessary in speech articulation as in the production of automobiles or cookies. Quality control requires that

- Information about the output continuously be fed back into the system. The feedback information be compared to a desired standard to determine discrepancies.
- A continual adjustment be made to the ongoing production process to ensure that the output remains within standard tolerances.

A production *error* is considered to occur whenever a discrepancy between what was intended and what was effected deviates beyond tolerance criteria. The self-regulating system, or *servosystem*, functions to hold output within the desired standards.

Feedback is an integral component of the speech communication system; without it effective communication is impossible. The rules of a given language set models for speech at the phonologic level. We internalize these models of sound as we develop an understanding of spoken language. As infants we refine our articulation to approximate those models as closely as our ear and neuroarticulatory systems are capable. Tolerances of deviance are evidenced by the fact that a speech sound varies acoustically with coarticulation; they also are to be seen in our ability to comprehend persons speaking with a regional or ethnic accent. The latter tolerance is, however, more a function of the built-in redundancy of the language code than the breadth of acoustic tolerance.

A model of the feedback system serving speech production was developed by Fairbanks in 1954. It remains helpful in understanding this process. The model (Figure 8.3) is divided into three linked units:

1. *The effector unit*, which converts neuromotor commands into speech sounds
2. *The sensor unit*, which serves to feed back into the system a continuous record of production
3. *The control unit*, which compares the flow of output to the intended production to determine whether it is remaining within acceptable limits of tolerance

The function of the system is as follows: The message exits from the phonological level of the language system as a patterned flow of neuromotor commands to the speech mechanism.

It flows, over time, through the controller unit, where a facsimile is recorded and held for a brief period in storage. This unit acts as a delay stage to ensure that the copy of the intended signal and the actual signal can be brought together later for comparison in the comparator.

The instructions for the production of the speech pattern flow through a mixer (which we will consider later) to the effector unit.

The effector unit comprises (1) the *motor* power of the breathing mechanism; (2) the *generator* of sound, the glottis; and (3) the *modulator* of sound,

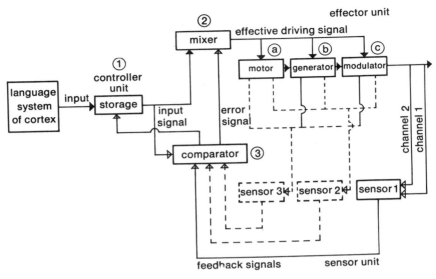

Figure 8.3 Model of a closed cycle control system for speaking. (Proposed by Fairbanks, 1954.)

the articulatory resonance system. It is the effector unit that transduces the neuromotor pattern into an equivalent sound wave.

The tactile and proprioceptive sensor units track the actual behavior of the speech mechanism, while the auditory system records the acoustic event as heard by air conduction (channel 1) and by bone conduction (channel 2).

The ongoing production pattern record flows back to the comparator where its arrival is synchronized with the delayed arrival of the original instruction pattern representing the desired output. The comparison between the desired and actual speech pattern will reveal any discrepancies. When an error is detected, it is used to calculate a correction factor to be applied to the continuing pattern production to prevent deviation of future units from the tolerance limits. The (predicted) *error correction signal* flows to the mixer to combine with the continuing pattern flow, thus serving as a correction of *anticipated* continued deviation in speech production.

Since coarticulation involves preplanning of speech sounds yet to be produced, the essence of the model is its feedforward mechanism. In Fairbanks's words:

> The essence of a speaking system however, is control of the output, or prediction of the output's future. In this kind of system the significance of the data about the past is that they are used for prediction of the future. (1954, p. 134)

Ling (1976) also has stressed the fact that the system serves to determine whether the desired articulation movements *have been made, not that they are being made*. He refers to Evarts's (1973) theory of corollary discharge, which suggests that the efferent (control) system sends a simultaneous discharge to both the sensory and the motor systems. The comparison between the intended and actual motor articulation is made by the comparator unit. If the two match they cancel each other out; if there is a discrepancy it is brought to conscious awareness. The impact of hearing impairment on this process is most serious when the condition is prelingual. Two stages of the process will be affected. First, the acquisition of models for the correct articulation of speech sounds will be impaired in accord with the severity and pattern of the impairment. Incorrect internal models lead to incorrect intended outputs. Second, the feedback will be deficient because of the hearing impairment. As a result the motor-kinesthetic, tactile, and auditory feedback will record a match between intended (but incorrect) and actual production accepting and ingraining the incorrect sound production.

For those who acquire a hearing impairment after speech articulation has been learned thoroughly, the internal models are correct. Although auditory feedback will be impaired, tactile and motor-kinesthetic feedback, except in a few cases, will prove sufficient to maintain articulation within normal limits unless the hearing loss is very severe.

In thinking about the process depicted by this model, the following concepts are important:

- The signal is an unsegmented neural pattern flow.
- The storage process should be envisaged as the passage of an echoic image from one side of a screen of limited width to the other. The signal trace is strongest as it enters from the left; it fades as it crosses the screen to exit from the right.
- The comparator synchronously displays the intended speech production instruction pattern as an overlay to the actual production to reveal discrepancies. This is also a continuous nonsegmental process with the two traces moving across the comparator screen. Cancellation occurs when the two images match. When they do not, our attention is drawn to the discrepancy.
- Errors already made cannot be corrected except by stopping and repeating the complete output unit.
- Adjustments to future output begin immediately production is commenced. This means that adjustments are being made to the planning of future speech sounds before they are articulated.
- All corrections are based upon *anticipated* error derived from past discrepancy.

The neuromotor command patterns to the articulatory-resonant system are direct equivalents of the phonetic values for the phonologic patterns. They are transmitted into the environment as acoustic patterns that carry coded information about how they were generated. If we know the code we can use this information to reconstruct the message through its various stages to achieve an *equivalent* thought. Before we consider the influence of the environment on communication, it is important to remember that the act of communication involves encoding information simultaneously into several channels. Thus, in addition to the transmission of orally coded speech information, visual and tactile message-related information also may be transmitted as depicted in Figure 8.1. This model includes the encoding of information through such means as writing, gesturing, facial expression, and body movements. The transmitters represent the organs of speech production (T^1), the hands and arms (T^2), the face (T^3), and other body parts (T^4). The coded message is transduced into a signal that differs depending upon which transmitter is encoding it, as does the channel into which it is transmitted. Thus the sending of a spoken message involves the simultaneous encoding of linguistic and nonlinguistic constraints related to the ideas to be communicated.

Finally, it must be remembered that whenever technology intervenes between speaker and listener, it becomes a part of the communication system. Telephones, radios, televisions, tapes, records, films, and slides are extensions of the transmission system, while any form of hearing aid comprises an extension of the ear. As such, the efficiency of these devices, whenever applicable, must be included in our assessment of the functional communication and learning capabilities of the hearing-impaired individual.

THE ENVIRONMENT

The patterns of information that carry the code for reconstruction of the message are broadcast into the environment by the transmitters. The primary media for transmission of the information between speaker and listener are air and light waves; we hear and see the speaker. Information also may be received through touch as in a handshake, an embrace, a reassuring squeeze of an arm, or a belligerent shove. Vibrotactile patterning of speech sometimes provides a valuable supplementary channel for transmitting speech pattern information to severely and profoundly hearing-impaired children. We already have considered in some detail in Chapters 3 and 5 the effects of the environment on the faithful transmission of the acoustic and visual signal from speaker to listener. We discussed the impact of noise and in particular signal-to-noise ratios; we considered the effects of distance and speaker-listener angle on both auditory and visual cues; and we saw how the level of contrast between speaker and background influenced the amount of visible speech cues received.

The environment is the bridge between speaker and listener. Its efficiency in carrying the coded message signal between the two communicants must be assessed as carefully as we assess the communicators. Each environment differs, thus it will be necessary to obtain some assessment of the particular environment in which each client must function.

THE LISTENER/RECEIVER

Peripheral Reception

We addressed some of the processes of receiving the spoken language signal when we discussed its encoding and transition by the speaker. Both speaking and listening were shown to require a need, which gives rise to motivation. In the listener the need motivates the behavior that we label *attention*. In the discussion of attention (Chapter 7, p. 78), I explained that it is an active process derived from expectancies. Expectancies set up the receptive system to process the incoming signal with the greatest ease. At the cochlear nuclei the complex signal is tonotopically analyzed allowing for replication of the acoustic components of the acoustic signal in terms of the frequency intensity pattern. This internal pattern replication, which involves echoic memory, is derived from the pattern of activity of the cochlear hair cells and their associated nerve fibers. The ability of the cochlea to replicate faithfully all components of the acoustic signal is dependent, therefore, upon the integrity of a full range of hair cells. Hearing impairment acts like a filter. The reduction or absence of hair cells anywhere along the basilar membrane will result in the filtering out of the finer details. Filtering means loss of the information that comprises the detailed instructions. These are necessary for the easy restructuring of the linguistic patterns, the equivalents of the conceptual message. Discrimination, particularly speech discrimination, depends upon the ability to use information about fine differences between patterns. Fewer and fewer of those details are reproduced as hearing impairment becomes more severe. Even though amplification allows us to activate hair cells not responsive to speech at normal intensity levels, it cannot replace the fine details recordable by the missing sensitive cells normally activated at low intensity. Thus, in the case of impaired hearing, even when speech is made audible by amplification, the replicated echoic pattern will lack many information-bearing details; there will remain distortion.

Pattern Analysis and Linguistic Reconstruction

Once internalized the echo is analyzed to decode the directions for reconstructing suprasegmental and segmental linguistic patterns. Identification of the acoustic correlates of articulatory features permits reconstruction of phonological, morphologic, and syntactic patterns, which are displayed in short-term memory. Sound patterns in this way initiate the reconstruction of linguistic patterns, which, in effective communication, are equivalent to those from which they derived. This occurs when two persons share a common set of language rules. To the extent that those two persons also share similar experiences, concepts will be activated by way of the semantic values associated with the decoded words and phrases.

Conceptual Reconstruction

The semantic values that culminate linguistic processing activate webs of experience. Semantic values call forth a repertoire of images and ideas relevant in some way to the language patterns. The meaning of the message received, therefore, is inherent in the listener. The choice of the assigned meaning is constrained by the nature of the language pattern into which it was encoded by the speaker, but the concept or idea finally experienced is highly individualized; it depends upon the nature and extent of the listener's experience.

SUMMARY

- We have discussed the value of models that help us conceptualize, integrate knowledge, and develop and rationalize our hypotheses for what is wrong.
- Communication was conceptualized as being dependent on a communicator, the environment, and a receiver.
- The basis of communication is need—need to communicate, need to listen.
- We communicate about direct and vicarious experience. Thus experience defines the limits of communication.
- Needs, ideas, feelings, and so on depend on the ability to encode them into a language shared by the listener.
- Language involves content and structure.
- Speech comprises vocal articulatory-resonant behavior that codes acoustic patterns to language.
- Sign languages involve coding by hands, face, and body postures.
- Communication systems require a quality control mechanism to ensure that actual output matches desired output.
- The environment degrades the signal to varying degrees.
- Fidelity of signal reception by the listener and the ability to reconstruct and interpret language patterns are essential to effective communication.

Conclusion

Reflection on communication models alerts us to their value in simplifying a complex process in a manner that allows us to make educated assumptions about what is involved. Models permit us to examine, hypothetically, various stages of a process and to think about how they may be modified when they appear to be causing a dysfunction. We must realize equally, however, that a model is speculative; it causes us to perceive *a* way things may function but temporarily prevents us from seeing other possible ways.

The process of communication is a holistic integrated one involving experiential, cognitive, linguistic, neuromotor, and sensory functions. It is affected by environment and by the compatibility of the sender and receiver. We must not fail to assess each of these influences when attempting to assess and ameliorate communication breakdown.

9

Hearing Impairment and Communication

We have devoted much attention to explaining how we use spoken language to cause others to know what we are thinking. This information is crucial to understanding the complex ways in which hearing deficiency limits verbal communication. The analysis of those limitations guides us in planning educational and remedial strategies to minimize the negative effects. Consider first what hearing impairment does to the acoustic information, and how that affects its processing by the individual.

REDUCTION OF PERIPHERAL INFORMATION

We have seen that the speech signal is an acoustic pattern resulting from the interaction of multiple vibrations. Each speech sound arises from a unique combination of acoustic features that gives the sound its perceptual identity. The diminution or exclusion of any feature by a hearing impairment will result in a distortion of the pattern. Because auditory processing of speech is based, at least initially, on the information pattern encoded by the cochlea, any distortion will reduce a person's competence to decode spoken language in this analytic manner, referred to as bottom-up processing. In an infant, such distortion will limit or preclude the learning of oral communication.

Boothroyd (1976) has demonstrated that different feature information in speech varies in its resistance to hearing impairment. He studied the ability of 121 hearing-impaired children to identify the temporal patterns of vowels and consonants as a function of the average hearing threshold at the frequencies 500–1000–2000 Hz. From his results, depicted in Figure 9.1, we can see that the feature information, which tells us where a sound is being produced in the mouth, is highly susceptible to information loss. An impairment of 60–70dB reduces correct identification of place of articulation to 50 percent, while an 80dB deficit provides only a 30 percent recognition. Vowel identification, the voicing feature, and the manner of production of a sound (e.g., plosion, nasalization, friction) show greater resistance to distortion, falling to the 50 percent level only for an average deficit of around 90dB. Most resistant of all is syllabic pattern information, which remains highly discriminable even for an average impairment of 90dB Hz.

These findings are understandable in light of what we know about where the different feature information lies on the frequency scale. Voicing derives primarily from strong low frequency vibrations in the 125–1550 Hz range with a median frequency of 500 Hz; manner-of-production cues extend into the middle and high frequencies, 335–2000 Hz with a median of 750 Hz; while almost all place cues, which are weak in intensity, fall in the 880–2650 Hz range with a median frequency of 1900 Hz (Miller & Nicely, 1955). This knowledge helps us to understand that a hearing impairment will affect the perception of different sounds in different ways. It also emphasizes the fact that information about a speech sound still may be of value to a child even though the sound may not be discriminable on the basis

Figure 9.1 Auditory identification of temporal patterns of vowels and consonant features by 121 hearing-impaired children shown as a function of mean hearing threshold level for 500–1000–2000 Hz. (From Boothroyd, 1976.)

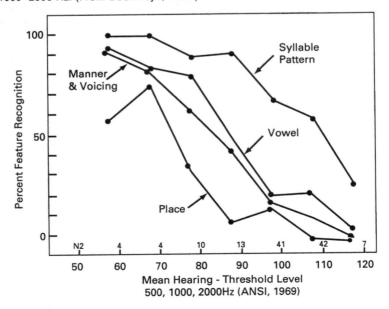

of acoustic information alone. Some sounds, because of their frequency composition, may remain sufficiently audible for all distinctive features to be discriminable; others, however, may be discriminable by manner cues but not by place. Thus the category to which the sound belongs may be identifiable (e.g., voiced stop consonant), while the place of production (e.g., bilabial /b/, alveolar /d/, velar /g/) may not. Such information can be of value in deciding whether analytic auditory training at the syllabic level has potential for improving discrimination accuracy. It is critical to deciding to what extent auditory emphasis will be effective in speech articulation teaching or correction. We will consider how this might be assessed when we discuss speech evaluation in Chapter 17.

The value in the Boothroyd data, indicating how many features remain potentially discriminable even with a hearing deficit, exceeds that which can be derived from the audiogram, for speech discrimination is an integrative suprathreshold perceptual task, while the pure tone data is based purely on threshold detection. There is, however, an obvious relationship between the severity and pattern of the audiogram and the probable acoustic information recorded by the cochlea. Research (Fletcher, 1953) has shown that the intensity range over which speech discrimination improves in normal-hearing listeners is 30dB. This range begins at the intensity level at which some word discrimination becomes possible. Word discrimination increases rapidly as the intensity of the words is increased until approximately 30dB above that discrimination threshold a maximum discrimination score is reached (Figure 9.2). Further increase in word intensity produces no further increase in discrimination. Eventually, if intensity

Figure 9.2 Articulation scores for three different types of test material (From Miller, Heise, & Lichten, 1951.)

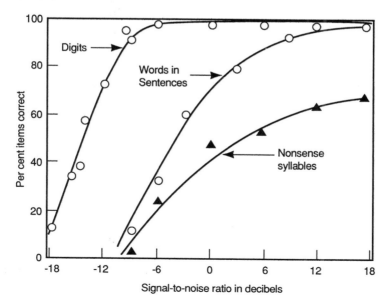

continues to increase, a rollover effect is observed as the maximum discrimination score begins to fall.

In persons with impairment of hearing, the intensity level at which word discrimination will begin will be raised by the hearing deficit. The growth of loudness with intensity growth above that level, however, will be accelerated, reaching discomfort and pain thresholds at or below the levels for a normal-hearing person. The most comfortable listening intensity likewise will occur at a lower intensity level than the degree of hearing deficit might lead you to expect. Thus the 30dB range for some hearing-impaired persons may be narrowed considerably by the raised threshold of intelligibility and by the lowered comfort level. This problem increases as the severity of the hearing impairment increases progressively above 60dB, making it more and more difficult to provide adequate intensity for discrimination without discomfort.

The pattern of hearing impairment as depicted by the audiogram also suggests the probable distortion due to loss of frequency information. We know that vowel sounds carry the greatest amount of energy but that it is the consonant sounds that carry the greatest information. We also know that it is the second formant transition that is crucial to recognition of both vowels and voiced consonants at the syllabic level. The second formant, together with much consonant production information, lies above 750 Hz (Peterson & Barney, 1952). If you consider the audiogram chart, you will note that the octaves from 125–750 Hz occupy a range of only 625 Hz, while from 750–8000 Hz they cover 7250 Hz. The contribution that various frequencies make to speech intelligibility is thus not equal. French and Steinberg (1947) investigated this. They determined the bandwidths of 20 frequency bands, each of which contributed equal information to the recognition of speech sounds. The data they produced indicate that as one moves up the frequency scale, the width of the frequency bands contributing equal amounts of information grows in the same way as the range of frequencies in the upper octaves of hearing grows. What this signifies is that while higher frequencies in speech contain more information, it is spread over a wider bandwidth. For example, to match the acoustic information contained in the range 250–375 Hz, a band which is 125 Hz wide, one needs a band 1280 Hz wide in the frequency range 5720–7000 Hz. However, at the basal end of the cochlea, where high frequency sensitivity is focused, a large number of hair cells are packed on a relatively small area of the basilar membrane. Damage at this end of the cochlea thus has a disproportionate effect on discrimination.

It has been shown (Risberg, Agelfors, & Boberg, 1975) that a sensorineural hearing impairment frequently reduces sensitivity to frequency changes even when tones are made audible. Risberg et al. (1975) studied children with various degrees of hearing deficit. Their findings reveal that for thresholds in the 30–60dB range, the ability to detect a change in pitch, the *just noticeable difference* (JND) or *difference limen for frequency* (DLF), in the 125–1000 Hz range was essentially normal, only about a 1–2 percent change. However, for deficits in the 70–90dB range, marked individual differences were found in pitch discrimination, ranging from 2–30 percent, while for deficits greater than 90dB some children required as much as a 40 percent change (e.g., from 500–700 Hz) before a pitch difference was noticed.

What does this imply? To understand the significance of DLF, you must remember that a speech acoustic pattern results from the interaction of multiple frequencies *changing over time*. These temporal changes in frequency and intensity generate the patterns of speech. The ability to record them at the cochlea is essential to speech. Consider the two patterns in Figure 9.3. The first illustration on graph paper depicts all the fine details of pattern change over time. The second illustration indicates what happens when it is not possible to record all the details. The pattern has lost many of the distinguishing features that differentiate it from other patterns. When the features eliminated are acoustic, speech sounds lose absolute discriminability. It still may be possible to categorize the sound as a voiced fricative or a voiceless bilabial, but it may not be possible to identify which sound in the category it is. Even vowels that are heard may sound so similar as to make discrimination between them impossible when hearing impairment is severe. Risberg et al. (1975) have demonstrated that frequency discrimination is an ability closely related to discrimination of spondee words, suggesting that fine frequency discrimination may be prerequisite to speech perception.

The effects of cochlear damage, therefore, are seen to be far more complex than a reduction of signal loudness. The acoustic signal is a direct representation of its articulatory production. Cochlear damage, by removing parts of this feature information, reduces the accuracy with which the pattern can be reconstructed by the auditory system. The vulnerability to distortion is greatest for place cues, while syllabic pattern information remains surprisingly resistant. The problem is aggravated further in many persons with severe to profound sensorineural deficits by a significant reduction in frequency discrimination, which reduces the recording and reconstruction of important frequency transmission changes.

PHONEME IDENTIFICATION

The unique combination of acoustic features that characterizes each speech sound ensures that each phoneme has a different acoustic makeup. It is not surprising, therefore, that a hearing impairment will affect the reception of the acoustic pattern of various phonemes differently. We will not consider the acoustic makeup of each sound since you already know that a person seldom processes individual phonemes. Some review of our discussion of the speech signal, however, is relevant to a consideration of the effect of hearing impairment on phoneme perception.

Vowels

We discussed the formant structure of vowels, stressing the importance to vowel identification of the second formant and, in particular, its transition. The second formant is keyed to the place in the oral cavity where the vowel

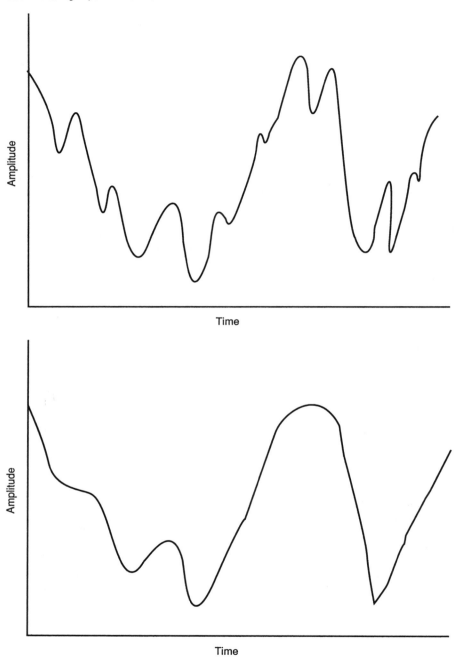

Figure 9.3 Reduction of pattern details by removal of information from intermediate points.

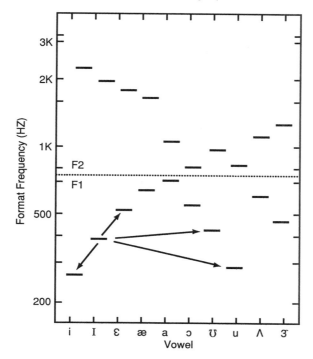

Figure 9.4 First and second formant frequencies of 10 American English vowels. Arrows indicate similarities in first formant frequencies, drawn to explain common auditory identification errors of severely hearing-impaired children in response to the spoken vowel /I/. (From Peterson & Barney, 1952.)

is being produced. From it we can determine whether the vowel is a front vowel such as /i/, which produces a high F2 (2300 Hz) or a back vowel such as /u/ in which the F2 is much lower (900 Hz) (Figure 9.4). As explained earlier (p. 23), it is not the absolute values of F1 and F2 that determine vowel perception since these change with the pitch of the glottal tone. It is the *relative spacing of the formants* (the *difference frequency*) that remains constant for all pitches that provides the information for identification. Vowels differ also in intensity, ranging from the /ɔ/ sound, which is the strongest, to /i/, the weakest, and in duration from /u/, the longest, to /I/, the shortest.

A vowel is subject to distortion when hearing impairment erodes acoustic information in the F2 range. Weak vowels and vowels of short duration, characteristics that for the most part coincide, are most prone to distortion. A severe hearing impairment, above approximately 1000 Hz, may so erode the F2 information as to make discrimination between some front and back vowels impossible even though F1 makes both audible. The vowels that are most vulnerable to distortion are, therefore, /a/ʌ/ə/ɜ//æ/ɛ/e/ I/i/, in progressive order determined by the higher frequency value of F2. To ensure positive discrimination of all vowels, hearing must be present to 3000 Hz (Ling & Ling, 1978).

Semivowels

Semivowels are very similar to voiced vowels in spectral composition but differ mainly in their shorter duration. They are, therefore, often misidentified as vowels by persons with severe hearing impairment.

Consonants

Discrimination of consonants derives from more complex information with the acoustic cues varying by consonant category.

Fricatives /f/, /v/, /θ/, /ð/, /s/, /z/, /ʃ/, and /ʒ/ are all frequency dependent for recognition, characterized as they are by the band of noise generated by the constriction of air flow that produces them. The voiced component of the /v/, /ð/, /z/, and /ʒ/, of course, will be in the low frequency range. This sometimes results in audibility though not discriminability. The identifying band of broad spectrum friction noise decreases in frequency as the point of constriction moves further back in the mouth. Thus the labiodental /f/ generates a band of noise in the 4500–7000 Hz range, /ʃ/ centers around 3000 Hz and /s/ around 5000 Hz. It is clear then that hearing loss in the higher frequency range above 2000 Hz will remove much, if not all, of the acoustic information by which fricatives are identified. The vulnerability is increased further by the relatively low intensity of voiceless fricatives.

Stop consonants are identifiable from a combination of rising F2 transition information, a burst of acoustic noise as air is released, and, for voiced plosives, the short duration of silence between the burst of air and the onset of voicing (i.e., *voice onset time*). The frequency pattern of plosives varies with the place of the stop in the oral cavity. In general, the more anterior the location of the stop, the higher the frequency of the noise burst. For /t/ and /d/ this may occur as high as 3000 Hz. Discrimination of stop consonants by persons with severe hearing impairment may be reduced to voice/voiceless decisions with confusions occurring between stop consonants and fricatives (Erber, 1981).

Nasal consonants depend upon both voicing and the resonance cues generated by primary resonation of the glottal tone in the nasal cavity. The nasality cue is so strong that even children with profound sensorineural hearing deficits can distinguish between nasal and nonnasal consonants (Erber, 1981). It is with the semivowels /r/, /l/, /w/, /y/, and the vowels that the nasal sounds most commonly are confused.

The purely acoustic cues we have reviewed comprise the basis for discrimination of speech sounds in combination with a consonant or vowel under test conditions. The information provided is valuable in so much as it helps us predict which acoustic cues a hearing-impaired person has the potential for receiving, given appropriate amplification. It provides insight into the probable effect of hearing impairment on the reception of individual speech sounds, suggesting those sounds that may be totally inaudible, and those that may be only partially audible and thus distorted. Finally, it helps us to anticipate and understand the auditory confusions that may occur between and among speech sounds if a person must depend primarily on the acoustic pattern for dicrimination. Figure 9.5 indicates the frequency and sensation levels of speech-sound components. An audiogram plotted

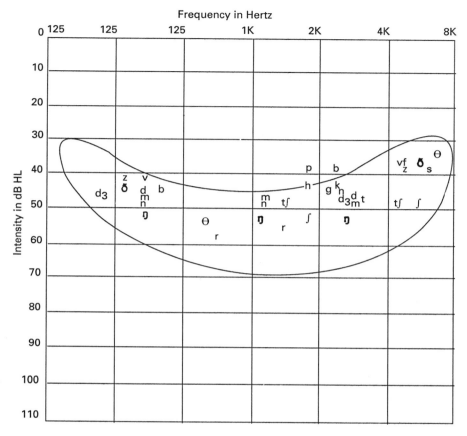

Figure 9.5 Intensity range of speech at various frequencies on an audiogram scale.

on this chart reveals which components fall above and below threshold. This information can be obtained from both unaided and aided pure tone audiograms. Such knowledge is invaluable in developing realistic expectations for speech development in hearing-impaired infants, in the teaching and correcting of speech articulation, and in developing strategies for improving receptive communication skills.

LANGUAGE AND AUDITORY DISCRIMINATION

When we consider the relationship of acoustics to the sounds of speech, it is important to realize that the acoustic signal is a continuous unsegmented pattern; it contains no discrete phonologic units. Phonemes exist only as *perceptual* linguistic values. Phonologic units are arrived at analytically only *after* we have processed the syllables of which they are an integral part (Levin, 1972). This fact emphasizes that we process the speech signal as spoken language once we are able to restructure the analog pattern of the acoustic signal in echoic memory into the segmental linguistic patterns that characterize short-term memory. From this point on, language knowledge permits expectancies to be developed and predictions made about the probable evolution of the structure and content of the message. This synthetic processing is referred to as top-down, in contrast to the analytic nature of bottom-up processing. Remember that top-down processing involves the use of one's knowledge of the language structure and rules to facilitate construction of anticipated linguistic message components. The process operates primarily at the levels of language processing that involve meaning, namely the semantic and syntactic levels. The listener, familiar with the language rules governing the speaker, is able to generate an evolving hypothesized linguistic pattern. The hypothesis is based on the subject and on situational and contextual cues already available. The actual signal received need not, therefore, be processed in detail. Instead, the incoming message signal is processed only so far as is necessary to check that it is indeed that which was expected. Detailed analysis is necessary only if the hypothesis proves incorrect.

Bottom-up processing, by contrast, is analytical. It operates when our ability to predict how the message will evolve is poor and occurs when we have not yet identified or are unfamiliar with the topic, when the vocabulary and concepts are unfamiliar, or when there is competition with, or distortion of, the message signal. Under these circumstances we must analyze the incoming signal in considerably more detail at the word or syllabic level to extract from it sufficient information for larger chunks of the pattern to be reconstructed. Thus the comprehension of spoken language consists of the continual interaction of incoming data with internally generated expectancies. Godfrey (1984) states:

> Psycholinguistic research has shown repeatedly that top-down and bottom-up processing interact in numerous complex ways, so that any change of acoustic input, or any change in available interpretive information, may have effects at any level. (p. 54)

The relative contribution of bottom-up and top-down processing shifts constantly depending on all the factors that influence predictability. The efficiency of auditory processing, however, is greatest when top-down processing dominates. Thus, processing moves rapidly to provide sufficient bottom-up information to permit predictions to be generated and a shift made to top-down processing. This begins at the syllabic level. At that level and above, a wealth of coarticulatory information becomes available to the listener familiar with phonologic rules. This means that auditory discrimination is no longer dependent purely upon the reception of all acoustic components of a speech sound. Clues to a speech sound can be found in the adjacent sounds that make up the syllable-plus section of the speech acoustic pattern being processed. The implication of this is that a sound may no longer need to be heard, or at least not heard in full, to be perceived. Perception derives from predictions which, at the phonologic level, can be made on the basis of the influence a sound exerts on the character of adjacent sounds in a given phonetic context. Ling (1976) stresses the need to determine not simply whether a child can hear a sound, but whether there is any phonetic context(s) in which she can discriminate (predict) it.

This requires that a child's discrimination of a sound be tested systematically in every combination (phonologic context) in which that sound can occur in the English language.

In addition to coarticulatory cues to speech discrimination and comprehension, a person familiar with a language draws heavily upon contextual constraints. These operate both within each level and between levels from the phonological to the semantic, allowing top-down processing. By processing the information in the acoustic signal within a contextual framework, we are able to formulate hypotheses concerning which phonemes, words, sentence structures, and meanings reasonably can be expected. Norlin states that

> through the awareness of relationships of an element with its context, we extract and assign its "meaning." In this way, context is especially obvious when we examine the oral, symbolic communication system. (1981, p. 90)

Bateson (1967) places such importance on the role played by context in language comprehension that he makes the claim that communication cannot exist without it.

Each contextual constraint utilized increases the predictability of the message and decreases dependence on the details of the acoustic signal. This can be seen in terms of how the amount of contextual information increases the rate at which discrimination grows as a function of intensity (see Figure 9.1). Boothroyd goes so far as to say that because of linguistic and contextual redundancy, "the acoustic speech signal is simply physical evidence that the listener 'consults' in the process of deciding what the talker has said" (1978, p. 129).

The point is that auditory discrimination and speech comprehension involve different processing strategies. One listens very differently when focusing on the acoustic details than when listening for meaning; the two goals are only loosely related. Bottom-up and top-down processing stand in an inverse relationship. When we can predict meaning or even language patterns, we do little analytical processing of acoustic features; when meaning is obscure, or a word or sentence unfamiliar, our dependence on auditory discrimination increases.

EFFECT OF REDUCED AUDITORY INFORMATION IN THE ADULT

When a hearing deficit develops after language rules have been learned thoroughly, the individual is not faced with a complete breakdown in auditory communication. The process, being primarily cognitive-linguistic in nature, has so much intrinsic redundancy that a surprising amount of information loss in the acoustic signal can be compensated for before communication breakdowns occur. The observable difficulties experienced in communication begin when the combination of acoustic information and contextual constraints fails to provide sufficient cues for pattern recognition. As the definitiveness of the information at the primary stages of processing decreases, the degree of confidence that accompanies a perception also decreases. Subtle deficiencies have been shown to occur even before the hearing impairment reaches a level that results in errors of discrimination. Pisoni (1981) demonstrated that samples of synthesized speech that were 100 percent intelligible nevertheless caused listeners to require longer time to make decisions on word tasks than normal speech. This reflects the inferiority of the synthetic acoustic stimulus. Commenting on these findings, Godfrey (1984) says:

> These results imply that all lost acoustic information has its price, not necessarily measurable in feature counts or specific misidentifications, but at times in effects as subtle as less time and/or information available for decisions about the tense of a verb or the intended references of a pronoun. (p. 55)

Hearing-impaired persons frequently complain of the stress involved in listening; "It's so exhausting" they say. This is understandable, for the reduction of information at the periphery lessens the accuracy with which predictions can be made. Salient pattern features often are missing, forcing a more detailed processing of primary data. This in turn, as Godfrey (1989) previously explained, reduces the time available for higher level cognitive-linguistic evaluation of the message. The listener no longer can cope easily with the high rates of information transmission characteristic of normal speech. Attention, usually devoted to evaluation of the meaning and intent of the reconstructed message, must be diverted to the process of reconstruction of the message itself. In everyday conversations, when person-to-person distance is short and the speech is comfortably above the noise levels and situational constraints present, a person often can manage. He does so in the way you manage in a foreign country where you speak the language, but not very well. You understand most of the time. However, you know that you let passages of speech go by without fully understanding them in the hope that you later will be able to piece the meaning together. However, if the details of the message are important—for example, in road directions or in an instruction on how to make an overseas phone call, or if you have to attend instructional classes in that language, you no longer can afford just to "get by." It is at a comparable point that a person with impaired hearing begins to adapt to the situation by making excuses for not catching what was said or, more often, by progressive withdrawal from difficult situations.

Impact on Memory Processing

The reduction of auditory information has an impact on all stages of perceptual processing including memory. The first stage, echoic memory, is directly affected since the pattern-analog it reproduces is dependent upon the capacity of the cochlea to record faithfully the acoustic pattern. Sensorineural hearing impairment results in a distortion of the echoic image. Thus it is from this distorted image that segmented linguistic patterns must be restructured into short-term memory. The fidelity with which the phonologic patterns can be reproduced, along with the subsequent morphologic and syntactic structures, will depend to a great extent, therefore, on how closely echoic memory reproduces the acoustic pattern at this intake level.

The loss of peripheral data has subtle effects even before intelligibility is effected, slowing down the rate at which information can be processed. This results in difficulty in chunking the signal into the larger units necessary for overcoming the capacity of short-term memory (STM) which is limited to 7 ± 2 items. Thus communication becomes too rapid to follow in detail, and the listener struggles to process as much as possible. For as long as it is enough to get by in a situation, the hearing-impaired person passes as having no difficulty. The price lies in having to pay greater attention, with the associated tiredness, and in a reduced feeling of communicative and social security. Long-term memory (LTM) will be affected similarly as hearing impairment increases because what is restructured into it is based upon depleted information.

Perhaps the saddest effect is when the memory problems arising from impairment of hearing are misinterpreted by older persons and their families as a deterioration in mental function. Information counseling should include, therefore, an explanation of how hearing impairment has an impact on information intake, processing, and storage.

EFFECTS OF REDUCED AUDITORY INFORMATION IN CHILDREN

The effect of hearing deficiency occurring prelingually is quite different from that occurring after language and speech are well established. All children are born with the human predisposition to develop spoken language. Studies have demonstrated auditory discrimination of place of articulation in infants as young as six weeks of age (Morse, 1972). Morse (1977) summarized the results of such studies thus:

> In sum, all of these studies in infant speech perception reveal that infants can discriminate almost every relevant acoustic cue(s) in those speech sounds that have so far been presented to them. . . . This research thus supports the position that *some aspects of processing in a speech mode are either a genetically endowed capacity in infants or they are learned within the first few weeks of life.* (p. 166)

However, the development of the sophisticated neural networks of the auditory system, which *are* the speech language system, is totally dependent on continuous exposure to sound.

Impact on Language Learning

Language and speech development are an integral part of cognitive and sensorimotor development, all of which are dependent upon the maturation and myelination of the nervous system. Thus, predictable periods exist for the emergence of various abilities. These include the acquisition of language skills. The importance of optimal learning periods for language has been stressed by McNeil (1966), Lenneberg (1967), and Fry (1978) among others. Once a critical period for learning has passed, the ease with which a function can be acquired decreases rapidly with the decreasing capacity of the brain to adapt and reorganize. The point is that the child's brain will organize itself neurologically as a natural function of maturation, but the organization will exclude the use of auditory information if it is not available. A watershed for language learning appears to occur around two years of age by which time a child has an organized internal model of its world. Many objects and events that make up the system now have names, and the basic rules by which language functions have been sufficiently deduced to permit comprehension. The foundations of language have been laid. After two years of age the development and use of that system accelerates dramatically. If the rules have not been established, the neural system continues to evolve in ways not compatible with the use of language. As a result increasing inertia to change develops.

It is important to remember that the acquisition of the mother tongue by the infant occurs without teaching:

> Every individual child learns the whole language system of his native community for himself and from scratch, and he does so by abstracting the information he needs from the mass of sensory inputs by which he is surrounded. (Fry, 1978, p. 16)

Language learning occurs, therefore, through induction. Deprived in part or in full of the essential information in the acoustic speech signal, the child has no accurate models from which to discover how language works. Significant reduction of the ability to hear spoken language results not simply in a delay of language development but, far more seriously, in the establishment of a biological perceptual posture in which verbal language has no relevance. Furth describes the deaf child with little hearing above 90dB HL who receives no special education until entering a program at age three or four:

> The deaf child has quite happily advanced in the development of his personality without the acoustic input which the hearing child has had. Language has no place in his development and biologically the deaf child has no need for it. (1974, p. 175)

Thus the reduction of acoustic information in the prelingually hearing-impaired child prevents or disrupts language acquisition and with it the manner in which the world is known and experienced. Cognition is heavily influenced by the possession of a sophisticated language system. The failure of speech development also affects thought processing, particularly memory, which is essential to the analysis, refinement, and storage of experience. Thus hearing impairment impedes learning:

> In addition to the evidence that ability to speak enhances speech reception there is also evidence that speech codes are normally used in all forms of verbal learning. They are used to rehearse and to organize linguistic material in memory and they shape our perceptual strategies. (Ling, 1976, p. 5)

REDUCED AUDITORY INFORMATION
AND ENVIRONMENTAL ACOUSTICS

We discussed the effects of environmental acoustics on normal speech perception in Chapter 3. We saw how the reverberated sound energy creates indirect sound waves that mix prolonged outdated information with the current information of the direct wave, resulting in distortion. The effects of poor signal-to-noise ratios and their relationship to distance from the speaker were also discussed. We saw the effects that these conditions have in further reducing speech discrimination by normal-hearing persons particularly when long reverberation and low signal-to-noise ratios coexist. As you would expect, the impact of less than optimal acoustics on speech discrimination, comprehension, and auditory learning are compounded when a person has impaired hearing. The effects are naturally most severe in children. The hearing-impaired child or adult faces the combined effects of distortion of the acoustic signal from noise and reverberation and from cochlea filtering and distortion. Furthermore, since tests of discrimination invariably use monosyllabic words or larger language units, any deficiency in linguistic knowledge will reduce the positive role of linguistic redundancy in compensating for a reduction of acoustic information.

Evidence of the severity of the effects of noise and reverberation on word discrimination by hearing-impaired children has been provided by Finitzo-Hieber and Tillman (1978). They made a comparison of the discrimination scores obtained by 12 normal-hearing children between 8 years, 8 months and 12 years, 8 months with 12 hearing-impaired children aged 8 years, 10 months to 13 years, 9 months. The hearing impairments in the latter group were mild to moderate, bilaterally symmetrical, with speech reception thresholds in the 35–52dB HL range. The maximum discrimination scores for the hearing group were in the 78–96 percent range. These were obtained using tape recorded Kindergarten Word Discrimination lists controlled for vocabulary. The words were presented at 25dB above each child's speech recognition threshold (SRT) at 12 feet from the speaker, either in a nonreverberant (anechoic) chamber or in a chamber in which reverberation times could be controlled. Competition to the signal (noise) consisted of a babble of eight talkers. Signal/competition (S/C) ratios of 0dB, +6dB and +12dB were used. A quiet, no-competition condition was identified as $+\infty$. The results obtained by Finitzo-Hieber and Tillman (1978) are shown in Table 9.1. Consider first the scores for normal-hearing children. Even in total quiet (S/C = $+\infty$) you can see that increasing reverberation from 0.0 seconds to 1.2 seconds reduces discrimination by 18 percent. At S/C +6, which represents the average S/C ratio in a classroom, the same increase in reverberation time decreased discrimination by 25.5 percent. Signal/competition ratios also were shown to have significant negative effects on the scores obtained by these hearing children:

- In no reverberation, a S/C = +12dB ratio allowed a score of 89.2 percent which dropped to 79.7 percent at S/C = +6dB.
- When noise and reverberation coexisted, the scores were 82.8 percent at 0.4 seconds and S/C = +12dB which fell to 71.3 percent at S/C = +6dB.
- For the more typical classroom conditions of a 1.2 second reverberation time and +6dB S/C ratio, the discrimination was reduced to 54.2 percent.

Thus, it is apparent that noise and reverberation, which always coexist, have a serious negative effect on word discrimination by children with normal hearing. This in turn increases the need for attention, reduces ease of comprehension, and thus can be assumed to have a negative effect on learning.

TABLE 9.1 Mean monosyllabic word discriminations scores of the normal-hearing children (loudspeaker-aided) and the hearing-impaired children. Children listening in the high-fidelity condition (loudspeaker-aided) and listening through an ear-level hearing aid (hearing aid-aided) for all combinations of reverberation time and message-to-competition ratio. Finitzo-Hieber & Tillman, 1978, p. 448.)

		GROUPS		
Reverberation Time (sec)	*Message-to-Competition Ratio in dB*	*Normal (Loudspeaker-Aided)*	*Hearing-Impaired (Loudspeaker-Aided)*	*Hearing-Impaired (Hearing Aid-Aided)*
0.0	$+\infty$	94.5	87.5	83.0
	$+12$	89.2	77.8	70.0
	$+6$	79.7	65.7	59.5
	0	60.2	42.2	39.0
0.4	$+\infty$	92.5	79.2	74.0
	$+12$	82.8	69.0	60.2
	$+6$	71.3	54.5	52.2
	0	47.7	28.8	27.8
1.2	$+\infty$	76.5	61.8	45.0
	$+12$	68.8	50.2	41.2
	$+6$	54.2	39.5	27.0
	0	29.7	15.3	11.2

The impact of the poor acoustic conditions on hearing-impaired children was found by Finitzo-Hieber and Tillman (1978) to be even more severe. The data for the hearing-impaired group revealed that

- Listening in quiet through a quality loudspeaker, the maximum score at comfortable loudness was 87.5 percent when reverberation was not present. A reverberation time of 1.2 seconds reduced discrimination by over a quarter, to 61.8 percent.
- Competing speech babble in nonreverberant conditions reduced scores to 65.7 percent at S/C = +6dB, a 21.8 percent drop from maximum. In the typical classroom condition of 1.2 sec reverberation +6dB S/C the score dropped to only 39.5 percent.

The performance of these children fell even more when they listened through a monaural hearing aid, an effect that became more marked as reverberation increased. As can be seen from the last column in Table 9.1, even under perfect acoustic conditions, listening through a monaural hearing aid reduced word discrimination scores a further 4.5 percent (87.5 to 83 percent). Under classroom conditions (1.2 second reverberation +6dB S/C), the score was a totally inadequate 27.0 percent. Remember that these results were obtained by children whose hearing deficit was not severe, in the 30–50dB range. The significance of the findings is serious, particularly when you realize that the ability measured was discrimination. In school the listening process serves the far more important role of providing information for learning. Later we will examine research related to the effects of noise on learning. It is appropriate first, however, to ask whether the poor performance of the hearing-impaired children in the study just discussed could be due to the fact that they were listening through a single hearing aid.

Monaural versus Binaural Listening

We talked in Chapter 3 about the importance of *directivity* in speech perception. The ability to localize sound and to focus auditory attention on one sound source in the presence of background noise is optimal only when using two ears. One might assume that binaural hearing would produce superior discrimination performance as a function of directivity and the ability to separate the signal from the noise background. Several researchers have addressed this question. Gelfand and Hochberg (1976) investigated the importance of binaural listening in combatting reverberation. The binaural discrimination scores obtained by a group of normal-hearing subjects was 90 percent at 1-second reverberation time. When reverberation was increased to 3 seconds, discrimination dropped to 64 percent. By comparison the monaural score for the 3-second condition fell a further 12 percent to 52 percent. The scores for hearing-impaired persons on the same task were 64 percent binaural at 1-second reverberation time, falling to 48 percent at 3 seconds. Comparative monaural discrimination scores were 55 percent at 1 second and only 37 percent at 3 seconds. These scores all were obtained in quiet. They indicate that binaural hearing plays a role in combatting the distortion effects of reverberation both in normal-hearing and in hearing-impaired subjects. For both groups the study evidenced a 12–15 percent advantage of binaural over monaural listening. Although the benefit was less for hearing-impaired subjects than for those with normal hearing, the significance of the improvement is greater for the person who is hearing impaired since the need is greater (Table 9.2).

Nabalek and Pickett, in two earlier studies (1974a, 1974b), reported the comparative discrimination scores obtained by hearing and hearing-impaired subjects listening under very short reverberation time conditions of 0.3 and 0.6 of a second. The test items were presented at various S/C ratios using speech babble as the competing stimulus. Subjects listened monaurally and binaurally through hearing aids. The results are also shown in Figure 9.6. Compare first the monaural (0) and binaural (x) curves for normal hearing subjects.

In Figure 9.6 note the rapid rise in discrimination scores for both conditions. Note also that the scores rise rapidly at negative signal-to-competition ratios even with monaural listening. Compare this to the very shal-

TABLE 9.2 Discrimination scores obtained by hearing and hearing-impaired subjects listening monaurally and binaurally in quiet under two conditions of reverberation. (After Gelfand & Hochberg, 1976.)

	Hearing Subjects		Hearing-Impaired Subjects	
Reverberation time	1 sec	3 sec	1 sec	3 sec
Binaural listening	90%	60%	64%	48%
Monaural listening	—	52%	55%	37%

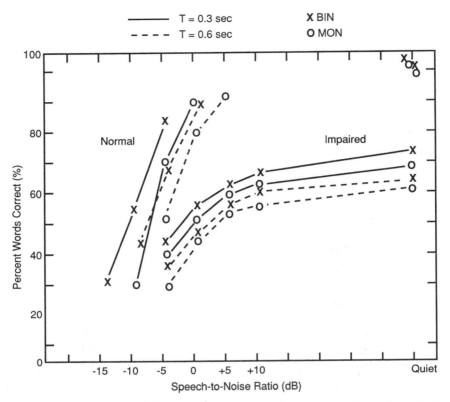

Figure 9.6 Mean percentage of words correct as functions of speech-to-noise ratio for five subjects with normal and five subjects with impaired hearing, binaural (crosses) and monaural (open points) listening, at reverberation times equal to 0.3 sec (solid lines) and 0.6 sec (broken lines). A babble made up of eight voices was used as the masker. (Nabalek & Pickett, 1974b.)

low rise of the discrimination curve for the hearing-impaired group, which under no condition approaches normal maximums. When listening binaurally at 0.3 seconds, the normal-hearing group reaches the 50 percent discrimination level at -10dB S/N and the 80 percent level at -6dB S/N. The figures for monaural listening are 50 percent discrimination at -7dB S/C and 80 percent at 0dB S/C. When reverberation is increased to 0.6 seconds, higher S/C ratios are required to achieve the same results. Now compare the scores obtained by the hearing-impaired group. Binaurally the 50 percent discrimination occurred at $+2$dB S/C while the maximum discrimination of 60 percent did not occur until $+10$dB at 0.3 second reverberation. Monaurally, 50 percent discrimination was reached at the $+7$dB S/C level while a maximum score of only 54 percent required $+10$dB S/C. It can be seen from this study that two aids did provide better discrimination than one even in short reverberation times. However, the hearing-impaired subjects do not show as great an improvement with binaural amplification as the normals. It must be remembered, however, how much greater is their need for increased information. This makes even a 10 percent increase extremely important. Remember also that word discrimination scores translate to much higher scores when related to equivalent sentence discrimination (see Figure 9.2).

Environmental Acoustics and Learning

The question remains whether exposure to noise, especially during preschool and early school years, affects the development of auditory skills, auditory processing behavior, and learning.

The number of studies that have investigated the effects of noise on preschool children are few. Wachs, Uzgiris, and Hunt (1971) included noise among one of the variables in a series of studies of physical environmental influences on psychological development of infants. They used trained observers to rate the "noise confusion" in homes included in the study. Noise confusion proved to be a significant variable in influencing cognitive development. Exploratory behavior, use of gesture, and extent of vocal behavior all were found to be depressed by noise confusion. On the basis of these results, one might expect that children from noisy home environments would experience reduced learning skills, particularly auditory processing skills, when entering school. Hambrick-Dixon (1980, 1982), in two conference reports, stated that a study of children in day-care centers revealed that the infants were negatively affected by noise. They found depressed performance on psychomotor tasks but not on perceptual or cognitive tasks. Following up on these children, the authors found that children in quiet centers showed consistent improvement on test tasks over time. Surprisingly, those in noisy centers at first scored better than those in the quieter centers. However, after two years of exposure to the noise, the performance of these children fell progressively behind that of children in quiet learning environments. Long-term exposure to noise, therefore, appears to reduce the neural system's ability to resist the negative effects.

More research results are available for children of school age. In 1973 Cohen, Glass, and Singer compared the auditory discrimination skills and reading ability of children living in noisy home environments (65dBA) with those living in quieter residences (55dBA). Even when the children living in the noisier homes were tested in quiet, they exhibited poorer discrimination and reading performance than the group living in homes with lower noise levels. Race, socioeconomic level, and hearing sensitivity were controlled for. Bronzaft and McCarthy (1975) tested children in a school adjacent to an elevated railway on which trains created noise levels of 89dBA every four to five minutes. They compared the reading performance of children in classes facing the tracks with those on the quieter side of the school. They found depressed reading abilities in the classrooms experiencing the recurrent high noise levels.

In 1981 Cohen, Evans, Krantz, Stokols, and Kelly reported on a longitudinal study of the aftereffects of noise on third- and fourth-grade children in school. Part of the study investigated the impact of prolonged noise exposure on attentional strategies. They wished to determine whether the adaptation strategies are continued in nonnoise conditions. Data were collected on inattention, auditory discrimination, and reading achievement. The results showed that children in noisy schools are more likely to fail on cognitive tasks than those in quiet schools and are likely to give up on a task before using all the time allowed. Children in noisy schools show more inattention, a problem that increases with the number of years spent in noisy schools. Surprisingly, neither auditory discrimination nor reading performance were found to have been affected. This latter finding was not supported in a later study by Lukas, Dupree, and Swing (1981). In a study of children in 100 classrooms in 15 schools located near California freeways, they found that the incidence of reading retardation increased as noise level increased.

The effect of noise on academic skills in hearing-impaired children appears not to have been studied. However, it appears justifiable to make a number of assumptions based upon what we know about these children:

- When amplification is worn, hearing-impaired children are not isolated from the effects of noise because both speech and noise are amplified.
- Increasing numbers of hearing-impaired children are now placed in mainstream classroom noise environments.
- Many children with impaired hearing are wearing only a single hearing aid, which decreases the ability to discriminate speech in noise.
- The reduced language knowledge of most hearing-impaired children is a handicap not present among the hearing children who demonstrated reduced auditory processing performance and depressed reading as a result of noisy environments.
- Hearing-impaired children frequently lack effective listening skills and attentional strategies even in quiet. They will be at an additional disadvantage in noise.
- The negative effects that noise has been shown to have on the reading abilities of hearing children will be magnified in hearing-impaired children. This is so because the reduced language knowledge that results from impairment of hearing already predisposes them to reading difficulties.

SUMMARY

- Hearing impairment reduces information at the cochlea, thus distorting the pattern recorded.
- Some features of speech, such as voicing, manner of production, and syllabic structure, have a higher resistance to distortion than others.
- Place of production of a sound is highly susceptible to distortion.
- Maximum discrimination occurs at approximately 30 dB HL above threshold. Further intensity decreases discrimination.
- Most information in speech lies above 750 Hz.
- The ability to detect fine changes in the speech pattern (different limen frequency or just noticeable difference) decreases with increasing hearing impairment. Small DLF is thought to be a prerequisite to speech discrimination.
- Vowels suffer less from distortion than consonants. Weak short vowels are most prone to distortion.

- High frequency unvoiced fricative consonants most quickly become inaudible or indiscriminable. Strong consonants often remain audible but may be indiscriminable within category (e.g., plosives).
- Spoken language usually is processed at the meaning level. This involves checking synthetic top-down linguistic predictions against input.
- When information is low, unfamiliar, complex, or distorted, analytic bottom-up processing is used until predictions can be made and top-down processing adopted.
- Thus language knowledge enhances speech perception.
- Loss of acoustic information can be absorbed to some degree by linguistic redundancy if the hearing impairment is postlingually acquired.
- Hearing impairment, however, always demands extra effort and may appear to affect attention, concentration, memory, and learning.
- Prelingual hearing impairment retards oral language learning.
- Poor acoustics reduce speech discrimination by normal-hearing subjects. The effect is far greater when hearing impairment exists.
- Binaural hearing increases tolerance of poor acoustics.

Conclusion

The effect of impairment of hearing is to reduce the amount of acoustic information received by the listener. The pattern that carries the instructions by which the listener reconstructs the linguistic message is distorted. Usually the person hears but cannot easily discriminate what is said. When the listener knows the language well, he/she can to varying degrees fill in the linguistic gaps by top-down processing. When the distortion is high or the content difficult or unfamiliar, top-down processing fails. Prelingually hearing-impaired children have little ability to use top-down processing due to language deficiency. They are, therefore, more seriously affected by hearing loss. For all hearing-impaired persons, poor acoustics will have a significant negative effect on speech discrimination. The acoustic environment thus is an important consideration in assessing hearing handicap.

10

Understanding Audiologic Test Results

Your responsibility to the child or adult you will be seeking to help demands a practical understanding of (1) the hearing impairment, (2) the amplification provided, and (3) the results that indicate the measured improvement in auditory performance provided by the hearing aid(s). Consider each of these categories of information that the audiologist can provide.

DIAGNOSTIC AUDIOMETRIC TEST RESULTS

To gain some appreciation of the condition with which your client is having to cope, you will want to know as much as possible about his/her hearing. Begin by asking yourself a series of questions.

Are the Pure Tone Thresholds for the Ears Symmetrical? You will see that the hearing impairment of Subject A, illustrated in Figure 10.1a, does not affect each ear similarly. Hearing in the left ear, while approximately equal to that in the right ear from 250–1000 Hz, is much better from 1000 to 8000 Hz. Subject B's hearing is approximately symmetrical for the two ears. The possibility of providing binaural amplification for both these persons nevertheless would need to be explored. Binaural amplification always should be recommended unless there are definite audiologic reasons for not doing so. This does not mean that the client should accept that recom-

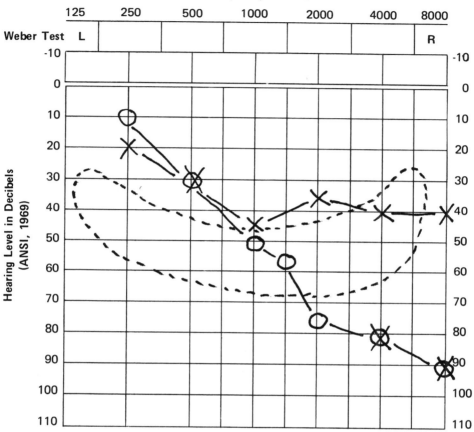

PURE TONE AUDIOGRAM
Frequency in Hertz

Figure 10.1a

mendation, for a number of factors must be taken into consideration before making that decision.

What Is the Configuration or Pattern of the Remaining Hearing? Residual hearing, which is the positive way of considering the audiogram, comes in all patterns. Some configurations are, however, common. One of the most frequently seen patterns is the falling pattern of residual hearing, which slopes with varying degrees of steepness from near-normal hearing in the low tones to various degrees of residual amounts in the high tones. This configuration, seen for Subject A's right ear (Figure 10.1a) means that even with amplification there still will be filtering of the high–information-bearing components of the acoustic signal represented by the second for-

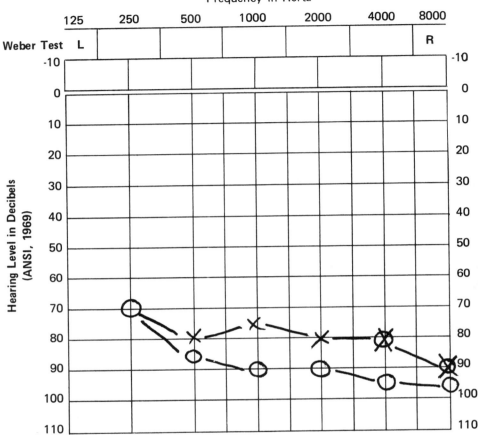

PURE TONE AUDIOGRAM
Frequency in Hertz

Figure 10.1b

mant and its transitions. Fricative information is also likely to remain distorted. By contrast, a mainly flat pattern of residual hearing (Figure 10.1b, Subject B) will enable the remaining hair cells to extract far more high frequency information from the amplified acoustic signal. People with inverted bell-shaped audiograms and patterns of hearing rising from low to high frequencies, though not common, can often further enhance potential discrimination when fitted with appropriate amplification. By referring to the speech spectrum map (Figure 10.2), you will be able to estimate which speech characteristics will be inaudible or weak at normal conversational levels.

How Much Residual Hearing Is There? This question really can be answered only in terms of the severity of the threshold levels. It is recom-

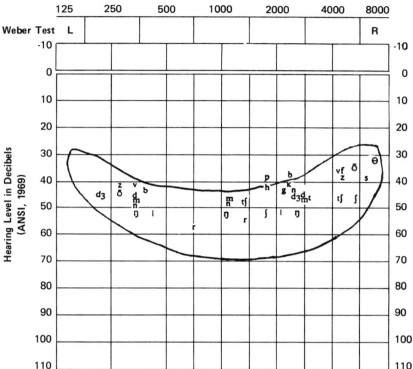

Figure 10.2 Intensity range of speech at various frequencies on an audiogram scale.

mended that the severity of hearing impairment be calculated in terms of the average of the thresholds at 500, 1000, 2000, and 4000 Hz in the better ear (Suter, 1980; AAO-ACO, 1979). The categories conventionally used are

mild		20–40 dB HL
moderate		45–55
moderately severe	thresholds between	60–70
severe		70–90
profound		90 and above

Difficulties arise when we forget that these categories define *only* the severity of the change in thresholds for pure tones. The labels we assign to the hearing threshold range often take on semantic implications beyond this. For example, individuals with thresholds in the 20–40dB range are not infrequently told by medical specialists that their hearing loss is "only mild" and that they are "not yet ready for a hearing aid," despite the difficulties they are experiencing in less than optimal listening conditions. The physician's judgment does not take into consideration the *effect* of a "mild" hearing deficiency on a person's ability to function normally on communication tasks of varying difficulty in a range of acoustic environments. Even the use of the so-called "speech frequencies" 500, 1000, and 2000 Hz in expressing the severity of impairment has been called into question. Research with elderly persons and with younger individuals with impaired hearing indicates that the severity of the impairment is best indicated by including 4000 Hz in the average. Suter (1980) in reviewing the results of her study to determine which combination of frequencies best predicted speech discrimination scores states:

> The results showed that the *500, 1000, and 2000 Hz* combination was the poorest predictor, and the *1000, 2000, and 4000 Hz* combination was the best predictor of those tested in quiet as well as in noise. Tests of the significance of differences among correlations of the various frequency combinations showed the 500, 1000, and 2000 Hz combination was a significantly poorer predictor than any of the combinations that included frequencies above 2000 Hz. (p. 207)

There exists a correlation between the severity of the hearing deficit and maximum auditory discrimination. The more severe the impairment, the less refined will be the hearing that remains, and the more carefully defined should be one's expectations for the role residual hearing will play in communication. In postlingually impaired persons, the knowledge of the language and experience with language enhance enormously the usefulness of even small amounts of residual hearing. When the impairment is prelingual and language is limited, one expects to have to augment maximal use of residual hearing by heavy dependence on other sensory information. Thus the 85–90dB HL impairment shown for subject B in Figure 10.1, if occurring in an adult with amplification, may allow for quite surprisingly good spoken language comprehension. The same deficit in a child, even with amplification, will make auditory oral communication very difficult.

Speech Audiometric Results

On the audiogram, you also will find speech test scores for each ear. Remember that these were obtained under headphones, in quiet. Look first at the *speech recognition threshold* (SRT), formerly known as the speech reception threshold. This provides an indication of the minimal intensity at which unaided hearing first makes a minimum of comprehension possible in a quiet listening condition. It is the intensity at which one just can grasp the general idea of a conversation—rather like being in a foreign country with a bare minimum of language fluency. Listening at this level requires great concentration and effort that cannot be sustained for more than a brief period. SRTs for normal-hearing persons fall below 10dB HL. The level of a person's SRT thus gives an idea of how much unaided hearing is contributing to comprehension and how much the person is having to depend on linguistic predictions, visible speech, and contextual and situational cues.

To feel comfortable when listening to speech in a favorable acoustic environment, you and I like at least 40–45dB of intensity *above* normal SRT. Thus Mr. Davis, whose audiogram is shown in Figure 10.3a, has an unaided SRT of 35dB HL in the better ear, his acoustic cushion is reduced to a mere 5–10dB, and hearing is contributing only minimally to speech comprehension in demanding circumstances. In Figure 10.3b we see Mrs. Pedrowski's audiogram. She has an 85dB SRT, which means that unaided speech is totally unintelligible, in fact barely audible.

Speech Discrimination Scores

Speech discrimination scores, too, will be provided on the diagnostic audiogram. They are derived from monosyllabic word discrimination at 40dB above SRT, measured under phones. This intensity brings loudness to an

Figure 10.3a

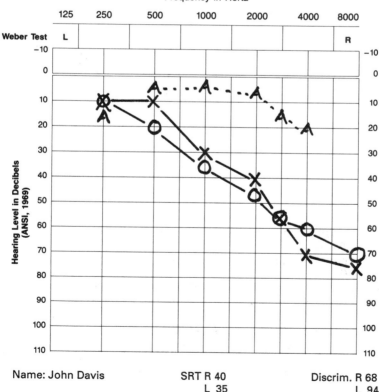

PURE TONE AUDIOGRAM
Frequency in Hertz

Name: John Davis   SRT R 40   Discrim. R 68
                          L 35   L 94

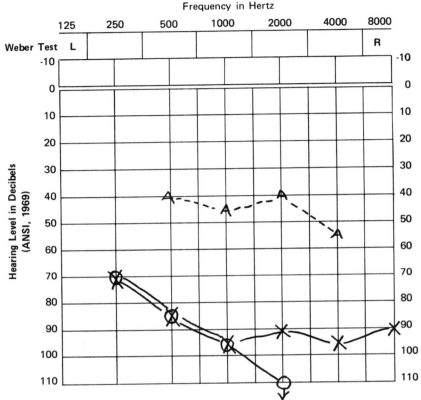

PURE TONE AUDIOGRAM
Frequency in Hertz

Figure 10.3b

acceptable, but not always optimal, listening level. Even at comfortable loudness under phones, the client's maximum hearing potential often is not reflected, since headphones do not shape the acoustic signal to provide for special amplification needs. Furthermore, the scores for monosyllabic word discrimination reflect auditory perception only. They minimize the opportunity to capitalize on contextual and situational constraints. The person's ability to follow a lecture or to understand a play or movie cannot be predicted from discrimination for words except when the score is very low. Remember that these were obtained under headphones, in quiet. Nevertheless, it is helpful to have some prior information concerning the clarity with which the speech signal is heard when amplified.

In the two audiograms, note that at 75dB intensity Mr. Davis achieves normal speech discrimination in the left ear but only 68 percent in the right. However, because of the steeply falling audiogram, we would hope for better discrimination with shaped amplification. Mrs. Pedrowski, who has basically a flat audiometric configuration, probably will not show better scores when aided, but nevertheless she has useful discrimination ability considering the severity of her impairment.

Test Results with Children

The test results we have discussed should be available for each adult referred to you. Test results for children often are difficult to obtain. The younger the child the harder it is to generate an audiometric profile and the more tentative must be the acceptance of the results that are obtained. Early audiograms often are little more than approximations of thresholds. These may have been obtained binaurally in a free field using a loudspeaker, and they often are confined to the critical speech frequencies. Even with older children, one requires repeated audiometric testing before reliability and validity can be assured. Results obtained from speech reception and discrimination tests should be treated with great caution since so many variables must be controlled. *Judgments concerning a young child's hearing potential must not be made on audiometric data alone.* The child's auditory learning potential must be explored thoroughly through diagnostic teaching coordinated carefully with audiologic management. We will discuss this when we consider the management of young hearing-impaired children.

RE/HABILITATIVE AUDIOMETRIC ASSESSMENT

An audiologist often will provide information beyond that already discussed. The most important findings for you will be what the audiologist can tell you about the benefits amplification shows. Aided test results should replicate the diagnostic tests to allow a comparison of unaided and aided performance.

The Aided Audiogram. An aided audiogram will allow you to see how much of the speech signal spectrum is brought within the range of residual audibility by the hearing aid(s) and which frequency components of speech still remain weak or absent. This information will guide you in your expectations for discrimination based upon the acoustic information of the speech sound alone versus discrimination based upon the coarticulatory effects of adjacent sounds. It will explain why a speech sound is recognizable in some phonetic contexts but not in others. The aided pure tone results for Mr. Davis (p. 145) show thresholds very close to normal limits for the left ear out to 4000 Hz, while very significant improvement occurs in the right ear also. Energy from 1500–4000 Hz is now within audibility though it remains softly heard. Significant improvement in sensitivity also is obtained by Mrs. Pedrowski; however, even with amplification, pure tones are not audible below approximately 50dB HL.

I cannot stress too strongly the importance of remembering that amplification does nothing to change a person's hearing deficiency regardless of improvements in test results; the actual sensory capabilities of the cochlea remain unchanged. What a hearing aid aims to do is to amplify speech so that the signal is intense enough to stimulate those remaining hair cells that are not activated by speech at normal intensity levels. Thus a severe hearing impairment remains a severe hearing impairment regardless of the improvement in audibility of pure tones and speech that we hope will result from amplification. In our earlier consideration of the relationship of the increase of speech discrimination with intensity (p. 121), we saw that the 30dB range within which speech discrimination increases in normal-hearing subjects narrows as hearing impairment increases. We must realize, therefore, that the goal of amplification *is not* to achieve aided threshold responses as close to normal as possible. This would result in a reduction of maximum discrimination due to amplification beyond the optimal intensity level. We aim to keep the amplified speech well within the level of comfortable loudness. A level of amplification (gain) from one-third to one-half the hearing deficit appears to provide the best discrimination results in most individuals. We will discuss this in the next chapter.

The Aided Speech Reception Threshold. An aided speech reception threshold will evidence the increase in the cushion of acoustic redundancy provided by amplification. The closer the aided SRT is to normal the greater is the potential for the child or adult to listen with reduced effort. The less a person must strain to reconstruct the message from the acoustic signal, the greater the time available for message content evaluation, response, and learning. Mr. Davis's aided SRT borders on normal for the left ear while the right ear permits topic recognition when voice is little above the intensity level of a whisper. For Mrs. Pedrowski the aid permits topic recognition at soft voice level rather than at the level of a shout necessary for unaided SRT. Her SRT indicates that at least in terms of loudness, normal conversational speech has been made highly valuable as a source of information.

Aided Speech Discrimination in Quiet. You should have an unaided discrimination score administered at normal conversational intensity (50dB HL) and an aided score for the same input level. This will show the person's optimal aided discrimination for the speech signal with minimal linguistic cues and with no visual, contextual, or situational cues. It is helpful if the audiologist then re-presents each word incorrectly identified by hearing alone, allowing the listener to watch for visible speech cues. The difference between the auditory and auditory-visual scores will suggest the person's ability to draw upon visible speech cues to clarify auditory confusions.

Mr. Davis discriminates 68 percent of words at conversational level even without amplification; with the aid he approximates normal scores (88 percent). This indicates that any visual speech-reading skills he has will provide resources he can draw upon in difficult listening environments or situations. The discrimination scores for Mrs. Pedrowski indicate that at normal conversation level (50dB HL), she derives no intelligibility from unamplified sound alone. With the hearing aids only 32 percent of speech is intelligible to her in quiet while the addition of visual cues raises her score to 56 percent.

Discrimination in Noise. Speech discrimination in noise is particularly difficult for hearing-impaired persons. Rehabilitative audiologic assessment, therefore, should include results of how well a person can discriminate against a background of speech babble or speech noise. Speech babble consists literally of the unintelligible babble of multiple speaker conversations; speech noise is noise with a long-term spectrum that matches that of speech.

Speech discrimination at 50dB first should be tested at $S/N = +5dB$ (S.50/N45dB), which is the average S/N ratio in a classroom (Sanders, 1965) and at $S/N = +10dB$ (S50/N40), which is a favorable but not optimal listening condition. The results will provide some insight into how much speech interference affects discrimination. You will recall, however, that the most serious threat to acoustic clarity comes from reverberation, which we are not normally able to assess except in real-life environments. The effect of reverberation can be assessed if a reverberation chamber or equipment to electronically alter speech stimuli is available. These, however, are not usually present in audiology clinics.

At a signal-to-noise ratio of $+5dB$ (S55/N50), Mr. Davis's maximum aided discrimination score by hearing alone drops from 88 percent in quiet to 68 percent in noise, indicating significant difficulty in listening in poor acoustic conditions. At $S/N = +10dB$, he still was able to score 84 percent. Remember, though, this is discrimination for single words with no contextual, situational, or visual cues. However, even when given the opportunity to see the speaker, at an S/N of $+5dB$, Mr. Davis's score rose only 8 percent to 76 percent, suggesting that visual cues in fact are not being exploited fully. This may be because once linguistic context and situational cues are available, this gentleman manages with minimal use of visible speech cues.

Mrs. Pedrowski (see Figure 10.3b) has a much harder time listening in noise. At $S/N = +5dB$ her amplified score of 32 percent drops to 12 percent. Even at the more favorable noise level of $S/N = +10dB$, she achieves only 24 percent. Visual speech cues, however, are helpful to her, restoring much of the masked acoustic information and raising her word discrimination to 56 percent.

You should begin now to see how the re/habilitative audiologic test results can provide insight into the limitations that the hearing impairment imposes on a given individual and the auditory potential that remains. Now consider the findings in the light of some background information and with the test results summarized.

Mr. Davis (Figure 10.3a)

Mr. Davis is a manager in a data-processing company. He is 56 years of age and works in a quiet office where he meets clients on a 1:1 basis. He attends group meetings held around a table in a committee room with favorable acoustics and spends part of his day with computer operators in a data-processing room where the printers generate quite a lot of noise. Mr. Davis occasionally experiences difficulty in a face-to-face situation when not close to the speaker or when not watching; this is true particularly when conversing with female speakers. He has difficulty mostly in group discussions and in noise.

The audiologic tests reveal the following:

- Type of impairment: bilateral sensorineural
- Configuration: sloping, left ear has borderline normal hearing for frequencies to 500 Hz with a steep slope from 10dB HL at 500 Hz to 80dB HL at 4000 Hz. In the right ear the slope is steady from 20dB HL at 500 to 70dB at 4000 Hz
- Severity: 500–4000 Hz averages 37dB for the left ear, a mild loss. In the right ear a moderate impairment of 53dB
- Speech reception thresholds: R 40dB L 35dB
- Speech discrimination: R 68% L 94% at SRT +40dB
- Most comfortable listening level: 65dB free field
- Unaided SRT: 35dB Aided SRT: 25 dB HL
- Unaided discrimination free field at 50dB HL: 68%
  Aided discrimination free field at 50dB HL: 88%
  at S/N +5: 68% + vision 76%
  at S/N + 10: 84%

These findings suggest that Mr. Davis's difficulties arise from the filtering of the high frequency information particularly affecting consonants. The reduction in information has minimal effect in quiet because of the client's ability to compensate linguistically. However, for ease of listening he does like conversation to be at a raised level. This increases the intensity of the weaker components of speech. The pattern of hearing accommodates binaural amplification, though the left ear required that the low frequencies be deemphasized and that high frequency acoustic be provided for both ears. With binaural hearing aids this gentleman achieves near-normal discrimination and does well even in noise. However, he does not appear to make use of visual cues in adverse listening conditions. The aids fitted provided moderate amplification and ensured that intense sounds did not exceed his comfort level. This was particularly important because he had considerable residual hearing for the low tones. The signal was shaped to limit low-tone amplification and to emphasize the high tones. The type of hearing aids that fits into the ear canal was rejected because of the need for considerable high frequency emphasis. Hearing aids that fit into the pinna and the canal were selected for cosmetic reasons.

Mr. Davis normally would not have been referred for rehabilitative management; however, he had a great deal of difficulty in accepting the need for amplification, particularly a binaural fitting. He felt the aids would be nothing but trouble. He also initially was set on having canal aids if he had to have any.

This client illustrates the need to consider more than the acoustic effects of amplification when deciding upon the need for counseling and rehabilitation services both before and after hearing aid fitting.

Mrs. Pedrowski (Figure 10.3b)

Mrs. Pedrowski presents a very different hearing difficulty. She is a 78-year-old widow who lives alone but close to a daughter and two grandchildren in their early twenties. Her family visits her often. Previously an active lady, she now does not go out very much. She no longer attends church, the women's group, or bingo games. She has difficulty hearing TV, which she cannot turn up loudly enough because the neighbors hear it. Communicating with her is both difficult and frustrating for her family.

Audiologic tests reveal:

- Type of impairment: bilateral sensorineural
- Configuration: flat in the speech frequencies in the left ear, gently sloping in the right ear
- Severity: severe bordering on profound in the right ear with no responses above 1000 Hz; limited residual hearing in left ear but hearing across full range of frequencies
- Speech reception thresholds: not obtainable for right ear; 85dB HL left ear
- Speech discrimination: could not test in either ear under headphones
- Most comfortable listening level not measurable without amplification but good tolerance at 110dB
- Unaided SRT and discrimination at 50dB: not measurable
- Aided with high-powered postauricular aid in the left ear: SRT 40dB, discrimination at 50dB 32 percent; with visual cues 64 percent

Despite the severity of the impairment and the poor discrimination score, amplification definitely changes Mrs. Pedrowski's hearing potential. From not hearing speech at all, her comprehension is improved to the point that she now is able to hear normal conversation.

AUDIOLOGIC FINDINGS ON CHILDREN

A re/habilitative audiologic assessment is not carried out routinely on each child or adult referred for help, as is the diagnostic audiologic evaluation, even though it is just as important. You, the speech-language pathologist or teacher of the hearing impaired, will need to explain your needs to the referring audiologist and agree on the components of a re/habilitative assessment. For children, it often is necessary to accumulate the information over time. The age of the child and his/her language competence will determine what information can be obtained and when the child can cooperate. You will be able to facilitate testing by assisting the audiologist in selecting for speech discrimination testing materials that are within the child's receptive vocabulary age. You can screen standard children's test items to eliminate those with which the child is unfamiliar and when necessary generate individual lists from the child's vocabulary. Tests that allow the child to point to the test item named facilitate assessment of young children.

David (Figure 10.4) is six years old. He has a congenital hearing deficiency and has worn an aid for two years. He had just been placed in a mainstream first grade even though he is nine months delayed in language development.

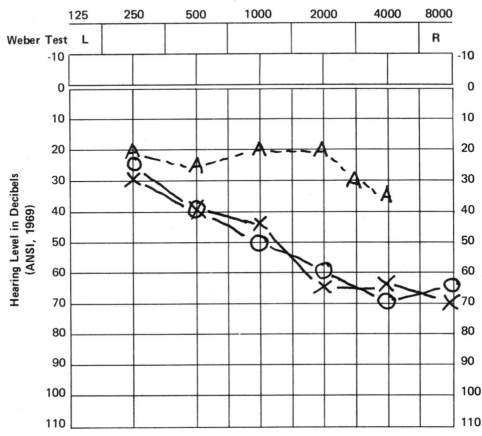

Figure 10.4

Audiologic tests reveal:

Type of impairment: bilateral sensorineural
Configuration: gentle slope from 40–60dB HL in the speech frequencies
Severity: moderate
SRT: 50dB right and left ears   Aided: 20dB
Discrimination: (PBK: children's Phonetically Balanced Kindergarten List)
R 96% L 92%   Aided: 92%
No other aided test results are available

David obviously has much usable residual hearing in both ears. His aided SRT borders on the normal range and his aided discrimination is within normal limits. The surprise is that he is wearing a single postauricular hearing aid in the left ear. He appears to be an excellent candidate for a binaural fitting. He has moved to the area recently. His mother said the audiologist who fitted the aid did not believe in binaural amplification for fear of further depressing the hearing. For almost two years, David alternated the aid between ears each week. He now wears it continuously in the left ear. This is clearly a question that needs to be addressed by an audiologist in your community. You make the appropriate referral and receive the following report:

> David's present hearing aid is in functioning order and appropriate as a monaural fitting. However, David is an excellent candidate for binaural amplification and was fitted with a second postauricular aid. David's unaided SRT was 45dB, with a binaurally aided level of 20dB. With binaural aids, he obtains a 92 percent discrimination at 50dB HL on selected PBK words presented in quiet. In noise (S/N = +5dB HL) his monaural score was 60 percent; with binaural amplification, this improves to 76 percent. This compares well to an unaided free field score of 28 percent at 50dB.

The evaluation of children's communication abilities requires a complete assessment of all aspects of auditory, cognitive, linguistic, and social skills. This we will discuss in a later chapter. Our immediate concern is to become familiar with the amplification devices that facilitate communication.

SUMMARY

- Audiograms should be examined to determine degree of symmetry of hearing between ears, pattern of remaining hearing across frequency, and amount and extent of remaining hearing.
- The hearing in the range 500–4000 Hz is the most critical.
- A correlation does exist between the extent of the residual hearing discrimination for speech, but it is not absolute.
- Amplification does nothing to change the hearing deficiency. It does allow sound to activate remaining hearing hair cells that respond only at higher intensity levels.
- Residual hearing is best activated by amplifying by one-third to one-half the hearing deficit at each frequency.
- Aided speech discrimination scores in quiet and in noise help indicate the amount of hearing handicap remaining after amplification. This guides your counseling and management strategies.

Conclusion

Hearing impairment cannot be restored by amplification. Our emphasis is on the extent and quality of residual hearing. Amplification brings sound within reach of the hearing that remains. It achieves this best by amplifying to approximately one-third to one-half greater than the deficit at each frequency. Each subject's impairment will differ as will the potential of his/her residual hearing. This is measured by aided speech discrimination in quiet and in noise. Although the importance of aided hearing performance cannot be emphasized too strongly, it is essential to remember that many variables will determine the impact of the hearing impairment on a given individual. Management begins with optimal amplification but continues with the application of other compensatory means.

11

Principles and Practicalities of Amplification

RATIONALE FOR COUNSELING ABOUT AMPLIFICATION

All of the problems arising from impairment of hearing derive initially from a reduction of auditory information. The information for reconstructing a linguistic message, or for identifying an environmental sound, is depleted or distorted by the damaged cochlea. It is obvious, therefore, that our first goal in rehabilitation will be to make available as much of the depleted auditory information as possible. This is what we attempt to achieve with amplification.

To plan a realistic program of management of resources for a hearing-impaired person, it is important that you understand what can and cannot reasonably be expected of amplification. You need to know what assessment data the dispensing audiologist can generate concerning the benefit the aid provides to an individual and how to interpret and use that information. Audiologists generally fit hearing aids in specially designed acoustic environments. As a result, there usually is little information in the hearing aid evaluation report pertaining to the extent to which amplification actually changes the ability of the hearing-impaired individual to meet the demands of daily living. As the professional responsible for the habilitation or rehabilitation of the client, you will need to generate such additional information. This process will serve three functions:

1. It will sharpen your perception of the difficulties the individual experiences even when wearing the aid(s).
2. It will target problem situations.
3. It will facilitate the formulation of appropriate procedures for problem reduction.

A cooperative relationship between you, as the audiologist, and all those responsible for helping the child or adult to function optimally will enhance greatly the possibility of success. As the audiologist you must assume responsibility for

1. Ensuring the most appropriate amplification
2. The quantitative measurement of the benefits it provides
3. The technical monitoring of the performance of the hearing aid(s)

The role of the individual who accepts responsibility for management beyond the hearing aid fitting also is threefold:

1. To help the child or adult to adjust psychologically and practically to amplification
2. To assess and monitor its impact on the individual's capacity to function in real-life situations
3. To integrate amplified sound into his/her management of communication situations

Thus it is important that all concerned feel comfortable in their working knowledge of hearing aids. While discussing the client's amplification needs with the audiologist and while counseling the client, you must feel confident. It is important to understand how much the present hearing aid is helping and to be familiar with special fittings for special needs. If you are a speech-language pathologist or teacher of hearing-impaired individuals, you may even find yourself asking the audiologist whether a different fitting might reduce the particular difficulties your client is experiencing.

It is my intent, therefore, to present in this chapter just as much familiarity with the principles and practicalities of amplification as you need to optimize its use in habilitation/rehabilitation.

AMPLIFICATION AND HEARING IMPAIRMENT

In trying to understand how amplification enhances a person's ability to function, it helps to reconsider the nature of hearing deficiency. An impairment of hearing arises from the absence of functional cochlear hair cells and nerve fibers in various sections of the basilar membrane. Generally speaking, the number of nonfunctional units will determine the severity of the deficit; their location on the membrane will determine which frequencies are affected. The combination of these two factors determines the pattern and severity of a hearing impairment as defined by pure tone thresholds.

We know that as the severity of the impairment increases, greater and

[handwritten note at bottom: # of nonfxnal units → severity; location on the membrane → affected freq. } determine the pattern & severity of HI as defined by pure tone thresholds]

greater acoustic intensity is needed to activate the remaining hair cell and nerve fiber units and, thus, to effect hearing. Furthermore, as the hair cell units are reduced in number, the capacity of the system to record the fine details of frequency, intensity, and changes in those acoustic parameters over time decreases. Thus both loudness and clarity are diminished by sensorineural hearing impairment.

Amplification increases the energy of sound waves to the point where they activate sufficient numbers of the remaining functional hair cell units to make the stimulus comfortably loud. There are limits, however. Despite the reduced auditory sensitivity, the sensitivity to the actual physical pressure of the sound wave remains unchanged. This means that for a person with a profound hearing deficit, the thresholds of tickle and pain may be little above the intensity necessary to activate the few remaining hair cells. Threshold levels for loudness tolerance also may be reduced in the damaged cochlea. Finally, in considering the effects of hearing impairment, it is necessary to remember that no matter how excellent the quality of the amplified sound we present to the ear, it must pass through the damaged cochlea to be perceived. I have mentioned already that damage to different sections of the cochlea causes frequency filtering, reducing or eliminating the availability of information in that range of the speech signal. In addition to this, we know that there is cochlear distortion that is not directly accounted for by the pattern of the audiogram. The audiogram, therefore, limited as a measure of the effect of hearing impairment on processing since it measures sensitivity of but two of the parameters of the speech signal, namely intensity and frequency. The third characteristic, duration, which conveys all the temporal information that the auditory system needs, not assessed. Thus, two matched audiograms may be shown to be accompanied by very different discrimination scores. This can arise from differing degrees of cochlear distortion and from differing capabilities of the central systems to process durational cues. The significance of understanding this information lies in the expectations that you and your client will have for amplification. Information concerning what benefits a hearing aid does and does not provide for an individual child or adult will influence your management strategies. It will help you decide how much you can depend on the auditory system alone as a channel for information, and how much supplementary channels must be developed. It can influence greatly the client's definition of "a successful fitting" and thus motivation and attitude. Successful amplification occurs when we are able to use all of the residual hearing potential. When that potential is limited we must tailor our expectations to be realistic.

Before we explore how hearing aids provide for amplification needs, consider the types of hearing aids currently available and the major characteristics of each type.

TYPES OF HEARING AIDS

1. Eyeglass and Body Hearing Aids (Figure 11.1). Very rarely will you encounter an eyeglass fitting. Only infrequently will a client wear a body aid. The need for these types of aids is confined to some infants and to

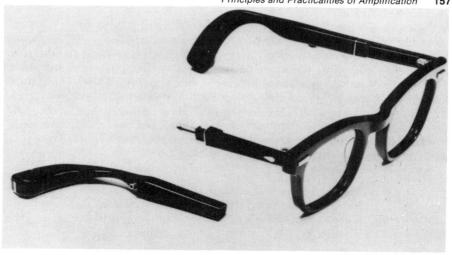

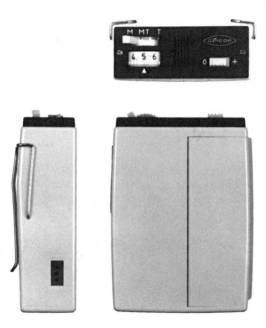

Figure 11.1 Eyeglass and body hearing aid. (Body hearing aid courtesy of OTICON, Inc.)

people with poor manual dexterity. Infants sometimes are fitted with the body aid when first diagnosed because ear-level aids do not fit tiny ears. The body hearing aid still affords the audiologist the greatest flexibility in selecting and changing the signal strength and the pattern of amplification. This is particularly important at an age when a child's exact threshold measures are not determined easily and speech audiometry is precluded.

However, once a pinna can accommodate a postauricular hearing aid and we have confidence in our assessment of the child's amplification needs, a postauricular behind-the-ear fitting usually is preferred. This fitting provides the advantage of true binaural amplification, which is very important to early development of speech and language.

2. Postauricular or Behind-the-Ear (BTE) Hearing Aids. These are the most common type of aid worn by children. They are worn by less than one-third of adults who use hearing amplification. The unit sits behind the ear quite snugly (Figure 11.2a, b). The casing houses the

- *Microphone*, which picks up the sound and converts it to an equivalent electrical pattern
- *Amplifier*, which magnifies the electrical signal
- *Receiver*, which converts the amplified electrical signal back into a sound wave pattern
- *Battery*, which provides power to the amplifier

The amplified sound leaves the aid by way of the *ear hook*. This is a plastic hook that serves to channel the sound and to hold the aid behind the ear. Attached to the ear hook is a length of clear plastic tubing that is connected to the earmold. The tubing allows the sound to pass from the ear hook to the custom-fitted earmold that sits snugly in the concha and ear canal.

3. In-the-Ear Hearing Aids. The in-the-ear (ITE) hearing aid now represents close to 75 percent of aids worn by adults and is increasingly becoming the style worn by school-age children with mild to moderately

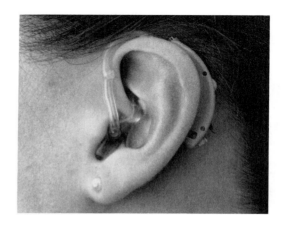

Figure 11.2a
The behind-the-ear hearing aid fits comfortably behind the pinna (Courtesy of Phonak, Inc.)

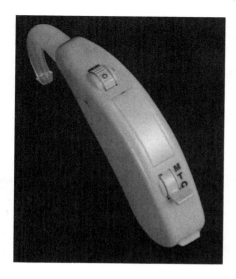

Figure 11.2b The controls on the BTE hearing aid usually consist of an OFF (O) telephone circuit (T), a microphone switch, and a volume control wheel. The battery compartment is in the base. (Courtesy Siemens Hearing Instruments, Inc.)

severe impairments, up to about 60–70dB. All components of the aid, microphone, amplifier, and receiver, are housed in the custom-molded shell that is worn in the ear just as an earmold would be worn (Figure 11.3). A major limitation of this and the canal type instrument is that they do not have external controls to allow you, the audiologist, to modify what the aid does to the incoming speech signal. In ordering an in-the-ear or canal hearing aid, the audiologist requests the manufacturer to adjust it to meet specifications that accommodate the individual person's amplification needs. Your ability to modify these specifications once the aid has been received is minimal. Furthermore, in most instances, when the instrument malfunctions it must be returned to the manufacturer for repair. Unless the client has a custom earmold, or can be fit adequately with a stock model, he/she will be left without amplification because these hearing aids are molded to the individual ear.

4. Canal Hearing Aids. Fitted to adults and increasingly to older teenagers with mild to moderate hearing impairments, the canal hearing aid is custom molded to be accommodated completely within the ear canal (Figure 11.4).

BINAURAL AMPLIFICATION

In the previous chapter, we reviewed the evidence indicating that binaural listening is superior to monaural in combatting the negative effects of noise and reverberation. We saw that binaural discrimination scores for both normal hearing and hearing-impaired listeners were superior to monaural scores. Binaural amplification can be provided for any of the types of aids we have discussed. Occasionally, because of a difference in the residual hearing in the two ears, a person achieves binaural amplification by using

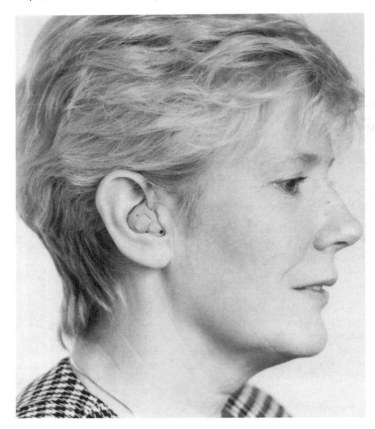

Figure 11.3 The in-the-ear (ITE) model hearing aid is housed in a custom-molded shell that fits into the concha of the ear. (Courtesy Siemens Hearing Instruments, Inc.)

aids of different types, for example, an in-the-ear aid and a postauricular aid. Later we will discuss some of the factors, other than audiological considerations, that the client has to take into account when considering a binaural fitting—factors that may need to be addressed in the rehabilitative management program. Surprisingly many adults still are fitted with a single hearing aid despite the convincing evidence of binaural superiority.

SPECIAL FITTINGS

CROS/BICROS

Two special fittings with which you should be familiar are the CROS (contralateral routing of signal) and BICROS (binaural contralateral routing of signal). *CROS* is a system designed to help persons with a unilateral hearing impairment in which the affected ear cannot use amplification. The client

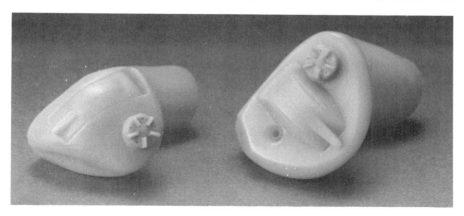

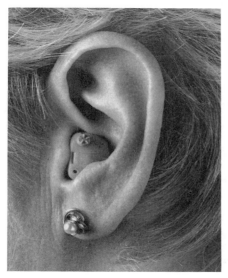

Figure 11.4 The canal model hearing aid is accommodated within the external auditory meatus. (Courtesy Siemens Hearing Instruments, Inc.)

wears two units. On the bad ear she wears a small behind-the-ear unit that houses a microphone and a transmitter. This unit is held in place by a skeleton earmold. The microphone unit sends the sound wave it picks up to a receiver unit on the good ear. The transmission usually is by an FM radio signal, though very occasionally one still encounters a wire connection worn around the back of the head under the hair. The sound from the side with poor hearing then is fed into the better ear through an open mold that does not block the ear canal. Miraculously the brain is able to sort out the two sets of information.

BICROS is an extension of the same principle. It is used when the better ear itself has a hearing deficit that also requires amplification. The signal from the ear that cannot be aided is transmitted to a hearing aid on the side of the better ear, where it is amplified along with sounds being picked up by the instrument on that ear.

Automatic Signal Processing (ASP)

Recent hearing aid technology has led to the development of the first generation of automatic signal processing hearing aids, which aim to suppress noise and thus increase speech intelligibility in noisy environments. To achieve this the ASP hearing aid circuitry is designed so that when low frequency sound energy reaches a preset intensity, a filter is activated. This reduces the amplification in the low frequency range relative to the amplification of higher frequencies. As the low frequency components in the noise increase, so does the amount of suppression provided by the filter circuit. Once the low frequency energy falls below the preset criterion, the hearing aid reverts to its normal pattern of amplification. In some ASP hearing aids, the actual filtering characteristics, which determine the sensitivity of the circuitry to noise, can be manipulated by the audiologist to determine the best fit.

Research (Stach, Speerschneider, & Jerger, 1987; Wolinsky, 1986) has shown that the benefits of ASP can be quantified clinically and that substantial benefits are obtained by some users. It must be stressed, however, that not all persons are comfortable with the sound changes that occur when the ASP circuit is activated. Furthermore, not all encounter enough adverse noise environments to merit the use of ASP. Some individuals who need amplification of the low frequencies in speech actually may experience poorer speech discrimination when ASP reduces amplification in this range. The presence of a conductive component in the low frequencies also may make an ASP fitting inappropriate.

Digital Hearing Aids

Conventional hearing aids process acoustic information in the form of an electrical analog, literally an analogy of the sound wave. Present digital hearing aids do not use this form of information coding at all stages of processing. Instead, digital processing recodes the acoustic information into a numerical digital code. This form of coding permits the acoustic information to be modified in ways that cannot be achieved by conventional analog circuits (Widin, 1987). In addition, the circuitry is more stable over time, tolerates temperature and voltage fluctuations better than analog circuits, and suffers less from internal noise and distortion (Schnier, 1988).

The term *digital*, as applied to hearing aids, is at present very imprecise. Ideally, every stage of processing would be digital and would operate in real time. That is to say, processing would occur instantaneously, obviating the need for storage. Such an aid, however, would require more power than it is possible to provide in ear-level hearing aids. Furthermore, as Schnier (1988) states:

> Digital design techniques are difficult to implement effectively in order to gain all the advantages without degradation of instrument performance. (p. 10)

As encountered in the literature, the *label* digital may describe a hearing aid in which the digital function simply replaces the mechanical control such as the volume control or those that modify gain, frequency response, or output. By contrast, the *adjective* digital may be used to describe an instrument in which a range of functions are controlled digitally. Most so-called digital hearing aids process the signal by analog but use digital memory storage to provide options and to control how the signal is processed. This involves the capability of the hearing aid to be programmed. Such hearing aids commonly are referred to as *programmable hearing aids.*

Programmable Hearing Aids

Advanced systems of programmable hearing aids permit a wide range of characteristics (e.g., gain, output, frequency response curve) to be programmed and reprogrammed by the audiologist while the aid is being worn by the potential user (Hodgson, 1988; Hodgson & Lade, 1988). The setting of such programmable hearing aids is made possible by use of an external computer system or "programmer" to which the aid is connected during the fitting. The audiologist puts into the computer complete audiologic data for the client and selects a preferred prescriptive formula. The computer then proceeds to generate an appropriate fitting that it programs into the hearing aid. Adjustments or reprogramming can be made at any time by the audiologist. In some aids as many as eight different performance curves can be stored in the hearing-aid memory bank. This feature enables the wearer to select, at any time, the prescription that proves most effective for a given listening situation. It is equivalent to having eight separate hearing aids built into one, since each memory is programmed independently.

Digital hearing aids offer you, the audiologist, greater flexibility and complete control in the selection and subsequent adjustment of the hearing aid characteristics most appropriate to the needs of the individual. This allows far more precise matching of the instrument to the client than is possible with conventional hearing aids. Early reports suggest that digital programming does provide measurable improvement in speech recognition in noise and that many hearing aid users prefer a programmable aid for listening to speech in quiet and in noise and for listening to music (Johnson, Kirby, Hodgson, & Johnson, 1988). It must be stressed, however, that caution is needed when considering what commonly are referred to as digital or programmable hearing aids. As I have explained, the terms may mean that much or very little of the process is actually digital, depending on the specific system. One must know what a particular system can do for a client and how much better a given system is than an appropriate analog hearing aid.

Digital technology in hearing aids is in its early stages. There is every reason to believe it will assume an increasing role in future generations of hearing aids. Meanwhile, its effective use depends on close cooperation among the audiologist, the client, and the person responsible for aural rehabilitation training. Clinical quantification and careful observation of the benefits of a digital aid in adverse listening environments, supplemented by the client's subjective ratings of sound quality for different sound inputs, should provide an adequate basis for fitting decisions.

HOW AMPLIFICATION ACHIEVES ITS GOALS

The three basic goals that amplification seeks to achieve are to

1. Increase the strength of the speech signal to make it audible
2. Shape the signal to meet the needs of a particular pattern of hearing deficiency
3. Protect the ear from uncomfortable loudness

1. Increasing Signal Strength. The amplifier of the hearing aid receives the *input* signal that the microphone has converted from an acoustic to an equivalent (analog) electrical pattern. Its role is to increase the intensity of this electrical signal across its full range of frequencies, which usually is from 250 Hz to approximately 5000 Hz. The amount of signal amplification stated in decibels is referred to as *gain*. The more powerful the hearing aid is, the greater gain it will have. The maximum gain for each aid is determined by its circuitry. The volume control determines how much of the maximum gain is added to the input signal. It would seem logical that a person would require the same amount of gain as the hearing deficit. As stated earlier, it has been found that the most appropriate gain tends to approximate one-third to one-half the hearing loss. Usually a formula is used to approximate half the hearing loss. For example, in my work at the Hearing Evaluation Services of Buffalo, New York, the targets for gain at each frequency are

250 Hz $\frac{1}{3}$ hearing threshold level minus 10dB
500 Hz $\frac{1}{3}$ hearing threshold level minus 5dB
1000 Hz $\frac{1}{3}$ hearing threshold level
2000 Hz $\frac{1}{2}$ hearing threshold level
4000 Hz $\frac{1}{2}$ hearing threshold level

This results in a deliberate shaping of the amplified signal in order to emphasize the high frequencies without overamplifying the lows. In this way we increase the potential for maximizing intelligibility.

A recent technological advance has made it possible for a hearing aid wearer to control the volume on the hearing aid remotely. The system uses an FM radio signal sent from a small hand-held unit to increase or decrease the gain level of the hearing aid. This operates on the same principle as the remote control device used to change channels or volume on a TV set. Its use would be particularly valuable, for example, to a businesswoman in a committee meeting. The remote control would permit her to adjust the volume to pick up the voice of a person sitting at the end of the table without frequently having to adjust the controls at ear level in a conspicuous and distracting manner. This feature also would be of help at a presentation in which a speaker's distance from the listener is not constant, or in a church service where the comparative intensity levels of a minister's voice and of the choir and organ demand different volume settings. The remote control also removes the problem of finding and manipulating tiny switches and controls. This is particularly helpful for those with finger dexterity problems and older persons with reduced perception of body image. Each such advance, *if shown to have practical application in real-life situations*, adds to the resource we have in adapting the hearing-impaired person to his/her world and thus reducing the handicap.

2. Signal Shaping or Selective Amplification. Even those of us with normal hearing require amplification at times. For example, in an auditorium or at a play in an outdoor arena, we need greater enhancement of the weaker higher components of speech than we do the strong low tones. This need for signal shaping is far greater when hearing deficiency affects the sensitivity of the ear to different frequencies unevenly. Current hearing aid technology allows us to achieve considerable *selective frequency amplification*. Shaping of the electrical analog of the acoustic input is achieved by the circuitry of the hearing aid. All hearing aid manufacturers provide aids that have a range of frequency characteristics. Hearing aids worn on the body and those worn behind the ear usually provide a tone control that allows the audiologist to modify the frequency shaping to fit a client's needs better. It is now possible for the audiologist to measure the exact shape of the amplification pattern of each aid (the *sensitivity curve*) by using an electroacoustic analyzer, a device that every dispenser of hearing aids should have. Even more accurate measures of the actual sound pattern reaching the eardrum at various hearing aid settings can be obtained using *real-ear measurements*. These involve the placement of a small microphone pickup in the ear canal alongside the earmold. This permits readings to be made of gain and output across frequencies while the client is wearing the hearing aid. A sweep frequency test tone of a measured 60dB input to the hearing aid microphone is used. The output of the hearing aid is then measured close to the eardrum while the aid is worn.

Acoustical Shaping by the Earmold. In addition to the electrical shaping of the speech signal within the hearing aid, it is possible to shape the amplified sound further after it leaves the hearing aid receiver. This is achieved through control over the design of the earmold, which serves the function of delivering the amplified sound into the ear canal. Earmolds come in different shapes and are made from different materials. The choice of the characteristics of the earmold will depend on the predicted acoustic needs of the impaired ear. Each earmold will have a specific reaction pattern to sound energy passing through it. Acoustic modification is intended to alter the signal passing through the mold in a predictable manner: this is achieved by controlling the shape and dimensions of the channel through which it passes. The channel, being a cavity, acts as a resonator. Depending upon the shape and size of the channel, the air within it will have a particular pattern of sensitivity to energy passing through it. It will vibrate readily in sympathy with certain frequencies in the sound wave, thus facilitating their transmission. It will be less sensitive at other frequencies, resulting in a reduction of energy in those frequencies. Through careful selection of the resonant pattern of the earhook, tubing, and earmold, energy in the amplified speech wave can be shifted to the particular frequency range where it most benefits a given client. The extent of this method of shaping the signal can be seen in Figure 11.5 which shows six markedly different responses from a single hearing aid. These are effected by changing the resonant characteristics of the channel through which the amplified sound passes on its way from the hearing aid receiver to the eardrum.

Techniques of Acoustic Signal Modification. There are three ways of achieving modification of the output signal of the hearing aid: (1) earmold venting, (2) damping, and (3) tapering or horn shaping. It is not necessary for you to know the technical aspects of these, but you will feel more confident in talking with the audiologist and your client if you understand what has been done in terms of the fitting.

1. *Venting.* This involves the provision of a channel in addition to the one carrying the sound through the earmold. The second channel runs from the tip of the mold, which sits in the ear canal, to the outside face where the tubing enters the mold. The vent may run parallel to the sound channel or cut into it diagonally. The opening of the vent on the face of the mold may have small changeable plastic plugs that have holes in them ranging from a pinhole to almost the full diameter of the vent itself. These "select-a-vent" (SAV) inserts (Figure 11.6) allow the vent size to be changed easily. The vent serves primarily to reduce or attenuate the energy in the frequencies below 1500 Hz, when hearing is much better in this range than in the high frequencies. Appropriate venting also can reduce or eliminate the echo or hollowness of the hearing aid user's voice, which sometimes occurs with amplification. Finally, a pinhole vent usually eliminates the sensation of fullness that amplified sound pressure in a plugged canal often causes. The importance of venting has been demonstrated by research (Cox & Alexander, 1983). It has been shown that appropriate venting results in better speech intelligibility and speech-sound quality ratings by hearing-impaired persons than is obtained by equivalent electronic shaping of the sound.

Figure 11.5 Frequency response of one hearing aid fitted with six different earmold plumbing arrangements. (Reprinted with permission from Killion, M., Problems in the application of broadband hearing aid earphones. In G. Studebaker and I. Hochberg (Eds.), *Acoustical Factors Affecting Hearing Aid Performance.* Baltimore, MD: University Park Press, 1980.)

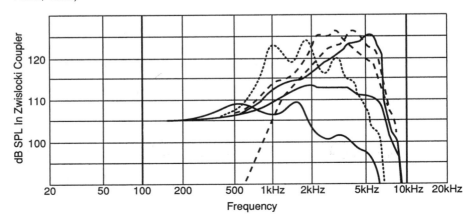

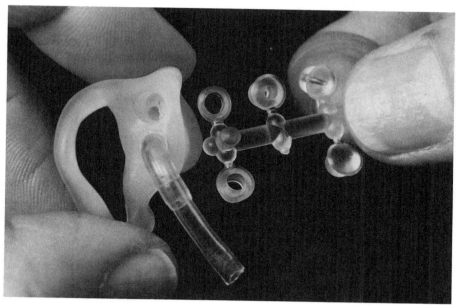

Figure 11.6 Select-a-vent earmold filter.

2. *Damping.* The placing of small plastic or metal filters in the ear hook of the postauricular hearing aid serves to impede the transmission of energy in the middle range of frequencies and to smooth out peaks in the output curve of the hearing aid. The choice of different filters, which are color-coded to indicate different degrees of damping, allows the audiologist to modify both the quality and frequency response curve of the sound entering the ear canal.

3. *Tapering or horn shaping.* This technique shifts energy into the higher frequencies, centering around 3000 Hz. It is a particularly helpful shaping device for the many people whose hearing impairment is much greater above 1000 Hz than below it. The effect is achieved by tapering the diameter of the canal from a wide mouth to the relatively narrow width of the standard tubing, in the manner of a horn. The commonly used design was created by E. Libby and is known as the Libby horn. Other types of earmold modifications further narrow the range of frequencies allowed to reach the ear. Even persons with normal hearing below 1000 Hz usually can benefit from amplification when it is coupled with a special earmold such as a Jansen type, which has a long narrow canal. This type mold is known as an *open fitting* mold, since it does not plug the canal. The sounds for which the person has normal thresholds pass unamplified into the canal around the mold. The high frequency sounds are amplified and delivered through the mold, which will only pass vibrations above 1000 Hz.

Even with appropriate electrical and mechanical shaping, there are psychological and physiological limits to how much amplification a defective ear can tolerate. Thus it is necessary to limit the maximum output of a hearing aid.

3. Output Limiting (Saturation Sound Pressure Level, SSPL 90). The signal leaving the receiver component of a hearing aid and entering the ear is known as the *output*. It is the sum of the input signal plus the amplification gain.

Input + gain = output

50 + 30 = 80dB SPL

One might assume that a severe to profound hearing loss would protect a person from the negative effects of very intense sounds. This is not the case. The physiological sensitivity of the ear to discomfort caused by high sound pressure levels remains unaffected by hearing deficit. Moreover, as I have pointed out already (p. 122), the tolerance of loudness often is affected by recruitment, a phenomenon by which loudness grows disproportionately rapidly as intensity increases. Our goal for amplification is, therefore, to bring the energy at all speech-sound frequencies to within the *most comfortable loudness level* (MCL) without allowing the overall sound pressure level to reach the *loudness discomfort level* (LDL). To achieve this, you, the audiologist, will select and adjust a hearing aid to limit the capability of the aid to put out sound that would exceed an individual wearer's tolerance level. This is called *output limiting*.

The technological ways of achieving this need not be discussed in detail. Simply put, two methods are used. The preferred method is to include in the design of the aid a circuit that is triggered immediately when the signal strength exceeds a preselected amount. Triggering of this circuit reduces output intensity by reducing the gain and compressing the whole signal to bring it within the comfort range. Once the excess input falls, the gain is restored automatically. Aids that incorporate this circuitry are referred to as having AGC (automatic gain control). The method of limiting is called *compression amplification*.

The second method of limiting output is by *peak clipping*. By this method those peak intensities in the acoustic wave that exceed the preset level are clipped—that part of the wave form simply is deleted, squaring off the pattern. This method reduces output without reducing gain. Unfortunately, peak clipping produces a distortion of speech that some patients find reduces their discrimination.

The four types of aids (body, postauricular, in-the-ear, and canal) all are capable of meeting these goals. The body and postauricular aids, however, make it possible for you, the audiologist, to change the response and maximum output of the aid and to modify the amplified signal further through earmold technology. Binaural amplification provides the best listening unless such a fitting is contraindicated; CROS and BICROS fittings accommodate the person with usable hearing in one ear only. The most recent advances of automatic signal processing and digital hearing aids hold promise of providing amplification that adapts automatically or manually to different listening conditions.

The implications this knowledge of amplification and shaping of the speech signal has for rehabilitation management are practical ones. Unfortunately, not all hearing aid fittings are made by audiologists experienced in current amplification technology. Achieving an optimal fitting for some adults and for most children requires familiarity with current hearing aid technology, a real willingness to listen to the patient's observations and those of people close to a child, and a willingness to cooperate in experimentation. You, the therapist/teacher, together with the hearing aid(s) user and his/her family should be part of the hearing aid evaluation team whenever the need arises. In counseling the client and in designing management strategies, it will be your task to make use of the information you can obtain or generate about the hearing impairment and about amplification.

Now that you are familiar with the basics of amplification and the types of hearing aids, we will consider some of the practical matters concerning the use and care of personal hearing aids. First, however, we will summarize our discussion to this point.

SUMMARY: PRINCIPLES

- Hearing handicap results from loss of information, usually at the cochlea.
- The result is deletion and distortion of pattern details.
- Our responsibility is to assist adjustment to amplification, monitor its effectiveness, and train the person to maximize its use.
- Amplification does nothing to restore hearing. It *does* make residual hearing potential functional.
- Pure tone audiograms indicate only threshold sensitivity; only speech discrimination tests reveal the effect on auditory processing.
- The most commonly used types of hearing aids are in-the-ear, canal, and behind-the-ear models.
- Binaural amplification is recommended unless contraindicated.
- Special fittings such as CROS and BICROS assist when only one ear has usable hearing.
- Automatic signal processing hearing aids (ASP) seek to improve speech discrimination in noise.
- Digital hearing aids use numerical coding of the acoustic signal instead of analog coding.
- The term *digital* is used imprecisely; it is necessary to determine exactly what processes are performed digitally.
- Most digital processing in current hearing aids involves storage (i.e., memory capacity).
- Programmable hearing aids permit tailoring of the aid's characteristics for individual needs while worn.
- Digital processing permits up to eight responses to be programmed into a hearing aid for selection by the wearer as appropriate to the situation.
- Amplification increases signal strength, shapes the frequency pattern, and protects from excessive loudness.
- The optimal signal increase (gain) is one-third to one-half the average hearing threshold.
- Further shaping is achieved through earmold technology.
- Venting reduces tones below 1500 Hz. Damping reduces mid-frequencies and smooths peaks. Tapering emphasizes higher frequencies, around 3000 Hz.
- Output is limited to keep sound in the most comfortable range using peak clipping or compression of the signal.

PRACTICAL CONSIDERATIONS CONCERNING THE PERSONAL HEARING AID

You need to be familiar with personal hearing aids for three reasons:

- They are the instruments that in part will determine what you and the client together can achieve through re/habilitation.
- You need to be able to ask meaningful questions concerning the optimal functioning of amplification.
- You need to be prepared to answer the client's questions about the hearing aid(s) and to ensure that he/she is knowledgeable and confident in the use and care of the aid(s).

First you need to know how to check a person's hearing aid(s). This need is obvious when working with a child, less obvious with an adult. However, not infrequently I have found problems or misunderstandings about the care and use of a hearing aid when I have made the fitting and counseled the client or a child's parent myself. So, we need to check these matters.

Body Type and Postauricular Aids

Consider these first because both require an earmold. Ask the client to remove the aid, then look carefully at the pinna. There should be no sign of soreness, redness, or pressure indents caused by the earmold. I have watched children wince from a sore spot as I remove the earmold. I have had adults tell me they do not wear the aid continuously because their ears become sore; *this is totally unacceptable*. Dry scaly skin accompanied by irritation may be caused by an allergic reaction to the earmold; it is a condition that needs relief either by medication or by using a hypoallergenic earmold or both. Any of these symptoms warrant referral back to the dispensing audiologist. Examine the earmold next; it must be without sharp edges or cracks. The mold should be free of wax which may block the canal opening. Sometimes the wax dries white in the borehole; wax must be removed, preferably through ultrasonic cleansing by the dispensing audiologist. Finally, if the mold is vented with a "select-a-vent" (see p. 166), check with the dispenser of the aid that the appropriate plug is in the vent opening: "Oh that little thing came out a long time ago," the client often says.

Body Aid. Now look at the receiver button of the body aid. It should be clear of green oxidization, have a clean plastic washer if used, and show no cracks or chips. The earmold should snap tightly onto the receiver. The cord that connects the receiver to the microphone and amplifier case should be unfrayed and its connecting prongs at both ends should be bright. They can be cleaned with an emery board. The prongs should insert *tightly* into the receiver and hearing aid; sometimes a small plastic washer assists the seal. Finally, examine the hearing aid and battery. The battery compartment will have a hinged door or sometimes a sliding lid; open it and remove the battery. Examine both battery and compartment for a damp leakage or

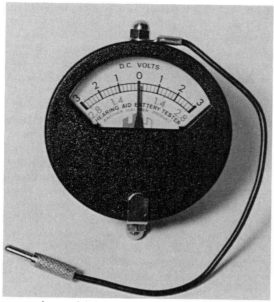

Figure 11.7 A hearing aid battery tester should be used to ensure adequate battery voltage. (Courtesy Hal-Hen Company, Inc.)

corrosion, which is usually crusty white or green; both merit attention. Note the battery contacts + and − which should be brightened with an emery board or end of a pencil eraser, if necessary. Check the battery using a battery tester—it is very important to have one available (Figure 11.7). If the battery in use is not charged, insert a new one.

The controls of the aid with which you are concerned are the *input selection control*, which selects the microphone (M), telephone (T), a combination (MT), or uses the third setting for ON/OFF and a *volume control* wheel that sometimes combines the ON/OFF switch. Now, bring the receiver button to the microphone, turn the selector to M, and turn the volume up full. This should cause the aid to squeal from acoustic feedback, indicating that it is operating. Finally, cup the receiver to the ear and evaluate the aid for clarity. Speech should be clear and without the intermittency caused, usually, by a defective cord. There should be a low level of background hiss of the type small radios often exhibit, and volume increase should increase loudness smoothly.

Postauricular Aid (BTE). Examine the postauricular aid (see Figure 11.2). Locate the battery compartment, which may be in the rear, side, or at the base of the aid. It opens as a hinged drawer and has a small ridge or flange to provide support for the ridged side of the battery. Usually a small (+) sign may be seen on the top side of the drawer to indicate the correct placement of the battery, with the positive (+) flat side up and the ridged negative side resting on the ledge of the drawer. The controls will consist of an OFF (O), telephone circuit (T), and microphone switch (M). There may be an M, M/T, or T combination, particularly on a child's aid, with the OFF position built into the volume control. There also will be a volume or gain control wheel. Other controls are for you, the audiologist, to set output and frequency shaping. These controls often are not visible to you. The earhook adapts the hearing aid to the tubing that connects to the mold. You may notice a small insert (plug) filter in the ear hook where it connects with the tubing. This is a damping device inserted at the time of the fitting.

Checking the postauricular aid involves much the same procedure as that used for the body type hearing aid. Examine the pinna on removal of the earmold; then check the earmold as described. Now check that the tubing connecting the earmold to the aid is clear, soft, and pliable and that it is not cracked, yellowed, pinched, or twisted at any point. There should be nothing in the tubing; occasionally wax intrudes and dries crusty white. Should any of these requirements not be met, the tubing should be replaced by an audiologist or hearing aid dispenser. The ear hook should be undamaged as, of course, should be the hearing aid, with no cracks or chips. Cup the hearing aid and earmold in the palm of your hand and turn the volume to full to effect acoustic feedback.

You can check a postauricular aid further by gently removing the tubing from the ear hook and then testing for acoustic feedback. If there is none, gently unscrew the ear hook from the aid and repeat feedback check. If feedback now occurs, the problem usually is a blocked filter or ear hook which must be replaced.

In-the-Ear and Canal Aids. These generally have no other control than the ON/OFF volume control. All you can check is the battery and the tiny borehole of the aid that has the microphone at the end, which is not visible to you. This opening must be free of wax. If wax buildup is a known problem, the opening may have been covered by a grill cap that is a wax-guard. This is replaceable if it becomes clogged. You may notice a small plastic ring in the tiny secondary venting channel in the canal aid; it is a venting tube helping to provide appropriate frequency shaping. The aid should be causing no pressure or sore points, nor should it be cracked or chipped. Check for feedback in the prescribed manner.

To facilitate listening to a hearing aid to check for clarity of sound, absence of strong background noise, and smoothness of volume increase, you can purchase a plastic stethoscope (Figure 11.8) available from the Hal Hen catalogue.* To use the stethoscope, just place the rubber end over the opening in the earmold or over the ear hook when detached from the mold. For in-the-ear and canal aids, place the rubber cap over the bore opening of the aid.

What the Wearer Should Understand about the Aid

The hearing-impaired person will have been given information about the hearing aid. However, often he/she does not understand, absorb, or remember it. You should review the following:

---

* Hal Hen Company, Inc., 35-53 24th St., Long Island City, NY 11106-4416; telephone 1(800)242-5436, in New York State 1(800)336-9786.

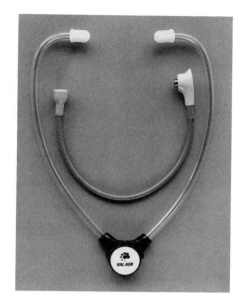

Figure 11.8 A hearing-aid stethescope facilitates listening checks. (Courtesy Hal-Hen Company, Inc.)

- The earmold must be wiped clean with a tissue each night and the openings kept clear of wax. Wax may be removed carefully with a special pick that a dispenser will provide or by using the end of a paper clip. Do not use a wood toothpick which may break off.
- In-the-ear and canal aids should likewise be wiped clean. *Never insert anything into the bore opening as the microphone is easily damaged.* A small brush usually is provided with the aid to remove wax from the bore opening.
- Always open the battery compartment when not wearing the aid—this conserves battery life.
- *Never allow the aid to get wet*; remember to remove it before taking a shower or bath or washing your hair, at the beauty parlor, before swimming, and so on. Do not leave a hearing aid in the bathroom as the steam from baths and showers can affect the circuitry adversely.
- Never place the aid in or close to heat (e.g., in the glove compartment of the car, on a radiator, on the stove).
- Remove the aid before going to sleep except in exceptional circumstances: "My husband has a heart condition; I need to hear him call." "I am a single mother; I need to hear my baby cry at night."
- Overnight it is wise to store the aid in a commercially available drying kit (see page 176.) Do not forget to remove the battery first.
- Set the volume control as instructed by your audiologist. If you do not know how to do this, use the following method: Have a person with normal hearing adjust the volume control on a radio or TV to comfortable listening. Set this level during a program, not a commercial. Then either mark the setting or leave the volume set. Using the volume control of the hearing aid, adjust the TV or radio sound to comfortable loudness. Turn off the TV/radio; then repeat out loud the days of the week saying them without pause—Monday, Tuesday, Wednesday, and so on. If your voice is comfortably loud and without echo, the volume setting is appropriate. If your voice echoes or sounds in

your head or chest, turn the volume down *very* slightly and then listen again. Repeat until the echo disappears and your voice sounds acceptable (Cornelisse, Gagne, & Seewald, 1991). Be sure to adjust the volume control with very slight movements to fine-tune the level.

When the Aid Is Not Working

- Check that the opening to the earmold (or microphone in ITE and canal aids) is not blocked with wax.
- Check that tubing is not crimped.
- Test or replace battery and ensure correct placement.
- Place aid for one or two hours in Superdriaid Kit available from Hal Hen.
- Check cord on body aid. This should be done first visually, checking for any fraying of the insulation of the cord. Then you should rub the cord between your thumb and index finger while listening through the receiver for any crackling sounds or intermittency of the signal. The length of the cord should be checked in this manner.

The most common and most easily remedied cause of hearing aid malfunction is a dead or inappropriately fitted battery. It is helpful to be familiar with the following information about batteries.

Batteries

There are two common types of hearing aid batteries, *zinc air* and *mercury*. *Silver*, a third type, seldom is required by today's hearing aids.

Zinc Air. Zinc air batteries represent the most recent development in batteries for use in BTE and canal hearing aids. The zinc air battery discharges by using air from outside its case to interact with internal chemical agents. By placing one reactant source (air) outside the case, the space released can be packed with more internal reactants. Thus this type of battery has a life expectancy two to two-and-a-half times that of a mercury cell. In addition to prolonged life, the zinc air battery affords clearer sound, less distortion, and a decreased need for volume adjustments than the mercury or silver cell types. When stored at room temperature, these batteries will retain 90 percent of their power for up to 12 months. The zinc air battery has a tab on it that closes the air channel. This keeps the battery inactive until the tab is removed, thus making air available to the internal reactants. Once the tab is removed the battery *cannot* be made inactive by replacing the tab. Placing the tab on a calendar records when you changed the battery. Tabs are color-coded to indicate battery size. The most common sizes are 13, 675, 312, and 41. Prefixes and suffixes to these numbers (e.g., R*13*ZA) are brand codes. The 13 indicates comparability of battery size among manufacturers.

Mercury Cell. Mercury batteries have half the lifetime of zinc air batteries, but they cost half the price. They are most appropriate for people who require a lot of power because of a severe hearing impairment. They offer reliable performance for high-powered hearing aids. Body type hearing aids, for which zinc air batteries are not available, usually use AA mercury cell batteries. Mercury cell batteries are available in all sizes compatible with ITE and canal hearing aids.

Silver. Silver batteries are used in few hearing aids. They provide even more power than mercury cell batteries; however, they are the least economical. Silver, mercury, and zinc air batteries are interchangeable, providing they are of the same size as denoted by the code.

When the Aid Squeals or Whistles

The signal or whistle is acoustic feedback. It is acceptable for this to occur when your hand or a telephone receiver reflects its output of sound back into the microphone. In the latter case, the receiver of the telephone needs to be moved a little further from the head. Feedback occurring when the aid is in normal use never should be tolerated. When it occurs, check for correct snug insertion of the earmold. A loose mold is the most common cause of acoustic feedback. The mold may be inserted incompletely or it may no longer fit snugly. The latter is often the case with growing children and with the elderly whose ears lose their cartilage tone. Wax in the ear canal also often will cause feedback. If feedback persists, an audiologist should be consulted. Never control feedback by turning down the volume control except on an interim basis until the audiologist is consulted. Such a practice reduces the signal strength necessary for hearing with maximum benefit.

Condensation Problems

Problems may occur from time to time in ear-level hearing aids as a result of moisture condensation. This occurs quite commonly on hot humid days and is aggravated by moving from outdoors into air conditioning. The client often reports that the hearing aid suddenly stops working, or works intermittently. The moisture condenses in the circuitry of the hearing aid, in tubing where it may be seen as steaming or water drops, and in the earmold. In-the-ear and canal hearing aids, which are constantly in the warm, moist environment of the ear canal, are particularly prone to moisture problems. The solution is for the hearing aid wearer to use a drying kit.

A drying kit contains a chemical agent that absorbs moisture. Placed in a container that can be sealed, the chemical provides an environment in which moisture is absorbed. One such kit, the Superdriaid Kit (Figure 11.9) supplied by Hal Hen, consists of a screwtop jar filled with little white pellets interspersed with blue pellets. A foam pad sits on top of the pellets. The hearing aid, *with the battery removed*, together with the tubing and earmold in the case of behind-the-ear hearing aids, routinely should be placed on the foam pad overnight or when not in use. The jar then is sealed. After several hours any moisture in the hearing aid will have been removed. When the pellets eventually become saturated, the blue ones turn white.

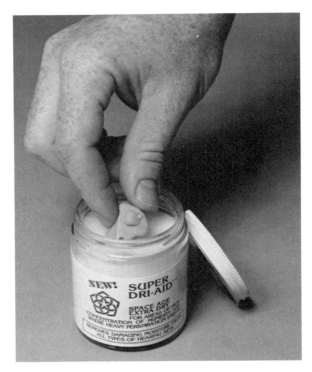

Figure 11.9 A drying kit such as the Super Dri-Aid Kit removes moisture from the hearing aid and from the earmold and tubing of BTE aids. (Courtesy Hal-Hen Company, Inc.)

The pellets then may be removed and dried out in a regular or microwave oven for reuse.

Maximizing Amplified Sound

- Always sit as close to the speaker as possible.
- If monaurally aided, place speaker on aided side.
- Usually it is inadvisable to sit close to hard reflective surfaces such as walls and windows as they may cause sound distortion and/or feedback. However, in some situations, such as in a noisy restaurant, a wall may actually help you to hear a speaker in a booth by reflecting the voice and acting as an amplifier while reducing the relative intensity of background noise. Only experience can teach you to make wise seating decisions.
- If monaurally aided, choose a seating position near the end of a table, placing those present on your aided side.
- Choose a seating position that provides good lighting of the speaker's face, rather than backlighting.
- For important communications, if possible, select a favorable acoustic environment or step out of a noisy reverberant setting for a private conversation.

- If noisy environments are unavoidable for important communications, discuss special fittings with your audiologist.
- Never give up monitoring technological advances. Check annually with your audiologist to try new fittings, but only when recommended by qualified audiologists in an established practice or agency. Studiously avoid door-to-door, telephone, or magazine contacts; they usually are high-pressure sales pitches.

Even the best hearing aids fitting will leave some situations and needs of some individuals not adequately satisfied. When this occurs, we turn to assistive listening and alerting devices for additional help. This is our next topic for discussion.

SUMMARY: PRACTICALITIES

- Hearing aids should be checked daily by the user or by parents.
- The components of a hearing aid system include the earmold, insert vents and filters, cords, and receiver depending on the type of hearing aid.
- The battery should be checked using a battery tester. Check with the audiologist about the best battery type.
- Zinc air batteries afford the best performance except for high-powered hearing aids that need mercury or, more rarely, silver cell types.
- The aid should be listened to for sound quality. A hearing aid stethoscope will facilitate this task.
- Check telephone circuit if available.
- Review instructions for care and operation of hearing aid, tubing, and earmold.
- Review how to select volume setting.
- Encourage use of a drying agent kit for overnight storage, first removing the battery.
- Determine causes of acoustic feedback.
- Review tips for maximizing benefits of amplification.

Conclusion

Amplification is the primary management tool. It aims to raise the input signal sufficiently to activate residual hearing while keeping intensity within comfort range. A further aim is to shape the amplified signal to provide appropriate gain at each frequency in accord with the pattern of deficit. Finally, it aims to provide the best quality of sound for different acoustic environments. Amplification cannot restore lost capacity, but it can help maximize the usefulness of residual hearing.

Amplification is the primary means of reducing hearing handicap except for the profoundly hearing impaired for whom it plays a supportive role in communication. Therefore, a hearing aid user needs to understand what the hearing aids can be expected to do and what they cannot do. Users need to know that hearing aids are prescriptive instruments and why a certain type is best. It is essential that we educate hearing-impaired persons about new technological advances so that they can decide about purchasing new hearing aids that might improve listening.

A range of different types of hearing aids and special fittings meet individual needs. The most recent development is digital processing, permitting in-use programming of optimal acoustic characteristics. Memory-storage capability permits the user to switch among characteristics within a single aid to select the one most effective for a given situation.

All hearing aids increase the intensity and shape the acoustic signal to the wearer's needs while protecting the ear from uncomfortable loudness. Earmold technology enables the process of signal shaping to be further fine-tuned.

Finally, we conclude that effective use of hearing aids depends on optimal fitting. Users need continued counseling and guidance in the use, care, and maintenance of their own hearing aid(s) in everyday situations. It is our responsibility to ensure that hearing-impaired persons are given adequate opportunity to become sophisticated users of amplification.

12

Special Amplification Systems and Assistive Listening and Alerting Devices

SPECIAL AMPLIFICATION SYSTEMS
FOR CLASSROOMS AND PUBLIC SPACES

The personal hearing aid constitutes the primary resource for surmounting the communication and learning difficulties arising from impairment of hearing. However, despite many technological developments, a personal hearing aid has yet to be designed that overcomes the problems of low S/N ratios and reverberation that occur whenever the speaker and listener are not close. Thus, in classrooms, meeting rooms, auditoriums, courtrooms, theaters, and places of worship, to list a few of the offending acoustic environments, listening usually remains very difficult for a person using a personal hearing aid. Learning under such conditions is even more limited. It remains the goal of the hearing aid industry to produce a personal hearing aid that provides a favorable speech signal even in noise; it is doubtful that an aid ever will combat signal distortion due to distance and reverberation. Nevertheless, technological progress already has blurred the distinction between amplification used in a classroom and that used outside through the development of systems that provide special sound transmission advantages. Some systems use separate units; others incorporate the use of the personal hearing aid. Totally portable special amplification systems are now very common.

MAJOR SYSTEMS

Four major systems have been developed to overcome the negative effects of room acoustics on speech and to provide a quality signal in special listening environments:

1. Hardwire systems
2. Frequency modulated radio systems (FM)
3. Electromagnetic loop induction systems
4. Infrared light wave systems

In the past, such special devices have been referred to as auditory trainers. However, the extension of their application to public meeting places and entertainment environments makes that term too limiting. When you read about these systems, bear in mind that the purpose of each is to:

- Receive the input signal with minimal acoustic masking or distortion
- Replicate the acoustic pattern as an electrical *analog* or copy
- Amplify the patterned signal well above the background noise level
- Convert the signal into a form that allows it to travel to a receiver sensitive to that medium
- Reconvert the signal to an electrical analog that can be amplified, shaped, and controlled to meet the listener's needs
- Convert the amplified electrical signal back into sound for delivery to the ear

The goals for each system are to

- *Provide wide frequency range amplification with high fidelity.* This is more easily achieved with the larger components of these systems than with the very small wearable aid.
- *Maintain at the listener's ear(s) a constant optimal S/N ratio and eliminate distortion from reverberation.* This is important in overcoming the effects of the distance between the speaker and listener. Consistency of signal also is essential to ease of comprehension and to attention.
- *Allow the signal to be controlled and shaped to the acoustic needs of each person's ear(s).* Without this the amplification system will fall short of that provided by a well-functioning personal hearing aid.
- *Allow mobility of both speaker and listener.* The unit should not demand that the normal communication behaviors for a given situation be restricted.
- *Allow the listener to hear not only the speaker but also himself and others.*
- *Accept special inputs such as TV, phonograph, and tape recorders.*

Not every system achieves each goal; thus, each must be assessed carefully in terms of the purpose for which it is to be used.

Hardware Systems

Hardwire systems were so named because a wire connects the microphone to the amplifier and the amplifier to the headphones via a control box. The large-group units are no longer widely used in special education; they have been replaced by other systems. The individual and small-group units, however, remain a valuable way of providing quality amplification that extends

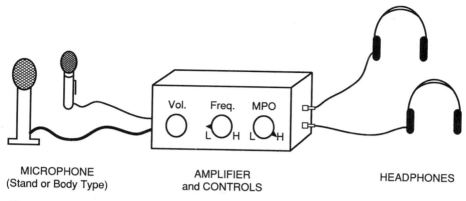

MICROPHONE   AMPLIFIER   HEADPHONES
(Stand or Body Type)   and CONTROLS

Figure 12.1

well into the high frequencies (Figure 12.1). The control box on group and individual units allows the amplified signal to be controlled and shaped for each child. Some units permit separate settings for each ear. It is imperative that the settings used be appropriate to each child's individual electroacoustic needs. A unit may be truly binaural with two microphone inputs and individual amplifiers. Many, however, are *pseudobinaural*, with a single microphone input split between the ears using a Y cord. The need for true binaural amplification is reduced when the teacher speaks directly into the microphone, since this ensures high S/N ratio with little or no reverberation. Movement of the teacher away from the microphone will limit severely a monaural unit's effectiveness. This requirement of proximity to the microphone constitutes a limitation of hardwire systems whenever teacher and/or child mobility is important in a learning or re/habilitation lesson. A further restriction is that many group hardwire units have only the teacher microphone. Thus, the child hears neither her own speech amplified nor that of her classmates. Some designs overcome this problem by providing each child with a microphone input attached to the headphones on a boom. This places the microphone within inches of the child's mouth, leaving her hands free. Teacher mobility also can be provided by using a wireless microphone to transmit the signal to a receiver unit in the amplifier.

The group hardwire system can be valuable for providing quality amplification individualized to each child in a structured learning situation that does not require the children to be mobile. Appropriate use of separate inputs accommodates TV, radio, record player, or tape recorder. Small portable units are very useful in working in a one-on-one teacher-therapist situation, as well as in the auditory perceptual training of the speech-language pathologist and in teaching speech production to individual children and small groups since an optimal acoustic signal always is of paramount importance for these activities. Once again, however, the controls must be set appropriately for each child's needs; the audiologist will need specific guidance in order to accomplish this. A further condition is that the microphone always must be close to the speaker's (child's or speech-language pathologist's) mouth when talking or the advantages of the system will be lost and the result may be amplified sound no better than and possibly inferior to the child's own hearing aid(s).

Electromagnetic Induction Loop Amplification (ILA)

This type of amplification system was developed with the goal of providing mobility to a child in a special classroom by maintaining a constant favorable signal-to-noise ratio that is unaffected by the child's distance from the teacher. The system was widely adopted until its limitations presented some significant impediments to its effectiveness in an educational setting. The limitations included spillover of the signal from one classroom system to another, variable signal strength in different parts of the room, and dependence on the child's aids being functional. The development of FM wireless systems soon led to the demise of loop induction as a common system of classroom amplification. However, the system has been used again recently mainly by adults in private and public meeting places, in churches and theaters as well as in private homes. For this reason, as well as the fact that electromagnetic loop induction provides one method of integrating FM systems with a person's own hearing aid(s), we will discuss it.

Consider first how the system works. It consists of a microphone connected by a wire to an amplifier (Figure 12.2). The connection also can be

Figure 12.2 Block diagram of an induction loop listening system.

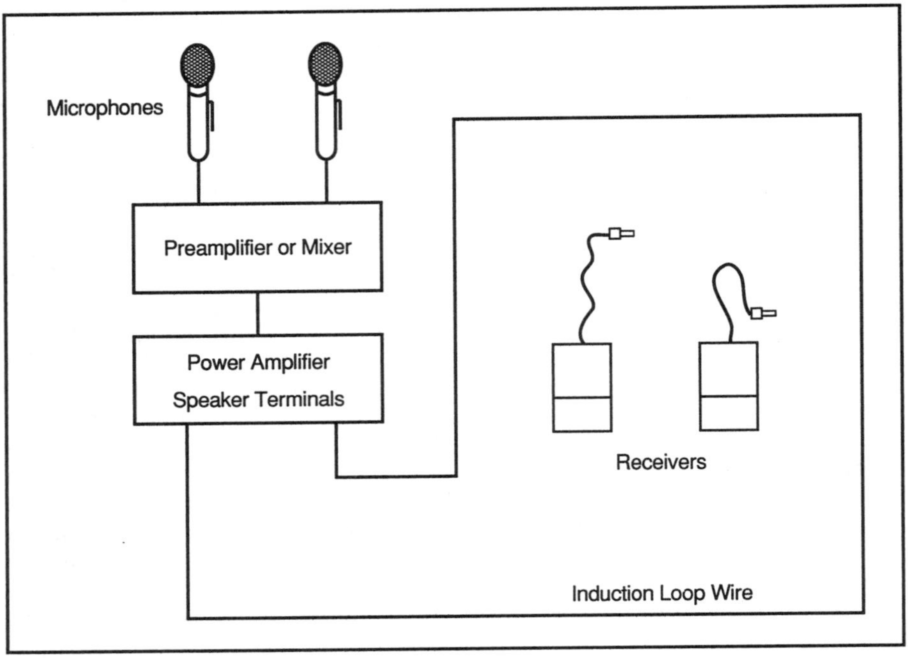

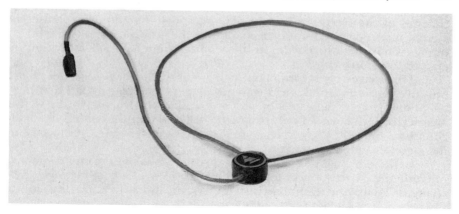

Figure 12.3 A neckloop for electromagnetic induction of a hearing aid(s).

made by an FM radio signal if a wireless microphone and an FM receiver are incorporated in the amplifier. A long wire extends from the amplifier. This wire may be looped around any area of space. The area may be as small as the head and shoulders of a person (a neckloop) (Figure 12.3) or an armchair in front of the TV (Figure 12.4) or it may be as large as a number of church pews, a seating section in a theater, or an outdoor space. The wire, under its insulation, is wound around a magnetic core. This magnetic core, as is characteristic of any magnet, sets up a magnetic field around it. When a current flows through the wire coiled around the core magnet, the pattern of its magnetic field changes, mimicking the pattern

Figure 12.4 With an audio loop wired to a television set a hearing impaired viewer can adjust volume on a hearing aid set on T-switch without disturbing the listening of another person. (Courtesy National Information Center on Deafness, Gallaudet College.)

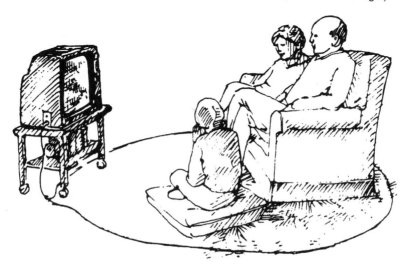

changes of the electrical current. These, you will recall, mirror the frequency intensity and durational changes in the acoustic event at the microphone. Thus the information in the acoustic event is broadcast within the area of the loop.

To receive this information, it is necessary to have a device that is sensitive to the magnetic field changes. A personal hearing aid that has a telephone circuit, indicated by a T-switch, has this capability, as well as any device with such an induction circuit. For example, conference halls, churches, and other large areas often use a wand-type receiver to pick up the electromagnetic pattern.

In the personal hearing aid, the T-switch cuts out the environmental microphone. It activates instead the circuit sensitive only to magnetic field changes. To use the telephone with this system and a BTE hearing aid, the phone receiver is placed *behind* the ear *against the case of the hearing aid.* This allows the special circuit to pick up the magnetic changes in the telephone receiver that cause the diaphragm to vibrate and convert them to sound waves. These magnetic patterns are fed to the amplifier of the hearing aid for amplification and shaping to the user's needs. The electromagnetic induction circuit will respond in exactly the same manner in an area looped for electromagnetic induction.

As I explained, the T-switch cuts out the environmental microphone. This is very helpful to a person listening on the telephone in a noisy environment. However, in a situation that incorporates a loop induction system, it frequently is important to hear both the teacher and the questions and contributions of others. It also is important to be able to monitor one's own voice. To make this possible, hearing aids may be purchased that have an M-T switch that activates the telephone circuit but does *not* deactivate the environmental microphone.

This system has definite advantages:

- Small and medium area loops are inexpensive to purchase and operate, but large area installations are not less expensive than alternative systems.
- Small area loops are easy to install; prepackaged kits are available.
- Small area units can be used anywhere and can be moved easily to different locations.
- The listener's mobility is not limited.
- High S/N ratios are provided when the speaker talks directly into the microphone.
- No special receiver equipment needs to be provided to the listener with an aid that has a T-coil circuit.
- The number of users is limited only by the number of persons with T-switches on their hearing aid(s).

At international conferences in particular, this system often is used to provide simultaneous translation services to hearing delegates. A receiver amplifier is built into a hand-held wand containing a speaker that is held to the ear. The output volume can be adjusted by the user.

Since the growth of the use of radio frequency (FM) loop induction systems in public places, many advances have been made in designing special loop arrangements to optimize the signal for a specific site. However, the system still has its drawbacks:

- It is neither as good as nor less expensive than FM or infrared systems when designed for large areas.
- The amplitude of the signal in the loop is not consistent; it changes as the listener moves within the looped area.
- Telecoil reproduction of the signal received by the hearing aid often differs in quality and characteristics from that of the environmental microphone input.
- All listeners must have a hearing aid with a T-switch; without it the system cannot be used.
- The system depends on the listener's hearing aid(s) being in good working condition.
- When worn on the T-setting, no sound is heard other than from the loop.
- To speak with another person, the listener must switch back to the M-setting.
- It is very difficult to prevent loop systems in the same building from interfering with each other.

Nevertheless, for small and medium areas, this is an inexpensive system that allows hearing aid users with telephone circuits in their aid(s) to understand more easily in audience situations and environments in which listening is otherwise difficult or impossible.

Radio Frequency Modulated Systems (FM)

The most widely used special amplification system in all types of educational settings is the FM system. This system also is available in an increasing number of public places. It exists both as a group system (Figure 12.5) and as a personal amplification system (Figure 12.6). The operational principle is the same for both.

The system is comparable to a miniature FM radio station. The teacher broadcasts to a child or group of children on a specific FM radio frequency; the children tune into the teacher's "station" on their wearable radio receivers (Figure 12.7).

The teacher wears a lightweight microphone hung high on the chest that picks up speech in close proximity to the mouth, ensuring a constant high signal-to-noise ratio approximating $+20$ to $+25dB$. The microphone is connected via a cord to a small body-pack transmitter that may be clipped anywhere on the clothing. Converted first to an electrical analog, the signal is amplified and then patterned onto an FM radio signal that is broadcast into the environment. The child or children wear a lightweight FM radio receiver tuned to the frequency of the teacher's transmitter. This picks up the signal, converts it first to an equivalent electrical pattern, and amplifies and shapes it to the child's needs. It is extremely important that the FM receiver be treated as a hearing aid. Its frequency response, gain, and output must be set specifically for an individual child's needs (Figure 12.8, page 188). This is the responsibility of the audiologist.

A variety of options are available to feed the signal to the ears. It may be heard using a lightweight Walkman-type headset, though this is usable

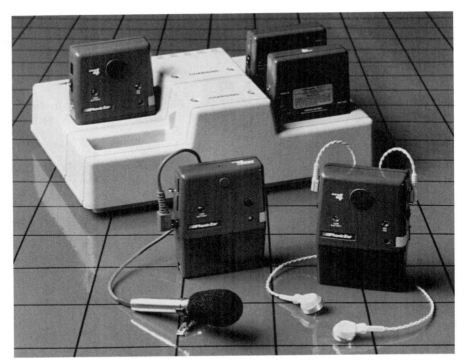

Figure 12.5 Group FM systems are available for special classes in school. (Courtesy Phonic Ear, Inc.)

only for moderate acoustic gain; it may be fed to button transducers clipped to personal earmolds, as with a body-type hearing aid; a silhouette inductor or teleloop may feed the signal electromagnetically to the induction coil in a personal hearing aid; or it may be fed by direct audio input into a hearing aid.

Simultaneous transmission of more than one transmitter on the same frequency is not possible. The need for two independent systems to permit, for example, a teacher-aide in a special classroom to work separately with an individual or small group using an FM system, while the teacher instructs the rest of the class using FM, is provided for. The use of removable color-coded plug-in receiver crystals, each tuned to a different frequency, permits the frequency of the microphone to be changed instantly from one transmitter frequency to another (Figure 12.9, page 188).

The advantages of a frequency-modulated system include

- *Teacher/child mobility.* The signal is broadcast by a radio beam from an antenna that is part of the teacher's neck microphone. The teacher, therefore, has complete mobility. The children also receive the signal by radio input so they have equal freedom.
- *Constant favorable signal level.* The constancy of the distance of the teacher's

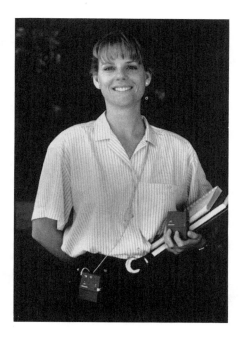

Figure 12.6 The Phonic Ear personal FM system can be taken wherever the student goes. (Courtesy Phonic Ear, Inc.)

Figure 12.7 Teacher-microphone-transmitter and child receivers can be seen in this group activity. (Courtesy Phonic Ear, Inc.)

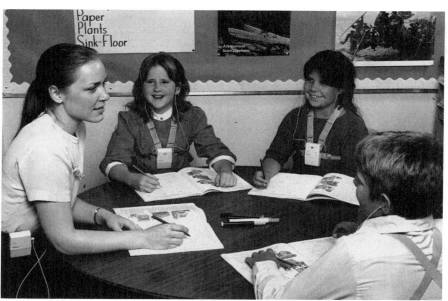

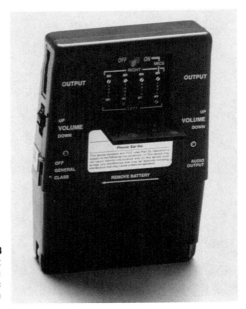

Figure 12.8
The frequency response, gain, and output of an FM receiver must be set for each child's specific needs. (Courtesy Phonic Ear, Inc.)

Figure 12.9 The use of a modular crystal insert permits the FM to be tuned easily to different frequencies.

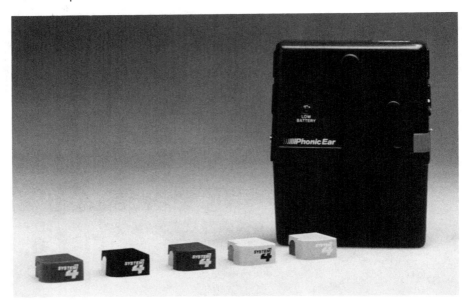

microphone to his or her mouth ensures that the S/N ratio is always optimal. Furthermore because signal strength varies little in the room the signal received by the child does not change as he or she moves from place to place in the room. This, you recall, was frequently not true with the loop-induction system.

- *Compatibility for use with personal hearing aid.* It is possible to feed the amplified electrical signal from the child's FM receiver into an induction coil worn around the neck. In this manner the child can listen to the signal through his or her own personal hearing aid set on T or M-T. Because the field of the loop moves with the child, variations in signal intensity are not a problem.
- *Self-monitoring.* Most FM units incorporate into the child's receiver pack either a single microphone or two microphones. This permits the child to receive the FM signal while listening to monophonic or stereophonic amplification of airborne sound. Thus the child may monitor his or her own speech and that of others around him or her while receiving the teacher's voice at a highly favorable S/N ratio.

The receiver can be switched to FM only, to external microphone only, or to a combination of both. This gives the teacher flexibility in conducting the class. For example, if the teacher desires to have only some of the children listen to FM transmission, he or she instructs the remainder of the class to switch to the environmental microphone. If children are reading out loud, or participating in discussion, they can monitor their speech and listen to others nearby yet still receive the teacher's comments or requests clearly by FM reception.

- *Multiple channels in a single classroom.* The receiver units may be tuned to different stations by a frequency selector switch or by color-coded modules that plug into the child's receiver. In this way, using two microphones broadcasting on separate frequencies, a teacher's aide or resource teacher can work independently with a small group of children in the corner of the room. The class teacher may then work with the remainder of the children using a different frequency. Further, as children change classes, they simply unplug the insert-frequency module, turn on their binaural environmental microphones, and listen to environmental sounds as they walk along the corridor. When they get to the next class, they plug in the colored module that matches the teacher's microphone.
- *Portability.* The units are perfectly portable. They may accompany the teacher and class on field trips where communication with a group wearing personal hearing aids is often difficult. The signal limits of the FM microphone are determined only by the strength of the microphone transmission. Power for these units is provided by rechargeable batteries. At the end of school each day the units are replaced in a charger, which ensures they are fully powered by morning.

The disadvantages are:

- *Limited choice of response curves.* With the current FM systems, the possibilities are limited for modifying the electroacoustic characteristics of either the FM receiver or the hearing-aid unit to suit the needs of individual children.
- *Lack of true binaural FM amplification.* Although the FM signal can be fed to both ears, true binaural amplification is not provided because there is only one input signal. The hearing-aid unit of the receiver may be monophonic or truly binaural with two separate microphones and amplifiers.
- *Cosmetic appearance.* The units are all body type, necessitating that they be

worn with a strap, neck cord, harness, or belt clip. Some children, particularly older ones who have become accustomed to ear-level aids, find this cosmetically unacceptable.

- *Need for checking operational controls.* Problems can arise if the teacher neglects to turn off the microphone when, for example, a parent or another teacher comes into the room to speak privately with him or her. In fact, the same situation can occur if the teacher steps out of the room for a moment to speak confidentially with someone. The result is that the private conversation is broadcast clearly to the whole class. In class the teacher must also become accustomed to controlling which group of children are tuned into the microphone. These, however, are teaching techniques that most teachers can accommodate without a great deal of difficulty. Similar procedural problems occur when the child is in a normal classroom rather than with other hearing-impaired children in a special class.

Infrared Light Systems

Infrared light systems are the most recent amplification system. They use an invisible light as the medium to carry the signal from a transmitter to individual light receivers. The input signal to a microphone is sent by hardwire or by a wireless microphone to the amplifier transmitter that floods the space with infrared light waves. These waves are patterned to carry an analog of the signal to a small infrared-sensitive light receiver worn by the listener. The receiver converts the light signal pattern to an equivalent electrical pattern that is then amplified and converted to sound at the ear. In large areas the light beam originates from an array of infrared diode emitters mounted on a wall or, less desirably, on portable tripods. A small portable unit that uses a single row of diode emitters is available for use in a home or office (Figure 12.10). For meeting halls, theaters, and other large areas, several arrays of emitters in different locations often are necessary to ensure that no part of the space is in shadow from the beam.

The advantages of infrared systems include the following:

1. The quality of sound is excellent.
2. The systems are free from electromagnetic interference since the infrared light waves cannot pass through walls.
3. The personal system can be completely portable.
4. Any indoor space can be equipped.

The disadvantages include the following:

1. It is the most expensive system to purchase and operate.
2. It is prone to interference from the infrared rays in sunlight; thus, it cannot be used outdoors or in rooms well lit by natural light.
3. The reception of the light beam is blocked whenever something (hand, program, book, pillar) or someone comes between the light emitter and receiver.

Comparison of Systems

It should be apparent from our discussion that there is no one system suitable to all needs. Each system has both assets and liabilities, emphasizing the importance of analyzing the situation for which amplification is to be

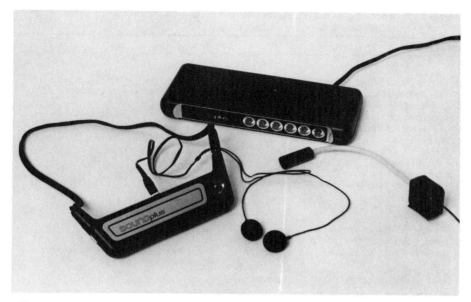

Figure 12.10 Sennheiser portable unit. (HES)

provided. The needs of the speaker and the listener must be identified and accommodated as well as possible. These needs include mobility, self-monitoring of speech, communication with others besides the person with the microphone, access to external inputs such as radio and TV, and the ability to integrate personal hearing aids into the special amplification system. In addition, such considerations as cost, portability of equipment, number of listeners to be accommodated, and area to be embraced by the system will influence the final choice. In keeping with the general philosophy of this text, the task is one of (1) problem identification, (2) analysis and definition followed by (3) identification of available resources, (4) selection and organization of appropriate resources, (5) application of resources, and finally (6) evaluation of effectiveness. This approach is equally important when considering other assistive devices that may reduce the handicap a hearing impairment imposes on a given individual. Williams (1984) has summarized effectively the advantages and disadvantages of each system (Table 12.1).

INTEGRATING THE PERSONAL HEARING AID WITH SPECIAL AMPLIFICATION SYSTEMS

Successful adaptation to the use of personal hearing aids results in the brain's becoming accustomed perceptually to the world of sound as heard through them. That perception becomes a person's auditory reality. Maintaining the consistency of sound received, and the perception of the audi-

TABLE 12.1 Advantages and disadvantages of four special amplification systems. (Williams, 1985.)

Advantages	Disadvantages
	FM Systems
☐ The users have the freedom to choose their own seating location. ☐ The system is not susceptible to electrical interference. ☐ It is usable in daylight and dark environments. ☐ It is simple and inexpensive to install. ☐ Prepackaged systems can be installed in a short time. ☐ The system has a low operating cost and is highly energy efficient.	☐ The system is slightly more expensive than hard-wired systems or AM radio systems.
	Infrared Technology
☐ The system is not subject to electromagnetic interference. ☐ It can be used anywhere in the world.	☐ The system is relatively complex to install and operate. ☐ It is vulnerable to interference from natural and artificial light.
	Hard-Wired Systems
☐ The simple technology permits easy installation and maintenance if only a few locations are needed. ☐ Freedom from electromagnetic interference.	☐ Hearing-impaired people are forced to sit in a few predetermined locations. ☐ Installation can be quite expensive in a completed building. ☐ Additional locations require redesigning of the amplification system to maintain proper impedance matching.
	Induction Loop Systems
☐ Relatively simple technology is employed. ☐ Prepackaged systems can be successfully installed in small- and medium-sized spaces.	☐ The system is vulnerable to interference fields that cannot be suppressed. ☐ Large-space systems are expensive to install and have complex installation requirements. ☐ A high-powered amplifier is required. ☐ Physical separation is required between differing program installations. ☐ Users not equipped with telecoils require special receivers that are relatively expensive.

tory world derived from it, is extremely important to the hearing-impaired person. However, we have seen that the personal hearing aid does not provide adequate clarity of amplified speech at a distance from the speaker or in a poor acoustic environment. Ideally, amplification for a hearing-impaired person would incorporate the advantages of both the personal hearing aid, which provides a prescriptive acoustic fitting, complete portability, and cosmetic acceptability, with the capabilities of special amplification systems, which combat noise, reverberation, and distance effects. To achieve this end, manufacturers of hearing aids and special systems have developed ways of integrating the two by providing another way for the postauricular hearing aid to receive the signal than through the external microphone. This was achieved in three ways:

1. *Direct audio input.* Using this method, the FM or infrared receiver worn by the listener is connected to the hearing aid by a very thin wire. The wire is plugged into a socket in the hearing aid or snaps onto a metal jack plate. Thus the electrical signal generated by the FM or infrared receiver is fed directly into the hearing aid where it is shaped and amplified appropriately (Figure 12.11).
2. *Silhouette inductor.* This device converts the electrical signal from the FM/IR (infrared) receiver into an electromagnetic field by means of a thin inductor plate. The plate, shaped like the case of the postauricular hearing aid, is worn between the hearing aid and the head. It induces a current in the hearing aid through the telecoil circuit (Figure 12.12).
3. *Neckloop induction.* The induction coil neckloop operates in the same manner as the classroom induction loop system discussed earlier in this chapter. An insulated coil worn around the neck is plugged into the FM/IR receiver. The changes in the electrical signal pattern entering the loop cause equivalent pattern changes in the magnetic field around the wearer's head. These induce an analog signal in the telecoil circuit of the hearing aid set on T or on a combination M-T position.

Each coupling method permits clear reception of the signal from a special amplification system while maintaining the individual acoustic shaping by the personal hearing aid(s). It also permits small, cosmetically more acceptable FM or IR receiver units to be used. With specially ordered hearing aids, it is possible to receive both the FM/IR signal and the hearing aid environmental microphone input. Thus, when appropriate a person would hear the speaker clearly yet still be able to hear his own voice, hear questions, and follow discussions.

Before we consider special devices to further enhance the listening and event awareness of the hearing-impaired person, it is appropriate to review our discussion this far.

SUMMARY: SYSTEMS

- The four major systems are hardwire, FM, electromagnetic loop, and infrared.
- All systems aim to provide high fidelity wide frequency range amplification, optimal S/N ratios, low acoustic distortion, mobility, and individual control over signal reproduction.
- Ability to hear self and to tap into accessory input are important requirements.
- Hardwire systems usually are confined to small-group or individual sessions.
- Electromagnetic induction loops are now almost exclusively used for home use and in public spaces.
- Electromagnetic induction systems depend primarily on personal hearing aids with telephone circuits, though special receivers can be purchased.
- FM radio systems are widely used in group and individual units. Their major advantages are cost, portability, and sound quality.
- Infrared light systems are used increasingly often in theaters. Their use in offices and homes is growing. They cannot be used in bright light environments and remain expensive.
- All systems can be integrated with personal hearing aids by direct audio input, with a magnetic induction plate worn under the hearing aid, or through the use of an induction coil neckloop.

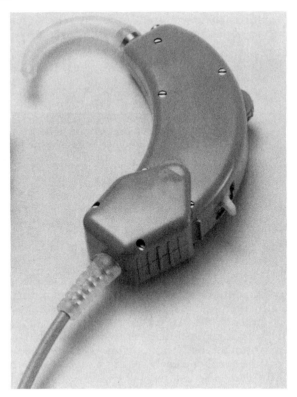

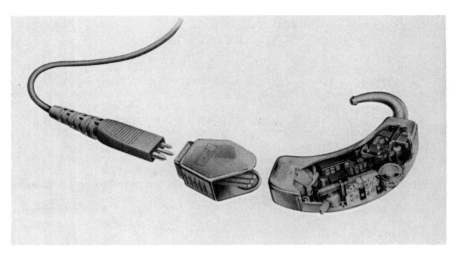

Figure 12.11(a) and (b) A direct audio input connection allows external sound sources to be connected directly to the hearing aid. (a,b Courtesy Phonic Ear, Inc.)

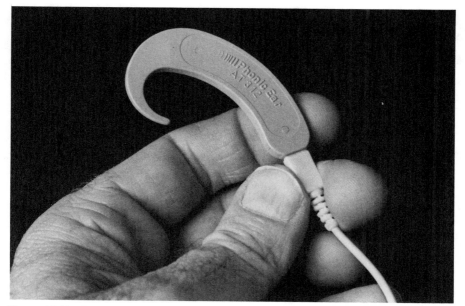

Figure 12.12 Silhouette Inductor plate.

ASSISTIVE LISTENING DEVICES

Systems Designed for the Individual User

The systems we have discussed so far were designed primarily as a means of providing improved sound quality for multiple users in classrooms or public places. In recent years technology has provided a range of devices and systems designed for individual users to supplement the capabilities and benefits provided by the personal hearing aid. These devices are identified as assistive listening devices and listening systems (ALDs). Some are designed to surmount specific listening difficulties that, as we have seen, arise from distance, noise, and reverberation effects. Others are intended to draw attention to events occurring in the environment or to provide means of receiving information other than through sound transmission. Thus, we can classify the devices and systems as those that:

- *Provide enhanced listening* in conjunction with personal hearing aids or may be substituted for the hearing aid in specific listening situations
- *Convey verbal communication information* by means other than the acoustic signal
- *Alert* persons to sounds that otherwise might be inaudible or not loud enough to attract attention

Enhanced Listening Devices

Enhanced listening devices utilize each of the techniques we have already discussed to overcome distance, noise, and reverberation effects—namely,

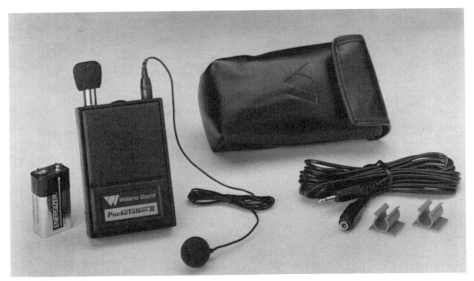

Figure 12.13 Hardware connections permit a personal amplification unit to be used with an external microphone placed some distance from the listener thus enhancing the signal-to-noise ratio. (Courtesy Williams Sound Corp.)

hardwire connections to a hearing aid or headphone, induction loop input, or FM or infrared light waves.

Hardwire and Direct Connections. These require that the speaker and the listener be connected by a wire from an amplifier to which the speaker's microphone is attached. An example of such a system is the Pocketalker® System (Figure 12.13). This consists of an amplifier that has a miniature microphone attached, a cord of appropriate length for person-to-person conversation, and a nine-foot extension cord. The extension cord is very useful in a conference situation; it permits either an omnidirectional or directional microphone to be placed closer to an individual speaker or in the center of a group around a table. When working with a child, a hand-held microphone reduces the speaker/microphone distance to an inch or so while still allowing the child to see the speaker's face. This is particularly useful to parents who are helping a child with homework or providing speech and language stimulation. In outdoor environments placement of a soft foam hood over the microphone is effective in reducing wind noise. The same hood improves listening in small-group situations and will help reduce environmental noise effects and the effect of table vibration on a stand-based microphone.

These and other similar units accept such accessories as miniature lapel microphones and TV adaptors and may incorporate an electromagnetic circuit that permits them to be used as audioloop induction receivers. The units may be powered by regular or rechargeable batteries. These hardwire systems are effective in situations in which the traditional personal hearing aid is compromised—for example, in a car, a noisy restaurant, or when talking through the window opening of a bank or ticket office.

Another application of the hardwire principle is *direct audio input* to the hearing aid, which was described earlier (p. 193). It can be used to provide optimal listening to tape cassettes and radio. Television sound can be received by direct input to the hearing aid either by a patch connection into the set or by a cord to an external adhesive microphone placed on the TV speaker. If desired, the loudness of the audio input signal can be controlled by inserting a hand-held volume control between the audio input plug and the attachment to the radio or TV set. A similar hand-held volume control can be inserted into the direct audio input to the hearing aid. This permits easy adjustment of loudness when, for example, listening to different speakers at different distances in an audience or around a large table.

Electromagnetic Loop Induction Systems. These systems represent an application to home and public environments of technology originally designed for classroom use (p. 193). Audioloop kits are available commercially. Small home kits, such as the Minicon™ (Figure 12.14), are completely transportable systems that are easy to set up at home. They use a direct feed from the radio or TV to an induction neckloop or a miniloop encompassing a chair or by looping a complete room around the baseboard or under the carpet. Some manufacturers provide adhesive microphones; others patch cords to the TV. It is also possible to obtain power cords that permit the induction miniloop to be used where AC current is not available. It can be run off the 12-volt car battery using a cigarette lighter patch cord.

Figure 12.14 Induction loop amplification is available for public environments and also for home use (Courtesy Oticon, Inc.)

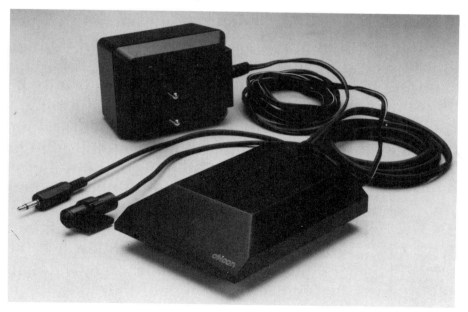

The basic units, such as the Oticon Minicon™ System, cover an area with a perimeter up to 100 feet. A patch cord allows direct connection to a radio, cassette player, or TV set. For persons who do not have an aid with a T-circuit, a loop transmission receiver amplifier, such as the Pocketalker II™, may be used instead of the hearing aid.

Sophisticated loop systems are high-powered units capable of covering a 200-seat area in a public space. Such units can be expanded to cover much greater areas. They also allow for multiple microphone inputs and permit control over the audio signal.

Telephone Amplifiers. These are available in several models. The portable battery operated type (Figure 12.15) may be used on any phone, with or without a hearing aid; a strap is used to fit it to the receiver of the phone handset. Modular, push-button, or rotary phones can be adapted for amplification. The regular handpiece can be replaced by one that houses an amplifier and volume control. A small portable in-line modular amplifier (Figure 12.16) that plugs directly to the phone base at one end and to the handpiece cord at the other end is useful in adapting a phone in a motel or when visiting friends or relatives. A volume control turns the amplifier on and off and allows for appropriate adjustment of loudness. Not all phone models will accept amplification devices. Note also that some public coin telephones do not emit a strong enough magnetic signal to make them compatible with the telephone circuit on a hearing aid. Such phones can be recognized by a small *dark grey* band or *grommet* where the cord and receiver are connected. These *are not* compatible, while those with a *blue connector* or with *no connector* are compatible. A device called Phonear™ manufactured by Phonak surmounts this limitation. It attaches to the receiver where it picks up the audio signal and converts it to a strong electromagnetic signal. Alternatively the phone call can be amplified by using a coupler such as the Telelink™, which links a hardwire pocket amplifier such as the

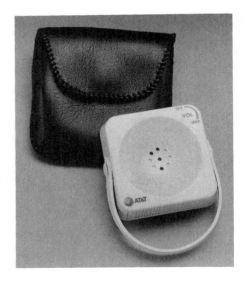

Figure 12.15 The pocket sized AT&T Portable Amplifier attaches to the earpiece of virtually any telephone to increase sound levels by 30% to help people who have hearing impairments. The two-inch by two-inch amplifier can be carried easily by people when they travel. It is compatible with inductively coupled hearing aids. (Courtesy AT&T.)

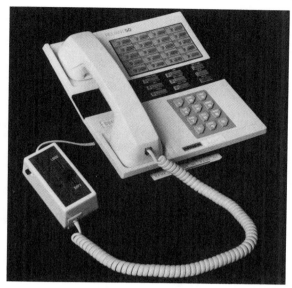

Figure 12.16 A portable modular telephone amplifier can be plugged into the telephone connection from base to handpiece.

Pocketalker™ to the telephone. The coupler links the phone and Pocketalker™ between the handset cord and the base. The person listens to the phone with one ear while using the earphone in the other ear. Up to 40dB of gain can be obtained this way.

FM Input. You will recall that FM radio transmission systems provide the greatest mobility and flexibility of all the systems discussed. Their attributes have been utilized successfully in the development of personal FM systems. The FM system provides an individual with the ability to set up a direct FM link to the speaker in any situation indoors or outdoors at ranges from 3 to 500 feet. The FM unit may be worn in a car, making any passenger audible from any seat, in a bus particularly when on tour, or in any other form of transport, even on bicycles. A personal FM system can help mother and child maintain voice contact both in the house and outdoors and can be used in sports instruction, such as riding or skating lessons. Inside, the unit can be used by an individual in the classroom, lecture hall, or church by having the speaker wear the microphone/transmitter or by placing it on a lectern or pulpit. A lightweight wearable belt-pack transmitter with a lapel microphone sends the FM signal to the receiver unit worn by the listener, just as in the classroom group FM units we discussed earlier. The signal is amplified and shaped and then fed to an insert receiver(s) or headphone(s) or can be integrated with a wearable hearing aid(s) in the ways already described. Both transmitter and receiver packs operate on either regular or rechargeable batteries.

For public institutions such as theaters, cinemas, or churches serving

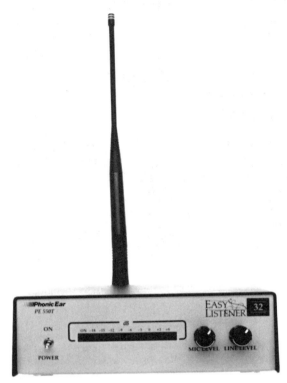

Figure 12.17 FM system transmitter designed for use in large public places such as halls and theatres provide hearing access to many events. (Courtesy Phonic Ear.)

a number of hearing-impaired persons, a base station FM transmitter can be linked to the public address system, thus transmitting the optimal input signal from multiple stage microphones to receivers in the audience (Figure 12.17).

The signal from the FM receiver may be fed to a hearing aid by direct audio input or via a neckloop induction coil. Alternatively the signal may be fed to the telephone circuit of the hearing aid by means of a silhouette induction plate. The signal also may be fed through a cord to a receiver snapped onto a personal earmold.

FM devices may be worn inconspicuously, are fully portable, have great flexibility of use, and provide excellent quality sound. As such they offer great assistance to listening in one-to-one, small-group, and public performance situations.

Infrared Systems. We have discussed the principles by which these systems operate (p. 190). They currently are used in many theaters where the light transmitters are mounted permanently above the stage. Members of the audience rent the receiver unit for the performance, using it with a headset receiver, an induction neckloop, an induction silhouette plate, or by a direct input into their own hearing aid.

For home use a small light transmitter (Figure 12.18) may be placed on a desk or table facing the receiver; the speaker wears a miniature microphone with a hardwire connection to the transmitter. For television watching the transmitter is placed on top of the console and connected by a listening jack to the TV set. Alternatively the microphone may be attached directly to the TV speaker using a Velcro disc. The receiver may have a built-in environmental microphone that allows the listener to hear his or her partner while receiving the infrared transmission. The receiver can be adapted for loop induction input to personal hearing aids with a T-circuit.

Nonauditory Communication Telecommunication Devices

Severely and profoundly hearing-impaired persons may be unable to use the telephone even with an amplifier. For these persons telecommunication devices for deaf people (TDDs) (Figure 12.19) provide a means of communicating typed messages by phone to a receiver that displays them on an LED screen. Current technology has made possible the conversion of the TDD message to a computer-generated voice message for hearing persons with advanced TDD receivers. It also is possible for messages to be communicated to hearing persons who do not have a TDD receiver through the use of a message relay service. The relay person receives the message on a

Figure 12.18 Infrared amplification systems designed for home or office can enhance many listening situations. (Courtesy Sennheiser-Siemens Hearing Instruments, Inc.)

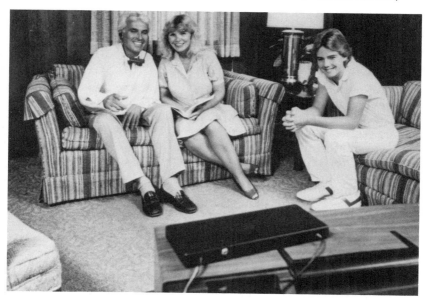

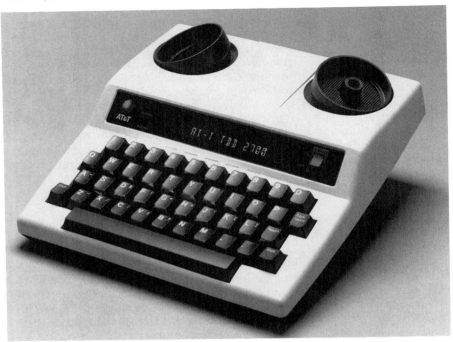

Figure 12.19 The AT&T TDD 2700 is a lightweight Telecommunications Device for the Deaf with a flexible acoustic coupler, a 20-character display, and a port for connecting to an external printer. (Courtesy AT&T)

TDD and reads it over another line to the person for whom it is intended; responses then are typed back to the deaf sender. This service is invaluable for making appointments or obtaining information.

Television Captioning. Television is a source of both enjoyment and information. However, its accessibility is limited by severe hearing loss. Access for persons unable to hear the sound even with amplification has been made possible by increasing use of *closed captioning.* Quite simply this means adding subtitles to programs. The subtitles are broadcast on a separate network. They can be received, decoded, and added to the screen. The subtitles (displayed by an adapter that is connected to the regular TV set) appear simultaneously with the audio and visual signal. Completely portable telecaption converter units are available.

ALERTING DEVICES

When we talk of auditory communication, we usually mean speech communication. Person-to-person communication is not, however, the only form of auditory communication we use in our daily life. Normal-hearing individuals usually take the ability to hear environment sounds for granted; such sounds keep us in contact with events around us that necessitate action. Think of your own environment; it generates such referential sounds all the time: the doorbell or phone rings, the alarm clock wakens you, the timer on the stove warns you to turn the oven off or remove a cake, while the noise of the washer/dryer informs you when it needs your attention. In the event of a fire it may be the audible signal of the smoke detector that saves your home or even your life. Alerting devices serve to make severely hearing-impaired persons aware of these information-bearing sounds. They greatly facilitate daily activities and also provide that fundamental sense of well-being and security arising from our contact with the auditory world (see Chapter 6).

Alerting devices (Figure 12.20) fulfill their purpose by listening on behalf of the hearing-impaired person and then drawing attention to the sound source by generating a visual or vibrotactile signal. An alerting device may monitor an acoustic event through a microphone attached to or placed close to the sound source, or it may be wired into a sound-generating source to monitor the electrical current or electromagnetic changes occurring in the phone when it rings. Whichever system of detection is used, the sensor activates a transmitter that sends a signal to a receiver plugged into a lamp or vibrator, causing it to flash or to vibrate. The transmitter-receiver link is

Figure 12.20 An array of alerting devices attract attention to sounds not audible to severely hearing impaired persons. (Courtesy Hal-Hen Co.)

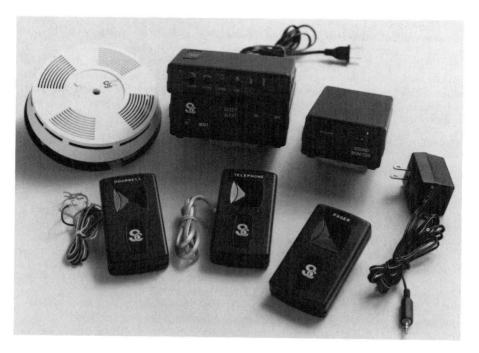

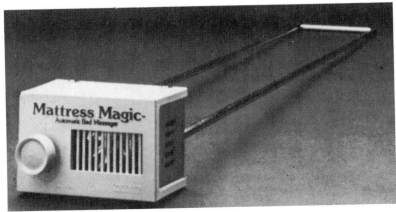

Figure 12.21 Wakeup devices may be visual or vibratory as this bed vibrator which plugs into an alarm clock. (Courtesy Hal-Hen Co.)

a wireless signal and thus can operate remotely, signaling a person in the kitchen that the washing machine has stopped or is on tilt, or that the baby upstairs is crying. Alerting devices that use wireless receivers can have additional receivers plugged into wall outlets in other rooms, thus allowing remote signaling. Sophisticated systems provide a personal receiver that, when activated by one of a number of sensors in different locations, signals the wearer by vibrating and provides a coded LED display indicating which sensor has been triggered.

Several methods are available for alerting the hearing-impaired person to the fact that the phone is ringing. The simplest is to use a bell amplifier. These are plugged into the phone or into the wall jack. Up to 100dB SPL sound level can be achieved by the loudest bell. Another device available from the telephone company transforms the energy of the ring into the low frequencies where it usually is more audible. Up to 90dB SPL of output can be generated by this unit.

Wake-Up Devices

Even with normal hearing, many of us have trouble waking up in the morning. Persons with even mild to moderate hearing impairment frequently need help in knowing when it is wake-up time. To facilitate this the systems we have considered can be coupled to a clock timer. The timer triggers a strobelight or flashes a bedside lamp at a preset time. An alternative means of waking the person is to create a vibration either by a unit that is placed under the pillow or by a heavy-duty bed vibrator that attaches to the bed or slips between boxspring and mattress (Figure 12.21).

THE COCHLEAR IMPLANT

Each of the assistive listening devices we have considered to this point has utilized the available residual hearing of an individual. Unfortunately, for some persons their residual hearing is so little or so distorted that it is essentially nonfunctional. Until recent years there was no way in which such people could receive the information conveyed by sound, regardless of whether it was environmental or speech. This situation is now in the process of change. Because of the pioneering research efforts of Howard P. House, M.D., and his brother William F. House, M.D., a breakthrough was made in the early 1970s that has enormous significance for those persons for whom no significant communication benefit can be derived from conventional hearing aids. For this relatively small group of profoundly hearing-impaired persons, hope has been provided by a prosthetic device called the *cochlear implant*. Before we examine what this device is and what it can do, it is essential to make quite clear certain important facts:

- The cochlear implant in no way restores or approximates normal hearing.
- The cochlear implant, in its present state of evolution, is not intended to replace a conventional hearing aid.
- Not every profoundly hearing-impaired person is a candidate for a cochlear implant.

The selection criteria recommended by Chute and Nevins for a cochlear implant follow:

Candidates for the implant must satisfy strict screening criteria. These include demonstration that benefit is not available from optimal hearing aid prescription, special CAT scan imaging, and for adults a determination of whether responses from the auditory nerve can be stimulated by placement of an exploratory electrode on the promontory of the middle ear between the oval and round windows. Documentation that the condition of the inner bone is receptive to an implant and a physical examination to approve surgery and cochlear implantation also are required. In addition, persons under 18 years of age must satisfy psychological evaluation.

Chronological age: From 4–10 yrs is a favorable age.
Teenage years are highly questionable.
Duration of deafness: Under 3 years is excellent.
4–10 yrs causes some caution.
10 yrs+ causes considerable concern.
Status of cochlear: Partial closure due to ossification causes doubt.
Complete ossification eliminates a candidate.
Multiple handicaps: Noncognitive handicaps cause some concern.
Cognitive difficulties or learning difficulties are definite deterrents.
Functional hearing: Good history of persistence with hearing aids and response to tactile discrimination training are desireable.
Limited experience is a deterrent.
Speech language abilities: Language should be close to chronological age.
Emerging language 1–3 yr delay requires caution; a 3-yr delay is a serious deterrent.

Family structure and support, school services on a frequent basis, and a positive cognitive and learning set in the child all are important factors in selecting candidates. (adapted from Chute and Nevins 1991)

In 1985, the U.S. Federal Drug Administration gave its approval for general use of the Nuclear 22 implant in adults. It now may be used as part of a standard operative procedure. Similar approval was granted for use with children in 1990. The use of this implant now is considered as accepted medical practice for management of profound hearing impairment in appropriate children and adults (Staller, 1991). By 1991 over 3000 devices had been implanted in adults and 550 in children worldwide.

The Nucleus 22 Channel Cochlear Implant

The Nucleus 22 implant consists of two major components:

1. An internal receiver/stimulator
2. An external transmitter and microphone attached to a micro speech processor (Figure 12.22)

The internal receiver/stimulator consists of a single unit surgically implanted under the skin behind the ear that has three parts:

The *receiver coil* is embedded within a silicone rubber covering and has a powerful magnet mounted in its center.

The *stimulator* consists of electrical circuits hermetically sealed in a capsule. Both receiver and stimulator are embedded in a casing that can be bent to fit the curve of the skull.

The third component is an array of 22 electrodes embedded in a stiff but flexible rubber casing resembling a tail.

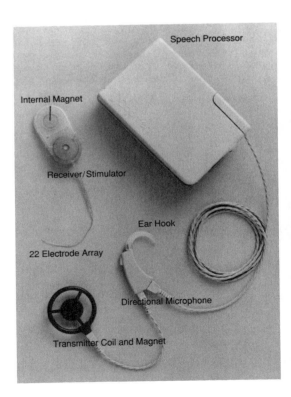

Figure 12.22
The Nuclear 22 channel cochlear implant device consists of an internal and an external component. (Cochlear Corporation.)

The electrode array is inserted into the scala tympani through the round window. The insertion places the tip of the electrode array some 25 mm

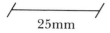

25mm

into the scala tympani with the most peripheral electrode 8–10 mm

10mm

inside the round window (Patrick & Clark, 1991). A ground electrode is placed along the eustachian tube, within the middle ear cavity, or under the temporalis fascia.

The external unit consists of

The transmitter. This consists of a coil housed in a wheel-shaped casing. It is held in place on the skin against the underlying receiver/stimulus by a magnet.

The microphone. This is unidirectional and is housed in a postauricular (BTE) casing. The case also accommodates part of the transmitter circuit, a wire connection to be made from the microprocessor to the transmitter, as well as from the microphone to the micro speech processor.

The micro speech processor. This is a miniature programmable computer powered by a single rechargeable AA battery with about a 16-hour charge. It is the size of a small body hearing aid weighing only 3.5 ounces and is worn on the clothing or clipped to a belt. Its function is to "mimic the normal function of the ear by stimulating different regions of the cochlear according to the spectral content of the speech signal" (Patrick & Clark, 1991, p. 7S). It does this by analyzing the acoustic information which has been converted to an electrical analog by the microphone. Having analyzed the features of the incoming signal, it recodes the analog pattern into a digital code.

Processing Scheme

Feature Analysis (Feature Extraction). The processor identifies voicing from frequency information below 350 Hz. Formant information is extracted from two frequency bands. Energy in the frequency range 280–1000 Hz identifies F1, while frequencies 800–4000 Hz signify F2. In recent models, extra cues to high frequency sounds are extracted from three additional bands, two in the 2000–4000 Hz band, one in the 4000–7000 Hz range. The intensity of formants is coded by varying the combinations of current strength and pulse width. From the frequency analysis, the micro speech processor determines which combination of the 22 electrodes to stimulate. Those close to the round window are stimulated in response to high frequency components; those at the far end of the electrode array will be stimulated by low frequency responses in accord with the tonotopical arrangement (frequency order) of the organ of Corti.

The sequence by which direct stimulation of the auditory nerve fibers occurs is illustrated in Figure 12.23. Remember, the auditory nerve fibers require an electrical impulse to fire. This has not been available in the deaf ear because the hair cells that usually provide it are damaged or missing. Their function must be replaced by the implant. To achieve this, the sound enters the system at the ear level directional microphone where it is converted into an electrical analog. This electrical pattern then travels, via the

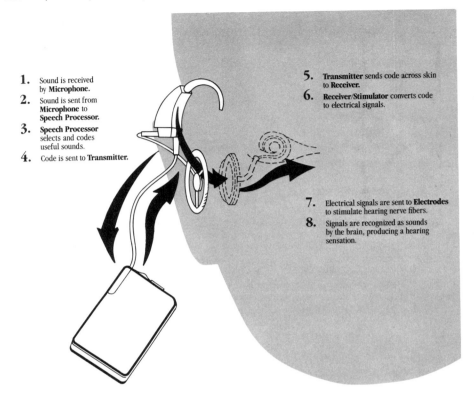

1. Sound is received by **Microphone.**
2. Sound is sent from **Microphone** to **Speech Processor.**
3. **Speech Processor** selects and codes useful sounds.
4. Code is sent to **Transmitter.**
5. **Transmitter** sends code across skin to **Receiver.**
6. **Receiver/Stimulator** converts code to electrical signals.
7. Electrical signals are sent to **Electrodes** to stimulate hearing nerve fibers.
8. Signals are recognized as sounds by the brain, producing a hearing sensation.

Figure 12.23 A depiction of the sequence by which a cochlear implant provides direct stimulation of the auditory nerve fiber. (Cochlear Corporation.)

connecting wire, to the micro speech processor. Here the signal is analyzed for its spectral features, as explained earlier, and the resultant information is recoded into digital form. The speech processor then selects and codes the appropriate sound information which then is sent via the microphone case to the external transmitter. The link to the internal receiver, embedded under the skin, is made by a radio frequency signal. The signal received is recoded by the receiver-stimulator into electrical impulse patterns that are sent to the electrode array. The electrodes in turn stimulate the acoustic nerve, which carries the information through the usual eighth nerve pathway to the auditory cortex where it is perceived as a sensation equivalent to hearing. This whole process takes only milliseconds, so sound is heard virtually as it occurs.

The Benefits of a Cochlear Implant

In Chapter 6 we discussed the role that sound plays as a conveyor of environmental information. This function was shown to serve both a preconscious need for ongoing monitoring, which contributes to a sense of well-being, and a conscious alerting and attention-orienting function. Cochlear implant devices hold the same potential for the user. Postlingually deafened adults, who have a memory of the acoustic patterns of environmental sound, find they are able to correlate many of the new stimulus patterns with those memories. Children, who without the implant device would have remained unaware of acoustic information, have the potential to acquire the correlations among sound, the neural stimulus patterns resulting from the implant, and the events to which they refer. Although the monitoring of the acoustic environment is fundamental, speech communication is the primary concern of those who seek assistive listening devices.

Speech Recognition Results: Adults

Data are available about the performance of a large number of cochlear implant users in North America and Australia (Cochlear, 1991). These data were submitted to the Food and Drug Administration, which must approve claims of patient benefit made by manufacturers of prosthetic devices. The data submitted were accepted and the claims approved. The claims state that when used in conjunction with visible speech cues (speech-reading), almost every user demonstrated improved communication ability. This was determined by assessing exact repetition of simple story or sentence material. Using audition-only to discriminate the open set CID Sentences of Everyday Speech, 82.3 percent of users were shown to evidence significant postimplant change (mean percent discrimination preimplant 2.27, postimplant 29.61). There were, however, wide individual differences (SD = 25.14). Fifteen percent of users experienced no significant change, while 2.4 percent experienced a lower postimplant speech recognition score.

Speech Recognition Results: Children

Since the majority of children chosen for cochlear implants were deafened before two years of age, concern for developing perceptual abilities has been great. In addition to speech recognition skills, a range of other auditory perceptual abilities has been studied in children using the cochlear implant. The effect of the device on language development and speech production also has been investigated.

In an analysis of the test results of 330 children monitored in over 30 centers around the world, data were collapsed into seven categories to indicate improvement of nonspeech and speech receptive abilities and speech production skills (Cochlear Corporation, 1991). The results are shown below:

	N	PERCENT SHOWING IMPROVEMENT
Sound detection	(80)	100
Environmental sounds	(58)	52
Pattern perception	(77)	66
Close-set word identification	(72)	63
Open-set speech recognition	(59)	46
Lipreading enhancement	(70)	47
Speech production	(61)	79

You can see that after the implant almost half the children could recognize open-set word or speech test items, while the usefulness of sound for learning correct speech improved in over three quarters of the subjects.

In a study of 28 children who had used the Nucleus 22 Cochlear Implant System, Osberger et al. (1991) evaluated the children on a battery of 20 tests of speech perception and sound effect recognition. They report that 61 percent of the children were able to achieve open-set speech recognition and 14 percent closed-set recognition. None achieved comparable performance with conventional hearing aids.

Staller, Dowell, Beiter, and Brimacombe (1991) reported on 142 children who had used an implant for at least a year. They showed average improvement in sound field thresholds to be 35dB at 500 and 1000 Hz. At 2K, 3K, and 4K responses were obtained at 50dB. No threshold responses were obtainable with conventional amplification.

In discussing the postimplant performance of prelinguistically deafened children, Staller et al. (1991) showed that these children develop perceptual skills more slowly than those deafened during or after language development. All, however, evidenced postoperative improvement, though achievements varied widely among children. As a result of the implant 23 of 32 children (71.8 percent) achieved better than chance scores on the Monosyllable Trochee-Spondee test (Erber & Alencewicz, 1976). Their scores ranged from 23–65 percent correct, versus only 4 subjects (12.5 percent) who scored better than chance preoperatively. For 9 subjects, deafened after birth but before 22 months of age, those whose scores exceeded chance increased from 2 (22.2 percent) to 8 (88.9 percent). The authors concluded that the most significant factors influencing performance by children wearing the implant are age of onset and duration of deafness. The same is true for adults. The more advanced the language development of a child at the onset of deafness, the more favorable is the prognosis for achievement of more sophisticated auditory perception. The study also reported continued growth in perceptual abilities with longer use of the device.

In assessing the impact of the 22 channel cochlear implant on speech production ability after one year of use, Osberger, Robbins, Berry, Todd, Hesketh, and Sedey (1991) reported that 67 percent of the utterances of subjects were recognizable as English phonemes. Tobey, Pancamo, Staller, Brimacombe, and Beiter (1991) and Tobey and Hasenstab (1991) demonstrated increased phonemic production in children after the same postimplant period as well as improvement in quality of suprasegmental imitation. Voice quality and control of vocal pitch and intensity also showed marked improvement.

Since oral language is developed through hearing spoken language, it is reasonable to hope that a cochlear implant will enhance the development of language sophistication in profoundly deaf children thus fitted. Clearly the age of onset and duration of deafness prior to the implant will exert a critical influence. In evaluating the potential impact of the implant on language development, Tobey and Hasenstab (1991) reported on the language development of four children fitted with the cochlear implant at age five or younger. The authors presented a case-by-case illustration of pragmatic semantic, syntactic and morphological, and phonological changes occurring after the implant. In summarizing the results they state that as might be expected performance ranged along a continuum. Improvements attributable to the implant device were observed in all four children at each level of the rule system, though the degree of change varied with each child, in one case quite significantly. They conclude that predicting exact benefits a given child will experience in language development after cochlear implant may not be possible. However, it is believed that a positive impact on spoken communication interactions will accrue from use of the device.

Whether we are dealing with a sensorneural impairment or a cochlear implant, only a holistic conceptualization of our responsibilities as audiologists and speech-language pathologists will ensure that all the listening needs of the client are identified and addressed. Our role is to increase the client's success in functioning within her personal environment. An important component of this task is to increase verbal communication performance under adverse listening conditions, which focuses our attention on assistive listening devices. However, we must not neglect the nonverbal functions of sound and its role as a communicator of important information. This requires that we survey with the client those circumstances in which significant environmental sounds are not adequately audible. Working together as audiologists, speech-language pathologists, and teachers of the deaf, we then must ensure that these needs are met to the maximum extent of current technology.

SUMMARY: ASSISTIVE LISTENING AND ALERTING DEVICES

- ALDs may use hardwire, electromagnetic, FM, or infrared links.
- Accessories such as extension microphones, TV, or radio jack connectors further increases ALDs' application to special needs.
- Special portable amplifiers for use with or without a hearing aid are available. A specially adapted phone handpiece with built-in amplifier can be purchased.
- Not all public phones are compatible with a hearing aid T-circuit. Incompatibility is signified by a dark grey grommet where cord and receiver connect.
- Hearing aids can be integrated with personal FM ALDs by direct connection or by electromagnetic induction using an induction coil neck loop or silhouette plate to activate the telecoil T-circuit.
- Portable infrared systems may be purchased for home and office use. These have accessory microphones and TV radio adapters. They, as well as FM systems can be coupled to hearing aids.
- Telecommunication devices for the deaf (TDDs) permit typed messages to be sent by phone to receiver-printers. Some convert to computer voice systems.
- Message relay services facilitate communication with non-TDD users.
- Closed captioning units print subtitles onto coded TV programs.
- Alerting devices detect sounds and activate a visual or vibratory stimulus. Some systems discriminate and code sound sources.

- Telephone bell amplifiers and frequency transformers are available.
- The cochlear implant makes available information about acoustic cues otherwise unavailable to persons with little or no useful hearing.
- The cochlear implant replaces neither hearing nor the hearing aid.
- Strict evaluation is essential for candidacy for a cochlear implant.
- Both adults and children have demonstrated significant improvement in sound-detection recognition, speech recognition, and speech reading performance post-implant training.
- In children, voice control and voice quality improved after implant, as did speech production and intelligibility.
- The limited information available suggests that cochlear implants have the potential to influence positively language development in young profoundly deaf children.

Conclusion

The best possible hearing aid fitting leaves some persons' listening needs in many situations less than optimally provided for. Assistive listening devices have been developed to provide for these unmet needs. They are available to optimize signal-to-noise ratios and to minimize the effects of reverberation in both public and private environments. All types of systems have been adapted to this purpose and coupling devices have been developed to allow hearing aids to be integrated with such ALDs. A range of accessories provides a means of adapting ALDs to accommodate the demands of special communication situations and environment, including group meetings, distance from the speaker, radio and TV listening, and telephone use. To accommodate those who cannot hear on the phone, even with amplification, telecommunication devices, augmented as appropriate by message relay services, have been developed.

The need for monitoring of significant acoustic events in the client's personal environment has been provided for by alerting devices that recode acoustic events into information detectable by other nonimpaired sensory modalities. The maximizing of the use of residual hearing must incorporate the capitalization of assistive listening devices as special situations demand. Where appropriate we also must address the person's need to hear important meaningful sounds around him by informing him about appropriate alerting devices.

For selected children and adults for whom conventional amplification does not afford useful benefits, the cochlear implant provides considerable potential for developing and improving speech communication. Not all severely hearing-impaired persons are suitable candidates, and those selected require special training in order to learn or relearn the relationships between the stimulus patterns provided and their referents. The full potential of the cochlear implant as technology advances has yet to be determined.

Audiologists and speech language pathologists have a responsibility to address each individual client's need for optimal listening in all situations and environments. While personal hearing aids remain the primary device for achieving this goal, they often prove inadequate in special listening circumstances and acoustic environments. In addition we must address a person's need to be alerted by acoustic referents to important events. Our professional and ethical responsibilities in this respect have now been augmented by law. The Americans with Disabilities Act (PL. 101–336) (see Chapter 20, p. 469), which became law in January 1992 mandates that access to a wide range of public environments, services, and events be provided to disabled persons. For people with impaired hearing this means the right to communication unimpeded by barriers. This necessitates that audiologists routinely assess a client's needs for special assistive listening devices and familiarize the client with available devices appropriate to his or her need. Palmer (1992) has provided an excellent short course on the types of interactive software and the types of evaluation and demonstration which need to be provided, and methods of promoting public awareness of such devices and services. She also provides an extensive bibliography on the topic.

An earlier publication, *Assistive Listening Devices and Systems: Professional Practices* (ASHA 1985), contains chapters and readings which provide comprehensive coverage of this topic. Also included in the ASHA 1985 publication is an illustrated compendium of assistive devices reprinted from *Hearing Instruments* (1985).

For those wishing to purchase devices, Clark School for the Deaf publishes a booklet illustrating those available from their Assistive Devices Center, which is open to the public. The Hal Hen Company supplies a wide range of devices, which are illustrated and described in their product catalog.

13

A General Model for Intervention Management

In this second part of the text, we will be concerned with intervention procedures designed to reduce the handicap imposed by the disability of impaired hearing. *The handicap is the gap between the communication and learning demands placed on a given individual and the resources that person has with which to meet those demands comfortably.* Remember, the actual demands will vary from person to person, from situation to situation, from task to task. Each age group will encounter demands related to that stage in life. Specific resources will be needed for each individual, as well as specific strategies. However, we can describe a general model that will accommodate those concepts of management appropriate to each age group.

THE GENERAL MODEL

The general model involves eight management steps:

1. Provide emotional and informational support
2. Review and interpret available test results
3. Ascertain present situation and needs
4. Supplement interview and test results
5. Determine primary and secondary goals
6. Identify appropriate resources
7. Develop a management plan
8. Monitor effectiveness of intervention strategies

214

1. Provide Emotional and Informational Support. The most pressing need of a person seeking help is reassurance. He wishes to learn what his problem is and to be reassured that it can be corrected simply and quickly. The immediate problem this person faces is anxiety—fear of the unknown. Unfortunately we rarely will be able to satisfy the wish of the client to eliminate the problem completely and immediately. Nevertheless, until we are able to address the unknown and the anxiety it generates, we are unlikely to have the client's maximum attention and cooperation in the habilitation process. Thus the first step is to acknowledge and legitimize the feelings of anxiety that the client and family often experience as a normal reaction. We then must attempt to reduce the stress. Three factors contribute to such a reduction.

Acknowledgment and Acceptance of Feelings. At each age level the clients with whom we work react emotionally to the disability and their perception of its significance. These feelings either are "bottled up" because the individual feels ashamed of them and feels she should handle them herself, or they manifest as frustration, anger, denial, or depression. To hear a therapist calmly acknowledge these feelings and state that they are understandable and normal often provides immediate stress relief. Not infrequently a client will have tears in his eyes and will "get all choked up" by such acceptance of what he may acknowledge as having considered foolish. Acceptance of the client's feelings contributes to trust, the second stress reducer.

Development of Trust. Trust must be earned; it is based upon experience. However, a client usually derives significant anxiety relief just from feeling comfortable with a helper. This usually is referred to as developing rapport. I feel confident and less anxious when a person helping me communicates through behavior and words that she is genuinely interested in my difficulty and wants to be of help. I want to know that she feels confident that I can be helped, that I can minimize my problems. A helper must be very careful, however, not to accept total responsibility for minimizing the problem. The helper should identify herself as a resource, a guide, an experienced partner. Given such a relationship most clients say that they "feel better already."

Imparting of Information. Information limits the unknown. The more tangible the client's perception of the problem becomes, the more likely he is to begin to feel competent to deal with it. Information counseling involves

- Clearly reporting what you know already about the problem
- Using the available data to explain how the disability impacts upon normal communication
- Explaining how others react to communication breakdown when they are involved with the client
- Explaining the side effects (inattention, memory problems, embarrassment, social withdrawal, etc.)
- Explaining the ways in which normal people attempt to cope with communication reduction

Provide an outline of how you plan to proceed, the additional testing you need to conduct, the information you need to obtain, and how, together, you will determine an intervention plan. This knowledge builds the client's confidence in his own abilities and strengths, engenders trust, and encourages him to feel that the problem will be brought under control.

2. Review and Interpret Available Test Results. Frequently the client will have been referred to you for habilitative/rehabilitative management. Whenever possible you should have available the audiologic test results prior to the first appointment. Review and interpret these in terms of the implications they have for understanding the problems and needs the individual is likely to encounter in communication and learning situations.

Your primary interest will be in aided hearing results that suggest the potential contribution aided hearing can make to recognition and comprehension of speech. If discrimination also has been assessed in noise, you can relate the results to difficulties that the client may report experiencing in certain work or social environments. Speech in noise results should be given particular attention in the case of children of school age, since we know that the S/N ratio in the normal classroom is very small, of the order of $+5dB$. What these results tell us may motivate us, for example, to do everything possible to obtain an FM system for a child or if one is available to make the acceptance of the unit and its consistent use a priority. In the case of an infant or preschool child, the evaluative test information will shape your expectations concerning the auditory behavior you should look for in the child with the hearing aids. It will help you predict the probable characteristics of developing speech and the need for the use of supplemental sensory avenues in communication stimulation. An evaluation of the implication of the audiologic assessment data will guide you in your determination of the client's present situation and needs.

3. Ascertain Present Situation and Needs. At the first meeting with the client or the parents of a hearing-impaired child, it is important to establish a positive relationship. This can be achieved at the same time that you try to gain a general picture of the client's perception of the problem. Emphasize to the client the importance of her perception of her difficulties and needs. Encourage parents to describe what they feel their needs are and their perception of their child's difficulty. In this way you communicate the partnership role you seek to establish. This approach makes individuals feel comfortable and encourages trust because you show respect for them. Seeking to understand the hearing impairment in the broad context of how it impacts on a person's life communicates concern for people as human beings. At the same time, a general profile serves your need to identify the most pressing problems, to place test data in context, and to form a general impression of the task you and the client will undertake. I need to stress that the problem to be addressed always is the one the client perceives, that is, his reality. That perception may be modified by our input, but even so the problem still will be as the client sees it. Thus, we try first to profile the present situations in which difficulty is experienced, the demands the client feels he is not adequately able to meet, his method of dealing with these situations, and how he feels about his ability to cope. We need to know what difficulties parents see their child encountering, what they see the most pressing needs to be, and how they feel about the present situation.

4. Supplement Interview and Test Results. The diagnostic assessment report for a client with impaired hearing falls short of the information you will need to develop a specific management plan. It will be necessary to supplement the report findings in accord with the needs of each individual client. The supplementary information can be obtained from the client or a child's parents, from the audiologist, or from the preschool/school, or it may be developed by the speech-language pathologist. The information you collect will allow you to diagnose problem situations, assess the side effects of the communication difficulty (educational, social, emotional), and explore resources (the client, family, school setting, other professionals, and technology).

5. Determine Primary and Secondary Goals. When you review the available data (see p. 140), you will gain a broad general picture of the difficulties the client and those closely related to her are having. It probably will be necessary to focus more sharply on these problems. You may need to know when, where, and under what circumstances the problems arise, how often they are encountered, and how important they are. The problems may be in communication; in the client's reactions to the communication breakdown; or the reactions of a spouse, boy/girlfriend, or supervisor; or they may have to do with making business or social plans. For parents of a hearing-impaired child, the problem may involve communication, education, or social or behavioral management situations. You need to be sure you have a complete picture and that you understand which problems the client/parents feel most urgently need attention. It will be necessary, through discussion with your client, to develop a priority list of needs and to set realistic short- and long-term goals for each individual.

6. Identify Appropriate Resources. The achievement of goals depends upon the careful selection of appropriate resources, which will be found in technology (amplification and assistive devices), in other professionals (teachers, psychologists, educators, social workers, vocational rehabilitationists, etc.), in the ability to modify the environment, in the family, and in the client.

Each resource chosen must reduce a particular component of the problems encountered by the child or adult and family.

7. Develop a Management Plan. After identifying the needs and the resources that can be used to address those needs, you must develop an overall management plan. This should comprise a series of *action steps*. Each step must be designed to engage a specific resource to reduce a specific need. This is the stage in which you decide *how* to go about mobilizing the appropriate resources. The plan should address needs in order of the priority you established when determining primary and secondary needs. For each need you will match a resource and state a plan of action to engage that resource. Responsibilities will be shared. If a personal FM amplification system is needed, you should assume responsibility for contacting the audiologist for support and for working with the parents in contacts with the Committee on Special Education and with the school authority that can purchase the item. If the need is to improve an adult's ability to communicate in group situations, you and the client become the primary resource. The action plan will be to analyze typical situations, to determine present communicative behavior, and to develop and practice a series of new communication management strategies.

8. Monitor Effectiveness of Intervention Strategies. Together with the client it will be important to assess the effectiveness of your intervention strategies. This should be programmed into your management plan. Objectives for a month or six weeks should be set in terms of strategies for the achievement of a series of short-term goals selected to achieve a reduction of the handicap in specific situations. Both objective and subjective criteria for evaluation should be considered.

We began the description of this general model by considering briefly the components involved in providing emotional support. The task of counseling is not one in which we are given much professional training (Luterman, 1984). It is helpful, therefore, to discuss in somewhat more detail the general principles of supportive counseling.

GENERAL PRINCIPLES OF SUPPORTIVE COUNSELING

Counseling in Our Profession

Few of us have had any formal training in counseling; our focus has been on the management of hearing, speech, and language needs. We have a strong need "to do something," to be seen as taking the situation in hand. This is understandable; after all, we are eager to take the necessary steps to minimize the handicap. My professional training taught me that I must assume responsibility for training/retraining the handicapped individual, that as a professional I should know what is best for the client, and that I should set goals and show him/her how to achieve them (Rollin, 1987). This view of my role excludes the client from the process; he becomes merely a recipient of "prescriptive therapy."

Unfortunately, with prescriptive therapy we do not know exactly how effective a given prescription will prove to be with a particular individual nor what side effects it may induce. Side effects in our field are seen in the form of a rejection of the prescription recommendations or a failure to "take them" as prescribed. We also may overload the person's system so that the requirements we prescribe make it difficult for the individual to cope with all his/her other responsibilities. The role I am suggesting you assume rejects the prescriptive approach and instead places you in an equal partnership with the client who will make the ultimate decisions. This runs contrary to the traditional view of professional responsibility but fits well into the definition of counseling.

The Nature of Counseling

Webster's New World Dictionary (1984) defines *supportive counsel* as "a mutual exchange of ideas, opinions, etc." while Fiedler (1950) views it as a variation of the practice of good interpersonal relationships. Those definitions are reassuring, for they encourage us to believe that we possess already the resources necessary to provide support to the client. Indeed, Tyler (1969, p.13) suggests that if we define counseling as "a service designed primarily to aid normal individuals to make the choices upon which their development depends," we will, in fact, find ourselves in harmony with what the client feels to be her real need. The point to bear in mind is that the persons who seek our help are as normal in their psychological makeup as we. Were it not for the hearing impairment, they would not be seeking our support. The abnormality lies in the hearing mechanism not in the individual. However, with a tangible disability, our clients feel insecure and apprehensive. They perceive a threat to the way in which they have their lives organized; they do not understand the nature of the problem nor its ramifications for their employment, their family life, or their social activities. If the client is a child, the parents often feel they no longer know how to be "good parents." They worry about the child's ability to learn to communicate, about his social development, and most particularly, about his education (Webster, 1977). In both cases the persons involved do not know how best to cope with the unfamiliar situation. Rarely does a person express for more than a brief period the conviction that he/she can no longer cope at all; if this does happen you will know immediately that a referral for professional counseling is essential. In such instances the hearing impairment is not the central problem but is an additional problem that threatens to destabilize a whole life structure.

Thus we *are* equipped to deal with the normal feelings and reactions to the abnormal situation caused by hearing impairment (Freedman & Doob, 1968; Goffman, 1969). Before we can be effective helpers, however, we must understand the nature of the counseling process.

Reactions to Impaired Function

The process by which we come to acknowledge that something is wrong with us, or with someone dear to us, is an agonizing one often spread over many months. Denial that anything is wrong, heightened awareness of minor behaviors, rationalizations, self-diagnosis both terrible and trivial, anxiety, even guilt for being suspicious, all often occur in a confusing flux of feelings. We struggle to maintain the reality that all is well, to convince ourselves that our concern is unfounded (Kubler-Ross, 1969). We want our spouse, our child, or ourself to be normal. Even when the disability is acquired traumatically, the apprehension of what has happened occurs slowly. Our mind protects us from the unthinkable through disbelief, slowly opening the window to reality as we feel capable of dealing with it. Recognition of the normality of this process, by you the helper, is critical; it should guide your perceptions of the client's needs through phases of rehabilitative management. Several authors writing about the process of adapting to disability in adult or child have used the Kubler-Ross model (Gargiulo, 1985; Moses, 1977; Seligman, 1979; Webster, 1977). It is helpful to be familiar with the three basic stages of adaptation that almost always occur.

Stage 1

Shock Reaction. This is a self-defense mechanism; it provides protection against the unthinkable. The person blocks out the evidence that threatens her reality. There is a genuine disbelief in the evidence, a strong emotional reaction, or emotional numbness and an intense feeling of loneliness.

Management of Shock Stage. We need to acknowledge the reasonableness of this reaction to bad news, to verbalize what is happening to the client. We must allow the client, parent, or spouse time to work through this stage. Avoid any attempt to force information or to stress the new reality. Ask, "Would you like me to explain anything right now?" Address the general situation not the details; give honest hope; keep communication lines open: "Please call me when you have talked with your husband." "I'll get back to you as soon as I can."

Stage 2

Defensive Retreat. When shock wears off we seek to avoid the pain of what we are beginning to recognize as the new reality. We feel inadequate and unable to cope, so we search for a rescuer. We seek someone with cures and solutions—someone who will give us instructions. Above all, we look for someone to assume responsibility for handling our problem.

Management of Retreat Stage. Do not accept the dangerous role of rescuer; identify the normal feelings of inadequacy and stress the cooperative model and your continuing support. Emphasize the client's resources, personality, education, and desire for action, or the parent/spouse's expertise and ability to give love, enrich experiences, explore, experiment, and support. Emphasize the importance of progressive understanding of the disability and the experience they will gain in facilitating coping behaviors.

Stage 3

Acknowledgment Stage. The earlier reactions do not disappear, but the need to live anew, to rebuild, becomes stronger than the need to defend the old reality that is no longer tenable. Disappointment, anger, and frustration all persist to a lesser degree, but action is possible. The client is ready for guidance, participative planning, and shared responsibility and is ready to learn about the problem and to explore ways to deal with it.

Management of Acknowledgment Stage. Restate the problem; identify immediate needs; stress the partnership; and negotiate shared responsibilities and together set goals and methods.

Remember always that no one fits a model exactly. Individual reactions vary; a person may experience overlapping stages or may regress at times to earlier stages.

The Goals of Counseling

The ultimate goal of the counseling interaction is the client's achievement of a genuine confidence in his ability to cope with the situations affected by the hearing disability. Counseling seeks an improvement in the quality of the individual's life through a reduction of the negative physical and psychological influences of the hearing impairment. To achieve this, we must assist the person in reducing the anxiety, frustration, guilt, feelings of inadequacy, and self-pity that understandably may arise from learning that one's normal self or one's normal child is "handicapped," "hearing impaired," or "deaf." A climate must be created that maintains and strengthens the client's personal integrity. Webster's dictionary defines *integrity* as "the quality or state of being complete." When one feels complete one feels secure, and trust can be extended. Respect for integrity demands that we see the *completeness* of the individual and the family. We must be interested in the hearing impairment, not as a clinical entity to be treated, but as a limiting influence that impacts in many ways on the person, her family, and her life-style, threatening the effectiveness of existing individual and family structures. The people with whom we work need our help in preserving that vital sense of wholeness. Sensorineural hearing impairment is incurable. Thus, in addition to the use of amplification and communication training, the preservation of personal integrity will require various degrees of reorganization of the client's self-perception or of the parents' perception of the child. As part of the management responsibility, you must be willing to understand and to assist in the reduction of the negative impact of the disability on the individual and her family.

The Counseling Relationship

We have defined counseling as a relationship in which two persons coordinate their resources to reduce the actual or potential negative impact of a communication impediment on a life-style. A relationship, by virtue of its ongoing nature, does not require that special sessions be set aside for counseling. It may well be that on any given occasion the need to talk through specific problems and feelings takes a full session. That, however, reflects no more than the flexible allocation of time to whatever is perceived to be the most pressing need. Counseling, therefore, refers to the way in which you, the client, and family members work together on all aspects of rehabilitation; it is a process inextricably woven into the fabric of problem solving. To this partnership we each bring special knowledge and expertise. Your contribution represents knowledge and experience about communication, hearing, and hearing deficits. You are familiar with ways in which the impact of hearing impairment on communication can be minimized. You know how a child learns to communicate and how hearing deficits restrict that learning. You also have expertise in ways to enhance the child's experience, his use of sound, and the development of language, speech, and general learning skills.

The expertise of the client and the family by contrast lies in their intimate knowledge of the total impact of the hearing impairment. It is the client and family who know the specific problems they face. They know in what ways they most feel threatened, what their most urgent needs are, and what financial, emotional, social, and time resources they have available. The ultimate choices of action and the carrying out of the problem-solving plans that have been drawn up cooperatively lie with the client. Only the client can make things happen; you can only help. Luterman (1984) says, "control is always vested within the client and not the therapist" (p. 14). The counselor informs, questions, and supports but never directs or decides except in areas of technical expertise.

Establishing the Relationship

The development of a relationship begins with the first contact and continues throughout all shared experiences. The primary goal in developing a relationship is to earn trust. To be trustworthy a person must be sincere, honest, sensitive to the perceptions and needs of others, open-minded, and flexible. Feel comfortable in presenting yourself as a warm human being rather than as an expert or an authority. *Teacher, speech pathologist, audiologist,* or *clinician* are only labels for your job; it is you the person, not the title, with whom the client will work; be yourself. Tyler (1969) urges the counselor to think of the initial contact requirements "simply as hospitality" (p. 50). Show consideration for the client, and be on time for appointments; if you will be late, take the time to advise the waiting client how long the wait will be, apologize for the delay, and tell her/him that you know how annoying it is to be kept waiting. Greet the client by introducing yourself, extend a handshake if appropriate, inquire if the accompanying person(s) is related, and introduce yourself. *Invite* the client and partner to come to your office. If the client is elderly and has trouble walking encourage her to take her time; if a child is to be seen, greet him by name, do not just address the parent. In fact, I make a point of greeting the child first, commenting on an article of clothing or a toy, and opening a conversation before introducing myself to the parent. With an older child, treat child and parent equally, both in the introduction and during consultations. These are simple behaviors that communicate the type of relationship you wish to establish at a time when the client is highly sensitive.

The Client's Feelings

Throughout your interactions with our clients, you need to remember that it is the client's feeling state that dictates how receptive she is to the practical aspects of management, how diligently activities are carried out, and how willing she is to change. As a fellow human being, you are capable of being sensitive to what the client is feeling. You know that it is common to dislike seeking help, to feel it is a sign of weakness. You understand a client's resentment at not being able to take care of her own problems. The idea of dependence on someone else makes her feel uncomfortable or even inferior to the helper, even resentful toward you—the helper is a reminder that the client or her child is no longer whole, that there is a problem. A client awaiting a rehabilitative assessment may be concerned about what you will tell her about her chances of getting back to normal or about her child's learning to speak or going to normal school. She may be worried about how she will pay for the sessions or manage to fit them into her busy schedule. If she is coming for another "therapy" session, she may be wondering whether it is worth continuing.

Because of her feelings or perhaps lack of time, she has not carried out her home assignments or those for her child very diligently. She may feel that you expect too much of her, that you do not understand how many other demands she has, or how alone and unsupported she feels. She may be feeling frustrated with little hope for the future, or she may feel angry about the whole situation. As the helper you need to be aware that although the client's attitudes and behaviors may be directed to you, they rarely are caused by you. Once you acknowledge this, you no longer need to feel threatened by them. You will have no need to label the client as unrealistic, unreasonable, a worrier, an angry person, a nuisance. Instead, you will be able to accept these emotions as manifestations of hope for future return of the normal self, and the constant search for a closer approximation of normality for the self or for a loved one. Before you can work effectively with the practicalities of communication difficulty, you must accept and help the client acknowledge, understand, and address the feeling reactions to the effects of the hearing impairment. The client needs to see these as normal rational reactions to an abnormal situation. She needs to be helped in directing the anxiety and concerns toward attaining effective ways of reducing the communication impedance resulting from the hearing impairment.

General Responsibilities

The general responsibilities you should assume in the counseling relationship include the following:

- *Create a climate of trust.* This is essential to the establishment of an open and cooperative approach to problems.
- *Establish a partnership.* This involves helping the client and family understand the shared responsibility of management with each partner contributing a different expertise.
- *Assist the client in describing the problems he faces.* Through this process guidance and support can be focused appropriately.
- *Help the client translate feelings into needs.* Only when this is done can effective intervention be planned.
- *Determine appropriate referral for professional counseling.* You are responsible for recommending and facilitating referral to appropriate professionals when the problem is interfering significantly with other aspects of the client's life (e.g., marital relations) or is of a severity or tenacity that exceeds your ability to help resolve it.

General Counseling Strategies

There are general guidelines that are helpful in any cooperative interaction between you and the client. They are valid in an interview, in therapy, or a separate counseling session.

• **Ask the Client to Describe the Problem as She Sees It at This Time.** You should encourage the client to help you understand the problem from her point of view. The cause may be the hearing impairment, but the problem may be perceived to be adjusting to amplification or the inability to understand speech easily in some environments despite the use of amplification. The client may feel her spouse or partner is unsympathetic to her difficulty or she may be worrying about whether she should discuss her hearing problem at an interview for a new position. A parent may be worried about a child's ability to cope with subject-specific language in school, about how to manage the frustration her child experiences when not understood, or about the fact that her oral child wishes to learn sign language. In each case, it is the problem the client perceives that needs your attention; your perception of needs is secondary to this.

• **Restate the Problem Described to Ensure Your Understanding.** When you feel you know the needs the client is expressing, *summarize the situation:* "Let me take a moment to see if I have understood your concern." *Restate the key points of the problem:* "You seem to be getting a lot of help from the hearing aid, but in noisy environments you still have trouble understanding. You seem to be particularly concerned that you can't understand what your wife says when your are driving." or "You feel that your biggest need at this time is how to handle the situation when you don't understand what Mary says. You're having trouble dealing with the frustration she shows when that happens. You feel guilty that you become impatient with her."

• **Ask for Clarification on Points You Are Not Clear About.** "You say you have trouble in noisy situations; does this occur at work? Can you describe such a situation and how you are handling it?"

• **Focus Discussion on the Central Concern.** Effective counseling strategies take a general problem and break it down into key elements. Through reflection, requests for more specific perceptions, and more information, the client is enabled to focus on the central concerns. Often this proves to be something different from what the person originally complained about, something underlying the earlier perception of difficulty: "Hmm, perhaps it isn't really my hearing impairment that I'm worried about. I guess I'm not sure I can handle the job I've applied for. To be honest, I don't think the employer will care whether I wear hearing aids so long as I do the job well. I know I can function in groups because I'm doing it now."

Note for example the client's posture (relaxed, tense, body turned away from you), eye contact (frequent steady contact, fleeting contact, avoidance of contact), and stress indicators (foot and leg movement, finger drumming, nervous laugh). You also learn about the client's perceptions from listening to whether the perceptions are self-directed: "I always seem to be worrying about Mary." "I have little patients with my wife"; or other directed: "The school doesn't seem to care about David's needs." "People are always mumbling; why can't they speak clearly?"

• **Offer Your Impressions of What the Client Seems to Be Experiencing.** "It seems you are most concerned about keeping David in the normal classroom."

"You seem to have experienced a lot of stress without much support."

"You seem to be worried that with your hearing impairment, you simply won't be able to cope with all the things you're responsible for."

"You still seem to be trying to deal with the anger you feel about how this whole situation has been dealt with."

The specific counseling needs of hearing-impaired clients and their families change with the age and circumstances of the person. We will discuss the more particular needs as we look at management strategies appropriate to each age group. In concluding this chapter, I wish to emphasize again that effective counseling is neither given nor received; it is an interactive process arising from a cooperative relationship. In that relationship you and your client each make a contribution, you from your expertise and knowledge about hearing impairment, and the client from knowledge about its impact on his/her ability to continue a normal life-style. It is true that in the early stages of your career, you will not know that you can be an effective counselor, but neither will you know whether you will prove to be truly effective as an audiologist, teacher, or speech-language pathologist. That awareness comes only through experience, and you gain experience through involvement over time. Your acceptance that you do not know what is best for your client, that you cannot make decisions on his behalf, should remove much of your feeling of insecurity. Your task is to help the client inform you about his needs and to assist him in selecting problem-solving strategies appropriate to those needs. Once he realizes that you truly mean what you say, he will play the role of your advisor and your partner quite comfortably.

These general principles of management and counseling apply across age groups. We will now fine-tune them to hearing-impaired persons at different stages of their lives. Each stage we pass through from infancy to retirement gives rise to certain predictable needs. These we will address. However, we must remain especially sensitive to the particular needs arising from the life situations of each person and family. These cannot be predicted; they require that our intervention model maximizes the client's input and emphasizes his/her role in planning and decision making.

SUMMARY

- A general model accommodates for each age group the principles and stages of management of hearing handicap.
- An accepting supportive approach is a prerequisite to effective management.

- Information needs to be presented in practical terms that relate it to the experiences of the client.
- Primary and secondary goals derive from our understanding of the client's present situation and needs.
- Goals selected must be refined to be met by available resources.
- A management plan must be defined in terms of specific actions to be taken.
- Progress should be monitored regularly in terms of short-term goals.
- Though counseling needs vary with each client, an adjustment process is experienced by all.
- Counseling is an integral component of management.
- Specific management strategies are required to assist clients to cope with the shock, disbelief, and acknowledgment phases of adjustment.
- The counseling relationship requires that we accept a facilitating role, not a directing role.
- Basic counseling strategies involve careful listening, problem restatement, and focusing on the central concern.
- Although each stage of life presents certain general needs, these must be examined in the light of the specific life experiences of a given family.

Conclusion

Management of impairment of hearing is a task that can be organized in terms of a general model regardless of the age of the client. A cooperative working relationship maximizes the expertise of client and professional while protecting the integrity of both. The assessment must focus on the actuality of problems; the resolution of those problems must focus on practicability. Targets selected for intervention should be short range and the degree of success assessed frequently. Counseling will constitute an important part of management. It will be inextricably interwoven into practical management reflecting a trusting relationship.

14

The Young Preschool Child and the Family: Assessment and Intervention

ASSESSMENT

The management of the very young hearing-impaired child, unlike that of older children, does not have a clear-cut assessment and habilitation stage. Even audiologic assessment and hearing-aid prescription are ongoing processes. We cannot wait until assessment is complete before planning intervention because these early years do not provide a great deal of evidence that can be used to predict future achievements. There are, however, emergent behaviors that we need to monitor and record carefully. These include

Responsiveness to sound
Development of receptive and expressive language skills

Responsiveness to Sound—Age-Related Behaviors

Auditory behavior is dependent upon the maturation of the nervous system. Therefore, the normal-hearing child's auditory behavior and response to sound is developmental. There is variability in the exact age at which a particular response becomes evident in hearing children with normal neuromotor development. The norms for different responses in hearing children, however, have been established, so we can guide the parents in their expectations concerning the time it takes for auditory behavior and to develop and the sequence it can be expected to follow after hearing aids have been fitted.

During the first four months of life, we observe that the infant with normal hearing will show response to speech at conversational loudness level but that noise maker toys will need to be somewhat louder to cause eye-widening or arousal (Table 14.1). The infant's responsivity to warbled pure tones, by contrast, is much less; these sounds do not attract attention until they are very loud. As the hearing child matures we observe lateral sound localization evidenced by headturning toward the sound source at 4–7 months. At the same time, listening behavior evidences the beginning of auditory attention. By the time the child is a year old, we can expect to see localization of a sound in all directions except directly overhead. Note also that attention is drawn to voice at only 8dB above normal hearing threshold levels and also to quiet noise makers. However, it will take another nine months before the responses to pure tones begin, at about 18 months, to approximate the units of normal adult hearing.

Comprehension of spoken language, the ability to identify a few common objects from the child's own environment, to follow some simple learned directions (e.g., "Where's David's eyes? Show mommy your eyes"; "Where's mommy/pussy cat/teddy bear?") usually develops around 2 years of age in the hearing child. Increasing sophistication in developmental abilities between 2 and 5 years of age permit the child to respond to an ever-widening range of object and picture identifications at quiet intensity levels and to follow increasingly complex directions. Pure tone audiometry using behavioral play activity can begin to provide fairly reliable responses at as young as $2\frac{1}{2}$ years of age, becoming increasingly valid as the child reaches 3 and 4 years.

Critical Periods. Knowledge of the developmental stages of hearing in the non–hearing-impaired child is important to the management of the

TABLE 14.1 Auditory behavior index for infants: stimulus and level of response*

Age	Noise Makers (Approx. SPL)	Warbled Pure Tones (Re: dB HL)	Speech (Re: dB HL)	Expected Response	Startle to Speech (Re: dB HL)
0–6 wk	50–70dB	78dB	40–60dB	Eye-widening, eye-blink, stirring or arousal from sleep, startle	65dB
6 wk–4 mo	50–60dB	70dB	47dB	Eye-widening, eye-shift, eye-blinking, quieting; beginning rudimentary head turn by 4 mo	65dB
4–7 mo	40–50dB	51dB	21dB	Head-turn on lateral plane toward sound; listening attitude	65dB
7–9 mo	30–40dB	45dB	15dB	Direct localization of sounds to side, indirectly below ear level	65dB
9–13 mo	25–35dB	38dB	8dB	Direct localization of sounds to side, directly below, ear level, indirectly above ear level	65dB
13–16 mo	25–30dB	32dB	5dB	Direct localization of sound on side, above, and below	65dB
16–21 mo	25dB	25dB	5dB	Direct localization of sound on side, above and below	65dB
21–24 mo	25dB	26dB	3dB	Direct localization of sound on side, above, and below	65dB

* Testing done in a sound room. (Modified from F. McConnell and P. H. Ward, *Deafness in Childhood.* Nashville, TN: Vanderbilt University Press, 1967.)

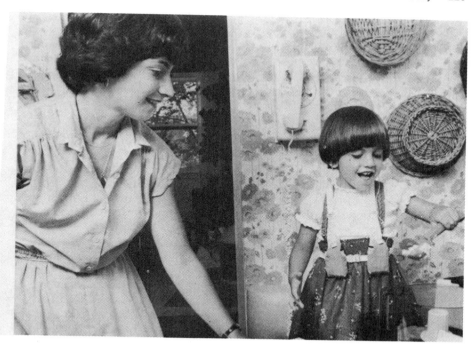

Figure 14.1 The parents should take every opportunity to reinforce and model the child's early utterances.

child with impaired hearing. The progressive stages of auditory development in the infant reflect the growing sophistication of the neural system. They also reflect neural learning—sensory systems evolve only in response to stimulation. Hearing impairment deprives the child of auditory stimulation. The result is an auditory system ill equipped to deal with stimuli even when amplification can make them available.

As a result, when sound is made available to the child's cochlear, it will at first evoke a minimal response. It takes 12–18 months of exposure to spoken language before the hearing child's system has developed the listening and cognitive processing sophistication for the spoken utterance of the first true word. Our hearing-impaired child is going to require time and a highly enriched spoken language environment if he is to make up for the lost stimulation.

Unfortunately, there is serious question as to whether the language delay resulting from auditory deprivation can be overcome completely. The concept of *critical periods* suggests that for an appropriate neural and cognitive ability to evolve, stimulation must be provided within a developmental age span when the system is programmed optimally to make use of it. Once this period passes, the system grows less and less capable of developing the ability:

The theory of critical periods states that there are certain periods in development when the organism is programmed to receive and utilize particular types of stimuli, and that subsequently the stimuli will have gradually diminishing potency in affecting the organism's development in the function represented. In the case of audition it means that a certain developmental stage auditory signals will be optimally received and utilized for important prelinguistic activities, but that once this stage has passed the effective utilization of these signals gradually declines. An analogous theory for language development holds that language input must be experienced at a certain stage, or it becomes decreasingly effective for utilization in emergent language skills (Northern & Downs, 1984, p. 106)

It would appear that the system is like play dough. When you first open the can, it is totally malleable; you can mold it any way you wish. As the days pass, particularly if the play dough is left out, it becomes less malleable, limiting the molding of fine details in the constructions you can make. To once more quote from Northern and Downs:

In the area of language for the signed deaf, where intensive training has been given in an attempt to remedy the language lag, only partial reversibility can be demonstrated when training is begun even as early as 2 yrs. But partial reversibility does not confer on the individual language functioning adequate to our complex life and its demands. (1984, p. 198)

In a cooperative working model with parents of hearing-impaired children, they too must understand the developmental stages in listening and the implications of the age of the child when intervention is begun. They join us as partners in stimulating, observing, assessing, and recording the child's auditory and early language progress following amplification.

Development of Auditory-Oral Language

Early vocal behavior appears to be driven internally rather than being externally stimulated. Around 2 months, the hearing child begins to utter strings of repeated sounds, apparently for pleasure. This indicates that the auditory feedback loop essential to further development has been activated (Northern & Downs, 1984). By 3 months of age the child is babbling, but not until 5–6 months do external models appear to influence the production of sounds (Northern & Downs, 1984). This suggests that hearing-impaired children will need, at a minimum, 6 months to activate and develop a system responsive to external models once those models become audible. We cannot rush natural development. Once this stage is reached, external stimulation forms the basis for natural language learning. Remember, however, that it will take yet another 6 months or more for the first word to appear in the hearing child. Two-word phrases will occur between 18–24 months while linguistic knowledge will continue to increase until about 5 years of age.

Determining the stage of language development reached by the very young child must depend heavily on careful observation, recording, and monitoring of the child's receptive and expressive language skills. This process can be facilitated by the use of such language scales and inventories as the Sequenced Inventory of Communication Development (Hedrick, Prather, & Tobin, 1975) with norms from $4-6\frac{1}{2}$ months, the Preschool Language Scale (Zimmerman, Steiner, & Evatt, 1979) and the verbal tests in the McCarthy Scales of Children's Abilities (McCarthy, 1972). Two tests, the Houston Test for Language Development Part 1 (Crabtree, 1958), which has norms from 6–36 months of age, and the Utah Test of Language Development (Mecham, Jex, & Jones, 1978) may help verify and qualify observations.

As we gather information about the child we need also to assess the parent's needs.

ASSESSING PARENTS' NEEDS

Any person confronted with a problem that affects her own health or well-being or that of a close family member experiences a need for support. This need is never more acute than when it is an infant or child who has the problem. A diagnosis of deafness or hearing impairment takes away from the "perfect child." It erases the parent's confident vision of parenthood and of their child's potential. They face instead an unknown future, or even worse, one constructed from a confusion of anecdotes and images based on information and misinformation. The first need of these shocked, confused, and anxious parents, therefore, is a sympathetic understanding of what they are experiencing.

Generally there is a gap between the time the audiologist or otolaryngologist informs the parents of the diagnosis and your first meeting with them to discuss what can be done for the child. In this time the initial protective numbness often begins to wear off, exposing the parents to the raw reality of an undefined but feared future. Any information given to them at the time of the diagnosis probably was not absorbed. Your first task, therefore, is to help the parents to understand, deal with, and modify in a productive manner the emotions resulting from the diagnosis. The guidelines for the initial management steps are

1. Provide Emotional Support. Whenever possible you should seek to provide a continuity of support from the time of the diagnostic evaluation. The parents need to know that they are not facing the problem alone, that sensitive caring professionals now share the seemingly awesome task of raising a "deaf child." I say "deaf" because many parents can think only of the category "deafness." They find it impossible, or at least difficult in the early stages, to focus on the fact that children with hearing problems are as different from one another as are children with normal hearing. Even when they know intellectually that there are many degrees of hearing impairment, parents often are unable to adjust their feelings to this reality. We, therefore, need to avoid the use of the term *deaf*, using instead *hearing impaired*.

At the initial visit you should strenuously avoid the temptation to tell the parents everything they need to know about impairment of hearing. Your primary goal should be to generate a feeling of quiet confidence.

Maliszewski (1988), the father of two profoundly deaf children, in his description of how the audiologist handled telling him of his second child's deafness, states with great simplicity: "Then he just sat with us and provided a sense of comfort" (p. 419). It is important that in your optimism about the potential that you know hearing-impaired children have for surmounting their handicap, you do not deny the pain the parents are experiencing nor their need to grieve. Do not try to be cheerful at a time when cheerfulness is inappropriate. Attempt rather to share the parent's feelings and to encourage their expression, which initially may be through crying or through a series of questions:

"Why did this have to happen?"
"What did I do wrong?"
"What caused this awful thing?"
"What am I supposed to do?"

These questions are rhetorical—accept them as such; accept them but do not attempt to answer them or, worse yet, to deny their justification. At this time do not attempt to reassure the parents that things really are not as bad as they seem, for to the parents, they are indeed as they seem. Avoid telling them of the great things that can be achieved, for in grieving the lost normality parents are not yet ready to even think about the future, certainly not to take up the challenge of a handicapped child.

A parent may make a series of statements such as

"We had such plans for David; now they're all spoiled."
"Everything's hopeless—I just can't cope with this on top of everything else. It's not fair."

The emotion that accompanies these statements, often with the lack of eye contact, should alert you to the fact that answers are not sought. The need to verbalize undefined emotions in the early sessions often is paramount. Just expressing those feelings and having them accepted without comment permits them to be vented and reduces their debilitating effect.

Beyond the common need to deal with feelings, the perceptions of parents confronted with this diagnosis will be highly individualistic. Maliszewski (1988) goes so far as to suggest that "the only shared experience understood by all parents of deaf children is an underlying sorrow often manifest throughout their lives" (p. 417). Therefore, avoid general statements or the giving of general advice; concentrate on listening and on helping the parents to express feelings, concerns, and needs.

2. Identify Resources. You and the parents must ensure that the intervention plan you develop is realistic, that it can be carried out. For this to be achieved, you must be sure that the necessary resources are available. As audiologists, speech-language pathologists, and special education teachers, we will provide a lot of specialized resources, yet these alone will not suffice. We must know what complementary resources the family can provide without undue strain. These will vary greatly from family to family, and from time to time for a given family. The goal is to ensure that demands stay within the limits of total resources. This process requires us to monitor circumstances carefully so that when demands exceed capacity we either locate extra resources or revise our goals. Resources include

Family Resources. No longer can we presume that a family consists of mother, father, and siblings living together with supplementary support from grandparents. We need to know how many persons will be contributing to family support.

- Is the father present in the family?
- Does he have an active interest in the child?
- Does he spend time with the child?
- Is the father on shift work?
- Is he at home during the day?
- Does the mother work full time?
- Is the child in day care?
- Is the mother remarried?
- Does the second husband relate positively to the child?
- Is there an unrelated male in the family?
- Does he provide support to the mother in the task of raising her children?
- Are there older siblings or stepchildren who relate well to the child?
- Are grandparents nearby?
- Are they supportive?

Do not fire these questions at a parent in the manner of an interrogation, but lead the discussion in ways that legitimize the topic being raised.

Financial Resources. Financial resources can contribute greatly to facilitate a program, while their lack may present difficulty in achieving goals. We are not entitled to inquire about actual assets. We do need, however, to ensure that bringing a child to therapy five days a week; purchasing appropriate toys, books, supplies, and hearing aid batteries; and getting a hearing aid repaired, a new mold made, or a second hearing aid do not represent financial demands that exceed resources. Such a situation will create guilt, sometimes shame, and even avoidance of the program.

Time Resources. Availability of time to bring the child for habilitation and for carrying out activities at home may be a problem for some parents who lack other resources. Time and financial demands often go together. Parents who have financial commitments to make mortgage or car payments, for example, often must work to meet those demands; single parents usually have no choice but to work. Work commitments may reduce time resources to the point where a parent cannot attend therapy sessions and time spent with the child at home may be limited. Both situations must be accepted as part of the parent's reality, and not condemned. We must help to explore productive ways of dealing with the need and avoid blaming the parent for limitations in meeting it.

Ability Resources. Not every parent has the good fortune to have well-developed intellectual, educational, and emotional resources. We must be careful to ensure that our plan for intervention does not ask more of the parents than they comfortably can understand, carry out, and accept emotionally.

Language Resources. With the heterogeneous population that constitutes our society today, we need to be prepared to manage situations in which English is not the language of the home. We need to know to what extent the parents/family are able and willing to communicate in English when the child is present as well as addressing the child in English. We need to be creative in working out ways to provide an English-speaking environment for the child while respecting the parents' language and culture. Regardless of our concern for the infant's needs, it is not our child. Until the child reaches school age, the parents will decide what course shall be pursued. We must give them the help to choose wisely and we must accept their choice even when it would not be the one we think we would make.

Legal Resources. The legal right to special education and related services constitutes a powerful resource for parents of disabled children of preschool age. Prior to 1986 the Education for All Handicapped Children Act (PL 94-142) mandated the special services that must be provided for all disabled children aged 3–18. This law was amended in 1986 to require that special education and related services be provided to children ages 3–21 in all states receiving federal support to education. A subsection of this act (Part H, Section VIII) passed in 1990 as part of Public Law 99-457 extended protection to infants and toddlers from birth through two years of age. The law gave states five years to establish statewide, appropriate early intervention services. Such services must be delivered through a system of coordinated comprehensive and multidisciplinary interagency programs. The services must provide for the child's physical, cognitive, language, speech, and psychosocial development, as well as self-help skills. Among the services that may be included are

- Family training, counseling, and home visits
- Special instruction
- Speech pathology and audiology
- Occupational therapy
- Physical therapy
- Psychological services
- Case management services
- Medical services confined to diagnosis or evaluation
- Early identification (Tucker & Goldstein, 1991, p. 13.20)

Case management is a particularly important service; Tucker and Goldstein (1991) describe it thus:

> "Case management" means activities conducted by a case manager to assist a Part H child and the child's family to receive the rights, procedural safeguards and services available under the states early intervention program. Under Part H, each eligible child and his or her family must be provided with a case manager who is responsible for (i) coordinating all services across agency lines; (ii) serving as the single point of contact in helping parents to obtain the services and assistance they need. (p. 13.21)

The case management services cited by Tucker and Goldstein (1991) include

- Coordinating the performance of evaluations and assessments
- Facilitating and participating in the development, review, and evaluation of individualized family service plans

- Assisting families in identifying available service providers
- Coordinating and monitoring the delivery of available services
- Informing families of the availability of advocacy services
- Coordinating medical and health providers
- Facilitating the development of a transition plan to preschool services, if appropriate. (p. 13.21)

For each child an Individualized Family Service Plan (IFSP) must be developed. This emphasizes the focus on the family. It accords perfectly with the model of management I advocate in this text. The IFSP must include

- A statement of the infant's or toddler's present level of development
- A statement of the family's needs, resources, priorities, and concerns
- A statement of the major goals for the child and family (as well as criteria procedures and time lines used to determine progress)
- A statement of specific early intervention services to meet the unique needs of the child and family
- A statement of the natural environments in which early intervention services are to be provided
- Projected dates for initiation and anticipated duration of services
- The name of the case manager (service coordinator)
- The steps to be taken to support transition to services available to three year olds and above. (Tucker & Goldstein, 1991, p. 13.22)

Parental consent in writing must be obtained before evaluation or service to the child and family may be initiated, though this requirement can be overridden if due process hearings are pursued successfully by a public agency. Parental objections or concerns may be resolved according to due process procedures established for disabled school-age children or by recourse to an impartial decision maker. The law thus insists on a family-centered management model for infants and toddlers with disabilities. It is not intended that the needs of these children be provided *in* agency-based environments. The act requires that

To the maximum extent appropriate, services should be provided in natural environments including the home, and community settings in which children without disabilities participate. (PL 102-119, 1991)

This is the model upon which this chapter is based.

3. Negotiate the Load. It is essential to allow parents to guide us in terms of the load they can bear effectively throughout the period during which we work together with their child. What we feel parents need or should do is, in reality, irrelevant. Effective intervention will occur only when it is in accord with what the parents understand, are able to support, and can manage. I have had the personal experience of having a mother pull a highly successful child out of a program because she felt left out of the process, shut off from her child, and, therefore, devalued as a parent. This does not mean that you should not offer guidance. Indeed your role is to assist the parents in finding a way through the complications and difficulties they will encounter throughout the child's preschool years. As you gain experience you will begin to be familiar with the general map of the preschool terrain across which the child with impaired hearing must travel. You will know where to turn for resources and ways to avoid or surmount particular obstacles. You will learn that for some children certain routes prove extremely difficult to navigate, while others progress easily. You will not know, however, which of several options available is most appropriate for a particular child until you know him and those who will support him.

4. Identify Need for Information. Explain to the parents that there is information you will want to share with them and information that they can provide to guide you. First, however, stress the importance of addressing their immediate concerns:

"There are so many things I want to share with you about hearing impairment, and in time and I'll do that, but first I want to know what your immediate concerns are. Perhaps I can lessen some of the anxiety you must be feeling."

The parents expressed concerns should be dealt with as simply, factually, and nonjudgmentally as possible. Luterman (1987) stresses the importance of recognizing that one of several needs may motivate a particular question. He urges us to "take a moment to determine the feeling behind the question" (p. 317). Webster (1977) helps us to do this by categorizing questions as

Requests for Facts.

Question: "Should she wear the hearing aid all the time?"
"Does Angela hear better with two aids?"

Try to respond to requests for facts and information concisely without the use of jargon or complex explanations.

Response: "Yes, the longer she wears the hearing aids, the sooner she will begin to understand speech."
"Definitely, the audiologist's results indicate that the aids really make a difference to her response to sound with the two aids. Try to see if you can notice a difference."

Requests for Opinions.

Question: "Do you think she can learn to talk?"
"Do you feel it would be a good idea to have another audiologist test her?"

If possible avoid giving opinions. Try to respond to seeking clarification.

Response: "Are you afraid she will need to use sign language?"

Or by interpreting a possible deeper question.

"You seem to be worried about Mary's progress in talking." "Do you feel the audiologic test results we have are not a true measure of Mary's hearing?"
"You seem to be dissatisfied with the way Mary was tested."

Requests for Clarification.

Question: "Do you mean I should move her around with me as I do the household chores?"
"Are you suggesting it might be better if I could leave her with a neighbor rather than at the day-care center?"

Answer these questions "yes" or "no"; then explain what you meant.

Response: "Yes, that way you can show her and talk to her about what you are doing."
"Yes, I think a willing neighbor would be able to spend more time with Jane and would talk to her more than the staff of a busy day-care center."

Requests for Discussion.

Question: "I need to talk about Michael's temper tantrums."
"I don't know what to do about enrolling him in all-day kindergarten."
"What do other parents do?"

These should be responded to by taking time out to talk about the situation.

5. Provide Informational Support. Parent questions are excellent guides to the information needed in order to deal with the situation as it is currently perceived. Giving information when you are not sure that the mother or father understands the need for it, or is not yet able to accept or make use of it, is a waste of time. Initially, concern will be for information that enables the parents to understand what the diagnosis of "deaf" or "hard-of-hearing" means in terms of:

- What their son can hear
- What effects the hearing aid(s) will have
- Whether the condition will improve
- How normally their daughter will function
- Whether their daughter will talk
- Whether their son will be able to go to a regular school

Since you can only speculate about the answers to these questions, it is important first to acknowledge the underlying need for reassurance. Then relate the question to the actions we and the parents can take to increase the chances of the child's achieving what is hoped for. For example, consider a response to the question, "What can my son hear?" This is a request for facts. We may explain briefly that environmental and speech sounds have a pattern of pitches, that is, frequency components, some of which are stronger than others. To hear the sound clearly it is necessary to hear all the parts of the pattern at a comfortable loudness level. Using test results, perhaps not yet an audiogram, you can indicate how well the child appears to hear low-, middle-, and high-pitched sounds without and with the hearing aids. You can point out, however, that there are other characteristics to sounds, both environmental and speech, that the child may well learn to use. Such characteristics include how sounds begin differently (onset), how long they last (duration), or how they repeat (pattern). Then you can relate this information to actions the parents can take. Urge them to begin to

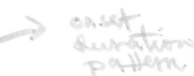

experiment with sounds, as we will consider later, developing a daily diary profiling their child's reactions.

In response to the question, "Will my daughter learn to talk?," you first must check that the question is a request for opinion rather than for a discussion of feelings. Often parents reject the threatening image of "deaf and dumb," seeking reassurance that this will not apply to their child. So you ask, "Are you afraid that Jenny may need extra support from signs?" This question opens up a discussion of supplementary or alternative means of communication. It leads to a(an)

- Exploration of what is necessary for spoken language to develop
- Review of resources
- Assessment of probabilities based on a comparison of needs and resources
- Discussion of sign language as a viable alternative to spoken language as the primary learning and communicating method

It is not possible to anticipate every question you may encounter, even less possible to consider them here. My purpose is to show you how to deal with questions, how to classify them, and how to provide information as appropriate, and whenever possible, how to address the issue in question with a plan for practical action in which the parents can follow or participate.

6. Address Audiologic Needs. As the speech-language therapist or special education teacher, you should expect to supplement the instructional counseling given to the parents of the preschool hearing-impaired child by the audiologist. Learning to take care of the child's amplification needs takes time and requires encouragement. Once the diagnosis of sensorineural impairment has been made, "it becomes essential that the focus be shifted from the hearing loss to the child's usable residual hearing" (Matkin, 1977 p. 127). As we have seen, the task of coming to terms with having a hearing-handicapped child places heavy emotional demands on the parents. You can understand how hard it is for many parents to broadcast their child's deficiency by having her wear the stigma symbol of hearing aids.

This particularly is true when a body aid is fitted. An initially negative reaction to the child's wearing a hearing aid should be accepted as normal and reasonable. Even hearing specialists, despite their knowledge, probably would experience the same feelings, though they would either conceal them or seek to work them through. Many parents also conceal such feelings. In some cases the aid may only be put on the child in the privacy of the home, or only when visiting the center for parent guidance. Any number of excuses may be offered to explain the child's nonuse of the aid, including: "It does not fit well," "She keeps pulling it off," "It hurts his ear," "It pulls on his clothing," "I am afraid she will lose it." Such objections most often are justified by a valid reason. Therefore, you must investigate and attend to each objection. When the complaints appear not to be justified objectively, then you can assume that equally valid subjective reasons lie behind them. You should, therefore, help the parents explore their feelings about the aid and what it signifies. Try to bring underlying attitudes to the surface. Accept the parents' feelings but do everything possible to separate them from the child's critical need for amplification. This particularly is necessary because you have shared responsibility for meeting the child's needs; failure to do so now will result in enormous feelings of guilt later. Make sure that the need for amplification as the keystone in the intervention program is both understood and accepted by the parents.

Perhaps the easiest way to try to understand needs in a general sense is to ask yourself what would you want for your child should you be told he were deaf or hard-of-hearing. Most probably you would want him to

- Be able to hear
- Talk
- Go to a regular school like other children

Assuming you attain these goals, you will want to

- Understand the nature of your child's problem
- Know the effects of the problem on what he can hear
- Know how his language and speech will be affected
- Understand how his learning will be affected

Finally, you will want to know what can be done to give him the best chance to hear, to speak, and to learn and what you can do to help. These identified needs provide us with a guide for intervention.

INTERVENTION PROCEDURES

The type of service we can provide to the very young hearing-impaired preschool child and family will be determined by the life-style of the parents. As has been discussed, family structure and the role of women have changed and continue to do so radically. It used to be true that mother was the primary person with whom the child spent the day until kindergarten age or even first grade. In today's world this remains true for less than half of all preschool children and that percentage continues to decrease. The complexities of present-day family arrangements include single-parent families, sometimes with the father having custody of the child, while other children live in families with stepparents and stepbrothers and stepsisters. This is why you need to know the nature and extent of family resources. It would be unwise, for example, to adopt a philosophy that insists that a mother should stay home with her hearing-impaired child. Although you may believe this represents the optimal preschool learning situation, it usually is unrealistic, impractical, even impossible. Therefore, in discussing how we can optimize the child's learning potential, we must adapt it to the family situation. We may need to guide and assist a grandmother or neighbor who cares for the child during the day. We may need to contact a daytime baby-sitter or day-care center. We should strive to develop a model that builds the parents' belief that what is being done is the best that can be provided, given the reality of the situation. However, regardless of who the main caregiver is, parent involvement will be important.

Ideally a parent guidance program involves the parent, child, teacher of the hearing impaired, and/or speech-language therapist in cooperation with the audiologist, in frequent regular learning sessions. Many preschool guidance programs have evolved to provide this maximal support. The sessions consist of the demonstration of child stimulation methods and of learning experiences for the parent under the supportive guidance of the professional.

For parents who find it difficult to attend such regular parent guidance sessions because of employment, transportation problems, distance, or other family commitments, the John Tracy Correspondence Course for Parents of Preschool Deaf Children can prove of great help. Indeed the course can be valuable as an enrichment source for parents of preschoolers who are in a program for hearing-impaired children. In such instances the speech-language pathologist or teacher of hearing-impaired children will need to integrate the Tracy program materials and activities with those planned in the preschool. The course is published in many languages, accommodating the needs of minority families. It maybe obtained from The John Tracy Clinic, 806 West Adams Boulevard, Los Angeles, CA 90007.

Goals of Parent/Caregiver Education

It is most important that the parents understand that you do not wish them to become teachers in the academic sense of the word. It is even more important to avoid working with them in a manner that might imply that this is your goal. The purpose of parent/caregiver education is to modify behaviors in everyday activities to optimize opportunities for the growth of thought, language, and communication in the child. Nevertheless, parents are natural teachers. The importance of "natural teaching" was stressed some 70 years ago by the Russian psychologist Vygotski (1962). His work is having a profound influence on current research into cognitive development learning and teaching. Tharp and Gallimore (1989a) state:

> It is now clear that long before they enter school children are being "taught" higher cognitive and linguistic skills. Their teaching takes place in the everyday interactions of domestic life. Within these goal directed activities the teaching consists of more-capable family and friends assisting children to do things the children cannot do alone. In such teaching, the subjects of direct instruction are the tasks themselves, not communication or thinking skills *per se*. Yet the pleasures of the social interaction seem sufficient to lure a child into learning the language and cognition of the caregiver. (p. 22)

Horton (1974, p. 483) defined five general categories of program objectives for early intervention with young hearing-impaired children:

1. To help parents learn to optimize the auditory environment for their child
2. To help them learn how to talk to their child
3. To familiarize them with the principles, stages, and sequence of normal language development and how to apply this frame of reference in stimulating their child
4. To demonstrate strategies of behavior management
5. To supply effective support to aid the family in coping with their feelings about their child and the stresses that a handicapped child places on the integrity of the family

Stimulating the Use of Hearing

This topic addresses the aspiration, "I want my child to be able to hear" and the question, "What does she hear?" It is difficult to document reliably the degree of residual hearing in many infants and toddlers; it is even more difficult to predict the potential use of residual hearing. Yet each of us involved with the hearing-impaired child seeks to optimize auditory potential. We have seen that the initial fitting of a hearing aid or aids on the very young child must be considered a trial. The prescription is tentative and exploratory. Adjustments will need to be made as more information about the amount and configuration of the residual hearing becomes available. Equally important to the assessment of amplification needs and the appropriateness of an exploratory prescription is observation of the effects amplification has on the child's behavior. This is where the parent or primary caregiver, the audiologist, and teacher/therapist all need to cooperate in a combined auditory stimulation and assessment program. Formal audiologic findings should be augmented and evaluated by you, the teacher/therapist, during parent/child guidance, and equally important, they should be supplemented by careful monitoring of the child's auditory behavior by the parents at home. Together, you and they will seek to stimulate and document the following behaviors.

1. Awareness to Sound. Infants and toddlers with severe to profound hearing impairment often are not aware of sound. As a result the auditory system develops neither neural networking nor the appropriate behavioral responses. Parents need to be sensitive to the child's response or lack of response. A baseline profile of auditory response behavior to sounds in the home, therefore, should be obtained. After explaining the picture you wish to obtain, identify the normally occurring sounds that comprise the child's acoustic environment. You might explain:

> What we need first is to know which sounds occur frequently at home, sounds Jane would be expected to be hearing if she had no problem. For example, your voice is a sound your baby will be close to often, talking, singing, calling. We need to learn if Jane ever indicates that she hears you when she has no other clues to your presence. That is, when she did not see you, feel you, or sense vibrations on the crib or highchair. Other sounds might be other people's voices, the dog barking, noise-making toys, appliances such as the dishwasher, washing machine, vacuum cleaner, the telephone, a car or truck outside. We need to know whether she ever responds to these sounds and if so were they loud or not so loud.

Awareness of sound may be indicated by several response behaviors. These involve changes generally evidenced by the child's becoming less active when busily occupied with something and more active when she is quiet at the time the sound occurs. The simplest is a change in the behavior state of activity, such as interruption of movement or sucking, or it may be the initiation of crying or sometimes a temporary cessation. More specific responses include eye widening, a turning of the eyes, or a rapid eye-blink. Ideally we would like to observe the difference between auditory response behavior without and with the hearing aid, though the latter information is, of course, the more valuable.

In addition to noticing the infant's response to naturally occurring sounds, we will encourage the parents to control sound sources, that is, deliberately causing the noise in order to note reactions. Voice is the most meaningful sound to the infant; it is also a stimulus for which intensity can be varied from loud to soft. Most controllable sound sources, voice included, can be varied in intensity by causing them to occur close to or at a distance from the infant.

Thus the question "Will she be able to hear?" translates into parent involvement in "Let's determine *what* she can hear." The observations we (the audiologist, parent, speech-language pathologist, and special education teacher) make then can be reexplained in terms of audiologic data. For example, we can compare observed behavioral responses to responses obtained to bursts of narrow band noise with different center frequencies, and at different intensities, to pure tones, to voice, and to noise makers with known frequency spectra. In this way the parents gain a realistic picture of what the child is responding to auditorily, and how the responses are increased by amplification.

2. Orientation to Sound. A somewhat more sophisticated yet still basic auditory response behavior involves orienting the auditory system to the sound. We achieve this through localization, which optimizes the signal to be processed. This also constitutes a low level of attention. Localization involves processing the difference or absence of difference in the acoustic signal arriving at the two ears. The perceived differences arise from the angle of each ear to the sound source and the distance between each ear and the sound source. When the signal is directly in front or behind the head, the signal will be identical at each ear. As the head or sound source moves out of this relationship, one ear will begin to be at an advantage to receive the signal. The advantaged ear will receive the sound sooner than the other ear. The signal will not have traveled as far to the advantaged ear, which means that it will be strongest at that ear. Moreover, the effect of the acoustic shadow caused by the head's being placed more and more between the nonadvantaged ear and the sound source will further reduce the intensity of the sound at that ear. For this effect to produce accurate sound localization, it will be necessary for the child to have at least some binaural hearing and to be fit with binaural hearing aids. The observed behavior will be searching with eyes and/or head for the direction of the sound. Turning directly toward the sound source, localization, is a more advanced and definitive response occurring in the normally hearing infant between four to six months of age. Once again the parents can supplement audiologic test results by observing the child's behavior. They should be encouraged to note the presence or absence of the auditory search response to naturally occurring sounds at home. Parents and teacher/therapist also can introduce sounds outside the child's visual field, to one side or the other, while suspending briefly other activity with the child. When an infant has a single hearing aid worn in one ear, he usually will search consistently to the aided side regardless of the location of the sound.

3. Seeking to Identify the Sound Source. Sound detection indicates awareness of an acoustic event exterior to the self. Overlapping and progressing from this behavior is a desire to locate the sound source and to know its nature. When this occurs the child has learned that sound is referential. The child hears a sound and wants to identify the object or person who is causing it. The response behavior may be suspension of activity in an expectant manner, or it may involve reaching of a hand or hands, excitement, and perhaps vocalization. Parents can stimulate the realization of the referential nature of sound by making objects (hand bells, rattles, noise-making toys, etc.) cause sound. This first should be done so that the child can see the source, then by holding the object out of sight and repeating the sound event again. Finally the sound making should occur again so the child can see its source. As the child grows we can help her to cause the object to produce sound.

4. Paying Attention to the Sound. Sound events, including speech, need to be paid attention to in order to be processed properly. We call this listening. Listening behavior in an infant or young child relates to information processing, to finding out about the sound source, to cognition. It is a behavior that should be looked for, noted, and encouraged. We need to show the parents how to model attentive listening, allowing the child to hear the sound and then to explore the object up close. Great interest should be shown in the sound source, which the child should be encouraged to handle if possible and to explore by other senses. We should verbalize what she sees and feels as well as what she hears. Boothroyd (1982) urges parents to be the child's "auditory watchdog" (p. 99) noting the quieter sounds occurring, such as water running, and the ticking of a clock. He tells us we must be alert to the sounds made by the child's own activities, such as banging a spoon or spinning the wheels on a toy. We should isolate these sounds from the activity as a whole and listen to them attentively.

Optimizing the Auditory Environment

This objective is worked toward first by focusing the parents' attention on the sounds that occur naturally in the home environment. Since early-language acquisition arises from events observed, objects that make noise in the home provide a natural basis for the child's early experiences with amplified sound. They also give rise to verbal comment:

> Listen. Oh, what a lot of noise! It's the blender.
> Oh, the telephone is ringing.
> That's the doorbell. Someone's at the door.
> Look. Mommy's going to turn off the alarm clock.
> Daddy's home. Listen, hear the car?

Parents should be encouraged to take the child with them when responding to environmental sounds. When the phone rings, suggest that they take the infant to the phone, let it ring several times while they point first to it then to an ear indicating that they hear it. Then they should say, "The phone is ringing. Hear the phone?" They should treat the dog barking, the water filling the bathtub, the toilet flushing, and the lawn mower being used in the backyard in the same way. Parents can anticipate or create environmental sounds for the child to listen to in the presence of the sound-generating object or event—they can wait for the clock to chime or make the whistling kettle boil, the alarm clock ring, the paper bag pop, the doorbell ring, the cup and saucer rattle, the spoon bang, the saucepan drop. The child needs to become aware of the world of sound, limited or distorted though it may be. The child needs to learn the referential function of sound. Your role is to convey to the parents that they need to orient the child to sound so that the child learns its value, begins to pay attention to it, and makes use of it in predicting events that he or she cannot see. You must guide the parents specifically in how to choose sounds that are likely to be significant to the child. This is why awareness of the child's daily experiences is so important. The sounds selected for special attention should

- Have a pitch and loudness that the child can hear
- Arise from experiences that have significance to the child
- Originate from objects with which the child is familiar
- Occur frequently in or around the house
- When possible, be capable of being started and stopped by the child

The parents must be shown how to respond to the sounds in a consistent manner that motivates the child to want to participate in the listening, discriminating, learning, doing activity. They can do this by visual and verbal communication. The parent ceases activity when the sound is made, adopts a listening attitude by placing a finger at the ear, pauses, gives a look of puzzlement followed quickly by happy enlightenment, then identifies the sound source. Initially it will be necessary to take the child to the sound source; later the child will begin to respond to the acoustic referent and to adopt recognition behaviors, indicating learning has occurred. Babies should be taken to the source of the sound and be allowed to observe the parents' response behaviors. Both parents need to be encouraged to become involved in these behaviors. Taking as an example a family in which the father works outside the home and the mother does not, when the father arrives home he should blow the car horn when he gets out of the car and the mother should try to anticipate the arrival: "Daddy's coming soon. Where's Daddy? He's coming. There's Daddy. I hear him. Let's go see." He should ring the doorbell, repeating long rings several times in a pattern code that will become identified with him. He should call loudly when he comes in, "Hello, I'm home, where's my Sarah?" The father should familiarize Sarah with the sounds of his activities around the house—for example, using an electric razor. Unfortunately fathers are too frequently not brought into the parent training, which is assumed to be the mother's responsibility. Because you are aiming to mold the family environment, you must involve the father in a manner compatible with his normal daily contacts with his children and in terms of his normal home activities.

Developing Auditory Discrimination and Recognition

Auditory discrimination and recognition means hearing the differences among sounds and using those differences to evoke the perception of the sound-making person, object, or event on the basis of the acoustic information. For the hearing-impaired child, the information will be incomplete. Some sounds may not auditorily be discriminable from others with similar spectra; however, durational and repetitional characteristics often make discrimination possible after much experience with the sound. Stimulating activities may be created using different sound-making objects or toys in a play situation. For example, when the doorbell rings, the parent can move toward the telephone with the child, shake his head to indicate the mistake, and then move to the door.

Developing Auditory Behavior

The goal of all the described activities is to attempt to develop auditory behavior in the child. Auditory behavior reflects a way of relating to the environment. It is predicated upon the usefulness of sound. I could not endorse more strongly Boothroyd's (1982, p. 104) reminder that every activity must ensure that the auditory behavior is productive, useful, and rewarding to the child. Listening for sounds that serve no purpose encourages the ignoring of sound. The guidelines for auditory stimulation are

Be particularly alert to naturally occurring sounds.

Exaggerate listening behaviors. Look attentive, puzzled; point to your ear; look around; express on your face enlightenment on recognition of the sound and pleasure in locating it.

Make a point of repeating this behavior often to commonly occurring sounds in the house.

Ensure something positive happens when a sound is located—this may be your obvious delight or pleasure, or it may mean a big hug for the child.

Arrange play situations that involve sound-making objects.

Compare and contrast sounds. Make exaggerated errors in sound discrimination then reject your choice to make the correct one.

Draw the child's attention to sounds made by her own activities (banging, splashing, spinning a toy).

THE COMMUNICATION DILEMMA

To this point in our discussion, the need to stimulate the use of residual hearing and the development of an auditory processing capability in the child has been our primary concern. Such a position needs no justification, for every child needs to know the world to the limit of his senses; this includes the deaf child. The development of awareness and meaningful response to the world of sound greatly enhances a child's total experience, since sound is an inseparable part of sound-making objects or events. This cannot be more true than when the sounds are made by people, particularly members of one's family. Stimulation of residual hearing is, therefore, not a contested goal. The problem arises when the parents ask, "But will my child learn to speak?" Consider first what the question implies. It suggests that the most obvious symptom of hearing impairment, other than visible hearing aids, is the inability of a child or adult to speak normally and to communicate effectively in the hearing world. People who cannot do this are unlike the rest of us; they are "not normal," "deaf." Second, the question embodies recognition that those who cannot communicate easily and effectively through speech must learn another language. Alternate language systems are seen by parents as separating their child communicatively, socially, and culturally from the mainstream of the hearing world. The parents realize that their child will be cut off even from them unless they and other family members become fluent in an alternative communication system. They worry that unless the child learns to talk, he will not be able to attend the regular public school with "normal" children, an aspiration most parents of hearing-impaired children rank highly. These are natural feelings experienced by almost all hearing parents who give birth to a child with severely impaired hearing. How should we react to them?

The goal, as always, must be to provide support to the parents as they struggle to learn about, make decisions about, and come to terms with the significance of a diagnosis of hearing impairment. You may have strong feelings about a particular method of communication for severely to profoundly hearing-impaired children. However, ethics demand that the parents, not you, decide what is best for their child. To achieve this, parents need as much information as possible about factors that influence the development of spoken language learning in hearing-impaired children.

The Auditory Verbal-Oral Method

The auditory verbal-oral method of education is based on the conviction that most hearing-impaired children, including those with severe to profound hearing impairments, can learn to communication orally and can be educated through the use of spoken language.

> Most hearing-impaired children can learn to speak and understand spoken language if they are given adequate opportunity to do so. (Ling & Ling, 1978, p. 1)

The method maximizes the utilization of residual hearing through optimal amplification. A few professionals advocate auditory-oral purism (Pollack, 1970), placing no conscious emphasis on speech-reading (lip-reading). They believe that stimulation of the deprived auditory system requires that it alone be the focus of emphasis until it has been established as the primary modality for speech processing. More commonly, oralists subscribe to a multisensory approach in which maximal use is made of all sensory modalities in the development of speech. In this method speech-reading assumes considerable importance as a source of information, while tactile and motor kinesthetic stimulation provides supportive avenues for spoken language acquistion. In both approaches rich intensive stimulation, drawing the child's attention to both naturally occurring and controlled events, is important. The parents are encouraged to narrate for the child in simple language what is happening to and around her. The benefits of effective auditory-oral communication are great. When the method succeeds with a child, the advantages include the ability to function and compete in the hearing world; to take advantage of most of the education, professional, and social opportunities that require oral communication; and to choose a hearing partner in marriage without causing family concern. Unfortunately such opportunities prove not to be realistic for many persons with severe to profound hearing impairment. When the auditory oral method cannot provide a viable communication system, the cost is extremely high. The profoundly hearing-impaired child receives only a very small part, and in some cases none, of the rich auditory information in which the hearing child is bathed constantly. The reality of sound, its referential function and its meaning, rather than being learned naturally, must be taught. Speech is a weak and distorted sound pattern decipherable only within tight situational constraints and with rich supplementary visual cues. Consequently acquisition of language through speech perception is slow and laborious. At a concrete level the child may show progress in naming people and objects, but those language constructs that enable us to acquire abstract thought present an extremely difficult learning task. Since experience, cognition, and language processing are symbiotic functions, a child delayed in language necessarily will be impaired in the ability to know and think about the world and himself.

The teaching of speech also represents a very demanding challenge to the child and the parent/teacher. To be useful speech must be intelligible. In the hearing child this is achieved through auditory and motor kinesthetic self-monitoring and by comparison with external models. Both are at best extremely limited for the deaf child, thus he is unable to acquire, monitor, and self-correct his speech without intensive help. The result may be speech that is difficult to understand. Lacking adequate spoken language skills, the profoundly hearing-impaired child faces difficulty in actively participating in the learning process, asking questions, offering perceptions, and recounting experience. Needs are difficult to express; failure leads to great frustration for parent and child with resulting emotional outbursts on both sides. The child needs to communicate about fears and anxieties; about being left alone unable to hear mother downstairs; about darkness, monsters, and big dogs, and about hurts and pains. Such difficulties suggest that all profoundly hearing-impaired children need something other than an oral system of teaching. That opinion is held by many. However, despite all the difficulties described, some severely and profoundly hearing-impaired children become effective oral communicators. It is to this hope that most hearing parents of such children cling during the child's early years. Predictions concerning whether a child will be successful in learning by an oral approach alone or whether supplementary use of sign in a total-communication approach are difficult to make since so many variables are involved. Downs (1974) attempted to take the significant variables into account in a scale suggested as a guide to a child's future potential for oral

TABLE 14.2 Suggested scale for deafness management quotient (DMQ)—total: 100 points

Residual hearing: 30 points possible
   0 = no true hearing
  10 = 250–500 < 100 dB   Add 10 points for conductive
  20 = 250–500–100 < 100 dB   element to hearing loss
  30 = 2000 < 100 dB
Central intactness; 30 points possible
   0 = diagnosis of brain damage
  10 = known history of events conducive to birth defects
  20 = perceptual dysfunction
  30 = intact central processing
Intellectual factors: 20 points possible
   0 = MR < 85 IQ
  10 = average 85–100 IQ
  20 = above average: >100 IQ
  Family constellation: 10 points possible
   0 = no support
  10 = completely supportive and understanding
Socioeconomic: 10 points possible
   0 = substandard
  10 = completely adequate
Auditory program leading to oral: 81–100 points
Total communicative program: 0–80 points

(Downs, 1974.)

success. The formula she used (Table 14.2) includes a weighted assessment of five contributing influences: residual hearing, central intactness, intellectual factors, family constellation, and socioeconomic level. Residual hearing and central nervous system intactness each have a maximum possible score of 30 points, the other three factors have a possible score of 10 points each with an extra 10 points added if there is a conductive component to the impairment making a possible *deafness management quotient* (DMQ) of 110 points. A score of 80–110 suggests potential for success in an oral program; fewer than 80 points suggests that a total-communication model should be used. In a study of the validity of the DMQ as a predictive device, Luterman and Chasin (1981) concluded that it was a valid tool for distinguishing oral from total-communication candidates. Geers and Moog (1987) also sought to develop a tool for predicting the potential of profoundly hearing-impaired children to develop functional spoken language. They recognize the importance of such a tool at the initial placement stage of a child when a decision must be made as to the most appropriate mode of communication to be used. They stress also the need for constant monitoring of the child's progress if the auditory-oral mode is chosen. Geers and Moog developed the *Spoken Language Predictor Index* in an attempt to surmount the following inadequacies inherent in the deafness management quotient developed by Downs (1974):

> The audiogram is not the best predictor of potential for use of residual hearing since it reflects neither potential benefit from amplification nor speech discrimination.

The identification of factors contributing to central dysfunction is inadequate, and objective evidence of dysfunction is absent.

There is no means for differentiating between mentally retarded (IQ < 70) and borderline (IQ 71–85) children, nor any extra credit for very high IQ scores.

There is weak definition of both socioeconomic status and parental support. There is a lack of intermediate educational recommendations between a pure oral method and total-communication method with no provision for a diagnostic teaching category.

The Geers and Moog predictor, like the deafness management quotient, assesses five factors, each with a weighted value:

1. Hearing capacity (30 points). Four performance levels are identified.
   a. No pattern discrimination of speech (i.e., cup versus lunchbox)
   b. Pattern perception ranging from minimal closed set discrimination to the ability to use suprasegmental information, but no vowel or consonant discrimination
   c. Limited discrimination of words in closed set
   d. Consistent discrimination in small closed sets (words, phrases, durational and stress patterns).

   Aided articulation score. Categories correspond to the ranges of the Monosyllable Trochee Syllable Test (MST) (Erber & Alencewicz, 1976).
   A child with an aided articulation score of
   0–20%   scores   0 points
   21–48%   scores 10 points
   49–69%   scores 20 points
   70–100% scores 30 points

2. Language competence (25 points). Determined from the percentile rank on a standardized language test estimated in relation to the scores of other similarly hearing-impaired children. Both signed and spoken language scores are used when appropriate. Appropriate tests are the Grammatical Analysis of Elicited Language (GAEL) (Moog, Kozak & Geers, 1983), the Scales of Early Communication Skills for Hearing-Impaired Children (Moog & Geers, 1975), and The Rhode Island Test of Language Structure (Engen & Engen, 1983).
   Points are assigned thus:
   10th percentile, 0 points
   11th–20th percentile, 5 points
   21st–40th percentile, 10 points
   41st–60th percentile, 15 points
   61st–80th percentile, 20 points
   81st–100th percentile, 25 points

3. Nonverbal intelligence (20 points). Any standardized nonverbal test may be used. Points are allocated thus:

Deficient or retarded range	0 points
(>2 standard deviations below mean)	
Borderline deficient range	5 points
(1–2 SD below mean)	
Normal range	
IQ 86–100	10 points
IQ 101–115	15 points
Above average	20 points
(>1 SD above mean)	

4. Family support (15 points).

No support or understanding	0 points
Minimal support	5 points
Adequate support	10 points
Above average support	15 points

5. Speech communication attitude (10 points).

Poor: Little or no effort to communicate	0 points
Fair: Use of speech only when prompted	5 points
Good: Consistently tries to communicate	10 points

Scores are recorded on the SLP Index Score Sheet and totaled. The results are used to facilitate educational recommendations:

RECOMMENDATION	SPEECH-LANGUAGE INDEX TOTAL SCORE
Speech emphasis	30–100
Provisional speech instruction	60–75
Sign language emphasis	0–55

Thus, for parents to reach a decision about the educational system with which they will feel most comfortable, they will need a means of assessing realistically the possible potential their child has for development of oral communication. They need to know how to monitor progress and they need to understand the cost of the delay if the auditory oral method proves inadequate to meet their child's communication needs.

Systems of Manual Communication

It is important for the parents to be familiar with other methods of teaching communication—with language systems that are predominantly manual rather than oral. They need to consider the advantages of providing the child with an unimpeded (visual sign) means of acquiring language at an early age and of establishing a comfortable communication bond between mother, father, and child. Through use of a sign system, the child will develop a viable language system early, and her ability to communicate needs will be provided for, eliminating or normalizing the frustrations that occur when needs cannot be expressed or anticipated. You may not be able to speak authoritatively on behalf of the manual systems of communication, particularly if you work in a program that uses an auditory-oral approach. You should, however, have a basic familiarity with the several systems.

American Sign Language (AMESLAN or ASL). This is the language of the deaf community and usually the language of the playground in schools for the deaf. It is a language system in its own right, fundamentally different from English (Bornstein 1973, 1979; Stokoe, 1960; Wilbur, 1979). ASL differs from English but not in the way that French differs from English, since direct translation between the latter two languages is possible. The difference is more akin to that between a physical concept, which can be expressed in the signs and grammar of physics, for example $E = MC^2$, and its verbal expression in English. Direct translation from AMESLAN in most instances is not possible since most signs represent concepts rather than English words. Furthermore, AMESLAN differs from English at all structural levels, having its own morphology, syntax, and lexicography. Finally, instead of being structured linearly in a single dimension as speech is in time, sign utilizes four dimensions, three of them spatial and relative to the signer's body, and the fourth the time dimension. AMESLAN, being a natural language, is dynamic. Signs, like words, evolve from new experiences. Having no access to the universal media of communication, namely print, television, radio, film, all of which are in English, new signs tend to be parochial, resulting in strong dialects in different communities. Problems also arise in representing precise technical information and in teaching abstract concepts and philosophies. For these reasons AMESLAN never has been the language of education for deaf students.

For many years pure oralism dominated deaf education. During the late 1960s reaction to the lack of success of oral education in the case of the majority of deaf children quickly led to the *total-communication* (TC) philosophy's becoming the predominant determinant of communication in the classroom.

Total Communication (TC). The philosophy of total communication is to provide the child with information using any of several modes of communication that proves successful in a given situation. Thus speech, natural gestures, finger spelling, and AMESLAN may all be used together with a system of signs. These signs support the spoken message constituting manual representations of the English language. This manual English has been formalized into systems such as *Seeing Essential English* (SEE) (Anthony & Associates, 1971), in which each word is signed, in contrast to the concept signs of AMESLAN. Word modifiers such as *-ly*, *-ing*, *-s*, *-ed*, and *-ous* also are signed along with articles, infinitives, pronouns, and so on. Two other similar systems, *Signing Exact English* (SEE) (Gustason, Pfetzing, & Zowolkow, 1972) and *Signed English* (Borstein, 1974) grew out of the Anthony and Associates system. All the systems of manually communicated English adhere to English morphology, syntax, and grammar.

It would seem that manual English systems would surmount most of the limitations imposed on auditory learning by hearing impairment. Nearly 20 years of almost universal education of profoundly hearing-impaired children by the total-communication method now have passed—a period during which early diagnosis, fitting of amplification, and preschool intervention have reached more and more of these children. Yet, as a population, children with profound hearing deficits remain significantly educationally retarded (Jordan, Gustason & Rosen, 1976). The typical profoundly hearing-impaired student today graduates from high school with an average third or fourth grade reading level (Allen, 1986). The problem according to Johnson, Liddell, and Erting (1989) lies in the failure of profoundly hearing-impaired children of hearing parents to develop sophisticated linguistic competence either in spoken or signed language by kindergarten age. Allen (1986) maintains that signed English systems, therefore, cannot tap into or build upon a natural language. For this reason some specialists are advocating that these children be educated from infancy throughout school years in American Sign Language and that a full family support system be provided to assist them in understanding and participating in this controversial educational model (Johnson, Liddell, & Erting, 1989). The philosophy of Johnson et al. advocates teaching AMESLAN as a first language and English as a second language, thus developing bilingual children. This philosophy has been advocated earlier by other scholars. Johnson et al. cite, among others, Woodward, 1978; Stevens, 1980; Quigly and Paul, 1984; Paul, 1988; and Strong, 1988. They also list a number of countries in which similar programs exist as national policy (Sweden, Uruguay, and Venezuela) as well as many schools in which "elements of bilingual experience have been instituted as part of the curriculum" (Johnson et al., 1989, p. 15). Four such schools are in the United States.

Finger Spelling. This method was developed by the Rochester School for the Deaf in New York State. It consists of a manually signed alphabet that allows letters to be seen on the hand; however, it is not a pure manual system since it serves to supplement rather than substitute for oral communication. It constitutes a form of visible speech if it is synchronized with the spoken message.

Cued Speech. Cued speech, a system developed by Orin Cornett, like finger spelling, is a supplement to oral speech. Using eight hand postures and four hand placements, it conveys visually phonetic information that supplements lip-reading cues to vowels and consonants. It is a system completely dependent upon lip-reading of spoken language. As such, though it uses a manual code, it is a modification of the oral method rather than a sign system.

Dealing with the Dilemma

The dilemma you share with the parents arises from the state of flux that education of the deaf has been in for many years. We face the statistics that indicate that when we consider the population of severely to profoundly hearing-impaired children as a whole, rather than the examples of success put forward by the advocates of the different methods, the evidence is far from encouraging. The problem is exacerbated by the conflict, even bitterness, that exists among the supporters of the different methods of teaching communication and knowledge to severely and profoundly hearing-impaired children. Yet we must support and guide parents in a manner that allows them to feel comfortable with the decision they make about the communication method they choose for the education of their child.

Guidelines for Resolving the Dilemma

I suggest that you consider the following guidelines when faced with this situation:

- Commend the parents for the concern they express about finding the best method of education.

- Explain that while you have your own opinions/prejudices, it is important that the parents reach a decision with as little outside influence as possible.
- Stress that there are several methods of educating deaf children, but that to this point none is without its limitations. Thus a choice always represents what is considered most appropriate for a specific child and his/her parents. It is not a question of finding the best system but the one all can feel most comfortable with.
- Point out that it will be necessary to make the choice from among those available in the community unless the parents are willing to relocate.
- Explain, as concisely and objectively as possible, the major methods and their advantages and disadvantages.
- Identify the alternative methods available in local programs.
- Encourage the parents to visit the different programs, discuss their philosophies, observe their teaching methods, and observe the children and their communicative interaction with teachers and peers.
- Review carefully all the information available that may be influential in determining the child's potential for oral language development.
- Make yourself available to listen to and discuss the parents' reactions, feelings, and concerns about what they saw and learned.
- Point out that a decision is not forever. A child who begins in an oral program can add or change to manual communication whenever the need is felt. Likewise a child in a total-communication program who demonstrates strong oral potential might move to an oral approach.
- Finally, when the parents make a choice, support them strongly, not in terms of the choice itself, but because of the considered process by which they made it.

MEETING THE INFANT'S COMMUNICATION NEEDS

We have discussed how congenital hearing impairment isolates children from the auditory world, cutting them off from the main channel through which we relate to each other. Rose (1987) points out that it is sensory experiences that promote the child's interaction with and exploration of the environment. When this process is diminished, she suggests, the very motivation to become involved with people, things, and events is affected. Rose quotes Stern's (1983) opinion that the hearing-impaired infant will be "at an enormous disadvantage in constructing a cohesive unified picture of the world of human behavior" and "in comprehending the basic fabric of human behaviors that constitute emotional expressions and verbal meanings and the material that makes school learning" (Stern, 1983, p. 12).

During the earliest months of the child's life, mother and child establish a special relationship through the mutual reading of and responding to each other's behavioral cues. This is a stage in what is referred to as the bonding process. Bromwich (1981) explains:

> The reciprocal reading and responding to each other's cues form the core of a complex interactional (or transactional) system between parent and infant. It is within that system that the child develops trust in the human and physical environment. This trust forces him to explore his environment. The child also becomes motivated to develop language as the communications between parent and infant steadily increase in complexity and sophistication." (p. 9)

We need to help the parent understand and maximize the behaviors that facilitate this bonding. The first goal, therefore, is to do everything possible to enhance the parent-child relationship. Parents and primary caregivers should be encouraged to emphasize the situations that increase human bonding. Whenever possible, the waking child should be moved around the house as the mother's activities move her from place to place. Explain that you appreciate that this involves extra effort in carrying the baby seat upstairs while you sort and fold laundry, or outside while you vacuum the car, or from room to room as you clean. However, it affords rich rewards. It makes possible the building of a relationship with the child, stimulating awareness of the shared events and providing a natural source of topics about which to talk in speech or sign with the preverbal infant. Language and communication are about what is happening, what is being experienced, what is being felt. These shared experiences help to facilitate a close mother-child relationship. Effort also should be made to compensate for the reduced auditory input by supplementing other sensory information. The mother, father, or any caregivers should be encouraged to increase their visual and tactile contacts with the child. Remind them that holding, hugging, touching, patting, stroking, and rocking while singing or talking to a child are soothing and reassuring. Likewise, lightly bouncing, gently swinging, or dancing while holding a child are stimulating and exciting. Such shared experiences should be reinforced by associated verbal stimulation. In this way, you are providing the language models that the child needs in order for her brain to sort out what language is and how it works. If the child is to use a total-communication model of learning, the parent should sign what he is saying whenever his hands are free. Remind the parent how important it is for the child to be able to see his face and/or hands when communicating. This means placing himself in an appropriate position relative to crib, playpen, or highchair.

Talking to the Child

The child's cognitive linguistic and sociolinguistic skills in this early developmental period derive from the models she encounters. The basis of language acquisition will be the semantic concepts the child learns (Miller & Yoder, 1974). First the child perceives objects, object functions, object relationships, and events conceptually—that is, the child attributes meaning to them. At the same time the linguistic commentary provides the appropriate language patterns associated with the object or event. When the concept is correlated to the linguistic pattern, the child has developed a semantic value for the experience. That semantic value, which is an abstract, then can be evoked by the appropriate spoken/sign language patterns. Later the semantic value can be correlated with its linguistic equivalent, allowing the child to communicate orally or manually. Parents must understand, therefore, the importance of talking about what is happening, about what they are doing, and about what the child is doing or experiencing. This, it should be pointed out, is a natural behavior exhibited by parents (Ling & Ling, 1978). You are seeking only to reinforce what they would do normally. The hearing-impaired child needs this even more than hearing peers. Early-language training, therefore, does not involve lessons, but the provision of appropriate linguistic commentary on events meaningful to the child. Turton (1974) states: "In terms of the hearing impaired child, the parents must be sensitive to his experiential background as it provides stimuli for language acquisition" (p. 497).

The use of language in context greatly enhances the potential situational redundancy. It is necessary to guide the parents in how to talk/sign to their child. This requires that you observe the rate, complexity, grammatical correctness, and articulatory clarity of the parent's communications. Explain to the parents that certain communication behaviors by them are known to be potentially very helpful to their child's development of language skills. These include using speech/sign directly related to what is happening; being physically and actively involved (sharing in) their child's experience; praising their child's signs, vocalizations, and verbalizations; verbalizing for their child what has happened and why and how it happened.

Research has shown that parents speak differently to young children than they do to older children and adults (Broen, 1972; Frayer & Roberts, 1975; Phillips, 1973; Snow, 1972). When we speak to very young children, we do so more slowly than to older children; we use more one-word sentences, more incomplete sentences (for example, "Go bye-bye?," "Come see Daddy"), and shorter sentences in general. The vocabulary and sentence structure of our utterances are simpler, and we often repeat or rephrase what we have said. It may be necessary for you to attempt to modify the parent's existing behaviors to reflect the natural characteristics just described. You may achieve this through demonstration and commentary on parent-child communication. This must be done cautiously so as not to imply rejection of the parent's speech. You should stress that speech that is acceptable for young hearing children often must be further modified to meet the special needs of the young child with impaired hearing. You will need to train parents to encode linguistic redundancy into their communication. They should learn to talk about events, not just to label them. For example, in bathing the child the parent might say:

Where's the soap?
Where's the soap gone?
Oh, here's the soap.
I found it. I found the soap.

or in a play situation:

There's the teddy bear.
List to teddy bear squeak.
Squeak, squeak, teddy bear.
Here, you hold teddy bear.
Squeeze it there.
Squeak, squeak, squeak.

Then, hiding the toy behind your back:

Where's teddy bear gone?
Where's teddy bear?
Squeak, teddy bear.

Then you squeak the toy:

I hear it, listen.
Do you hear teddy bear squeak?
There it is.
Hi, teddy bear.

Communication with the child should be worded simply but not distorted into baby talk. Statements should be linked together in a constructive, supportive manner:

Let's put on your shoes.
Here are your two shoes.
One shoe, two shoes.
Now we'll tie your shoes.
First tie this shoe—now tie this shoe.
There, all done. Your shoes are tied. Down you go.

Guidance should be given to the parents to ensure that they use natural, melodic speech, clearly articulated but not exaggerated, and that they do not speak unnaturally loudly to their child. Before a hearing aid has been fitted, the parents should be encouraged to talk and sing to their baby with their mouths within an inch or two of the baby's ear. This raises the intensity level of normal voice to 95 to 100dB HL without distortion. It also encourages close physical contact between parents and child.

Most important, however, the parents should talk/sign to the baby whenever they are with her during waking hours. The closer the parents are to the child, both physically and psychologically, the better the learning opportunity. The sooner the parents can assume the role of natural habitual commentators of events an experience, the sooner the child is likely to become speech and/or sign oriented. The younger the child is when this pattern of parent communication is established, the greater will be the optimal potential for the learning of communication. It takes time before the effects of talking to the child begin to be rewarded in terms of early attempts at speech. Parents need support and encouragement during this long period of waiting. Counsel them to look for reassurance in the child's nonverbal responses to auditory-visual speech input, in the increased attention span, and in the child's signs of pleasure when stimulated. In most cases the child will give observable evidence of processing the auditory-visual input. Eventually she will give signs of spontaneous vocalization and imitation. This calls for reinforcement behavior by the observer.

Responding to the Child's Communication

The vocalizations of hearing-impaired babies, even those with profound deficits, do not differ from their hearing peers during the first five to six months of life. Northern and Downs (1984) report finding the vocalizations of deaf infants to be identical with those of hearing infants of the same age. It even has been shown that when parents talk to profoundly deaf infants, the same increase in vocalizations occurs as with hearing babies (Downs & Akin, 1984). Northern and Downs (1984) state:

> It is obvious that the reason for this increase in vocalizations is not the baby's hearing the parents voice. We postulate that it is a pre adaptive reflexive response stimulated by the presence of the parent's face much as the smile response which appears at the same age. It may be that the increase in vocalization is as necessary a psychic organizer for ultimate communication integrity as the smile response is to ultimate psychic integrity. (p. 103)

If deafness precludes the child from hearing parental speech beyond the first six months of life, a decrease rather than an increase in vocalizations and speech-like sounds will occur (Mascarinek et al., 1981). Beyond the innately preprogrammed stage of vocalization and babbling, auditory feedback from self and others is critical to the activation, development, and shaping of linguistic precursors. For this reason parents need to be taught and encouraged to reinforce the child's earliest vocalizations. Both auditory and visual reinforcement should be given. When the infant vocalizes, the parents should respond with pleasure that can be seen by the child. The child should be responded to verbally: "Are you talking to Daddy? There's a good girl. Ah ba ba ba ba [repeating the utterance]. Come on, tell me some more. . . ." Touching, patting, or stroking the baby can help to reinforce such early vocalizations. The parents should echo the child's babbling patterns, allowing pauses for the child to begin to babble again. The idea is to encourage consciousness of those vocalizations, which in the hearing-impaired child tend to die out if not strongly reinforced. As soon as the child begins to attempt linguistic utterances, words, sentences, and meanings also should be reinforced by pleasurable responses.

Early stimulation of spoken language, as distinct from vocalization, is related directly to experience and to thought processes. The child's first use of words can be prompted, reinforced, molded, and expanded. If the parents have received early training, or if they have perceived the importance of talking to the child about what is happening, the child will have heard natural object and event-related language repeatedly. As soon as the child attempts to imitate the parents, either by vocalization or by spoken words, the communicative behavior must be reinforced. These early utterances can be molded by the parents, who should provide the child with several repetitions of the correct model:

Parent: *Here's your milk. Don't spill it, don't spill your milk.*
  Child: *ma ma*
Parent: *Good,—milk—say, milk, milk.*
  Child: *ma ma*
Parent: *Good girl, you said milk.*

Next time milk is given to the child, the parent should prompt the child to name it, asking, "What's this? What have I got for you?" If the child does not respond, the parent should name the object: "It's your milk—you say it—milk, milk—come on, tell me, milk."

Always accept the child's attempt to imitate even if it is only an approximation or indeed if it is no more than a vowel sound, but always reinforce by providing several repetitions of the correct model. Encourage, but do not pressure, the child to say the word. Do not overload the child by continuing the interchange at the expense of the child's willing participation in this language game.

Once the words or word approximations become consistently associated with appropriate objects, the parents can begin to expand on the child's utterance. According to Schumaker and Sherman (1978), an expansion is "a parent utterance that uses what the child has said to form a more adult-like utterance" (p. 300). For example, when the child volunteers "ma" for milk the parent may expand the one word to include an extended but better-defined experience with the milk—Parent: Yes, that's milk—drink your milk—drink it up. The word *drink* will be used with other liquids; thus, a concept begins to emerge through association.

Similarly when an infant playing with a doll says "bei-bei" the parent smiles and says:

Yes, that's baby—baby.

Sarah has a baby—love the baby.

Oh nice baby.

On a subsequent occasion the parent may expand the semantic content:

Look baby's crying—poor baby, she's crying.

Don't cry baby—love her so she doesn't cry.

Look, Mommy's crying (mother pretends to cry).

Don't cry Mommy (Mother smiles again, takes child's hands, puts them to her eyes, and speaks) Poor Sarah, Sarah's crying, don't cry Sarah.

Research by Slobin (1968) and Schumaker (1976) has shown that parents of young hearing children use expansions following 30 percent of their children's utterances. In reviewing this research Schumaker and Sherman (1978) recommended that this form of modeling should be used frequently with children who are potentially linguistically handicapped.

The role of parents in the stimulation and molding of the child's language development is paramount. We should stress again, however, that facilitating their child's language growth calls for comfortable, productive interactions rather than skilled teaching. Such interactions arise from parent-infant closeness and from an increase in transactions generated by naturally occurring events. Associated with those transactions should be natural language arising directly from the social circumstances. The development of a natural interactive communicative behavior with one's infant forms the basis of future exchanges. These become more sophisticated and exploratory in nature as cognitive and social learning interacts with language.

Familiarizing Parents with the Principles and Stages of Language Development

Parent education will be most effective when the language-stimulation activities of the parents are underpinned by an understanding of the principles involved. Parents should be helped to understand why they are learning certain behaviors and how they relate to the child's cognitive and linguistic development at each stage. They must be taught the manner and order in which language forms are acquired and must be shown the direct relationship between what the child is capable of and what they are doing with the child. Later the parent must learn to relate the child's early utterances to what the child is experiencing at the time.

Obviously, formal instruction of the parents in developmental linguistics is inadvisable, though parent discussion groups are often helpful for explaining the nature of the developmental aspects of language acquisition. Mostly, however, you will explain principles as you guide the parents in relating to their child. Describe what the child is doing, identify the cognitive-linguistic stage this represents, explain the next stage, give examples of what the child will progress to, and demonstrate the techniques for facilitating the gradual introduction of the more advanced language form. It is important to stress the difference between comprehension and use of language in the presence of the subject or event, and understanding and use of the same language form in the absence of context (Bloom, 1974).

Parents need to be helped to understand that language is a tool for dealing with experience. It enables us to think about what we are experiencing—to clarify, evaluate, and store knowledge about what is happening to us. Language enables us to relate events both present and past, forming and tapping into webs of experience. Parents can play an important role through encouraging their child to explore the many ways of using the language tool to examine, learn about, and question what is happening. Such parental involvement will continue through the learning years. It will be supplemented but not replaced by the somewhat more controlled learning environment of the special preschool program for the older child.

SUMMARY

- Assessment of very young hearing-impaired children is an ongoing process.
- Auditory responsiveness and emergent receptive and expressive language skills are the most important behaviors to monitor.
- Parents need to be familiar with age-related norms and developmental sequences.
- It is essential to assess parents' needs and family, financial, time, ability, and language resources.
- The management plan must be negotiated to avoid parent overload or expectations that cannot be met.
- Parents need guidance in how to optimize the auditory environment of their home.
- Specific guidelines for auditory stimulation should be provided.
- Guiding and supporting parents in the choice of a language-teaching approach requires provision of maximal information and unbiased support.

- The goal in the resolution of the communication dilemma is informed decision making by parents based on the documentation of the child's needs and predicted potential.
- Parents should be guided in how to maximize communication with their child.
- Parents are central to the management of the infant; our role is as educators and facilitators.

Conclusion

Assessing the residual hearing of infants and toddlers requires careful observation of the child's behavior in structured test situations and, equally important, in natural parent-child interactions. The task is, therefore, one of parent-professional cooperation. To this end we need to familiarize parents with the ages and stages of prelinguistic auditory-oral development. Natural parent behaviors with their child need to be reinforced and augmented to maximize auditory stimulation. The emphasis is on parent confidence through understanding and support. This is particularly true in the sensitive task of selecting the approach to communication, oral or total communication, selected for the child. Our role is one of informing, explaining, guiding, and supporting parents. We are not justified in making decisions for them.

15

Intervention for the Older Preschool Child

REVIEWING NEEDS AND RESOURCES

The division of intervention practices for preschool children into those for the very young and those for the older child is to a great extent an academic convenience. The needs of the child and the family change gradually as the child grows, but different needs occur at different times for different families. The major developmental factor that influences the model of education is the ability of the child to participate in cooperative learning. The ability of a child to interact socially with adults and children allows her to benefit from a more controlled and planned learning environment. When this stage is reached, usually around age three, the educational model changes from parent/caregiver-centered to child-centered. The child to this point has been gaining experience and language stimulation from naturally occurring events in the home or caregiver's environment. She now is ready to enter a "preschool learning environment" in which events and activities, to a large extent, are planned with particular goals in mind. The change needs to be effected gradually. The preparation of a young child for separation from mother, or primary caregiver, and for the change to a new learning model and environment is particularly important when the child has been in a home-based program. Handing the responsibility for the child's speech, language, and learning to a teacher/therapist without a transition

261

can leave the mother feeling bereft of her role. This is understandable when you realize how hard she has worked to become effective in that role. The potential for the parents to feel unneeded or unwanted when their child is "handed over to the school" emphasizes the need for ongoing support. We must continue to provide guidance to the parents as their role evolves. An excellent local program, the Language Development Program of Western New York, arranges this stage of child management very effectively. The home-based program involves two two-hour sessions weekly from each of several preschool specialists, including a special education teacher, a teacher of the deaf, a speech-language pathologist, an educational audiologist, and as appropriate, an occupational therapist, physiotherapist, and social worker. To withdraw all this support from a family suddenly when the child enters a preschool class would be unthinkable. Thus, for several months before class enrollment, mother/primary caregiver and child visit the class together for a half day a month. The second stage is for the child to attend the class program one or two half days a week for a month or so while home visits are continued. This leads finally to school enrollment for five half or full days. The gradual transition also supports the continuity of preschool educational philosophy and programming.

The Controlled Learning Environment

The preschool learning environment represents a hybrid between the normal everyday environment of children and the structured environment of the primary school. There should be little difference between the philosophy and goals of an excellent preschool for hearing children and one for children with impaired hearing. The differences lie only in the special qualifications of the teachers and therapists, the heavy use of amplification in auditory-oral programs, and in the emphasis placed on stimulating language and communication. I wish to stress that enrollment in a half- or full-day preschool program never should be viewed as a replacement for parental home stimulation. We and the parents should see it as an expansion and a focusing of what has been occurring since home guidance began. We must strive to achieve a truly integrated home-school model in which each reinforces the other in a symbiotic relationship. We must stress to the parents that the preschool program is not assuming the responsibility for educating the child—it is sharing it. To achieve this highly desirable mutual relationship, parents need to be reminded throughout the home guidance program that their role always will be a major determinant in the child's progress.

The actual amount of parental time spent with the child will be less when he enters preschool, but the importance of the continued parent input is in no way reduced. To ensure that parents' activities pertaining to the child's development and education remain significant, you must establish a model for cooperation that requires a

- Commitment by the teacher, speech-language pathologist, and other professionals to the philosophy that school and home need to interact

- Means by which information about events occurring at school and at home can be communicated easily between the staff and parents
- Means by which the staff can continue to provide support and guidance to parents concerning how to reinforce and expand on experiences occurring at school
- System for mutual monitoring of the child's behavior, knowledge, and communication growth
- System for mutual identification of problems and needs evidenced by the child and for shared exploration of coordinated ways of addressing these
- Means for the parents to continue to express and discuss their anxieties and concerns to a sympathetic professional

Review Available Resources

One advantage of the child's entering a preschool program is that the demands upon parental resources are reduced. However, you still need to be sensitive to existing resources in order to ensure that requests and suggestions are compatible with them. For the parent who is new to your program, you will need to explore the resources that we discussed in the previous chapter.

Family Resources. These change from time to time: Couples separate; child custody is determined; live-in partners change; men and women remarry; much needed grandparents move away at retirement or die. These represent changes in the support system of the parent(s) to which you should be sensitive.

Financial Resources. These, too, can change positively or negatively. The mother may take up employment when the child is enrolled in preschool, or she or the father may become unemployed. A move to a new home or a medical problem may place increased burdens on finances. Changes in financial resources may increase or decrease time resources and impact on the dependence on family resources.

Time Resources. These are probably the most subject to change. In addition to the effects of finances, the time parents have to devote to the child will be affected by changes in family composition such as divorce, remarriage, the birth of a child, or the mother's taking part- or full-time employment. You need to be sensitive to such changes in order to ensure that your expectations for parent involvement are commensurate with their resources.

Ability Resources. If the parents have been receiving guidance in the home guidance program, you will have an understanding of their level of sophistication concerning the problems of hearing impairment. Effective counseling should have increased the parents' confidence in their abilities to manage the child's developmental needs reasonably, comfortably, and effectively. This resource should, however, be discussed with them again as the child moves into the more controlled educational setting. Monitoring the parents' abilities to meet demands, intellectually and emotionally, shows empathy and ensures the appropriateness of our requests and guidance.

Language Resources. The demands of the child for English language enrichment at home will grow in extent and sophistication as the child's cognitive-linguistic skills develop. A linguistic barrier between parents and child will represent a brake on developmental progress. With the very young hearing-impaired child, the impact of parents' limited knowledge of English may be offset by the child's limited and concrete needs. Predictions can be made, needs anticipated. Simple English may be quite adequate for parent-toddler communication. However, the growing child soon may outstrip both need predictions and the parents' English language competence. A similar and equally serious gap in language resources can occur when a child's sign language ability outstrips that of the parents and other family members. For a communication system to be effective, both partners must have equal skills in the language used. You should monitor this resource lest the parents feel inadequate and guilty. Parent guidance must not be withdrawn when the child enrolls in a preschool program—the need for support is ongoing.

Needs of the Child

Provide for Experiential Needs. Thought and language arise from experience. We encounter people and things in different contexts, functioning in certain ways; we observe events happening; we participate in events and we experience what happens to us. *Experience is interactive, not passive.* Even when we are an observer of an event, we participate in terms of how we organize what we see, hear, feel, taste, or smell as a result of what occurs. Thus, the first need to be met by a preschool program is to ensure a rich experiential environment that provides the children with direct involvement with things, people, and events (Weikert, Rogers, Adcock, & McClellan, 1971). To experience it is necessary to be a part of what is happening. Relevant stimulating events must occur in which the children are actively involved. The activities that generate experiences need to be planned to ensure that appropriate materials and general scripts are available. They may evolve from seasonal events, such as the planting of seeds; growing carrot-top ferns in water; or collecting, sorting, and arranging autumn leaves. They may center around foods, making snacks, or playing shop, or they may relate to experiences with animals. Experience may be provided by bringing pets into the classroom. Kittens, puppies, hamsters, gerbils, and baby chicks all provide stimulation and encourage curiosity as well as a need to relate to and communicate about what is seen, felt, touched, and heard. This prepares the children for an outside visit to a pet shop, farm, or zoo. These experiences need to allow you, the teacher/speech-language pathologist, to explore with the children a range of other experiences that relate to some component of the original.

Related experiences comprise expansions or contractions of what the child has just experienced. Consider, for example, a visit to a local bakery. The sequence might begin with snack time. The teacher/therapist brings in breads for the children to help make jam or peanut butter and jelly sandwiches. She has brought slices of several types of bread: white, soft white, brown, pumpernickel, rye, raisin. The children are given small pieces of each to examine; they are encouraged to look, smell, and taste the different breads. This experience is followed by finding out about the bread. The children are given some grains; if it is autumn it may be possible to have the actual stalks of wheat, barley, and rye, supplemented with pictures of wheat fields ripe for harvest. The grains might be ground in a coffee grinder to produce a flour-like substance. Actual flour can be felt, smelled, and tasted and mixed with milk and water to produce dough. A simple bread recipe using yeast will allow the children to experience the ingredients that go into the bread. They can knead and pummel, slap and roll the dough and then experience its rising to twice its bulk. A small oven will allow the bread to be seen to bake. All the time appropriate language is provided to describe the experience. The expansion of this personal experience of bread could be a visit to a local bakery to observe what the children "know" about and to see the full-size process. A visit to the bakery shop allows them to see the many shapes in which bread is made. Finally, back in school, other bread forms such as toast, melba toast, hamburger buns, hot dog rolls, bread sticks, croutons, and breadcrumbs can be experienced at snack times.

Reinforce Experiences. To ensure reinforcement of these experiences, the parents must know what is planned, when it will happen, and suggested ways to reinforce the experience. A brief synopsis of planned activities can be sent home on a ditto sheet along with suggestions about shopping at the bakery section of a supermarket, using different breads, and baking cookies or making pastry. All these activities can involve the child and reinforce stored memories. Reminding hearing-impaired children of events experienced is particularly important since language deficits limit storage and recall of experiential memories. We need to supplement and strengthen the child's ability to "abstract," that is, to represent the experience apart from the concrete reality, to take it away in imagery that can be re-created and re-presented.

The most effective and motivating reminder of experience is to see it as it happened. This is possible now with small portable video cameras that can record and re-present to the children images of themselves and their friends in the process of the experience. Polaroid cameras capture experiences more simply and less expensively, if less dramatically, while color slides provide an enlarged photo image. Photographic images allow the experience to be relived, reexamined, talked about, learned about, clarified, and expanded. Books and pictures depicting comparable events should be readily available. These can be used to reinforce the experience at story time.

Materials that allow context-related free play are essential. For example, a ministore with a collection of empty cartons, jars, and packages of food items allows for play reenactment of a supermarket experience; toy animals and minicages allow for zoo play, farm animals and machinery recreate a country trip, and mixing the two encourages memories of the two experiences to be categorized and sorted. The real experience of the bakery can be re-created by the children if they have available play dough to knead and shape, pans to put it in, and a cardboard box with a cut out lid to serve as an oven. A long flat stick can be used to place the bread in the hot oven; gloves can be worn to protect hands; a mesh tray can be provided for cooling. Later the "loaves" can be bought at the minimarket and sliced for "snacks." Such situations enable the child to reexamine and creatively explore experiences to enrich and rework them. Play allows the child to control events, to assume different identities, and to explore new roles. At the same time, play re-creates the need for language as a tool for analyzing, molding, personalizing, and storing experience (Corsaro, 1984; McCune-Nicholich & Carrol, 1981). Since play often is interactive, or even cooperative, at the older preschool age, it encourages the development of social cognition and sociolinguistic skills (Corsaro, 1984). Children learn from experience that they cannot all talk to each other at once. This creates the need for them to explore the structure of dialogue, turn taking, commenting, asking questions, disagreeing, and so on. The guidelines for providing experiential learning are, therefore, that

- Experiences must be relevant and stimulating.
- The children must be actively involved.
- The objects and materials must be explored by the children with their senses.
- Whenever possible, the experiences should be extended into the outside world through visits after classroom preparation.
- Parents must be kept informed about planned experiences and given guidance in how to reinforce and extend those experiences at home.
- Visual records should be used when possible to re-create memory images.
- Play materials should be available to stimulate participative re-creation of the experience in free play.

ASSESSING AND PROVIDING FOR LANGUAGE NEEDS

Experience creates a need for language, whether it be oral or manual in form. It is recognized that children must learn language in order to encode cognitive knowledge. Boothroyd (1982, p. 119) states: "The central ability that hearing-impaired children must acquire is that of representing thoughts, internally, by language patterns." Furthermore, both cognition and language occur in social interactive situations that give rise to associated experience (Friel-Patti & Lougea-Mottinger, 1985). Experience, understanding (cognition), and language acquisition occurring within a social context are, therefore, interdependent. Just as experience gives rise to a need for language to define it, exposure to new language patterns directs attention to the persons, things, or events to which they refer. Language not only begets experience, it qualifies, relates, and refines it (Church, 1961). It is upon this perception of a complex relationship among social experience, cognition, and language that the current cognitive-linguistic approach to understanding language development in both hearing and hearing-impaired children is found (Moeller, 1988).

Use Language to Describe Experience

Reflect upon our discussion of the need to create concrete experiences for the child. We saw that the experience of the child derives from external and internal factors.

EXTERNAL FACTORS
- People, objects, and occurrences
- Relationships among these components
- Order in which they occur
- Situation or context in which they occur
- Effects they produce

INTERNAL FACTORS
- Ability to record the occurrence through the senses
- Ability to perceive identities and functions
- Ability to perceive relationships
- Ability to be aware of cause and effect
- Ability to integrate and perceive occurrences holistically
- Ability to symbolize linguistically the experience and its effect on self, others, and other components
- Ability to relate the experience through inner language to past experiences
- Ability to communicate the experience to others
- Ability to interact linguistically with others about the experience

For language learning to occur, a further set of factors must be in effect:

- The language must be coded into a form that is compatible with the child's sensory modality or modalities.
- The occurrence must be relevant to the child in order that attention be paid to it and a need for language generated.
- The relevant language must be provided as the experience is in progress.
- The message must have a high level of redundancy.
- The language must be developmentally age appropriate.
- The message should address both the occurrence and the child's involvement with it.
- The communication should comprise an interchange between you and the child.

Awareness of these influential factors and conditions and of the reciprocal relationship between experience and language allows us to develop a model for facilitating language learning. Our creation of structured but not rigidly controlled experience provides the essential need for language. Consider now the role language must play and the structure that can provide that function. Our model accommodates the factors we have just discussed.

Meeting Language Learning Requirements

First, *the message must be compatible with the child's sensory capabilities*. This requires that you have as much information as possible concerning the child's aided residual hearing. You cannot expect language to be developed through a purely auditory input when there is a severe auditory deficit.

Therefore, if the child is to learn through the auditory-oral mode, your first concern is to optimize the speech signal. To achieve this you will need to ensure fidelity of the acoustic signal. (You may wish to review our discussion of this in Chapter 11.) Hearing aid fittings should be binaural and preferably integrated with an FM system. If FM is not used, reducing the speaker-child distance is essential to preserving the fidelity of the acoustic signal. The acoustic speech signal for all children must be enhanced by visible speech cues, which means that the child always must be able to see you when you speak. Your face should be well lit and the child should watch you. You and/or the child should perform a component of the activity, talk about it, then repeat it. For children with severe to profound hearing impairment, it will be necessary to decide whether the message should be encoded into manual form and whether the manual code should be exclusive of associated spoken language. If a combined method is to be used, you will need to have clear answers to these questions:

> Which method will be primary?
> What guidelines are to be used for signing when speech is the primary mode?
> Are speech and, for example, signed English to be used simultaneously?
> Are signs to be used primarily to convey or to reinforce the spoken message?
> Is the complete message to be signed, or only key words?
> Is signing to be used only when speech comprehension fails?

Each of these decisions contributes to ensuring the compatibility of the message code with the child's sensory processing capabilities.

Create a Need for Communication

The next task is to generate a need for communication. Boothroyd (1982) states emphatically: "Your first and most basic responsibility in relation to language development is to establish dialogue between yourself and the child and more importantly between parents and child" (p. 133). The importance of dialogue as the critical form of facilitating learning is stressed also by Tharp and Gallimore (1989):

> But for the development of thinking skills, in particular the abilities to form, express and exchange ideas in speech and writing, the critical form of assisting learners is through dialogue, through the questioning and sharing of ideas and knowledge that happens in conversation. (p. 23)

Our understanding of experience accommodates the role of dialogue comfortably. Dialogue is the mutual give and take of communication that allows perceptions to be evoked and compared through use of language. Thus, just as experience derives from an interaction with the environment, language derives from an interaction with experience. It must arise from a relevant occurrence in which child and adults are cooperative participants. The topic of the dialogue, therefore, is the ongoing experience or the recreation of it. The experience is the structure; the control is how you interact with the child linguistically. You can guide his/her observations in ways that enable you to label, describe, compare, contrast, and relate what is happening or what can be seen, heard, felt, tasted, or smelled. To the extent that you guide or lead the child, you are the language resource. You are molding the experience and bringing essential components to the child's attention. At the same time you are relating the experience to other experiences using language to compare and contrast. You stimulate dialogue by asking questions:

- What are you doing?
- Where shall we put this?
- What color is the flour?
- What else do we have that's white?
- What do we need to mix the dough?
- Can we mix it with our fingers?
- Shall we use a spoon or fork?
- What shall we use this [a rolling pin] for?

In this way we satisfy also the requirement that language be provided as the event is in progress, weaving language into the experience. We encourage the child to associate words, phrases, and sentences with the meaning he is deriving from the experience. For all this to occur the child must be involved in an activity that excites and encourages curiosity. You stimulate communication by providing the words and phrases that describe what is happening and what the child is doing. It is equally important to address what the child is experiencing, what is happening to him:

Is that sweet or sour? Taste it—it's sweet, the sugar is sweet.

Taste this, ugh that's sour, lemons are sour.

Feel the dough—is it soft or hard? That's right, it's soft.

Can you find something that's hard? Yes, this piece of bread is hard, squeeze it. It's old bread. Old bread is stale, the bread is stale, stale bread is hard but the dough is soft. You can squeeze the dough because it is soft not hard.

The goal is a shared experience about which you can communicate.

BEGINNING STRUCTURED COMMUNICATION TRAINING

Provide Experiences and Associated Language

The hearing-impaired child approximately three years of age and older needs selected and structured learning experiences. You should choose these experiences to teach the child to deal with the basic concepts of the world in which she must function. Be sure that the conceptual and linguistic experiences you select are appropriate for developmental norms. When structuring activities remember that the development of cognition and language are intimately related. Together they follow a progression from concrete to abstract experience. At first the child is aware only of things present, things that can be experienced directly through the senses and through manipulative involvement. First we know, then we know about. Language provides the information that permits us to know about experience. It is first understood and used to describe immediate experience. Later the child learns to relate to toys, pictures, and models that represent the real things in their absence. Language becomes more important in filling out this less concrete type of experience. Finally verbal language alone permits experience to be restructured in complete abstraction. At this level experiences can be evoked and manipulated purely linguistically. It is this stage that presents the greatest difficulty to the hearing-impaired child. Through structured activities you will control experiences, highlight relationships, and provide appropriate language models for the child. You will create opportunities for the child's mind to test the validity of the hypotheses she will begin to make about ways to use language.

The child also needs to be exposed to peer-group situations, which generate communication needs and stimulate the growth of social-interaction skills. These two needs—structured learning and social interaction—appropriately are met by including the child in group activities. Initially these may consist of small groups of preschool hearing-impaired children. As far as possible the children in the group should be compatible for age and communication abilities. Mixing children with widely differing communication skills makes it hard for the teacher to accommodate individual needs. However, if it is not possible to match children fairly closely, a mixed-ability group may derive benefit under the guidance of an experienced teacher. The availability of a trained aide or experienced parent is also essential to permit the teacher the flexibility necessary to individualize influence. Placing a child in an integrated or even a normal nursery school is also a possibility.

In the home, situational language—that is, language in natural context—arises from the ongoing activities of the parents and other family members. Language is provided when events occur. In contrast, a structured learning environment controls experience. You choose the cognitive and linguistic experiences you wish the child to have and then you create specific situations to generate the appropriate language needs. In Mecham's (1969) words, you should aim to

> create an atmosphere of specific geographic locations or events which would be similar to particular experience units for the child in daily life. Structure experiences which might approximate the normal environment. The advantages of structured experiences in the classroom or therapy is that labels can be supplied at the moment of experience and therefore can more easily become part of the experience concept. (p. 53)

Even though you are structuring experiences, they are generally seen by the preschool child as play, which indeed they will be. But play is work when the child learns through doing. Choose activities that foster an awareness of the properties of things—color, size, shape, quantity, texture, and so on. Have the child match and group objects by color and then color pictures of things that are, for example, green (trees, grass, familiar green vegetables) or red (tomatoes, ketchup, fire, fire engines, and perhaps city buses or the child's sweater). Let the child distinguish big and small objects: making oneself big and then small, opening the small box, finding the big apple, filling the big glass, emptying the little one. Then let the child choose, match, and group pictures according to these properties. Expose the child to experiences of quantity by pouring water into big jars and little jars, putting beans or beads into big boxes and little boxes, choosing a large pile of candies instead of a small one. Each experience you provide must be stimulating and meaningful, and it must create appropriate language models. Seek to stimulate the child's awareness and attention to spoken language as it relates to concrete experiences. For example, when you involve the children in activities aimed to teach the concepts of size and quantity, verbalize what is occurring, emphasizing the relevant language vocabulary and forms:

Look the jar is full—it's full of water—you have too much water. Put some in the little jar. Now the big box is full—you have no more beans—the beans are all gone. This little box has no beans, it's empty. The little box is empty. Let's put some beans in the little box. There, now it's not empty. Is it full? No, it's not full, look we can put some more into it. The big box is full, we can't put any more beans in the big box, it's full. Let's make it empty—you empty it. There, now the big box is empty. Let's put all the beans in the little box—now the little box is full— the little box is full, the big box is empty. Give me the empty box.

You can also teach categories of objects by grouping them according to *function.* Center play activities on washing and dressing a doll, for example, by letting the child choose what one uses to wash:

Let's find the bath—here it is. Where's the water? We have to get some water to fill the bath. Come, we'll get some water to fill the bath. There, now the bath is almost full. We need some soap. Can you find the soap, Mary? We need the soap to wash the baby. Good, you found the soap. Now we need a cloth and a towel. Where is the towel, John? Can you see it? That's right—that's the towel. Now we can wash the baby with the soap and cloth.

Similar categorization along with associated language can be structured around dressing, eating, cooking, and so on—all activities with which the child has become familiar at home. New activities may be centered on such categories as animals and birds, fruit and vegetables, people who help us, things we use when we cook, garden, fix the car, or build a play house, ways we travel, types of buildings (schools, hospitals, libraries, firestations).

Children also need to be aware of the concept of roles in society. Roles and functions are related to categories. Each has associated vocabulary and language expressions. In the family the child learns the names and roles of mother, father, brother, sister, grandma and grandpa, aunt and uncle. Outside the family the children should be taught the language associated with the people they are most likely to encounter: teacher, letter carrier, doctor, nurse, shop assistant. Thus, you should develop activities that deal with "Who does this? What does he/she use?" By coordinating activities with the parents, you can reinforce experiences the child has had outside the class, such as a visit to the doctor or shoestore. Use such visits as the stimulus for teaching the concepts and language appropriate to roles and events. Similarly, planned visits to the zoo, circus, a children's play or parade or taking someone to the airport can provide further relevant language units. When you plan or recreate these language-stimulation experiences, try to capture not simply the vocabulary but also the event. Imagine yourself in the experience so that you can react as if you were actually there. You need to think in terms of natural language even though you will ensure redundancy through repetition and rephrasing. If you are talking about a visit to the airport, talk about more than the planes. Airports are busy places with parking lots, taxis, buses, luggage, check-in counters, coffee shops, bookstores. Encourage the parents to let the older children experience these broader aspects of a central concept in order to expand cognition and to provide an extended base for language needs.

Planned activities should be deliberately structured to provide such *expansion of concepts* over several sessions. This ensures that vocabulary and language structures can be reinforced and presented naturally in different forms. For example, the topic of food can encompass types of foods, categories of food, meals, what we eat at each meal, which foods we cook, ways of cooking, what we use to cook with, shopping for foods, ways of preparing food, and so on.

Lesson experiences should use real objects, play objects, pictures from commercial kits (for example, the Peabody Language Development Program), cutouts from magazines, and even photographs of the child visiting places being talked about or participating in activities at the center. Whenever possible, illustrate new vocabulary by acting it out or by using pictures. For example, you can demonstrate verbs such as fall, run, laugh, hit; adjectives such as angry, sad, happy, hungry, big, square, hot; adverbs such as quickly, quietly, loudly; prepositions such as in, under, behind, on top of. Exaggerated demonstrations that are funny and make the child laugh are always well received. Use examples in which the child can participate and can later copy and imitate. The visual images you create are hooks on which to hang concepts to keep them tidily placed with an appropriate experience. These examples provide the keys to generalization and categorization.

Use pictures only when real experiences are not possible, when concepts and vocabulary have been well learned, or as a record to remind the children of what they experienced. Things that can be illustrated should go into a scrapbook (workbook), which the parent(s), who should participate in lesson activities, can use with their child at home. The book should remind the parents of the concepts, vocabulary, and language structures that need to be reinforced and generalized to other similar objects and events at home. The integration of activities in the structural sessions with those of the child's daily experiences is essential to rapid learning. In the structured sessions draw on parental information about what the family has been doing. Likewise, the parents should reinforce what occurs in the preschool program.

Ensure That Language Is Appropriate

To facilitate language development, it is necessary to relate to the child's developmental language age rather than his chronological age. Your language structures should reinforce correct existing structures and model for the child at the next developmental level. Words not yet in the child's receptive vocabulary should be taught or should be used only in a context or situation in which the meaning of the word can be predicted. New words always should be used in sentences in order to develop knowledge of contextual relationships. If the child is at the one-word sentence level, that is, "Mommy" ("Where's mother?," a question; "Mommy gone," a need for reassurance; "Mommy come," a prediction), you need to respond with a simple sentence:

"Mommy's gone shopping."

"Yes, mommy's gone. She's coming back."

rather than "Mommy's gone shopping, but she'll be back in a little while."

Maximize Redundancy

In each of these teaching activities, we need to provide a high level of redundancy. I explained in Chapter 8 that information refers to all message-related cues from all sources. A minimum amount of information will be necessary in each situation for the threshold of comprehension to be crossed. Any cues in excess of the minimum are available to facilitate processing and to provide resistance to distortion or competition. The cushion of redundancy makes communication easier. As we have seen, hearing-impaired children seldom have the luxury of redundancy when learning. They need every cue/constraint we can provide. Thus, when we work with them we must strive constantly to provide as many cues as possible.

Teaching the child the relationship between what is happening and what we are likely to say about it is essential to increasing the chances of his understanding what actually is said. The ability to predict what will be said involves

- An understanding of the event (experience) or a described event
- The possibilities related to the event
- The sequence in which the experience evolves
- The language (words and phrases) associated with the occurrence

It is an accepted fact that a higher amount of information is necessary to learn something than to identify the same thing once learned. Thus, when new experiences and ideas are presented, you must ensure that you provide as many constraints or probabilities as possible. Sensory contact with the object, person, or event should be maximized. Looking, listening, touching, smelling, and tasting create the need for the words and phrases that identify those experiences. Draw attention to relevant properties or attributes of objects and people and then provide the language that communicates them. Statements should be simple in content and structure. They should be repeated and rephrased as you guide the child's awareness of what he is experiencing through his senses. Presenting spoken and/or gestured or signed language concurrently with the experience greatly increases the level of constraints affecting further communication. Try to build those cues into your dialogue. With flour in a bowl, sift it between your fingers. Then hold the bowl out to Mary. "Feel the flour, Mary." Do not cue David by holding out the bowl but look at him and say,

You feel it, David. The flour is dry. [Wet your finger, touch the flour, then taste it before turning to David.] Taste it David, taste the flour. Does it taste good? [Encourage David to reply.] Do you like it? Does it taste good? You don't like it, David. David pulled a funny face. Why doesn't he like it, Mary? You don't know? He doesn't like it because it's dry. Does it smell, Mary—smell it, smell it with your nose—no, it doesn't smell. David, what color is it? [No clues except that it is another experiential question. Provide constraints] Is it black? No. Is it green? No. What color is it? Right, David, it's white. What else here is white? Mary? Good, the milk—the milk and the flour are both white. Taste the milk, Mary—does that taste like the flour? [Mary fails to understand—dip a finger into the flour and another into the milk, taste them both and repeat your question] Does the milk taste like the flour? Do they taste the same? Taste them again, Mary. Do you like that taste, Mary [milk]? You like milk, it tastes good, but you don't like the flour.

As vocabulary is learned and language structures acquired, we can begin to reduce the constraints. This places greater demands on language as the source of information. We can use our photographs or cutout pictures rather than the real things to set constraints. We re-create the experience in abstraction; we recall memories of it; then we use language to discuss those memories. We recall, practice, and reinforce the language that now stands for the memories that stand for the real experience. Boothroyd (1982, p. 136) advises: "Withhold nonlanguage cues until the child has had an opportunity to process the language cues." You should quickly add more cues until the child understands, since communication always must result in success, not in frustration.

Mold Language

In the examples given, the children already are using language. Their communications, whether they use speech, sign, or both, should be accepted and responded to. It is essential that the child's communication meet with strong acceptance and encouragement. Being understood means success to the child. She never should be interrupted in the attempt to communicate since communication is about understanding. Language and speech patterns, however, can be molded within parameters of communicating. Acknowledging the child's communication by restating it provides acceptance but also provides an example against which the child's brain can compare and modify its own model.

We can increase the child's awareness of specific language use through activities that focus on particular linguistic structures or forms. For example, you can facilitate the acquisition of language function as part of auditory-visual communication activities. These might concentrate, for example, on selecting pictures to represent the subject-verb-object construction or the present continuous tense:

- The boy is running.
- The bird is flying.
- The fish is swimming.
- John is crying.
- Mother is cooking.

Are you ready, David, listen well. The bird is flying. [David responds incorrectly.] No, listen again; you thought I said, John is crying, <u>crying</u>—but I said—flying, the bird is flying. Try again, listen well. The bird is flying—good. The bird is flying. What is the bird doing? Right, flying, good for you. It is flying.

When an item is correctly identified, or has been identified for the child, you should ask the child to repeat the sentence after you. You can reinforce the model for the child by giving look-listen-and-interpret tasks that hold part of the sentence constant while you identify the remainder:

- Mother is cooking.
- John is cooking.
- Father is cooking.
- or Mother is cooking
          is reading
          is laughing.

This structure can be reinforced by instructing Mary what to do (cry, hop, smile, clap, etc.) and asking David to tell what she is doing.

Formal drill is not appropriate. The goal is to mold the language the child is using, to influence by restating in an enriched, correct form the idea the child is expressing. You also should manipulate the activities and situations to create a need for a category of words and for various structures to provide many examples and opportunities to use them. These must arise as part of general communicative interactions so that their use by the child derives from a meaningful context. In this way he will receive the rewards of effective communication.

If a child has difficulty formulating questions, you may choose to develop a lesson plan that combines the use of question forms with, for example, listen-look-and-interpret training on the topic of "People Who Help Us."

DOES	**DO**	**CAN**
Does the letter carrier bring us letters?	Do cats climb trees?	Can an elephant fly?
Does the dog say meow?	Do we eat turkey for breakfast?	Can a fish swim?
Does a ball bounce?	Do we wear a banana?	Can a cat bark?
Does a cup have a handle?	Do mice have tails?	Can children laugh?
Does a bird have four legs?	Do chairs have legs?	Can a dog laugh?
	Do trousers have sleeves?	

You can use photographs to identify the nouns used, or you may draw pictures to illustrate both the truth and the absurdities. Encourage children to ask the question by repeating it with you, then later by asking a question about a picture with minimal prompting by you. Similarly, use *who-what-which*, and *where-when-how* questions to structure a look-listen-and-interpret activity. Things and people can first be classified into *who* and *what* categories. The children listen while you name an object or person, and then give a sentence. "Ball—the ball bounces." They then find and place the picture in the "What" category. Later you can expand to Who *does* what and Who *has* what. *Which* can also be introduced to identify the appropriate category.

"Which bounces—the ball or the egg?"

"Who brings letters—the doctor or the letter carrier?"

Where, when, and how can be taught in the same way.

Remember, your role is to reinforce language use. Your primary concern is to increase speech understanding through listening and watching and to improve speech articulation through speech training. However, because both are performance skills based upon the child's language competence, it would be illogical to use materials or activities for speech perception and production training that are not supportive of cognitive and linguistic needs.

FOSTERING AUDITORY-VISUAL PERCEPTIONS

Paying attention to auditory and visual cues is a process intimately related to the language and concepts to which they refer. Auditory and visual training, therefore, must be an aspect of language stimulation. We need to consider listening and watching and interpreting as integral components of the process of comprehension rather than as separate skills to be isolated and trained. Thus in working with these children you should include techniques for focusing attention on words, phrases, and sentences within context, drawing attention to how they sound and look.

The aims of training in listening, watching, and interpreting should be to

- Make the children aware of sound made available to them by amplification
- Establish listening (attention) behavior
- Make the children aware of the referential function of sound
- Train the children to discriminate between and among sound patterns
- Make the children aware of speech as communicative behavior
- Encourage the children to pay attention to speech
- Relate speech patterns to conceptual values, thus forming semantic values
- Increase the children's ability to use auditory patterns to identify semantic values
- Integrate new auditory perceptual skills into the language-acquisition process by fostering the development of feed-forward competencies (that is, using cognition—linguistics and auditory perception—in an integrative manner to predict meaning)
- Develop awareness of the visible characteristics of speech behavior
- Train the children to watch for visible speech cues
- Train the children to discriminate among the visible patterns of units of speech
- Facilitate integration of auditory and visual constraint patterns
- Develop strategies for processing auditory and visual information

You must assess each child's needs carefully to determine at what stage she is functioning. The amount of residual hearing and the age at which amplification and intervention begin will greatly influence the child's acquired abilities. However, you do not know what a child needs until you have carefully observed her behavior and have assessed the level of function at each stage. You first should emphasize the utilization of residual hearing. However, naturally occurring visual cues to speech should be suppressed only for short periods during an activity; this concentrates listening and highlights the acoustic characteristics of the speech pattern. What you have isolated temporarily should very soon be fitted back into the total integrated conceptual pattern. Even the strongest advocates of a unisensory auditory approach to training do not suggest eliminating visual information. Pollack (1970) writes: "His energy is directed towards listening, and the rewards and reinforcements are for listening. True, he is not blindfolded, and visual perception can take place, but only in the same natural way it occurs during a normal hearing child's activities" (p. 87).

Listening and watching should, therefore, be treated as a single behavior. You should not deny the child the visual cues to speech, but you should focus attention on them only when the child appears to need more information than can be derived from auditory cues.

Listening, Watching, and Interpreting (Environmental Sounds)

Motivation is a prime factor in focusing and sustaining attention. The children should enjoy the activities you select. For this reason gross-sound discrimination provides an excellent way of introducing children to listening and watching behaviors. Recorded environmental sounds are most appropriate for this age group. These may be taken from commercially available records, or they may be recordings that you have made yourself. It is important to make recordings on a good quality high-speed tape recorder. Select the sounds on the basis of how commonly they may be expected to be encountered in the children's environment. Your choice will also be influenced by how easily you will be able to find an illustration of the object, person, and/or event that gives rise to each sound or group of sounds.

Your first task is to ensure that the children are aware of the sounds you have recorded and to check that each child is familiar with them. In the first session present each sound three or four times with a short pause between each presentation. For example, the first sound may be a telephone ringing. As you play and repeat the recording, show the children a picture of a telephone. You listen, point to the picture, and say, "telephone—the telephone's ringing—telephone." If you have any doubts whether a particular child can hear the sound, play the game with that child alone. "John—listen, point to the telephone when it rings—that's right, it's ringing—listen again—good boy." Repeat the procedure for a small group of different sounds that you should present one by one—for example, telephone ringing, dog barking, fire engine siren, vacuum cleaner going. These then constitute the sounds for a first lesson in listening and watching. Put all pictures of all four sounds on a stand and play the next part of the tape, on which the sounds are recorded several times in different order. Ask the children to listen, then point to the picture associated with that sound. It is helpful with the older preschool children to be able to move from single pictures to clear drawings on ditto sheets, or better still, to individual photocopies of professionally drawn illustrations so that each child can point to the object on her own sheet. To increase auditory attention, vary the interval between the sounds. Sometimes plan for two presentations to follow each other closely in time, but pause before the next one, encouraging the children to listen carefully:

Wait, listen (pointing to your ear). No (shaking your head and frowning as you listen hard). Ah, there it is (smiling and rewarding the child for a correct identification).

It is important to note if any of the children appear to be having difficulty in paying attention, or in correctly identifying the sounds. Do not let a child become discouraged in the group. It may be necessary to provide individual sessions for such a child to bring that child up to the level of performance of the group. An individual session frequently provides the same stimulation and success necessary for the child to gain confidence in the use of residual hearing.

Some children entering the preschool program late, particularly those with limited residual hearing, may need to work with actual noise makers rather than taped sounds. Drums, bells, keys, or rattles may prove more stimulating initially than recorded sounds, because the child experiences the actual noise source, can see and hold it, and can make the sounds herself.

Remember that discrimination of nonspeech sounds does not directly influence the ability to discriminate speech. However, both involve the perceptual processes of expectancy, attention, reception, trial and check, and perception, which we discussed in Chapter 7. Furthermore, because you use relevant spoken language during the listening and responding activities, you are providing the natural stimulus of speech in context. You will increase that context in the next stage of listening, watching, and interpreting training when you present sounds grouped according to activities or events. Once the children are responding well to short sessions involving individual sound recognition, move to the recognition of sounds in situational context. At this stage of training, you will integrate gross-sound recognition, concept building, language training, and speech. To do this, group sounds according to a common context. For example, you may select sounds usually associated with mothers (cooking, cleaning, drying hair, sewing, washing dishes), or you may use the sounds usually associated with fathers (hammering, sawing, mowing the lawn, taking out the garbage cans). It is not intended that mothers and fathers be characterized in stereotyped roles. However, the sounds the young child hears around the house during the day are most likely to be made by the mother or mother substitute. You may select sounds animals make, or sounds that occur in the home (telephone, doorbell, alarm clock, radio or television, clock). Encourage the children to listen to, identify, name, and talk about the appropriate sounds. You can use pictures depicting, for example, mother working in the kitchen, father building something at the workbench, male and female police officers or fire fighters at work, to provide the basis for explaining and talking about the activities to which these sounds relate. As the children learn the names of people and objects that generate the sounds, they listen to those sounds again. You want to develop a level of performance at which the sound cues the appropriate semantic values and evokes the associated linguistic structures.

Listening activities can progress from "Who or what makes this sound?" (mother, father, baby, dog, telephone) to "What is happening?" (mother is sweeping, father is hammering, the telephone is ringing). A child may respond by pointing to the appropriate picture of the sound source (for example, father) and then may choose from among pictures showing that person (father) doing different things that make sounds. Each time a correct response is made, provide the child with a language model appropriate to the event:

That's right, Mother is vacuuming *the carpet.*
Good, baby is crying.
Yes, the dog is barking.

Building a Bridge to Speech Perception

The next step is to have the children learn to listen, watch, and respond to the language structures that identify the sound in its absence. First, train the children to identify the objects and people by name. Select one picture representing each object or person. In the beginning, put only three pictures on the stand. Ask the children to listen and then to point to the appropriate person or object. In order to avoid separating words from spoken-language forms, present the person or object in a sentence as well as alone:

Dog—dog *is barking*—dog. *Mary, show me the* dog. *Where's the* dog?

As the children begin to gain confidence in their responses, increase the number of pictures to which you refer. When a child experiences difficulty, the first thing to do is to draw attention to the visual appearance of the spoken word. Require the child to watch carefully as you name the object or person that is difficult to identify auditorily. Frequently the child has already made use of the additional visual cues. In this case drawing attention to them may not result in correct identification. You need to increase the extrinsic redundancy by providing situational constraints. Say the sentence: "Dog—the dog is barking," play the nonspeech cue of the dog barking, then repeat the sentence. More concentrated auditory-visual processing within tighter constraints may help the child gradually build the level of expectancy, permitting him to predict the meaning of the communication from the minimal speech, auditory, and visual cues received. This may take many auditory exposures while listening intently. Do not rush into deciding that the auditory and naturally processed visual cues are insufficient for comprehension to be possible. *Auditory-visual perception of speech is so linguistically and cognitively related that what a child cannot perceive today may be perceived tomorrow if appropriate holistic stimulation fosters growth.*

Always try to provide the children with experience in listening to and identifying the nonverbal auditory and visual situational cues to speech. However, most listening and watching training will involve recognition and interpretation of spoken language. Always keep in mind that the tasks you are asking the children to perform must be useful, relevant to their experiences, correlated to their cognitive and linguistic levels of function, and related to their ability to model the sound they hear. Hearing, language, and speech are interdependent processes and should always be treated as such. When you focus on one of these three components, your purpose is to enrich the sophistication of all three. You must avoid training procedures that treat one component independently to ensure that your efforts do not prove disruptive to the integrity of the whole.

Listening, Watching, and Interpreting (Spoken Language)

Listening, watching, and interpreting are activities that cannot be separated from cognitive and linguistic growth. We listen to spoken language, which identifies relevant concepts. This activity consists, therefore, of auditory-visual stimulation to reinforce the child's cognitive and linguistic experience. Your aim is to focus on the auditory and visual components of the language related to these experiences. In so doing you will

> Provide repeated examples of the relevant spoken language, reinforcing the child's perceptions
> Provide the necessary structure to refine those perceptions
> Build the child's confidence in the ability to understand speech

To do this you need to be familiar with the unit that is being worked on in school, and it is hoped, reinforced at home. The teacher may be concentrating on foods we eat (when we eat them, how we cook them, how things taste), on colors, or action verbs, on prepositions, on people who help us, or on the experience of a class trip. Seasons and holidays, outdoor activities, and clothes we wear are all frequently occurring topics, too.

The level of language of the children in the group will influence your approach. First you will need to reinforce key words and phrases. When you do this, emphasize listening. Have the children close their eyes as you say the name or phrase appropriate to the picture; then have them open their eyes and watch your face as you repeat it. Now have them close their eyes and listen again very carefully to the same message. The children should be encouraged to listen and attempt to repeat what you say. Link listening to speech production whenever possible because listening and watching aim to develop the most accurate internal image of the spoken message. It is from this internal model that speech will be generated.

Your activities with very young or severely language-delayed children of necessity may be confined to auditory-visual recognition of primary concepts. These may be built around physical activities in which the children participate—for example, walking, jumping, hopping, running. They may involve such basic concepts as up and down, in and out, under and over. The activities may be accompanied by played or recorded music (Whitehurst, 1971). After physical involvement you can present the constraint cues in the form of pictures. Then ask the children to listen, watch and listen, and listen again as you say about the picture:

The little dog is under the table.
The little bird goes hopping, hopping, hopping.
Pussycat's up on the roof.

Then ask the children to choose the relevant pictures, or to make the appropriate cutout picture animal perform the described activity. Children learn by action (Menyuk, 1976). Whenever possible, use activities in which the child does something in response to speech. For example, first place a box, a hat, a toy bird, a cardboard ladder, and a toy dog on a table.

Lisa, come and find the hat—hat—hat—put it on your head—put the hat on your head. Good girl, you put the hat on your head.

David, the bird hopped into the box. Bird—make the bird hop—hop, hop, hop into the box. Make it hop into the box. That's right, into—into the box.

Sarah, the dog goes up the ladder—listen, dog, dog, the dog goes up—up, up—up the ladder—the dog goes up the ladder. Here I'll help you. Here's the dog—dog, dog—listen and watch—dog. Make the dog go up (pointing up) up, up, up the ladder (guiding Sarah's hand). Good girl, you made the dog go up the ladder—now make the dog come down—down, that's right, down. Up and down.

You will need to modify the cues and support you give depending on the capabilities of individual children in the group. Concentrate on listening and watching behavior. Increase auditory attention by having the children wait in anticipation for a few seconds before you give the message. Tell them:

I'm thinking (adopt an exaggerate thinking pose)—about—the pussycat. Are you ready? Are you listening? Are you listening, Jane?

The pussycat—jumps—into—the box. Pussycat into the box. Make the pussycat jump into the box, David.

Keep sessions short enough to hold the group's attention, ensure success and reward by providing appropriate redundancy and support, and repeat short lessons several times during the school session.

As the children show increasing conceptual and linguistic growth, listening and watching training can become more complex. It will be possible to have the children listen to simple descriptive sentences and then to act out the descriptions.

This morning when I got up I
- *rubbed my eyes*
- *stretched my arms*
- *brushed my teeth*
- *combed my hair*
- *put on my socks*
- *put on my dress/shirt and trousers*
- *put on my shoes*

The children can listen and participate as a group. Sometimes an individual child can be named to listen, watch, and interpret. You can modify the game to ask children to listen for absurdities.

I stretched my teeth. No we don't stretch our teeth (shaking our head and laughing). What do we stretch, Mary? That's right, we stretch our arms. Stretch everyone, stretch your arms.

I put on my hair. We don't put on our hair. What do you do to your hair, John? You comb it. Good boy. Comb—let's comb our hair.

I combed my shoes. Do we comb shoes, Dena? No. What do we comb? Right, we comb our hair. What do we do with our shoes? We put them on. We put our shoes on our feet.

David, did you put on your dress? Do you wear a dress, David? No. Mary wears a dress. What do you wear, David? A shirt—good.

In a unit on Thanksgiving you would first review vocabulary to ensure understanding; then, using pictures identifying key concepts, you can ask the children to identify the picture that is the topic of your message.

The Pilgrims first celebrated Thanksgiving. For Thanksgiving we have a big turkey. We eat cranberries with our turkey. Mother makes pumpkin pie. We sit around a big fire at Thanksgiving.

Other special holidays can also be identified by auditory or auditory-visual recognition of such statements as

I have a big chocolate egg.
The presents are under the tree.
We get dressed up in funny clothes and we collect candy.
We watch the fireworks.

Progressively developing an idea by feeding more information to the children will help hold interest and attention and will thus encourage good listening and watching behavior. For example, you can place an object in a paper bag and then progressively name its characteristics:

We eat it.
It is oval (show the oval shape with your fingers and repeat—oval, it is oval).
It is sour (pucker your face).
It is a fruit (point to illustration of various kinds of fruit).
It is yellow.
(If a child cannot identify the fruit ask:)
Is it an orange? No, an orange is not yellow. An orange is orange. An orange is not oval. An orange is round. Is it a banana? (And so on.)

Let the child feel the content of the bag without looking. If the child still does not guess correctly, first show the fruit, then name it. Finally, repeat what you said about it while the child listens and then listens and watches carefully. You may then show the lemon contrasted with an orange. Help the child compare orange to oval, feel the shapes, draw the shapes, discriminate between the shapes, learn the words. Then choose round or oval to describe: like a lemon, like a ball, like an orange, like an egg. Expansions of this lesson could involve auditory-visual discrimination of the names of tastes: sweet, sour, salty, juicy, dry, hot, cold; and of shapes: round, oval, curved, square, all as related to foods and food packages.

In another activity you may encourage the children to listen, watch, and interpret by giving each child two objects or pictures. You then tell a simple story involving one of the objects. When you name or tell about the object, the child who has it must give you that object. Receiving the object you say, "Good, Mary, I was talking about the egg. I said, The robin had three eggs in its nest."

As the child begins to acquire the perceptual behaviors that permit correct prediction of meaning from samples of spoken language, your concern will be for finer discrimination. You will wish to assess ability to discriminate between similar sounding words and eventually to discriminate between syllabic units. The perception of individual speech sounds is not essential to speech comprehension. In fact, we are seldom aware of the phonological components of speech because we perceive at the level of meaningful units—morphemes, words, or phrases. Sometimes we listen for a sound that has morphological value (for example, lady: lady's, ladies; laugh, laughed), but it is not often that we need to perceive an individual sound to resolve ambiguity. Nevertheless, improved discrimination between sounds similar in acoustic structure will contribute to redundancy. Even more important, when successful it greatly facilitates teaching correct speech articulation. We articulate speech in order to enhance the transmission of the message intent. Once again, therefore, we must remain cognizant of the inseparable relationship between language and speech.

We have stressed the importance of structuring listening, watching, and interpreting training around school and home experiences and language. A session that concentrates on these receptive skills differs only from a general class activity in the amount of emphasis placed upon them. In the classroom situation, overall communication is the main concern. Concepts and language are presented; experiences are provided and talked about. Total learning is taking place. Although the teacher will encourage watching and listening, it would be disruptive to concentrate on how a word or phrase sounds and looks when spoken. Spoken language must flow with the experience. The listen, look, and interpret session allows you to intensify perception of the auditory-visual characteristics of the spoken message. It permits you to build internal perceptual images at a time when a child can pay full attention to watching and listening within the framework of well-structured language and content. Yet listening and watching are part of the larger task of experiencing learning and communicating. It is an ability essential to full classroom participation. You are seeking to improve each child's ability to participate fully so that when the teacher says, "Are you listening David? Watch me," David will have the perceptual organization that permits him to attend closely.

ASSESSING AND IMPROVING SPEECH PRODUCTION

For children with some residual hearing, you as a speech-language pathologist or teacher will feel great pressure to have the child produce intelligible speech. Quite understandably, speech is seen by parents as the most significant evidence of their child's potential to survive in the hearing society. Even for children of this age who have severe to profound hearing deficits, the desire of most parents will be for them to achieve oral intelligibility, at least at a level that permits essential communication with hearing persons. For some parents, the period of structured preschool education represents a final opportunity to ensure the child will become oral and enter the mainstream of education. To them this is a now-or-never time. It indeed will be a deciding period for those children for whom the most appropriate method of education has not yet been determined. It is important, therefore, to make certain that the contract between you and the parents is understood thoroughly. Frank exploration and acceptance of the feelings of all influential family members, including, if appropriate, grandparents or live-in partners, are crucial. You should carry out the following steps at this point:

- Discuss the parents' current feelings regarding methods of communication for their child.
- Discuss thoroughly the ease or difficulty of communication of child to parents and parents to child.
- Discuss the level of frustration experienced by child and parent. Include discussion of the child's symptoms of stress or absence of such evidence.
- Review the communication abilities of children with normal hearing who are entering kindergarten. Encourage the parents to observe one or two kindergarten classes.
- Discuss the child's ability to communicate with people outside the immediate family and with hearing children.
- Review the communication and learning demands of regular kindergarten.
- Provide and discuss a current assessment of the child's speech production abilities and intelligibility.
- State frankly your interpretation of the assessment results. Do so in terms of the level of oral communication the child might reasonably be expected to achieve by the age of entry to public education.
- Set reasonable goals that are acceptable to the parents. Explain methods for achieving those goals.
- Describe and discuss the role the parents can play in contributing to goal attainment.

A Speech Teaching Model

I have stressed the importance of accepting a child's spoken communications since his primary motivation is to have his needs or ideas understood. I have discussed with you techniques for stimulating auditory behavior and vocal production. We talked also of the role that restating and modeling the young child's early oral communication plays in establishing optimal speech models in his brain. We can expect that by the later preschool years, those children with some residual hearing, who have received early amplification and oral stimulation, will be using spoken language, either as a primary or supportive means of communication. We can assume that since his first vocalizations, an up-to-date record has been kept of the child's progress in using speech as a communication tool. Only for hearing-impaired children identified late will the enhanced base for speech production that results from early stimulation be absent. For these children a complete ment will be necessary.

When considering how to make a complete formal assessme _ or speech production, one system stands out like a beacon; it is that of Daniel Ling. His book *Speech and the Hearing Impaired Child* (1976) comprises a thoroughly researched and philosophically sound rationale for systemic evaluation and teaching of all components of speech. Anyone working to teach or improve the speech of hearing-impaired children, or indeed of any child with a speech articulation problem, should be familiar with the method advocated by Ling. The text and full supporting materials are commercially available from the Alexander Graham Bell Association for the Deaf. Fundamental to the Ling method are the following principles:

- Speech production comprises a set of motor behaviors that are distinct, rapid, finely tuned, and coordinated.
- In normal speech production these motor behaviors are automatic.
- Normal speech is dependent upon auditory kinesthetic feedback.
- Monitoring of present output by feedback permits fine tuning of planned motor speech patterns to reduce error in ongoing production.
- Teaching of speech sounds requires that speech articulation be separated from spoken language in the early stages.
- Phonetic level activities precede phonologic use of speech sounds.
- Hearing-impaired children acquire speech sounds most easily when they are taught in the normal developmental order.

Ling believes that a child cannot learn to produce speech naturally before control of speech breathing and vocalization has been mastered and all the articulatory movements involved in speech can be produced. The control must be such as to allow smooth rapid and accurate motor behavior patterns at a level of automaticity. The particular combinations of these skills, requisite for a particular speech sound in a particular phonetic context, then can be taught. To achieve this, the child is helped to develop an internal perceptual model of the correct sound. This requires careful listening to auditory models and careful observation of visible articulatory cues supplemented as necessary by tactile information and special teaching strategies. We seek also to maximize the child's auditory and motor kinesthetic awareness of his own production.

By detaching speech-sound production from meaning, we avoid contamination from established faulty word articulation patterns. Further, we can control phonetic context to avoid difficult sound combinations during the learning stage. The sound is taught in nonsense syllables in all its phonetic contexts and raised to a level of automaticity before it is introduced into meaningful words (i.e., into the child's phonology). At the phonological level, since the sound now can be produced correctly, strategies are directed toward restructuring the auditory-motor-kinesthetic models of established word patterns. Assessment is dictated by this teaching model.

Assessment

The essential components of speech production to be assessed are

- Integrity of the oral-peripheral mechanism
- Phonologic performance
- Vocal control (intensity, pitch, duration, quality)
- Vowel production
- Consonant production

We wish to determine the child's present production of speech at the phonologic level, that is, his normal speech communication. We wish also to assess his ability to articulate each speech sound in all its phonetic combinations when uninfluenced by word production patterns.

Oral-Peripheral Assessment. It is essential to identify any significant deviancy that warrants referral for medical examination. Many syndromes with which hearing disability is associated also produce head and neck abnormalities. Any suspected deviancy upon referral may result in a revision of etiology and medical treatment and thus a modification in management plans. A physical deviance also may require special compensatory teaching strategies.

Phonologic Assessment. This is an assessment of the child's ability to articulate all sounds correctly in all phonetic contexts occurring in spontaneous speech. Ling (1976, p. 145) states that samples of 50 utterances representative of the child's oral communication provide an adequate basis for phonologic analysis. These samples are subjected to the same analysis as the elicited responses used to complete phonetic analysis.

Phonetic Analysis. This is made by having the child imitate your production of nonsense syllables or patterns. It should be conducted using optimal amplification. Analysis begins with the nonsegmental aspects of speech dependent on the control of the voice.

Voice. The control of voice is necessary for the management of suprasegmental, or prosodic, characteristics of spoken language. Since voice is the basis of all vowels and voiced consonants, it also is a critical component of speech articulation. Vocalization for speech is a complex process. It requires adequate breath and breath control to power and sustain vocalization as well as the ability to coordinate vocalization and breathing for clean initiation and termination of sounds. During vocalization, the vocal folds must make complete vibratory contact or air wastage will result in breathy speech. Finally the speaker must plan and execute speech breathing patterns appropriate to the syntactic structure of the linguistic message and must control pitch intensity and duration to generate the suprasegmental patterns that clarify meaning. Disruptance of one or more of these control abilities will interfere both with speech intelligibility and speech acceptability. Since voice monitoring by a hearing person primarily is achieved through audition, interference with the process will occur when impairment of hearing in the frequency range of the voice is severe. Children with hearing impairments exceeding 75dB HL in the frequencies below 500 Hz not uncommonly exhibit voice production and/or control difficulties. When the spontaneous speech evidences any deviancy in the control or quality of voice, a thorough assessment should be made once it has been determined that no physical anomaly is present to account for the deviance.

Assessment of voice production and control involves checking the ability of the child to

- Vocalize on command
- Coordinate breathing and vocalizing
- Sustain vocalization
- Produce nonbreathy sustained voice
- Vary and control intensity
- Vary and control pitch
- Plan and control appropriate patterns of breathing for speech
- Produce vocal patterns of intensity, pitch, duration, and rate appropriate for speech

Vocal duration. The child should be able to imitate sustained vocalization for three seconds or more [a————], brief vocalizations in series [a – a – a – a] and a stream of at least four vocalizations varying in durational pattern [a—a–a—a-a].

Vocal intensity. The child must imitate a loud vocalization, a quiet vocalization, and a whisper, each sustained for three seconds. The child must be able to do the same with several syllables.

Pitch control. The child must be able to imitate vocalization that changes in pitch pattern over at least eight semitones from low to high. She must be able to do this in both directions—low to high, high to low—using both continuous voice, and interrupted vocalizations. The pitch change should flow smoothly for continuous vocalization without abrupt shifts. The production of interrupted vocalization should produce true pitch shifts without slides.

Quality control. The quality of vocalization relates to breath control, laryngeal action, synchrony of breathing and vocal fold vibration, and control of oral-nasal resonance. Thus, in addition to pitch, intensity, and duration, you should listen for evidence of

- Breathy voicing caused by inadequate adduction of the vocal folds during vocalization of vowels and voiced consonants
- Breathy voice onset, caused by poor synchrony of voicing with consonant production
- Poor vocal arrest of vowels preceding unvoiced stop consonants: at-at-at, up-up-up
- Hyper- or hyponasal resonance resulting from inadequate velar-pharyngeal control for speech and/or inadequate oral resonance.

Segmental Assessment. This involves evaluation of the child's ability to produce speech sounds consistently, inconsistently, or not at all. Further, Ling (1976) stresses the need to assess the child's ability to

Correctly articulate repeated sounds /babababababa/ at normal rate
Alternate sound patterns batabatabata at regular rate
Vary intensity [ta ta ta], duration [tada . . . a tada . . . a], and pitch

da   da   da
[ta   ta   ta   ]

Vowel Dipthong Articulation Assessment. The criteria for appropriate vowel production as listed by Ling (1976, p. 150) include the ability to

- Sustain the vowel/dipthong for three seconds or more without quality change
- Repeat the sound at three per second in whisper and in quiet and loud voice
- Alternate any two target vowels
- Vary vocal pitch of a vowel over eight semitones while maintaining quality

Each criterion is assessed in terms of the child's ability to imitate the model you provide.

Consonant Production. Consonant production criteria include

- Correct consonant production in single and repeated syllables [di] [didididi]
- Ability to alternate consonants in syllables [badabada]
- Ability to produce consonants in whispered, quiet, and loud syllables
- Ability to produce consonants while varying pitch over eight semitones (Ling, 1976, p. 153)

Initial and final consonant blends are assessed in sets (Ling, 1976, Appendix B, pp. 166–168), omitting the test of alternating in syllables.

Ling provides in his text and in the kits available, all the necessary forms for recording a child's performance. It is obvious that this assessment procedure takes time and requires the child's attentive cooperation. It is a process that should be spread over several periods in order to ensure the validity of results. Several short assessment sessions, each well within the child's cooperative attention span, can be sandwiched among other activities. This should allow the assessment to be completed in two or three sessions even for a child with a well-developed phonetic system. Once a ceiling in the child's phonetic assessment has been reached, a teaching plan can be followed. The model presented by Ling is an extension of the model you used for assessment.

Teaching Speech-Sound Production

Ling (1976) uses the normal developmental pattern of speech acquisition as the frame for his model, which governs the teaching of classes of sounds and the target behaviors within each sound. The model delineates seven stages of speech acquisition for both the phonetic and phonologic levels. These are shown in Figure 15.1 (p. 290–91).

Target behaviors are the vocal articulatory requirements for the production of the sound. For example, the targets for /t/ and /d/ are tongue tips to alveolar ridge with lateral closure against upper gums and molar teeth, neutral lip and jaw, raised velum. To achieve the target appropriate to a particular sound, a set of subskills are a prerequisite:

> Orderly teaching demands that training result in the cumulative acquisition of subskills, each subskill providing some immediate gain compatible with later achievement. (Ling, 1976, p. 109)

The subskills for /t/ and /d/ are identified as

Subskill 1: Production of [d] or [t] releasing various vowels including [a], [u], and [i] (e.g., [da], [du]).

Subskill 2: Production of [d] or [t] in a series of repeated syllables, formed with one vowel or another (e.g., [dadada], [dididi]).

Subskill 3: Production of [d] or [t] in a series of repeated syllables, with various vowels (e.g., [dadidu], [dodida]).

Subskill 4: Alternation of syllables released with [d] or [t] and syllables released with other consonants taught in Steps 1 and 2 (e.g., [dono], [widi]).

Subskill 5: Production of [d] or [t] in syllables varying in intensity.

Subskill 6: Production of [d] or [t] repeated in intervocalic position with either the first or second vowel stressed.

Subskill 7: Production of [d] or [t] in repeated or alternated syllables varying in pitch over a range of at least eight semitones. (Ling, 1976, p. 320)

For each stage of speech acquisition, from speech breathing and voicing to the production of consonant blends, Ling identifies the target behavior, the prerequisite subskills, and the specific strategies for teaching. He also explains strategies for correcting faulty speech behaviors such as inadequate breath control, tension of articulators, exaggeration and prolongation of movements, and so on.

The teaching of speech should be quite separate from language at the phonetic level. The goal is to

> Persuade the child to focus intense attention on the auditory-visual sound stimulus
> Establish a new internal model
> Articulate that model
> Monitor and assess its production

These goals cannot be achieved in the traditional 30- to 45-minute speech therapy session, even with a school-age child. With preschool children it would be patently absurd to try. Thus teaching sessions must be very brief, no more than three or four minutes at a time. Instead of a lesson devoted to speech teaching, small units of teaching are spread throughout the day. Ten three-minute sessions of high attention and effort are infinitely more productive than a 30-minute session of progressive boredom and frustration. If you are bound by the 30-minute model, sandwich the mini–speech sessions within a larger language and experiential training unit, allowing seven two-minute periods of concentrated speech teaching. The two-minute sessions can be enriched by play activities that incorporate a particular

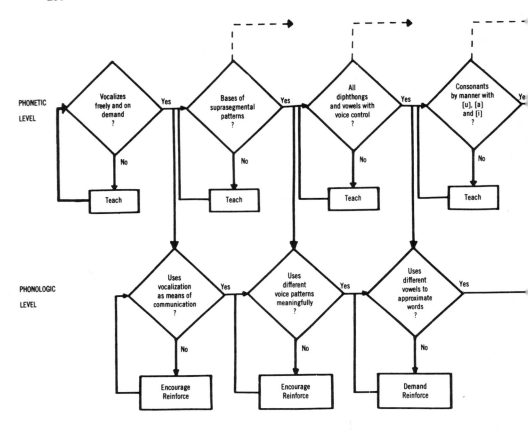

Figure 15.1 A seven-stage model for speech acquisition in hearing-impaired children. Diamonds represent evaluation and oblongs represent intervention procedures. Dotted lines indicate that when 70 percent of the work at a particular stage is completed, work at the next stage may be initiated. (Ling, 1976, p. 174–175.)

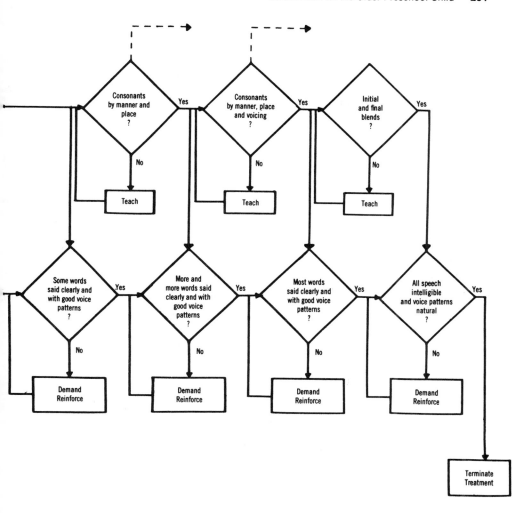

vocal articulatory pattern already learned. For example, if sustained and interrupted vocalization is the subskill, use or be an airplane that makes the sound only when it flies.

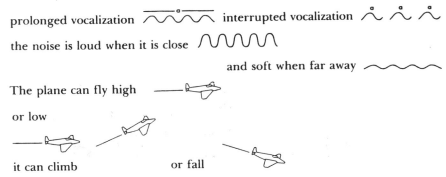

Similarly big tugboats chug fast, slow, high, low, soft, and loud; cars or subway trains hum, mmmm; little boats putt, while animals make all manner of sounds high and low, soft and loud, long and short (baa, moo, me-ow). In this way we can provide training in listening (auditory attention, discrimination, recognition), visual-speech recognition, auditory-visual processing, and object/activity identification, all as a relevant underpinning for speech.

Phonetic to Phonologic Transfer

> At the phonologic level speech and language come together. The model accords with the view that teaching at the phonologic level should be concerned, not so much with speech production per se as with spoken language development and with the integration of lexical, morphological, and syntactic development into the speech system. (Ling, 1976, p. 173)

At this level, our concern is only with those vocal-articulatory patterns that already have been acquired to automaticity. There should be no question about the child's ability to produce an aspect of voice control (intensity or pitch modulation, for example) or an articulatory behavior pattern for a given sound. Having acquired these, the goal now is to give the learned sound pattern appropriate linguistic value: To achieve this we must place the acquired vocal-articulatory pattern and its associated internal motor-sensory (auditory-tactile motor-kinesthetic) image pattern in linguistic contexts. This is necessary for the child to perceive the value of that particular speech behavior in terms of communication effectiveness. Both suprasegmental patterns (stress and intonation) and segmental units (speech sounds) need to be incorporated into the child's natural utterances. For example, pitch variations taught phonetically using nonsense syllables now can be transferred to meaningful words and sentences:

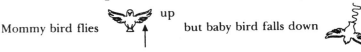

Stress and intonation patterns can be learned for a given word or phrase first using nonsense syllables (ba baba ba-ba) (bababa ba -ba). Tapping out these rhythms and stresses helps establish the image. The child can imitate the tapping, or you can tap with her hand. The pattern once learned can be transferred to an enjoyable language play.

> A small square of colored paper is stuck on the first finger of your left hand—its name is Peter.
> A piece of another color is stuck on the first finger of the right hand—its name is Paul. The two finger tips then are placed next to each other on the table and the following rhyme is said:
>
> *Two* little *dickie* birds *sitting* on a *wall*
> *One* named *Peter, one* named *Paul*
> *Fly* away *Peter, fly* away *Paul*
> *Come* back *Peter,* come back *Paul*

On "fly away" the hand is thrown over the shoulder and replaced, but now the second finger is on the table showing no colored paper. The first fingers with the paper are curled out of sight in the palm of each hand. "Come back" reverses the procedure to make the paper visible again. Soon the child is persuaded to give the "fly away" and "come back" commands.

Nursery rhymes provide an excellent source of material for rhythm and stress training in a language context. These can be reinforced by tapping or as in "pat-a-cake" by clapping, as you and the child/children say them in chorus.

Stories allow children to participate in vocal modulation, as, for example, in a father-bear voice, a mother-bear voice, and a baby-bear voice. Stress and intonation are encouraged in "Who's been sleeping in my bed?" Similarly, individual speech sounds can be focused on experiential language activities. Each child listens for his particular sound, which initiates or arrests a word illustrated by one of a series of pictures. The child must listen, watch, interpret (discriminate), and choose the picture with his sound in it. Once the child chooses a picture correctly, we tell an interesting piece of information; "The *f*ire engine is going *f*ast to the *f*ire. The people are *sh*outing. The firemen *shoo* them away, *shoo-shoo*." The child first repeats with stimulation, then is asked to say what the card illustrates. When all the cards are identified, the sequence is reorganized into a ministory. Each child describes his component with emphasis on correct articulation of the target sound. Thus the lesson involves experience of fires and firefighters, auditory and visual training, conceptualization, vocabulary and syntax, sequential logic, and spoken language training.

Speech and language are separate processes. Language is a set of rules for embodying ideas for communication; speech is one means of articulating the language pattern. Acquired separately as a set of vocal-articulatory skills, these new patterns must be applied to spoken language as they are mastered by the hearing-impaired child. We achieve this by creating communication situations and activities that facilitate and reinforce the use of new skills in meaningful communications.

MOLDING SOCIOLINGUISTIC BEHAVIORS

The ultimate goal of language and speech-development training is communication. This requires not only that children learn the rules of language, but that they also learn the social rules governing its use. Society has expectations concerning when and how we may communicate in a variety of different situations. We use different communication strategies to achieve different goals. In the early preschool years we are so delighted to find a hearing-impaired child attempting to communicate that we set aside the normal rules. We encourage the child to communicate orally in any form at any time. However, as the child grows older, she must learn the social rules for communication—when to speak and when to remain silent, how to ask a question, how to make a request in an acceptable manner, and how to use language manipulatively (Wood, 1976).

Acceptance of the hearing-impaired child by normal-hearing peers and adults will be determined not only by the intelligibility of what the child says, but also by how it is said. The pragmatic value of the communication skills acquired by the child becomes increasingly important as the school years approach. This is particularly true for children mainstreamed into normal school classes. Thus, during the later preschool years, we must begin to help the child gain the experience necessary to cope with a variety of communication situations in ways that will be socially acceptable. As Meers (1976), puts it:

> "The fuller the range of language uses and styles available to the speaker, the greater the number of informed choices that are open to him; thus he is able to influence his environment as well as knowing himself to be subject to its laws" (p. 147).

In his book *The Presentation of Self in Everyday Life*, Goffman (1959) views social behavior in terms of a wide range of roles that we learn in order to cope with others. Knowledge of these roles and the associated sociolinguistic behaviors is acquired by hearing children through daily exposure to people in context. The children observe the subtleties of communication and learn from the nature of the verbal interaction. They learn from the different ways in which they are addressed, as well as by the occasions on which they are all but ignored, sometimes even when they are the topic of conversation. They also learn from the control exerted on their verbal and nonverbal behavior by adults who reward and punish such behavior differently in different situations. Hearing-impaired children will need training to develop this sociolinguistic awareness acquired naturally by hearing peers.

Sociolinguistic behaviors cannot be taught formally (Darbyshire, 1977) for as Boothroyd (1982) points out, such functions as expressing feelings, asking questions, complaining, or protesting "are inherent, not in the nature of language, but in the nature of humankind" (p. 139).

Wood (1976) advocates that the social-communication competence of language-delayed children be developed through a situational approach. Attention must be paid to (1) the *goal of the communication*—to effect a course of action (for example, to gain praise, sympathy, understanding, or affection) and (2) the *critical-communication situations* that the child encounters. It is necessary to identify these situations for preschool children. As the children grow older, they will need to begin to assume responsibility for identifying and seeking help in dealing with such critical situations themselves.

Wood (1976) analyzes communication in terms of the following four categories:

1. *People I talk to*: parents, siblings, playmates, teachers.
2. *Places I talk in*: school (classroom, playground, hall); home (my room, family room, kitchen, garden); public places (church, library, supermarket, children's theater, or movie theater). These two categories are further broken down into the times of the communication—at breakfast/lunch/dinner, when I come home from school, before I go to bed, when Daddy comes home.
3. *What I talk about*: objects, events, people, ideas.
4. *How I talk*: how I use my voice, how I say things, whether I must wait my turn, whether I can call out.

Thus, to help the children use language to serve socioemotional needs, we must

GOAL	METHOD
Be alert to situations occurring naturally in the child's play or activities that create socioemotional needs.	Allow the child to experience the need before helping him resolve it linguistically.
Take advantage of such situations by resolving them through sociolinguistic behaviors.	Verbalize the need of the child, then model for the child/children language behaviors that are helpful in resolving the situation or relieving the emotion through verbal expression.
Recreate the situation soon after it occurs but when feelings are no longer dominant.	Recreate through use of doll or puppet play the situation the child had to resolve. Have the child work through the experience using appropriate language models.
Create similar situations.	Use doll or puppet play or older children to act out examples of social or emotional situations through small vignettes.

We learned in Chapter 8 that in communication, we transmit information with our voice, our articulators, and our bodily gestures and postures. Wood (1976) presents the options for communication for young children in illustrated form (Figure 15.2). By using charts such as Wood's, you can stimulate a child's awareness of the behavior of others during communication, thus enhancing understanding of message intent. At the same time, you can begin to foster awareness of the child's own behavior and you can teach the child how to mold it to be appropriate to the demands of various communication situations.

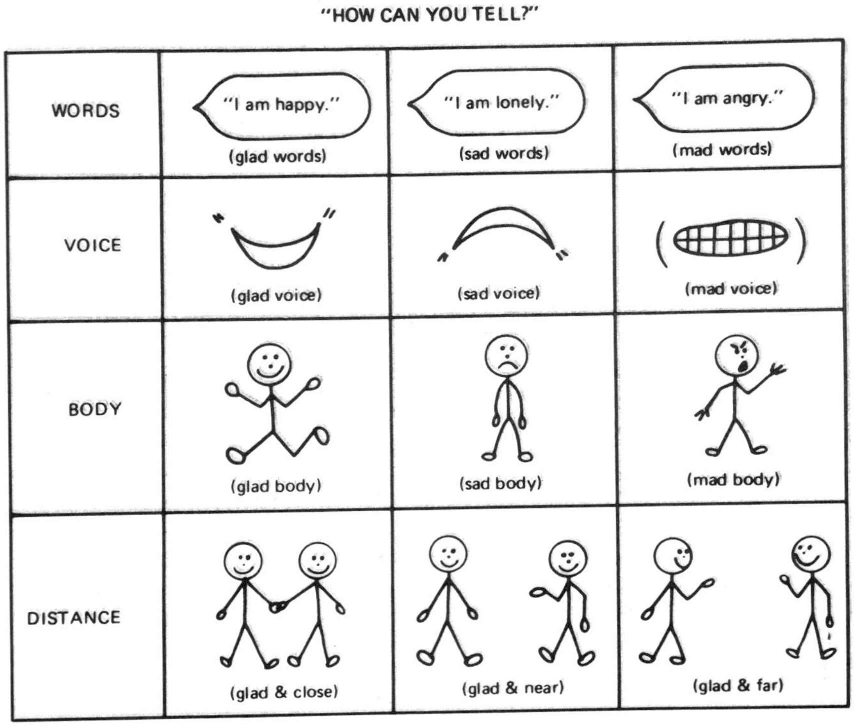

"HOW CAN YOU TELL?"

WORDS	"I am happy." (glad words)	"I am lonely." (sad words)	"I am angry." (mad words)
VOICE	(glad voice)	(sad voice)	(mad voice)
BODY	(glad body)	(sad body)	(mad body)
DISTANCE	(glad & close)	(glad & near)	(glad & far)

Figure 15.2 Illustrations can stimulate the child's awareness of options for communicating feelings. (Wood, 1976, p. 296.)

For example, you might have the child consider the times *when* we try to be quiet: for example, when someone is sleeping, when people are already talking, when someone is talking on the telephone, when you have special quiet work to do in school. The child can also learn *where* to be quiet: in a movie theater, in a library, in a doctor's office, at a concert. The child can then learn *what types of voices* are appropriate in different places: quiet voice in a movie, library, and so on; ordinary voice at dinner table, in the classroom, in the hallways; loud voice in the playground, on a busy street, at a fair. Attention can be focused on behaviors, such as taking turns to talk, waiting until someone has finished talking, raising your hand in a group when you wish to answer or ask a question, addressing a teacher by name to attract attention. Communication behaviors appropriate for various situations can be illustrated and practiced by small groups of children preparing for school. Play activities can be introduced that help the child learn how to manipulate people acceptably through spoken language: how to obtain someone's attention politely, how to make a request, how to ask a question in a group, how to refuse, how to communicate displeasure.

Feelings, bodily postures, gestures, and words and phrases also can be identified through pictures illustrating different situations. Recognizing the feelings experienced by others can help the children work out some of their own feelings. Hand puppets may be used to help children express their feelings both nonverbally and verbally. Happy, sad, angry, puzzled, and surprised paper faces can be pinned to the puppets to reflect appropriate feelings. Then, each child can select the faces that represent particular feelings. You should verbalize for the child the feelings being expressed through the puppet. Similarly, during classroom activities you should verbalize the feelings of a child when possible—pleasure, sadness, surprise, excitement, impatience, puzzlement, as well as anger. You should provide the child with the vocabulary with which to express those feelings.

"I'm sad/cross/angry."
"I don't like her."
"She's not nice to me."
"Don't do that."

It is even more helpful if you can identify and express the cause of the feelings:

"You're very angry. John took your boat.
That was your boat, you had it first.
That was not nice of John. John says he is sorry."

Parents should be encouraged to do the same at home. The acceptability of forms of expression of feelings also can be communicated by depicting children in situations to which they react in different ways. In this way, positive strategies for dealing with anger, disappointment, impatience, and fear can be reinforced while inappropriate strategies can be modified. Children with adequate levels of language should be encouraged to verbalize their feelings.

In summary, we can conclude that your concern as a hearing teacher/ therapist is the effectiveness of the child as a communicator of information, ideas, and feelings in a variety of situations. To achieve effective communication behaviors, it is necessary for the child to have adequate receptive language to permit understanding of what is happening in those situations, and to have sufficient language and adequately intelligible speech to be able to meet the demands of the situation. Furthermore the child must have available a range of communication behaviors and the ability to select strategies appropriate to the situation at hand.

We can do much to help the child learn effective ways of using language to satisfy needs and to express feelings. However, do not forget the needs of the parents. They are faced with many problems in dealing with the expressions of child's frustrations in situations at home, while shopping, visiting friends, or at the doctor's office.

Unlike you, they feel fully responsible for the child's behavior and judged by others who do not know or understand the effects of hearing impairment. In the final section of our consideration of the management of the preschool hearing-impaired child, we discuss the management of behavior and the feelings connected to it.

IDENTIFYING AND PROVIDING FOR
SOCIOEMOTIONAL NEEDS

Behavior Management and Parental Feelings

Any child's preschool years are characterized for parents by periods of great pleasure and delight interspersed with spells of extreme frustration. The child's rapid growth and development and the progressive demands of the world in which the child is maturing make for some difficult situations and periods. For example, the normal two-and-a-half-year-old is in a period of great disequilibrium, a period that may be overwhelming to both parents and child. The period is typically one in which the child is uncooperative, inflexible, demanding, and highly emotional. The third year of a child's life by contrast usually represents a quiet stage, a period of relative security and an easygoing approach to life. However, it does not last, for by four years the child is again in a rapid growth stage. The disequilibrium of the four year old results in behavior that is definitely "out of bounds," often shocking. Four year olds do all the wrong things. They kick and scream and run away when it is essential that they come quickly. They refuse to cooperate in dressing and are generally defiant and rude. Consider how the parents of these hearing children manage these situations.

Parents have expectations for the behavior of their child, a set of standards they feel he should meet at his age level. These are heavily influenced culturally both from within and without the family circle. The expectations may or may not be age appropriate. When they are not, the discrepancy may be due to

- Inexperience, as often occurs with a first child.
- An overly strict concept of how a child should behave.
- An inability or unwillingness to accept responsibility for disciplining the child ("Just wait till your father/mother comes home"). This may occur when the unacceptable behavior happens at a time when a parent cannot cope with all the immediate emotional pressures of the larger situation. It also may result from a conflict of unresolved needs, as for example, in the case of the mother who is ambivalent about her responsibilities as a career woman and as a mother. As a result, she experiences a conflict between her feelings of resentment over the demands her child makes on her time and guilt over not spending enough of it with him as she pursues career interests (Bromwich, 1981, p. 158).
  Fear for the child, a concern that is managed by overprotection and acceptance of socially inappropriate behavior.

Two-to-five-year-old normal-hearing children have well-developed receptive and expressive language abilities, which provide the parents with the primary means of behavior control. Parents can explain, reason, negotiate, cajole, bribe, and threaten. Language enables the parents or primary caregiver to modify much of the child's behavior through explanation of what has happened or is happening to cause frustration: "It will only hurt for a minute, then it will feel all better"; through reassurance: "Daddy's coming with you"; through negotiation: "When you have put your toys away you may have some ice cream"; or by warning of consequences: "If you don't hurry up you won't have time to play."

Likewise the child's expressive abilities permit him to express verbally feelings that otherwise would be vented through behavior, such feelings as anger, "I hate you"; unfairness, "I didn't do it," "I didn't know"; rejection, "I'm going to run away"; objection, "No! No!" "Don't"; refusal, "I won't." Similarly, through language the child appeals his case, "Please, Mommy," "I promise," "I'll be good Daddy." Thus language is the interactive tool for negotiation.

The relationship in the immediate situation breaks down when language fails. Now each party, child and adult, with various degrees of conscious awareness, seeks to control the situation in order to impose his will. The child resorts to behavioral defiance, a sort of civil disobedience—he goes limp, lies on the floor, backs away sulking, or runs and hides. If the emotion is strong he pulls, tugs, kicks, throws things or has a temper tantrum.

How would you react to a child of your own who behaved in this manner in a supermarket or in the presence of a critical relative? Just, I suggest, as most parents. The behavior must be stopped; you must take control, otherwise what kind of a mother/father will people think you are? How do you do it? By force, since language will no longer work. In situations outside the home, in order to be in control, you have two options: you can remove the child (kicking and screaming) and yourself from the scene, or you can administer pain to the child by smacking his legs or hands. Neither solves the problem; the second almost invariably makes it worse. If you are in your own home or with relatives or friends, you have the further option of isolating the child or yourself in another room.

These situations, along with the associated ways of reacting to them, are experienced more or less by all parents. At various stages of development, normal-hearing children exhibit all of these frustrations and behave accordingly. The rapid growth of language, however, quickly reduces the need for behavioral expression of frustrations and hurt feelings. This allows both parties to relate verbally, even though it may be to express strong negative feelings.

Behavior Management and the Hearing-Impaired Child

It is important for you and the parents to understand and keep in mind the behavior patterns of hearing children and the ways in which their parents attempt to deal with them. Knowledge that the behaviors evidenced by the hearing-impaired child are quite normal and the parental responses typical of how we all react in such situations does much to alleviate guilt. Of course, the behavior problems of the hearing-impaired child often are more acute and usually continue longer than those of his hearing peers. This, however, is understandable given the unusual level of frustration these children experience due to communicating insufficiently.

Because the child's language is delayed, the parents are forced to exert more direct control over their child's behavior than parents of hearing children (Schlesinger & Meadow, 1971). As a result they have been shown to be less flexible in the way they respond to the child's behavior, to allow the child less freedom, and to give less encouragement and reward than parents of hearing children. Difficulty in communicating with the child often results in an autocratic model of behavior control. The parents are unable to explain to the child why he must behave in certain ways. They cannot persuade or console the child into the desired behaviors. The child has, therefore, to adopt patterns of behavior simply because the parents demand them. This type of control is usually achieved through punishment. To minimize this, the parents often do for the child things the child should be capable of doing. Such a solution does little to foster self-confidence through self-reliance.

A less frequent reaction to the difficulty of molding the behavior of the nonverbal child is to become overprotective and overly accepting of the child's behavior. The family that adopts this model tries to accept and adjust to a child's increasingly unsocial behaviors at an age when linguistic bargaining should be modifying such behavior. The parents accept the aggression and temper tantrums, yielding to demands and rearranging family priorities in an understandable but misguided attempt to solve the problem. Both models of behavioral management arising from the difficulty in parent-child communication almost always exaggerate the normal development behavioral problems of the preschool years of any child (Vernon, 1969). The child, reacting to the conflict and frustration he experiences, often converts the resultant stress into symptoms of irritability, temper, aggression, or eating and sleeping problems. All of these are quite normal reactions to stress.

The effects of behavior-management problems also frequently give rise to secondary problems of interpersonal relationships among family members. Parents often disagree over how the child should be handled. One parent may feel that the other does not share responsibilities, avoids the problems and blames him for the child's unmanageable behavior. The working parent may feel that after a day's work he should not be expected to deal with problems the parent at home should have worked out during the day. Siblings resent the family disruptance caused by their handicapped brother or sister, object to the amount of parental attention the child receives, protest about the way in which meeting the child's needs interferes with what they see as their family rights, and are often embarrassed to bring friends into this atmosphere.

The importance of the emotional climate in the home cannot be stressed too strongly. Ross (1964) states:

> Parental harmony has a favorable effect on a child's adjustment and parental disharmony or disagreement has an unfavorable effect. The emotional atmosphere in a family would thus seem to be far more important for the understanding of the personality development of the child than the specific attitudes held by either father or mother. (p. 27)

The child's behavior problems cannot, therefore, be viewed in isolation; they are as much problems of the family as they are his own

(Altschuler, 1974; Northcott, 1975). They can be understood only in terms of an action-reaction model based on family expectations, management strategies, and reactions. Similarly, help can be provided only in these terms. The problems that arise do so because the parents feel they lack the experience necessary to cope with what they believe to be the child's abnormal behavior. You have the information and objectivity necessary to help them to understand what is happening. In almost every case the parents have the capabilities to make the adjustments necessary to reduce the conflicts they are having in dealing with their child.

Guiding Parents to Effective Behavioral Management

Your first aim is to communicate the normality of the situation. The child's behavior is understandable in terms of the frustrations she experiences. Similarly, it is equally easy to appreciate the parents' reactions to the situation. They have attempted to cope with the situation, but the methods they have used have not effected the desired results. The situation has become increasingly more difficult, and they now find frustration, even resentment and anger, affecting their behavioral management of their child. They feel badly about this but seem trapped in the situation. You should communicate to them that the difficulty is not in their failure as parents, but in the management strategies they have adopted. The solution lies in techniques that reduce the frequency of stress-creating situations and in identifying alternate ways of reacting in those situations when they occur.

In an excellent resource text, *Working with Parents and Infants*, Bromwich (1981) points out that actual behavioral management practices often fail to reflect the expressed philosophy of a program. To bring intervention processes closer to avowed aims in her own program, she formulated ten guidelines (pp. 20–24) that I recommend to you. They are just as applicable to our work with parents, given some minor adjustments. The recommended guidelines adapted to our needs are

- *Enable the parents to remain in control.* In so doing, parents are encouraged to be active partners in the management of their child and dependency is minimized.
- *Avoid the "authority-layperson" gap.* View the intervention process as a cooperative undertaking. Emphasize the importance of the parents' knowledge of their child by seeking their information and opinions. Suggest approaches; do not tell them what to do. Solicit their input all the time; never be judgmental.
- *Deal with parent priorities and concerns.* Encourage the parents to guide you in ensuring that you address what they perceive to be their most pressing needs. Consider their total situation as it relates to helping their child. Be sensitive to their need to discuss broader problems that affect their parenting abilities, and help them obtain other support services as needed.
- *Build parents' strengths.* Observe and comment positively on all parenting behaviors that are helpful to the child. On first contact with the parents, speak well but honestly of such behaviors as affection, warmth, attention, assistance, support, and so on that already are part of the parenting practices.
- *Respect parent goals.* Seek to learn and understand how the parents are managing their child, what they are attempting to achieve. Accept their goals as a

foundation for discussing effective management techniques. Do not impose new goals and techniques; instead explore, discuss, and negotiate acceptable modifications.

- *Involve parents in planning.* Encourage the parent to share responsibility for deciding how to achieve intervention goals in all aspects of management, including choosing appropriate activities—for example, toys, visits, or topics for discussion.
- *Respect individual styles of parenting.* Seek to know and understand how the parents relate to their child. Then strive to adapt your intervention activities so they are accommodated easily by the parents' individual parenting practices. Reinforce and build on the activities they enjoy with their child.
- *Explain praise; do not just give it.* Provide positive feedback to parents about actions and behaviors that are helpful in managing the child and meeting her needs. However, ensure that you describe clearly *what* you are praising and explain *why* you feel it was so effective.
- *Provide the parents with an "out."* Make clear your suggestions are just that. Explain that you want the parents to evaluate them for their usefulness and to question or reject them when the parents are not comfortable with them or when they simply do not work for them. Make clear that there is no right way, only ways that work and ways that do not.
- *Share how it feels to get no response.* Share in the activities you suggest and talk of your own feelings when the child fails to respond or the activity is a disaster. Emphasize that such lack of success is not the parents' fault. Explain that techniques fail, not parents.

Steps in the Management Program

With these guidelines clearly in mind, we now can consider the specific steps in a management program.

Encourage Analysis of Problem Situations. To objectify behavior it is necessary to understand it within the context in which it occurred. Use actual problems that the parents "recall vividly" in order to develop information about the event:

Where it occurred: at home, at a friend's house, in a supermarket, mall, bus, or in a park. Each location imposes different constraints on management options.
The situation that triggered the behavior: "I told her it was time to put her toys away." "I took away her toy duck before taking her out of the bath." "He wanted a cookie at the supermarket but I told him no." "I had to get him dressed for nursery school."
The child's behavior: "He lay on the floor kicking; he just went limp"; "she kept trying to pull away; she just made it impossible to dress her."
How the parent dealt with the situation: "I got angry and yelled at him; I smacked him hard"; "I picked her up and carried her out of the store kicking"; "I simply walked away and left her though I could still see her."
How well the strategy worked: "It didn't, she behaved worse"; "She was frightened and stopped for awhile"; "He stopped screaming and began to cry."
How the parent felt: Awful, angry, embarrassed, guilty, a cruel parent, judged badly by others present.

This stage of information gathering achieves two goals: it communicates to the parent your desire to understand and it gives you the information necessary to be able to discuss real occurrences in context. To achieve this, you must recognize clearly that you do not know how this parent should or could have managed the situation. To assume that you could have avoided or resolved the problem better is to be presumptuous. The solutions to problems lie within the parent not with you. In Luterman's (1984) words:

> Wisdom lies within the individual and the therapist's role is to help the person find out and tune into her own wisdom. (p. 14)

Identifying and Understanding Goals. Such parental wisdom can be tapped through self-understanding. The parents need to have clear in their minds what the desired goal for a situation was, to what extent it changed, and how the change affected the event. Goals can be either short or long term. Short- and long-term goals may be compatible or they may conflict. Helping parents to know their goals and to understand what is occurring as they deal with behavior situations strengthens their ability to cope with problems.

Long-term goals in general represent the desire to normalize the child's social behaviors, to develop in him the ability to express negative emotions such as frustration, fear, and anger in ways that are socially acceptable. As you can understand, the ease with which this can be achieved is greatly influenced by the child's capability to work out problems linguistically before the emotion builds to the frustration level. It relates also to the child's competence in use of the sociolinguistic rules of language. However, even before adequate language develops, we need to help him deal with situations in ways we will explore.

Short-term goals vary considerably for each situation. They are affected by the nature of the behavior; where it occurs; who, besides the parent, is present when it occurs; the time available to manage the situation; and other pressuring needs to which the parent must pay attention.

> Consider Mrs. Andrews. She has stopped off at a supermarket to pick up a few essential items on her way home from nursery school with Michael, her four-year-old severely hearing-impaired son. She feels under pressure because her daughter Julie, age seven, will be home from school soon and she must be there when Julie gets off the school bus. One of the items she picks up is a box of chocolate cookies. Michael reaches for the box and proceeds to open it. When his mother takes it away from him, Michael begins to cry loudly and then to shout protest. Kicking the shopping cart, he draws the attention of other shoppers. Mrs. Andrews's long-term goal is for Michael to learn acceptable social behavior; she is working to teach him this. However, she feels she managed the situation badly. Because of the pressure she felt to be home in time to meet Julie from school, and the disapproving looks she received from other shoppers, she gave in to Michael to gain his cooperation. "It was only one cookie,," she says, "I even showed him by holding up one finger." It worked, but Mrs. Andrews feels badly that she failed.

It is difficult for parents not to feel judged by us. We must do everything we can to put aside our apparent need for dominance and control in working with people (Gregory, 1963). We must help parents to accept full responsibility for their own decisions. In this case, we need to accept Mrs.

Andrews's evaluation, seek an explanation as to how she reached it, and explore and evaluate what options she had. Her actions were dominated by her need to get home quickly. Through our discussion, Mrs. Andrews begins to realize that she could not change this primary need. She was in a situation in which her short-term goal was incompatible with her long-term goal. The short-term goal was, moreover, at that time the primary goal. In discussing this, Mrs. Andrews, on reflection, decides that the supermarket was not an easy place in which calmly to enforce her rule about no cookies before lunch. Michael's behavior already was attracting unwanted attention.

"Given the time, how else might you have handled it?"

"Well—uhm—I think I would have parked my shopping cart, picked him up, and taken him out to the car. I'd probably have put him in the carseat till he calmed down."

"Do you think you would have felt angry with him?"

"Oh yes, well cross—but I would have been calm and firm with him. I would have had to have worked out a way to distract him from the cookies when we returned. I guess I should have left that item until last."

"But you couldn't do any of this in the circumstance."

"No—I guess what I did wasn't so bad."

Without our judgment, Mrs. Andrews has been able to reevaluate her actions. She is firmly in control of her goals and is beginning to understand they must be flexible in the short term.

Consider another situation Mrs. Andrews handled. Michael always has trouble changing activities. Ending his play when it is time for his evening bath has always been a problem. Mrs. Andrews wants to teach him to put away his toys at that time and not to put up a big fight every bathtime. We talked about how she handled the situation.

"Well I used to tell him it was time to put the toys away. I would show him, but he became quite angry and would throw toys. I ended up by picking him up and taking him upstairs, but it was always a big battle—I dreaded it. I always ended up putting the toys away myself."

"But it's not like that now?"

"Well I won't say it's perfect, sometimes he still gives me a hassle, but mostly it's no real problem."

"How come?"

"Well I thought about what we had talked about, you know, how it's important not to be hard on ourselves for the way things went but that we should think about what we want to achieve and other ways to get there. I'm rather proud about what I came up with. I really thought this would be a good time to teach Michael. I suppose I was able to make the long- and short-range goals the same. I made sure I had plenty of time. Oh, one thing I did that really helped was I brought Michael's bath toys downstairs and put them among his toys. I also bought a new one, a boat that floats. When it was nearly bathtime, I got things ready; then instead of telling him it was time to put things away I joined his play."

"That sort of broke up his concentration?"

"Yes, I thought that was good; we also were doing something together. Then I pointed to my watch and explained it was almost bathtime. I got together his bath toys—he found one of them. Then I said 'Let's play a game—I'll put one [toy] in the box, you put one in.' He thought that was fun. When we'd finished, I gave him the boat. He actually was upstairs before me. Oh, I also have him help me get the bath ready now—he finds the soap and towel and the

washcloth and helps me turn the water on. I used to have it all ready. I can't believe it works, but he's been good about it all week."

Mrs. Andrews is gaining confidence in her ability to have control of situations and, to an increasing extent, control over how she perceives and feels about them. Through sharing her perceptions and accounts of her management behaviors, she has clarified her long- and short-range goals and understands how situational properties determine primary and secondary needs. She is beginning to feel good about her management of Michael because she has growing confidence. Her feelings of guilt have lessened considerably since she began to evaluate situations, actions, and reactions objectively.

A MODEL OF INTERVENTION

Rose Bromwich (1981) has explored extensively intervention approaches for modifying parent-child interactions. She identifies eight modes of intervention. These accommodate and apply the principles of counseling we have discussed in earlier chapters. Thus, they offer a helpful model for guiding parents toward effective behavioral management. Bromwich's eight possible modes for intervention can be summarized and translated into the following actions that we can take.

Listen Empathetically

To do this, we must sincerely want to understand how the parents perceive the problem. We must try to do this within the framework of their perception of themselves and their relationship to each other and to their child. For us to come close to this requires a complete suspension of our tendency to evaluate and judge what they say and do. Webster (1977) says:

> When one listens in this way, one is not set to agree or disagree. Rather one is set to attend to and try to glimpse more fully the ideas, attitudes and emotions expressed by the other (p. 34).

This type of listening conveys to the parents the value we place on their feelings and perceptions. It emphasizes how important we believe it to be that we work within their framework rather than one we might impose. It also ensures that the parents do not feel pressured to answer questions about or discuss feelings they are not yet ready to share.

Empathetic listening is not a completely passive form of listening. It allows us to communicate our understanding of what is being shared; we can identify with the parents' experience. For example, when Mrs. Andrews felt embarrassed by the unwelcome attention Michael's behavior was attracting from other shoppers in the supermarket, we might quite naturally express understanding:

"I can imagine what you must have felt. None of us likes to attract those stares; you know exactly what people are thinking when that happens."

Our empathy with positive feelings also is helpful and appreciated reinforcement. For example, Mrs. Andrews clearly felt good about her achievement in molding Michael's behavior around bathtime. You can reflect your empathy by commenting:

"Oh, I know how good it feels when your efforts really pay off like that."

This mode of intervention provides us with information about the problem as it appears from the perspective of the parents. It is from that perspective that we must approach it. At the same time, it enables the parent to view him/herself in relation to the problem.

Empathetic listening also allows us to build or strengthen our relationship with the parent and to put into practice our belief that we and the parents are equal partners in problem solving.

Observe Carefully

Parents' observation skills relate to all areas of their child's growth and development. We discussed them earlier in relation to auditory behaviors and to speech and language growth. Careful observation of the child's social-affective behavior, both when he is in a state of equilibrium and when he is upset, can be equally productive. The parent and child always are communicating in an interactive relationship, regardless of whether verbalization occurs or not. By increasing parents' observational skills as well as our own, we increase our ability to understand their child's behavior and the situational influences that affect it. Similarly, as the parents' understanding of the child's behavior grows, so will their capacity to reflect on their own feelings, reactions, and behaviors. At this stage they begin to view events within a dyadic framework. Once this occurs, the parents, with increasing skill, will be able to read and respond to the child's behavior as communication about his feelings. They begin to see themselves as active-reactive participants in their interactions with their child, rather than seeing problems purely in the light of the child as causative agent.

Equally important is the role we can serve as an observer of the parent-child dyad. Once again, we do not observe to evaluate or judge, but to share with the parent what we notice or "observe" in interactions we witness in the preschool or home situation. This allows the parents to reflect on their goals for a given situation, to consider how they reacted both emotionally and practically, and to evaluate the effects of their management strategies for the purpose of improvement. The use of videotaping can be invaluable in this process, but it should be used cautiously and not at all until you have a comfortable trusting relationship with the family.

Comment Positively

Bromwich (1981) stresses the importance of communicating to the parents the strengths they already have, allowing them to build on those strengths and to gain self-confidence. Positive comments must offer more than praise; they must be quite specific in describing what is being recognized positively and why. They should identify skills and behaviors that prove effective in influencing the child's behavior favorably. For example, we would comment positively on Mrs. Andrews's handling of the prebath situation:

"That was very clever of you to understand the need to break up Michael's play concentration in such a positive manner."

"Buying a new toy was a really effective motivator for him."

"Involving Michael in preparing the bath really changed his attitude—he obviously enjoys being part of the process instead of just having it happen to him—that was a really good move on your part."

Other positive comments might be:

"I noticed you show a lot of affection for Mary. You showed it even when she was angry. Your gentle holding of her really seemed to calm her."

"You laugh a lot when you play with Mary—she really enjoys that; it seems to have a relaxing effect on you both."

"Mary's behavior really changed when you showed her how interested you were in her attempts to fit the puzzle together. She was much more relaxed when you pointed the pieces out to her but let her put them in herself."

Positive comments always must be justified, but even parents exhibiting a lot of difficulty with their child deserve encouragement for their willingness to attempt new ways, for their cooperation with you, and for their persistence.

Discuss Problems, Issues, Observations, Actions

As we have seen, discussion pervades all aspects of our relationship with the parents. Discussion is in itself a process of examination, exploration, and theoretical experimentation—one that is interwoven with all other modes of intervention. Through discussion, we share information with each other, suggest options, evaluate alternatives, and develop a cooperative approach to problem resolution. In particular, it is a primary mode in which the parents come to understand what is happening between them and the child and to understand their child's behavior within the normal developmental process.

Ask for Information

We use this mode of intervention in many ways. Like discussion, it is a thread that runs through all the other modes. Questions arise informally in our interactions with parents. The questions are of various kinds. We may ask

For information: "When did she first begin to wake up crying in the night?"

About parents' feelings: "When she cries like that, do you feel angry or anxious?"

About intervention techniques: "What do you do when this occurs? How effective does that approach seem to be?"

In order to focus a parent's observations: "Has her behavior changed during the daytime? How long does she nap in the afternoon? Does she have a nightlight on? Do you have trouble getting her to sleep?"

For evaluation of contributing factors or possible approaches: "Do you think she is ready to give up her afternoon nap? Do you think she is going to bed too early? Is she getting too wound up just before bedtime? Have you tried looking at books with her after she is in bed?"

Asking, therefore, is a mode of intervention in which questions are used as tools to achieve specific results.

Model Actions and Behaviors

Although modeling may at first seem a highly desirable mode of intervention, for it can be a powerful tool, Bromwich (1981) points to some important reservations concerning its use. We need to be alert to these.

Modeling should be considered as distinct from demonstration. In demonstration there is an expectation that the parents will attempt to replicate the demonstrated behavior, technique, or way of handling the child. Modeling, by contrast, encourages the parents to assess and critique what they observe. They are encouraged to express how comfortable they would feel trying a similar management approach. There is no implication that "this is how you should handle the situation." It helps to discuss with the parents what is happening as it occurs, or to do so immediately after the session. In this way, assessment of what was observed is made with insight and in context.

"I think Kevin feels insecure having so much freedom. He seems afraid of his own anger. That's probably why he accepted so easily the limits I set clearly for him. He may well be feeling the same at home when it seems to him that neither you nor he can control his aggression. That's a pretty frightening feeling."

It is the understanding that makes it possible to reevaluate a modeled behavior later. Although they may not respond positively at the time, parents may find the model helpful after they have had time to reflect. It is surprising how often people report later that they tried a technique that they observed and found that it worked:

"You know I was sure I couldn't be as firm with Kevin as you were, that he wouldn't accept it from me, but I tried it and it really worked—I was really surprised."

Care should be taken to avoid the danger of intrusive modeling. Bromwich (1981) stresses that it should not be used with such intimate interactions as feeding or putting the child to bed unless the parent specifically asks for help in these areas. Other intervention modes are more appropriate in such situations that are likely to be highly emotionally charged for parent and child. This is particularly true in home-based programs in which you are the invited guest in the domain of the parents. Modeling in this situation may be seen as "intrusiveness and possible interferences with the parent's sense of control in her own home" (Bromwich, 1981, p. 183).

Experiment

Experimenting at first may seem identical with modeling as an intervention mode. It may indeed be employed as a part of modeling, but Bromwich (1981) offers it as a separate mode of intervention for getting to know the child and for developing a relationship. We experiment with different activities and ways of engaging the child in a search for techniques that prove effective. We may experiment with techniques for holding the child's attention and for increasing her self-confidence or willingness to take risks. We also may experiment with techniques for reducing or expressing frustration, anger, fear, or overdependency in ways acceptable to parent and child alike. For example, anger that cannot be vented acceptably against people or animals can be released through gross physical acts such as pounding a pillow or hammering pegs through a board, throwing bean bags, breaking bubbles as soon as they are blown, or smashing small play dough people. Doing this *with the child* acknowledges and accepts her feelings. In the case of fear or apprehension, provide support, hold the child protectively, pick her up, view the feared situation together from a safe distance, approach slowly, and do not pressure the child. Since we do not know how best to handle a particular child's problem, experimentation communicates our partnership with the parent; it removes the aura of expertise that creates imbalance in our relationship. The parent will see that many approaches and techniques fail for us as indeed they do for them. They will see that failure is part of the process rather than an inadequacy or inability on their part, that it is not caused by them. Thus, potential guilt can be avoided or minimized. Experimentation is, therefore, particularly helpful in exploring ways to cope with difficult behavioral situations in a cooperative manner. Experimentation always should be preceded by careful analysis of the problem to be resolved, observation of the child's behavior, and discussion of how it presently is being managed. There should be full acceptance by the parents of the need to explore other ways of dealing with the problem and a sharing throughout of the appropriateness and acceptability of new approaches. Evaluation also must be made together as equal partners.

Encourage the Parents

Encouraging, the last of Bromwich's (1981) modes of intervention, occurs when the parent is trying to apply what you have discussed together or what has been modeled. She recommends its use for motivating and reinforcing effective intervention techniques or for involving parents in experimentation. It is tied closely to giving positive comments to and encouraging self-observation. The latter modes are particularly relevant when the parent lacks self-confidence.

Bromwich's text provides an invaluable source of guidance for those of us seeking to support parents as they strive to understand and manage the behavioral problems of their infants and preschool children. In addition to her clear presentation and discussion of issues, she presents 135 pages of problems and specific intervention responses in social-affective cognitive-motivational and parenting-caregiving behavior. These are guides, not recipes. In the same vein, I wish, in conclusion, to stress that there are no cookbook answers to the resolution of problems of behavior. Each parent and each child represents a unique dyad within a family. Expectations, attitudes, values, and resources differ widely from family to family. Your experience and confidence as a helper will grow as will your effectiveness. Desirable as this may be, it will not happen until you are prepared to shed the pseudo-professionalism that creates the authority-layperson gap and recognize the inestimable value of a true partnership with those other authorities, the parents.

SUMMARY

- The management approach for the older preschool child supplements home training with a controlled learning environment.
- Parent involvement in the nursery school experience is critical for maximum success; participation should be cooperative.
- Reassessment of family resources should be made.
- Assessment of the child's needs and resources should be ongoing.
- Language should be nurtured through controlled experiences that foster a need for communication.
- Highly redundant verbal commentary about events as they occur will facilitate comprehension and acquisition of concepts and the language to describe them.
- Listening, watching, and interpreting nonverbal and verbal information stimulates cognitive development prerequisite to communication.
- Sensory perception, linguistic processing and cognitive deduction are stimulated in concert through experiential learning.
- Speech teaching as opposed to spoken-language training should be viewed as developing controlled articulatory skills.
- Subskills for speech targets must be firmly established.
- Speech teaching should follow a normal developmental model.
- Speech articulation can be taught through vocal play activity. Sessions should be short, frequent, and intensive.
- Transfer of speech to spoken language should occur only after production of a sound is automatic (i.e., possible without thought or effort).
- Communication is a social act and requires adherence to sociolinguistic rules.
- Pragmatics, the use of sociolinguistic rules, plays an important part in the development of the older preschool child.
- Children in this age group need language to express feelings.
- Parents need to learn how to resolve their own emotional reactions to unacceptable behavior.
- Parents need support in learning how to manage the child's behavioral expressions of emotion.
- The Bromwich (1981) model for molding parent-child interaction involves

  - Emphatic listening
  - Careful observation
  - Positive comment
  - Discussion
  - Information solicitation
  - Modeling
  - Experimentation
  - Encouragement

Conclusion

Placement of the child in the planned activities of the preschool nursery represents an expansion of, not a substitute for, the educational model already discussed. Continued parent involvement in preschool education is critical to optimal success. In this respect, it is essential to establish the extent and means of parent involvement within the limits of family resources. The school experience provides for learning in a range of activities with various degrees of structure. Parallel verbalization of the children's activities as they are ongoing, re-creation of experiences, and interactive conversation constitute the essence of cognitive-linguistic learning. These activities foster observation, interpretation, and communication in the child. Speech training is seen as separate from spoken language. Vocal articulatory skills and control are taught intensively through frequent short speech play activities. Sociolinguistic knowledge can be taught through role modeling and through verbalizing of situations as they arise. Parents need to know how to do this and how to deal with their own reactions to child behavior. The suggestions offered by Bromwich (1981) provide us with guidelines as to how to work with parents to achieve the desired cooperative relationship.

16

Planning for Educational Placement

LEGALLY MANDATED APPROPRIATE PUBLIC EDUCATION

Enrollment in full-time structured education is the event for which the years of preschool education have been preparing hearing-impaired children. Regardless of the type of placement chosen as most appropriate, the years ahead will be characterized not only by increasing complexity of demands, but also by the rate at which that increase accelerates. The closer the placement is to the regular classroom for hearing children, the greater will be the expectations and the faster the pace. Matching the child to an appropriate educational setting, monitoring his progress in that setting, and ensuring continued availability of supportive services are the crucial tasks now mandated by federal law.

It was the passage by Congress of the *Individuals with Disabilities Education Act* (IDEA) in 1975 that empowered the advocates of the rights of handicapped children to demand a wide range of free public educational opportunities. That act is known as Public Law 94-142 (the 142nd act passed by the 94th Congress). It gives handicapped children from ages 3–21 the right to free public education in an environment determined to be the least restrictive to the child's development. Furthermore, the act stresses that the educational environment provided must approximate as closely as possible

312

the environment in which the nonhandicapped child is taught. Through specifying strict procedures for classifying the child's handicap, and by guaranteeing due process of law, the act ensures that each child's needs are assessed systematically without prejudice. For each child designated as handicapped, the law then requires that an Individualized Educational Plan (IEP) be developed. This plan must address the child's specific needs and how they will be addressed. The right of parents to have their opinions heard and their requests given weight also is guaranteed by PL 94-142.

Although the process by which a decision is made about the educational placement of a child is now well defined, the appropriateness of the initial placement will depend upon the amount, relevance, and accuracy of the information used by those who must make the decision. Your input can be extremely valuable. For this reason you should understand what the alternatives for education are, and how the decision process operates. At this point in our discussion, we focus attention on the initial educational placement. Progress must be assessed yearly, and a complete reevaluation of the child must be made every three years. Whenever a change in educational placement is under consideration, the legally defined process must be followed.

The Decision Process

A child approaching, or having reached, school age who is known or suspected of having a handicapping condition will be referred to an interdisciplinary team for evaluation. This team is established by the child's local educational agency or school district; each is required by federal law to create such a team. These teams are known by a variety of names such as the Committee on Special Education or the Individual Educational Planning Committee.

Before any child is identified as handicapped or placed in special education, full and individual assessment of the child's abilities, development, and current educational needs must be conducted. Tests and other evaluation material must meet certain requirements. They must be administered in the child's native language or other mode of communication, must have been validated for their specific purpose, and must be administered by trained personnel and tailored to assess specific areas of educational need. For example, just a single psychological measure of general intelligence is not adequate; several measures must be made. The assessment must include all areas that may relate to the suspected disability. These might include health, vision, hearing, social and emotional status, intelligence, academic performance, communication skills, and motor development.

For children with impairments that affect sensory processing, communication, or motor skills, the tests must reflect aptitude or achievement, not the impact of the disability.

Parental Rights

Procedural safeguards are provided for parents of handicapped children and are defined as *due process* procedures. The first of these requires that the multidisciplinary school committee have the *full and informed consent* of the parents, in writing, before evaluating the child. The parents must be advised how the child will be assessed and must be informed of the tests to be used. Written notice also must be given to parents prior to any subsequent placement or change in a child's educational program, initial evaluation, or reevaluation. The parents have the right to withhold or withdraw their consent for the evaluation or planned action. They may not feel the child's problem warrants her classification as hard-of-hearing, or they may object to the type of tests proposed. In that case they may discuss their objections with the chief school officer. If this fails to satisfy their objections, they then have a right to an impartial hearing and resolution of their complaint.

Given the parents' consent for assessment, the Committee on Special Education must determine

- Whether the child has a handicap
- How the primary handicap is to be classified
- Whether special services are necessary and if so which services and to what extent
- Which placement would be appropriate
- What degree of mainstreaming the child should receive

If parents feel that the assessment of any aspect of the child's status was not adequate, they have the right to request a reassessment by another agency or professional. If the local educational agency does not challenge the request, or fails to show at an impartial hearing that its assessment was appropriate, then the cost of a second assessment must be borne by the agency. Furthermore, whenever parents make a request or inform a school district authority that they intend to initiate the impartial hearing process, the educational agency must advise them where they can obtain free or low-cost legal aid or other relevant professional services within the area. One area of testing that often prompts a request for an independent evaluation is intelligence testing.

Intelligence Testing

One or more intelligence tests are almost always included in the test battery administered to the hearing-impaired child. Intelligence testing often causes the parents greatest concern. This concern is justified because the hearing impairment and its effects on language and communication can often cause a child to function below capacity on standard intelligence tests. Moreover, parents have legitimate reason to wonder whether the psychologist who administers the evaluation has the necessary experience with hearing-impaired children to ensure valid test results.

In 1974, Levine investigated the extent of the special qualifications of 172 psychologists working with children with impaired hearing in 48 states.

She found that 83 percent of the psychologists surveyed had no special training to work with the hard-of-hearing or deaf children whom they tested. Sullivan and Vernon (1979), psychologists with extensive testing and research experience with the hearing-impaired population, in discussing Levine's findings state, "The obvious conclusion from Levine's study is that psychologists lack the necessary training, skills, and specialized knowledge to provide adequate psychological services to hearing-impaired children" (p. 272). These authors emphasize that failure to be aware of certain crucial considerations in making psychological assessments of hearing-impaired children "can result in gross psycho-diagnostic errors of tragic consequences to the child, parents, and educational personnel" (p. 172).

You should be prepared to provide the parents of a hearing-impaired child with the information necessary to determine whether an intelligence evaluation meets the criteria identified as crucial to obtaining valid results. Vernon (1970, 1976) and Vernon and Brown (1964) have carefully described and explained the essential components for valid test administration. They have also identified and evaluated appropriate intelligence tests, achievement tests, and neuropsychological tests for use with hearing-impaired children. Sullivan and Vernon's assessment of intelligence tests appropriate for preschool and school-age populations is reproduced in Tables 16.2 and 16.3 at the end of this chapter.

Make a concerted effort to establish a working relationship with the psychologists who serve the children you work with. Usually you will find that a psychologist will appreciate an offer from you to work with him in obtaining an accurate measure of the child's intellectual capacity. Offer your services by informing the psychologist about the child's communication skills. Describe her language level, auditory comprehension, auditory-visual comprehension, and ability to follow directions. Discuss the mode of communication by which the child is most likely to comprehend, and how much the hearing aid contributes to the child's communication ability. Offer guidance concerning the conditions and methods that optimize the child's performance in a communication situation. It will be a long time before all psychologists who assess hearing-impaired children have had the training and experience necessary to ensure accurate test results. Until such time, you should make what contribution you can to ensure that the gross psycho-diagnostic errors to which Vernon refers are avoided.

When assessment has been completed, the findings reviewed by the multidisciplinary team, and the parents have been consulted, a placement decision is reached.

TYPES OF PLACEMENTS

Basically, we wish to treat the hearing-impaired child as normally as possible. Thus it is desirable to allow the child to be educated with little deviation from normal educational procedures. *It is important to realize, however, that no type of educational setting is intrinsically better than another. The criterion by which a placement decision must be judged is the degree to which it achieves compatibility between the child and the learning environment.* The intent is for the child to be educated in the least restrictive environment that approximates as closely as possible that of the child's nonhandicapped peers.

It is helpful to view placement alternatives for the hearing-impaired child as lying along a continuum from no special support services to a highly specialized learning environment. The task then becomes one of matching the child's needs to the alternatives available in a search for an educational placement. The ideal placement will

- Provide the specific services needed by the child
- Exert only minimal limitations on the child's ability to learn and to grow socially
- Stimulate growth of self-sufficiency
- Provide for the development of abilities, skills, and behaviors appropriate to functioning in a less-specialized educational setting

The types of educational settings on the continuum are identified in Table 16.1.

Normal School With or Without Special Services

Two broad categories of placement exist within a normal school setting: *mainstreaming* and *integration/inclusion*.

Mainstreaming. A mainstreamed child is in a special educational setting and spends part of each day in regular education. The child is expected to be successful in the regular subjects when mainstreamed but may be accommodated with testing modifications, a reduced number of written requirements, assistive listening aids and devices, etc.

Integration/Inclusion. A child in this model is in a normal, regular educational setting but is not expected to succeed in the regular curriculum. The child will have his educational needs met through curriculum changes to meet his specific requirements; i.e., if the hearing children are doing algebra, the integrated student in a regular classroom may be adding and subtracting via a computer with assistance from a special education teacher. The integrated student may spend part of the day in a special education group or class.

Northcott (1973, p. 3) has identified four characteristics that a hearing-impaired child must evidence if he or she is likely to be successful when fully mainstreamed into a normal school setting:

- Active utilization of residual hearing and full-time hearing-aid usage if prescribed
- Demonstrated social, academic, cognitive, and communicative (auditory and oral) skills within the normal range of behaviors of hearing classmates at a particular grade level
- Intelligible speech and the ability to comprehend and exchange ideas with others through spoken, written, and read language
- Increased confidence and independence in giving self-direction to the tasks at hand

If these are not all present, the child will need to be provided for by the integration/inclusion model. This model seeks to provide the child with

TABLE 16.1 The continuum of options and services

MAXIMAL SUPPORT	EDUCATIONAL PLACEMENT OPTIONS				MINIMAL SUPPORT
Specialized Residential or Day School	Special Classes Housed within a Normal School	A Single Special Class at Primary or Secondary Level	Normal School Placement with a Special Resource Room	Normal School Placement with an Itinerant Special Teacher or Consulting Special Education Teacher	Normal School Placement with Only Those Special Services Available to all Children

INCREASED SERVICES	SERVICES PROVIDED				DECREASED SERVICES
Full-time special education by specialist teachers. Small classes 6–15 children. Full range of audiology services usually available; hearing-aid monitoring and basic repair. Educational amplification systems. Special curricula. Specialist services in speech and language. Oral or combined oral/manual teaching. Social and activity clubs. Possibility of some mainstream experience for selected children. Career education. Augmentative communication systems (i.e. touch talkers).	Full-time special education by specialist teachers. Small classes 6–15 children. Education amplification systems. Special curricula. Access to services of speech, hearing, and language therapist. Teaching may be by oral or total communication method; choice sometimes available. Mainstream experiences where appropriate. Augmentative communication systems.	Full-time special education by special teacher. Small class size but usually up to 3-year age spread. Special curricula. Speech, hearing, and language services from regular speech therapist for school. Teaching usually oral. Educational amplification. Mainstreaming as appropriate. Augmentative communication systems.	Normal educational program among hearing children. Possible use of FM amplification in selected cases. Daily services of specialist teacher of hearing impaired for at least 1 hour per day individually or in groups no larger than 5 children. Services of school speech, hearing and language therapist. Augmentative communication systems.	Specialist resource teacher available at prescribed times. Usually provides individualized support or in groups of 2 or 3 children. Services of school speech, hearing, and language therapist. Use of special amplification integration/inclusion model.	Only such services as are available to all hearing children. These include the speech, hearing, and language therapist and in some schools a nonspecialist resource teacher or remedial reading teacher. Use of special amplification.

317

such supportive aids and services as assistive listening and learning devices, augmentative communication systems, note takers, sign language interpreters, and/or a consulting special education teacher or teacher of hearing-impaired children.

In considering a normal school placement for the hearing-impaired child, it will be necessary to provide a profile of her abilities in each of the previously mentioned areas. The child with a mild to moderate hearing impairment who has had early successful preschool guidance may be able to manage in the local primary school with support only from the speech, hearing, and language therapist. Some schools also have on staff a general resource teacher and/or a remedial reading teacher who helps hearing children with learning problems. The services of these teachers will increase the hearing-impaired child's chances of success.

The Resource Room or Itinerant Teacher Service

The child who has a more severe handicap, but who has the potential for meeting, or already meets criteria for mainstreaming will need the additional help of a specialist teacher of the hearing impaired. Help may be provided on an itinerant basis, or the child may be bused to a school that has a specialist resource room with a teacher of the hearing impaired on the staff. This teacher will not only be able to provide tutorial support and language enrichment, but will also serve as the manager of the child's academic needs. The specialist will be able to aid the classroom teacher, modify the child's curriculum appropriately, and coordinate the child's individual work with that of the classroom teacher. This child may have sufficient problems of understanding speech in the classroom to merit the use of FM amplification.

Separate Classes for the Hearing Impaired

For children who do not yet possess the characteristics important to success in a normal school, such a placement would limit their potential for learning. These children need continuous specialized teaching, intensive language and speech training, the use of educational amplification, and auditory-visual communication training. Such education should be available in special classes for hearing-impaired children that are usually housed in normal schools. It is important to know whether the special classes in a school district use a purely auditory-oral method of teaching or a total-communication approach, which accompanies speech with manual signs. Some urban school districts offer both types of education; other districts offer only one of the two methods. Ideally a child capable of learning by the auditory-oral method should not be placed in a total-communication environment, which is intended for children who need a supplementary or alternative communication system. This ideal may, however, not be achievable in a particular district.

For children with appropriate communication-learning skills, partial mainstreaming into selected subjects in the regular classes is often possible, thus exposing them to the normal educational environment into which some of them may later enter given appropriate resource support.

The advantage of the special class is that the child remains at home, maintains normal social interaction with neighborhood children, and has at least some contact with hearing peers in school. Although the child does not receive the constant spoken-language stimulation of the normal classroom, he is exposed to the hearing world for most of the day.

Residential/Day-School Placement

The number of hearing-impaired children attending residential/day school has dropped considerably since school districts have been required to provide increased local services. The population of residential/day schools now consists mainly of children from rural communities, where low-density population makes provision of a full range of special services very difficult, of children who need a total-communication teaching method when one is not locally available, and of children with multiple handicaps for whom severe or profound hearing impairment is a major factor. Despite the disadvantage of living away from the family and being separated from the hearing world, a residential placement provides many children with an opportunity for an education of which they would otherwise be deprived. For some children it truly represents the least limiting environment for learning. Such a placement may provide the only opportunity for the child to learn and to develop socially to his maximum capacity. It also makes available specialized preemployment training from teachers trained to educate young severely or profoundly hearing-impaired persons.

Residential schools may be state operated or state supported, or they may be approved private school programs. In either case no charge is made to parents for room, board, and tuition.

THE INDIVIDUALIZED EDUCATIONAL PLAN (IEP)

Once the placement decision has been made, the law requires that an Individualized Educational Plan be in effect before special education and related services are provided to a child. The following individuals must be included in the IEP planning meeting:

- A representative, other than the child's teacher, who is qualified to provide or supervise the provision of special education
- The child's teacher
- One or both parents
- The child, where appropriate
- Other individuals at the discretion of the parent or agency

At the initial IEP meeting it also is required that someone from the evaluation team, or someone who can serve the function of such a person, be present. Before each meeting the committee is required to make every effort to have the parents attend. If they cannot, then evidence of attempts to persuade them must be in the child's record. Of particular importance is the requirement that interpreters must be provided when parents are deaf or when English is not their native language.

The IEP is a required written statement of the intended educational program for an individual child. It is required of the school district at the time the child enters special education. Ideally, for a child entering school the IEP should be developed as soon as the placement decision has been finalized. Because the parents have a right to participate in the planning conference, you should discuss with them what you feel would constitute appropriate goals. Justify your opinion by referring to your report.

The IEP should include the following data:

- *A statement of the child's present educational performance level.* This consists of descriptions of language development, communication skills, motor development, social development, learning behaviors, and information about number skills and prereading skills. The preschool teacher will have this information. Working through the parent, or through direct contact with the primary school or special-class teacher (with written permission of the parents), the preschool teacher should ensure that what is already known about the child's performance is available at the IEP planning meeting.
- *The short- and long-term goals and objectives for the school year.* These should be related to the child's identified areas of learning and performance deficits. They should consist of general objectives to be aimed for over the long term and specific objectives whose attainment should lead to the achievement of the long-range goals. These goals should relate to the areas listed in the preceding paragraph. They should also include such specific areas as, for example, increasing the amount of time the hearing aid is worn, increasing the amount of time the child watches the speaker, improving the production of fricative sounds, improving sentence structure in written and spoken communication, increasing the number of communications the child makes in class. Because these goals should be based on needs that will have become apparent during the preschool experience, it is important that the teacher have the information you can provide.
- *The specific support services and teaching materials to be provided.* This should include specification of the amount of specialized tutoring the child will receive from the itinerant or resource room teacher, the amount of speech-improvement training and special remedial reading instruction that will be provided. Also included should be the recommendation about the child's need for educational amplification. These are clearly specialized aspects of IEP planning about which the audiologist and the preschool staff can offer valuable help to the teacher.
- *The amount of mainstreaming the child will experience.* The IEP must identify whether the child will participate in regular classes with hearing children, for which subjects, and for how many periods. The preschool teacher and hearing therapist will be able to advise the school district about the child's known learning capabilities and the extent to which the child can keep up with normal children. The likelihood of success in a full or part-time mainstream placement can be addressed by the preschool personnel.
- *The way in which the progress toward goals can be objectively determined.* The classroom teacher will have her own methods for evaluating the progress of a child. However, she is usually very receptive to suggestions as to how to assess the handicapped child in a manner that provides a fair evaluation. Certainly,

it would be helpful to suggest guidelines to help to ensure that the method of test administration will be appropriate for the child's communication abilities.

The guide for parents of handicapped children published by The University of the State of New York (1978) suggests that the parents make a list of questions and concerns about the program being proposed. Among the questions parents should ask are

- What do the test results show about my child's abilities?
- What academic subjects will my child be studying?
- What services will be provided to my child to help him reach these goals?
- What type of physical education will he be offered?
- What regular classroom experiences will be available to my child?
- What extracurricular activities will my child participate in?
- How do other children in the class react to my child?
- What behavior problems has my child shown?

The Audiologist's/Speech Language Pathologist's Input to IEP Planning

Prior to the parents' meeting with the IEP planning committee, you should provide them with a carefully written description of the child's performance at the preschool level. All formal test results including audiologic data, measures of aided hearing function, language level, and speech intelligibility should be given and explained. Pay particular attention to the child's ability to understand spoken language when wearing the aid(s). Comment on the effect of distance from the speaker and poor signal-to-noise ratios if possible, as well as the child's dependence on visual cues to speech. Include an overall statement about the child's ability to communicate effectively with others. Discuss the child's speech intelligibility when communicating with adults not familiar with his speech patterns and when talking with other children.

Describe the child's social behavior in structured activities and in free-learning/play situations, as well as his interaction with other children. Assess general behavior and personality, noting the child's level of curiosity, motivation to understand things, perseverance, friendliness to children and adults, self-sufficiency, and contentedness. Include copies of preschool progress reports in your case summary.

You should also communicate your evaluation of the anticipated support needs. Discuss whether the child will need intensive cognitive and linguistic training, whether special amplification will be necessary for learning, how much supplementary teaching will be needed, whether full-time special education will be necessary. You should relate your assessment of support needs to the description you have given of the child's preschool performance.

It is necessary for you to carefully go over the report with the parents to explain the significance of the information given and the nature of your recommendations. The parents will then have information that they understand to present to the Committee on Special Education.

The parents may request that you accompany them to their meeting with the committee, and that you present their case. You may perform this service as an audiologist, speech and hearing therapist, or teacher. Whatever your profession, if you agree, you should become fully familiar with the federal and state laws governing the educational decision process. Write to your State Education Department's Office for Education of the Handicapped to request all literature pertaining to special-educational placement and particularly to request materials written for parents. It is especially important for the parents to know their rights to an independent evaluation of their child's educational needs, and to know the process by which the committee's recommendation can be appealed.

SUMMARY

- Educational placement procedures for disabled children are delineated by the Individuals with Disabilities Educational Act (IDEA) of 1975, commonly known as PL 94-142.
- PL 94-142 provides for free public education for disabled children 3–21 years in the least restrictive environment.
- The decision process requires the establishment by each local education authority of a Committee on Special Education.
- The committee determines a classification of the handicap, identifies appropriate placement, determines services to be provided, and the degree of mainstreaming that will occur.
- The assessment must be comprehensive and administered in the child's native language or mode of communication.
- Parents have the right to due process; their written permission must precede evaluation, and they must be fully informed concerning the testing and intent to make placement.
- Parents may request independent assessment. If not objected to by the local authority, or if in an impartial hearing the authority fails to defend its test results successfully, the cost must be borne by the authority.
- Parents must be directed to impartial evaluation resources or legal aid on request.
- Placement possibilities provide a continuum of special services from minimal to maximal in mainstream, integration/inclusion, partial mainstream, and separate facilities.
- An IEP committee (qualified special education person, the class teacher, the parents, the child if appropriate, and invited professionals) determines the child's educational performance, the goals, support services, the degree of mainstreaming, and method of goal attainment.
- The audiologist, speech-language pathologist, or teacher of the hearing-impaired child should contribute information to the committee. They should be willing to assist parents who choose to appeal a placement decision.

Conclusion

The educational rights of children with disabilities are protected by federal law, which spells out the due process to which parents of disabled children are entitled. The assessment of the child, as well as the placement decision, are subject to challenge by the parents. In such instances the cost of impartial reassessment must be borne by the local education authority unless it can defend its own testing procedure and results. The main purpose is to ensure the placement of a child in an educational environment that fully meets demonstrated needs while approximating a normal school placement as closely as possible.

A placement must be supported by appropriate devices and services that are identified in an Individualized Educational Plan. This must involve parent input and requires the parent's approval. As an audiologist, speech-language pathologist, or teacher of hearing-impaired children, your input into this plan is important. Your guidance and support to parents involved in IEP planning, and your assistance if they request an impartial hearing, constitute the service offered in the educational planning process.

TABLE 16.2 Assessment of intelligence tests for infants and preschoolers (Sullivan & Vernon, 1979)

Test	*Age Range*	*Publisher*
Bayley Scales of Infant Development (Bayley, 1969)	2 mos.−30 mos.	New York: Psychological Corporation

Evaluation

The Mental Scale, Motor Scale and Infant Behavior Record are well standardized developmental measures for hearing children and meet satisfactory reliability standards. Although not valid for predicting later functioning or achievement, the three scales provide valuable estimates of *current* developmental status that may be used with hearing-impaired infants. Approximately 36 of the 163 items on the Mental Scale require auditory and/or language skills. These items should be corrected in final scoring according to the procedure employed on the Merrill Palmer Scale of Mental Tests (Stutsman, 1931). The items should be attempted to gain data on language skills using the child's communication mode. However, many hearing-impaired children may be expected to fail most auditory/language related items. All items are arranged developmentally. If the child passes a performance item at a higher level than a language item, the language item(s) should be credited that precede the successfully completed performance item.

Developmental Activities Screening Inventory (DASI) (Du Bose & Langley, 1977)	6 mos.−5 years	New York: New York Times Teaching Resources Company

Evaluation

This is a valuable performance *screening* measure of cognitive development. Test items tap a variety of skills including fine-motor coordination, cause-effect and means-end relationships, number concepts, size discrimination, and association and seriation abilities. Limitations include an inadequate description of normative data and procedures in the manual and the composite developmental quotient in a psychometrically weak quantification of test performance. Concurrent validity appears to be adequate but reliability data are not reported. Items are untimed, easily administered, and do not penalize children with auditory impairments or language disorders. Administraton adaptations are also available for visually impaired youngsters. The test appears to be appropriate for use with multiply handicapped hearing-impaired children. Instructional suggestions for the concepts assessed are included.

Hiskey-Nebraska Test of Learning Aptitude (Hiskey, 1966)	3−17 years	Lincoln, NE: Union College Press

Evaluation

The Hiskey is one of the best tests available for use with hearing-impaired children. Hearing-impaired and hearing norms are provided and comparisons, when appropriate, can be made of a given child's performance. Deaf norms are to be used, regardless of the child's degree of hearing loss, when pantomime administration directions are employed. Hearing norms should be used when the verbal subtest directions or total communication are employed. The discrepancy between scores using hearing and deaf norms is most probably due to the use of pantomime instructions. Although useful at younger age levels, the Hiskey should be supplemented with another measure on this table at 3 and 4 years of age. Pantomime subtest directions are easy to master. However, the test should be administered by skilled examiners familiar with its administration procedures. Although normative data are inadequately described, reliability and concurrent validity data are adequate.

TABLE 16.2 Assessment of intelligence tests for infants and preschoolers (Sullivan & Vernon, 1979) (*continued*)

Test	Age Range	Publisher
Merrill-Palmer Scale of Mental Tests (Stutsman, 1931)	2–5 years	Chicago: Stoelting Company

Evaluation

This test requires a skilled examiner with a thorough knowledge of the psychology of hearing impairment. Although the norms are dated, the variety of items have interest appeal for both language-impaired and hearing-impaired children. Adjustments in scoring can be made for items that are refused, omitted, or failed because of language difficulties. The time factor in scoring some items, however, is a weakness with hearing-impaired children. The Merrill-Palmer is a useful screening test to ascertain developmental functioning and may be used as a supplemental performance measure with another test on this table with young hearing-impaired children. This is one of the few tests with an adequate number of 2- and 3-year-olds in the standardization sample. Subtest instructions may have to be given in pantomime or total communication.

Smith-Johnson Nonverbal Performance Scale (Smith & Johnson, 1977)	2–4 years	Los Angeles: Western Psychological Services

Evaluation

This is an excellent test for use with young hearing-impaired children. Sex, hearing, and hearing-impaired norms are provided. However, the hearing norms are somewhat dated (1960) and the hearing-impaired normative sample included 36% with profound hearing losses and 64% with mild and moderate loss. The majority of hearing-impaired subjects were hard-of-hearing rather than severely and profoundly deafened. The test may be more appropriate for use with the hard-of-hearing. Subtest directions are presented in pantomime and many repetitions may be given. Although not recommended by the authors, total communication is suggested in the administration of this test to children who use this communication mode. Fourteen categories of subtests are presented and the child's performance level is categorized as below average, average, or above average in comparison to peers of the same sex and chronological age. As may be expected in preschool measures, test-retest reliabilities are low. Both reliability and validity data with hearing-impaired children are inadequately described in the manual. This test might also be used with hearing children who exhibit language difficulties.

Wachs Analysis of Cognitive Structures (Wachs & Vaughn, 1978)	3–6 years	Los Angeles: Western Psychological Services

Evaluation

This test is based upon Piagetian theories of cognitive development and is primarily nonverbal in format. It appears to have promise for use with the hearing impaired although they were not included in the normative sample. This test might be used to supplement another measure on this table.

Wechsler Preschool and Primary Scale of Intelligence Performance subtests (Wechsler, 1967)	3 yrs., 11 mos.– 6 yrs., 8 mos.	New York: Psychological Corporation

Evaluation

This scale is not recommended for use with hearing-impaired children. Most subtest directions are difficult to explain either orally, in pantomime, or in total communication.

TABLE 16.3 Assessment of intelligence tests for school-age children

Test	Age Range	Publisher
Arthur Adaptation of the Leiter International Performance Scale (Arthur, 1950)	2–18 years	Chicago: Stoelting

Evaluation

The Leiter is not appropriate for use with very young and preschool hearing-impaired children because norms for these age ranges are extrapolated from those for older children. In general, the test is psychometrically inadequate, inappropriately standardized, and lacking in reliability and validity for use with all hearing-impaired children. These limitations offset the ease of pantomime administration. See Ratcliffe and Ratcliffe (1979) for a review of these issues.

Hiskey-Nebraska Test of Learning Aptitude (Hiskey, 1966)	6–17 years	Lincoln, NE: Union College Press

Evaluation

This test is excellent for use with all school age hearing-impaired children.

Progressive Matrices (Raven, 1948)	9 years to adulthood	Los Angeles: Western Psychological Services

Evaluation

Raven's Progressive Matrices are most appropriate for use as a second test to substantiate another more comprehensive intelligence test. The matrices are easy to administer and score. However, care should be taken to ensure that the child is not responding impulsively to subtest items.

Wechsler Intelligence Scale for Children—Revised Performance Scale (Wechsler, 1974)	6–16 years	New York: Psychological Corporation

Evaluation

The WISC-R Performance Scale is an excellent test for use with school-age hearing-impaired children. It is ideally used with the Hiskey-Nebraska Test of Learning Aptitude as a supplementary performance test. The Performance Scale has been standardized with a hearing-impaired sample (Anderson & Sisco, 1977). However, research is needed to demonstrate the efficacy of these norms. A variety of sign systems and administrations were used in the standardization procedure, which may account for the population mean IQ of 95 and standard deviation of 18. These parameters must be considered in interpreting scores. Previously recommended administration modifications such as pantomime and visual aids should not be employed if the child is instructed in total communication. All six subtests should be administered. If the child has undue difficulty with Picture Arrangement and Coding only, which is frequently the case with hearing-impaired children, the PIQ may be prorated from the other four subtests. If the child has difficulty with Coding only, Mazes may be substituted and the PIQ computed from 5 subtests. However, these procedures affect test reliability and underscore the importance of administering more than one performance intelligence measure.

17

Assessment of the School-Age Child

ASSESSMENT OF CLASSROOM DEMANDS WITH CASE HISTORIES

It is common to think of assessment as a systematic process by which we determine the cause of a problem experienced by a child or adult. When we are attempting to ascertain a diagnosis, that is our goal. We assess the capacity of various sensory, motor, and cognitive systems to approximate normal function. Our concern in diagnosis is to determine which systems are not normal and how much they deviate from normal.

Rehabilitative assessment is an equally complex but rather different diagnostic process. It is important that we consider carefully the purpose for which we are making this assessment. We already have a confirmed diagnosis of hearing impairment, and we know the severity and pattern of the hearing deficit. Our concern now is to determine, as accurately as possible, the limitations imposed on the child by the reduced and distorted hearing. Further, we must assess the effects of reduced language, speech, cognition, learning, and socioemotional functioning secondary to the hearing deficiency. When we consider "limitations," it is essential that we know exactly what the demands are that the child will have to meet. This is necessary because the limitations imposed by a hearing impairment are not absolute; *they represent a relationship between demands and the resources available to*

326

meet those demands. As the demands decrease or increase, the resources will prove more or less adequate. What we are dealing with then is an assessment of the degree of impedance between the child and a range of demands arising in situations she will encounter in school and in school-related activities. In other words, we need to assess the compatibility between the child and the world of the classroom. Our evaluation of the child, therefore, requires that we

- Be familiar with the expectations for children in a particular classroom
- Ensure that as far as possible, we assess the child's capacity for meeting these expectations
- Identify the demands we anticipate the child will have meeting problems
- Translate our findings into an interpretive report intended to help the teacher understand the child's difficulties and needs arising from the hearing impairment

Assessing Classroom Demands

Consider the nature of the demands a child may have to meet. These demands arise from the nature of the

1. Physical environments
2. Prerequisite levels of knowledge
3. Mode of information transmission
4. Level (complexity) of language used
5. Teaching method
6. Prerequisite level of reading

1. The Physical Environments. In Chapter 9 we examined the negative effects of poor acoustic conditions on speech discrimination by hearing-impaired children. In the early grades of primary school, the child often spends all her academic learning time in a single classroom. This may be a new acoustically treated room with acoustic tile ceilings and carpeted floor. The school itself may be situated in a quiet suburban neighborhood and may stand back from the road in its own grounds. The behavior of the children in class may be orderly and quiet. The acoustic demands, that is, the expectation that a child can cope with the noise and reverberation, are relatively low. By contrast, a classroom in an old urban school situated on a busy thoroughfare at an intersection places far higher demands on the child. The walls, ceilings, and uncarpeted floors are highly sound reflective; desks and chairs have metal feet; class enrollment is high, as is the level of noise created by the children. We learned that such poor acoustic environments exert a negative effect on both auditory discrimination and on reading ability in children with normal hearing (see p. 137). The negative impact of poor room acoustics on a hearing-impaired child's ability to meet other classroom demands will be greater. Therefore, you should try to obtain observational or descriptive information concerning the type of listening conditions under which the child must learn.

As the child moves into the higher primary grades and into the middle and high school, the situation becomes more difficult. The demands become greater and more varied. Instead of having to deal with the acoustics of a single room, the child moves to different rooms for different subjects. Post–primary school learning environments include laboratories, home economics rooms, industrial arts areas, and typing rooms, as well as the auditorium, gymnasium, and swimming pool, all involving various degrees of oral instruction. In a workshop teaching environment, for example, the student may have difficulty understanding under the low signal-to-noise ratio conditions, since the high noise level may send her hearing aids into compression—further reducing the speech information received. The seating plan, lighting, and position of blackboards are additional physical factors that will exert an effect on how easily the child can understand what is said in class. We must determine in which of these environments significant difficulties in learning are experienced.

2. Prerequisite Levels of Knowledge. At each grade level there exists an assumption concerning minimal basic knowledge—that body of information prerequisite to the acquisition of new skills and further knowledge. The teacher does not plan to teach this information in his class. For example, in a fifth-grade class it is assumed that all children will have been exposed to the division of the world into countries and know that people in different countries have different life-styles. They will have acquired the necessary criteria for identifying separate countries—a name, geopolitical boundary, language, self-government, set of laws, flag, and national anthem. These criteria may be reviewed briefly but will not be taught as part of a lesson series on "Culture and Customs." Similarly a high school chemistry class may presume a working knowledge of elements, compounds, mixes, catalytic agents, and so on as the basis for describing, carrying out, and evaluating a laboratory experiment. I am not suggesting that you are responsible for teaching academic content, but you are concerned with attempting to raise language knowledge, linguistic skills, receptive and expressive auditory-oral (or signed) language competence, and cognitive reasoning to a level commensurate with lesson content. You should assume the task of determining to what extent a child's academic difficulties derive primarily from needs in these communication-learning areas. When you do so, you will wish to structure your intervention procedures to impact directly upon communication-learning requisites of the child's classes.

3. Mode of Information Transmission. Information in school is presented in a variety of ways. The dominant mode is through direct oral communication or in special classes through the total-communication method, which includes manual communication. A major concern in our assessment of the child will be his level of competence in receiving information through the primary mode of instruction. We must not forget, however, that important secondary modes of information are used increasingly in education. Almost every mainstream classroom today has a television monitor, usually with video playback capability. An increasing amount of information is presented by way of the television screen. This creates a different set of demands upon the child's receptive communication and learning abilities. Every attempt should be made to assess what these are and, wherever possible, to increase the child's ability to receive the information thus presented. In addition to video many classrooms have special learning stations with programmed audio-instruction tapes keyed to printed materials. Unless you are aware that a particular child is expected to use this method of learning, he may be deprived of its advantages or may struggle with it unnecessarily.

Another means of information transmission occurs in the school auditorium, where the speech signal reaches the child by way of the stage amplification system. When lectures are given to large audiences or there are guest speakers or school plays, our hearing-impaired student may find this means of information transmission inadequate because of poor acoustics.

4. Level of Language Used. When we work with children with significant communication difficulties, we often lose sight of the complexity of language that their nonhandicapped peers are capable of processing at a given grade level. Although observation of the child in the classroom provides the most accurate picture of what language demands are made, this method usually is not practical. You can obtain a helpful insight into language complexity at a given grade level by examining several of the textbooks used in class. Consider the vocabulary used, the syntactic complexity, length of sentences, and general clarity of language. This will provide you with a helpful yardstick in assessing the language impedance reflected by the child's measured performance on various subcomponents of standardized language tests.

5. Teaching Method. The method or methods of teaching that the child encounters throughout the school day will impact on her ability to learn, since different styles and methods affect the manner of information transmission. Consider the types of teaching methods that may be encountered:

- Direct oral instruction, teacher to whole class.
- Oral instruction to whole class combined with information on a blackboard. The written information may have been put up earlier or may be written simultaneously with the oral presentation
- Oral instruction to whole class related to textbook material to be examined concurrently with the teacher's information.
- Small-group instruction, teacher to children.
- Whole class discussion and question and answer.
- Small-group projects—children only.
- Video presentation using TV monitor.
- Filmstrip or slide and audiotaped instruction.
- Practical demonstration in laboratory classes.

The spacial relationship of the child to the information source influences the difficulty of learning in each of these various methods. The teacher may be standing at the blackboard in a classroom with traditional row seating or with rows of benches between him and the children, as in a laboratory. If it is a small group, the children may sit in a half-circle around the teacher and blackboard. In class discussion the source of information will vary constantly as contributions are made by children around the room and by the teacher. The factors here will be the variable intensity of the spoken information resulting from variable distances changing the signal-to-noise ratio, the variable distortion resulting from the relationship of the direct to the indirect speech wave, and the effect of directivity (p. 38). Visible information will vary also depending on whether the child can see the teacher. Visual information will vary as the teacher moves around the room, teaches from behind the child, turns to face the blackboard, or cannot be seen constantly because other children or laboratory bench shelves, faucets, and equipment interrupt the view. Visibility of the children making contributions in a class situation, even in a half-circle, often is poor. Video, filmstrip, slide, and audiotape presentations mean that visual cues to the spoken message usually are absent. They also usually mean that lighting is dimmed. This makes any comments by the teacher difficult or impossible to see, while his voice may be masked by the noise of the equipment or by the sound track. Thus the ease of learning will vary considerably with the method of teaching.

    6. Prerequisite Level of Reading. At first glance, it would seem that reading is an academic subject and thus falls outside our realm of responsibility. Indeed this is so if you consider only the specific skill of reconstructing messages from the printed page. However, that skill is predicated upon language knowledge. It is the two subskills essential to reading, namely, word knowledge and verbal reading, that are of particular concern to us. Together these two component skills account for 90 percent of the variability in reading abilities demonstrated by hearing children (Davis, 1972). Classroom learning demands call upon the child's knowledge of the experiential concept that a printed word identifies. Learning depends increasingly upon the ability to deduce the meaning of new words from other words in context. Even a dictionary does not provide meaning; it simply taps into other related words to facilitate the derivation of meaning from your existing knowledge. Meaning also is encoded into the syntactic patterns. The recognition of these patterns reveals relationships between and among component words, thus permitting the reconstruction of the meaning of the message. Beyond the sentence the child is expected to construct in her memory an ever increasingly complex web of ideas that together comprise what is being taught. Thus, the ability to see word relationships, to recognize sequences, to condense and summarize information, and to use verbal language for cognitive reasoning is fundamental to learning from the printed word. The importance of reading in learning is further increased by the interweaving of the teacher's information with that presented in the text. Your responsibility for improving the child's language knowledge and use, therefore, will need to encompass the cognitive linguistic components of reading.

    It should be clear from the factors we have just considered, namely, the physical environment, knowledge expectations, mode of information transmission, complexity of spoken and written language, and method of teaching, that we need more information than a conventional diagnostic assessment provides. Success in an educational placement cannot be predicted from an audiogram and a word discrimination score. It also should be apparent that each child experiences a variety of different demands that change throughout his school day and from year to year. What we must develop and monitor is a profile of that pattern for a given child. His unique profile will serve as the basis of an individualized targeted intervention program.

Look for example at the types of experiences two children with impaired hearing may have during a typical school day in two different school buildings.

Jessica is eight years old; she has just entered third grade in a regular school. Her classroom teacher is Mrs. Burwick. Jessica attends a suburban school in a quiet residential area. Set well back from the road, it has a play area on two sides and a parking lot separating it from public tennis courts at the rear. The school was built some 30 years ago, and new energy-conserving double-glazed windows have just been installed. Acoustic tiles in the ceilings and industrial carpeting throughout the building create a pleasant, quiet, damped sound environment.

Anthony's school is very different. Anthony is 17; he attends the high school in the district. Built some 20 years earlier than Jessica's school, it stands just back from a main road into the city, quite close to the expressway, which can be seen from the rear of the school and heard everywhere. Slated for renovation, it remains an old-style building with sash windows, hard composite floors, half-tiled rooms and corridors, and painted plaster walls and ceilings. The building echoes with the noise of the students. The general noise level is raised even more by traffic noise from outside, a particular problem in warm weather.

Now follow Anthony and Jessica through their school day. Today Anthony has not one but six different teachers in six different locations in the building. He starts in his homeroom for general announcements over a public address system, which, because of reverberation and competing noise, he has difficulty hearing. He does not like having to ask friends about notices thus given.

Anthony enjoys his social studies class. The alphabetized seating plan the teacher used places him in the left front row. An additional attraction is Susan, who sits next to him. Since Mr. Keriac rarely goes beyond the first row of desks and almost always teaches from that half of the room, Anthony finds he hears well. Mr. Keriac's deep rich voice and firm hand with the class make it easy to follow the material. The teacher rarely asks questions but illustrates many concepts by relating them to everyday situations and events. The textbook is new and attractively produced; concepts are explained clearly in excellent English with ample illustration. Anthony finds the text easy to learn from and appreciates the clear review sections. He does well in social studies.

Miss Lee's English class is very different. Anthony sits with his friends near the back of the room. A newly graduated teacher, Margaret Lee has trouble with classroom management. There is much talking and giggling going on while she is teaching; notes are passed from desk to desk when she is not watching. Miss Lee's high-pitch voice and nervous rapid speech are very hard for Anthony to follow. The text of *Julius Caesar* is impossible, difficult to read, with many unfamiliar words and phrases. Anthony is barely obtaining passing grades in this subject.

Chemistry is taught in the chemistry laboratory, a long room lined with work benches. There are blackboards on the front and left walls, a row of windows on the right. Anthony's group assignment places him at the next to last bench. Mr. Davis lectures from the front and sides of the room, using the blackboard extensively. He moves rapidly through the material, explaining formulae as he writes them on the board, depriving Anthony of visual cues. When experiments are assigned, he moves from group to group. This is very helpful to Anthony since he then understands what Mr. Davis explains and can ask questions. The text is rather hard to learn from, giving only one example of each process. The vocabulary and verbal reasoning are difficult for Anthony who particularly dislikes "thus . . . therefore" and "it therefore is obvious that. . . ." (when it is not!). Anthony's companions in the group are of little help—Mike understands no better than Anthony, while Maud, who always gets As, does all the work and has little patience with her group mates. Anthony is obtaining passing grades in class thanks to Maud's efforts and extensive help from his father, who is a chemical engineer.

The next two subjects are physical education, which Anthony enjoys and is successful at, and art. In physical education, he follows most instructions visually. Oral instruction in games usually occurs with students gathered around the instructor. By ensuring he is in the front of the group where he can see and even hear quite well, he has little difficulty. When in doubt he feels comfortable checking with his friends. Art, like physical education, is a subject that Anthony enjoys, but he does not excel at it. The teacher moves from student to student giving guidance. Understanding Anthony's needs, she stands close to him on the side that puts the light on her face. He has no difficulty understanding her.

The final subject of the day is mathematics. For many of us this never was a subject we looked forward to. Anthony is an exception; he excels in math. He has a natural ability, can follow mathematical reasoning, and appreciates the minimal number of verbal concepts involved. He has a seat close to the teacher, who uses the front blackboard only. The teacher encourages questions and makes a habit of repeating them. He repeats also any answers to questions or comments made by students. The only time Anthony has trouble in math is when the curriculum deals with verbal problems. He never can conceptualize trains traveling in opposite directions, leaving at different times, traveling at different speeds, and meeting at unknown destinations. Other than that he has consistently obtained A grades in math.

Anthony does not have German class today. He is managing the language requirement quite well. He chose German because its pronunciation is quite systematic as are the structural rules. The teacher has agreed to weigh his written work more heavily than oral performance.

Meanwhile Jessica is well into her day. Like Anthony, she had some difficulty with the general announcements on the PA system fed to the classroom. She is well seated at the front center of the room, which is good for her since she wears binaural postauricular hearing aids. The first subject was English. Jessica has trouble with this subject. She encounters many unfamiliar words in the reading book and in the teacher's discussion. She struggles with the compound and complex sentences that imprison the meaning for her; thus she often has but a general idea of the content of a passage. In class she misses the questions and comments from children sitting behind her since she requires visual cues to supplement the auditory cues to speech. Of particular concern to Jessica are spelling tests since she often is not sure of the target word even when she can spell it. She does not enjoy reading even when it is not school related.

Social studies provides a relief from the difficulties of English. The children are working on group projects dealing with American Indian culture. Jessica finds the other children supportive and feels a member of the team. At such a close distance to the group members, she is able to see, hear, and, therefore, follow the discussion easily. The book is much easier to follow than the English textbook. It is well illustrated with excellent review sections. Mrs. Burwick works with groups individually so Jessica follows her guidance quite easily. She completes written components of the project in short, simple, but correct English.

Music, which follows social studies, is enjoyable for Jessica. She can read music and plays the piano quite well. In school she plays a xylophone.

This class is followed by arithmetic. She is now experiencing the difficulties that Anthony has since the class has begun simple word problems. Jessica finds it difficult to deal with the linguistic part of these problems. It is not so much vocabulary as verbal conceptualization of sequences and relationships. Given the mathematical equation derived from the written statement, Jessica can find the answer. Mrs. Burwick feels that Jessica does not really try in arithmetic.

The science class also is difficult for Jessica, in part because much of it is illustrated by video presentation. She finds the narrative difficult to follow since the instructor is rarely seen as the camera focuses on the illustrations or activities. When she reads the text, she lacks the conceptual understanding that the video was chosen to provide. New vocabulary is difficult to learn and remember without a knowledge of what it identifies.

Jessica is fortunate in that she does not yet have to adapt to different teachers' styles of teaching, has a generally sympathetic teacher willing to help, and stays in a single room for most classes. That, of course, will change in fourth grade when children begin to be streamed for major subjects.

These two pupils illustrate some important concepts:

- Hearing-impaired children vary as much in abilities as hearing children.
- They have special abilities and aptitudes for certain types of subjects.
- Subjects that are heavily language based present the most difficulty.
- They are more quickly overloaded by demands than hearing children because they must always cope with reduced information.
- Their support needs vary from subject to subject, environment to environment, teacher to teacher, textbook to textbook.
- Support services must be prescriptive, determined by specific needs.

In looking at one school day, we can see certain problems that confront Anthony and Jessica—problems that will need specific intervention strategies. Do not forget, however, that these two young people will need support in other areas of communication. You will need to consider those needs arising from their personal relationships with their peers and their social activities and their need to come to terms with their hearing handicap. This very personal aspect of support underpins their educational performance and thus should not be neglected. All this may seem to be a rather overwhelming task, and certainly the needs are enormous. Your role, however, is to contribute to the overall well-being of the child, not to assume responsibility for ensuring it. Knowing the scope and the content of your responsibilities, and knowing ways to maximize your effectiveness, should ensure that you feel good about your contribution. We can begin our discussion of assessment by considering what resources are available to maximize the child's performance.

ASSESSING THE CHILD'S AUDITORY-VISUAL RESOURCES

We need to think of assessment of resources very practically. For each child you will have developed a profile of the demands that he must meet if he is to function adequately in the learning situation. To meet those demands resources must be identified and made operative. In most cases, various resources will need to be pooled if the demands are to be met.

Resources in the Child

Residual Hearing Resource. The greatest resource for the hearing-impaired child is residual hearing. Given that the audiologist has provided an optimal binaural hearing aid fitting, our task is to understand what the child's aided hearing potential is. The aided hearing thresholds on the audiogram have implications when we compare them to the intensity ranges of speech as a function of frequency. This area, referred to as the "speech banana" by virtue of its shape, is depicted by shading on the audiogram (Figure 17.1). If amplification fails to bring the child's threshold of detection in any particular frequency band to within this area, those frequencies of speech sounds containing components within that band will not be heard. Some sounds, such as /s/, /f/, /ʃ/, may be inaudible; others, though audible, may be distorted and indistinguishable from sounds with similar acoustic patterns. This occurs because the upper frequencies do not fall within the range of residual hearing, while the vocal tone and lower frequency components do. Thus, a sound will be perceived clearly only when all its frequency pattern falls within the shaded area.

By plotting the child's aided thresholds onto the speech spectrum, you can obtain some idea of what speech the child can hear. Compare the audibility that speech-sound components have for David (Figure 17.1a) and Margaret (Figure 17.1b). David has a moderate hearing impairment in the low tones sloping to a severe deficit at 4000 Hz. His aided audiogram indi-

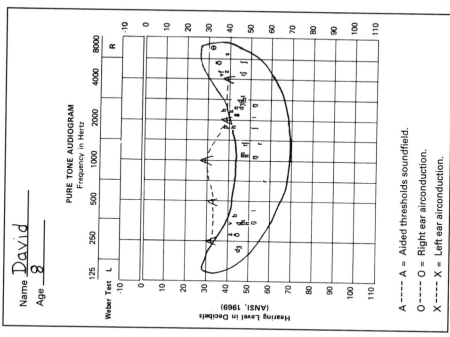

Name David
Age 8

PURE TONE AUDIOGRAM
Frequency in Hertz

A ---- A = Aided thresholds soundfield.
O ---- O = Right ear airconduction.
X ---- X = Left ear airconduction.

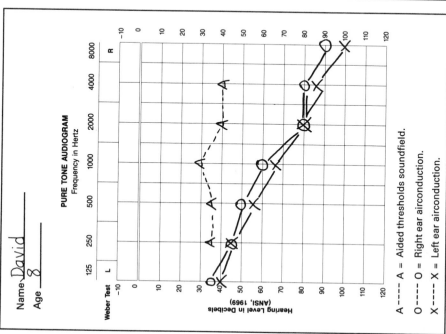

Name David
Age 8

PURE TONE AUDIOGRAM
Frequency in Hertz

A ---- A = Aided thresholds soundfield.
O ---- O = Right ear airconduction.
X ---- X = Left ear airconduction.

Figure 17.1a Audiogram for David.

335

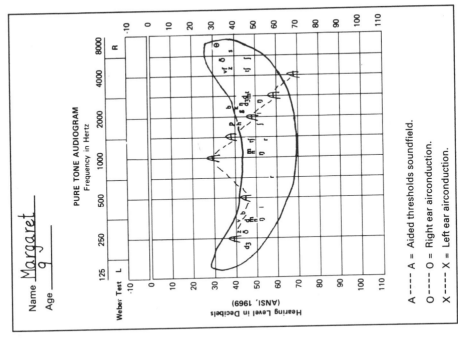

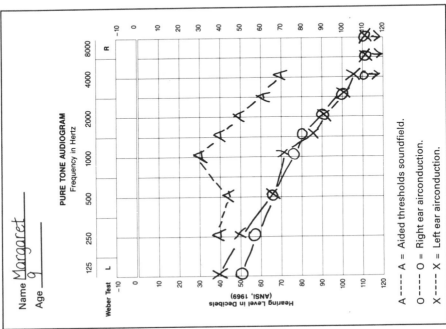

Figure 17.1b Audiogram for Margaret.

cates that amplification raises all of the frequency thresholds from 250–4000 Hz to well within the boundaries of the speech spectrum area. Thus, David's *potential* for speech discrimination is excellent with the hearing aids he is wearing. However, you must remember that the spectral area depicted was determined at one meter from the lips of a male speaker in quiet (Richards, 1973). There may be some decrease in actual discrimination when David has a woman teacher; there most certainly will be a decrease at greater distances from the speaker, and there definitely will be a decrease as a function of noise and reverberation. On the other hand, this prediction of potential for auditory discrimination calculated for one meter may be an underestimate. Considerable improvement may occur for speech at no more than four to six inches from the input microphone, as in the use of an FM system.

Margaret's hearing impairment is more severe than David's. She has a moderate deficit in the low frequencies and a severe to profound impairment in the high frequency range. Without her hearing aids, Margaret will hear only the vocal tone and the first formants of low back vowels, but few, if any, of the components above 1000 Hz. When amplified many more low and middle frequency speech components become audible, though most of the consonant sounds still fall well outside her range of hearing, as do the second formants of the vowels /i/, /ɛ/ and /æ/. Bear in mind the fact that these predicted abilities are based on frequency information only. In words, even in nonsense syllables, missing or distorted information often is compensated for by other acoustic cues such as intensity, duration, and voice onset time,* permitting that which is not heard to be predicted, even perceived. Probabilities deduced from linguistic, contextual, and situational constraints will enhance auditory perception even further. However, our present concern is only for what can be derived from the acoustic signal.

Another way of estimating which frequencies lie within the range of audibility for the child before and after amplification has been suggested by Ross (1982). He recommends plotting the unaided and aided free field audiogram on a sound pressure level chart that essentially is an inverted audiogram referenced to SPL instead of HL (Figure 17.2a,b). He also plots on the chart the reference level of average hearing threshold and the threshold of discomfort at each frequency. Next the output curve of the hearing aid is plotted, which is an SPL per frequency measure of a 60dB input signal. You now can compare the child's unaided threshold at each frequency with the output of the hearing aid. The difference in decibels between the two figures is the benefit the child receives at that frequency. The area between the two curves tells you the sound pattern the child hears when wearing the hearing aid, that is, the *aided residual hearing*. Ross also records these results numerically beneath the chart, computing gain by subtracting aided from unaided thresholds at each frequency. The average

---

* Voice onset time (VOT) is that interval between the release of a stop consonant and the first vocal fold vibration for the following vowel. For voiced stops the VOT is between 0–21 milliseconds; for voiceless stops, between 20–40 milliseconds.

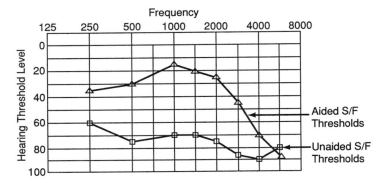

Figure 17.2a An unaided and aided free field audiogram for a child with a high frequency hearing-impairment. (Ross 1982).

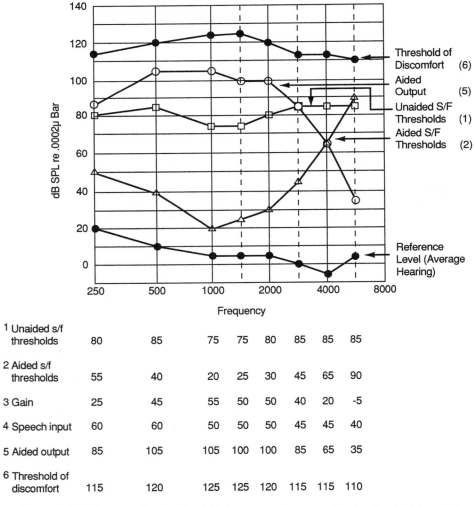

1 Unaided s/f thresholds	80	85	75	75	80	85	85	85
2 Aided s/f thresholds	55	40	20	25	30	45	65	90
3 Gain	25	45	55	50	50	40	20	-5
4 Speech input	60	60	50	50	50	45	45	40
5 Aided output	85	105	105	100	100	85	65	35
6 Threshold of discomfort	115	120	125	125	120	115	115	110

Figure 17.2b The same thresholds plotted on a sound pressure level scale which involves an inversion of the curves. (Ross 1982).

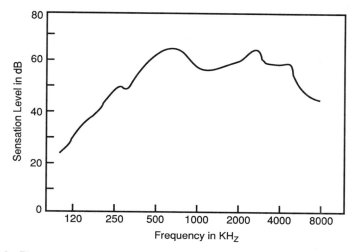

Figure 17.3 The perceived spectrum of speech in a normal ear. The speech spectrum is modified by the head, pinna and ear canal and the threshold frequency response of the normal ear to produce the sensation levels indicated in the illustration. (Ross 1982).

speech input indicates the average intensity occurring at each frequency, that is, frequency distribution of the energy in conversational speech (Pascoe, 1978). (Figure 17.3) Output and gain also can be read from the output of the hearing aid at each frequency. The difference in decibels between those curves is the *aided residual hearing*—what the child hears when wearing the hearing aid. Ross uses these results to compare how well aided hearing approximates the normal speech sensation levels of a 60dB SPL speech signal.

Analyze the results in Figure 17.2. The unaided and aided (SPL) free field thresholds, obtained through the loudspeaker in the sound-treated room, are simply plotted on an inverted audiogram instead of a regular one and show the improvement resulting from amplification. The numerical data below the audiogram indicate

Row 1: *Unaided* sound field thresholds
Row 2: *Aided* sound field thresholds
Row 3: *Functional gain* of the hearing aid (aided minus unaided thresholds per frequency)
Row 4: *Approximate level of sound pressure* in conversational speech at each frequency
Row 5: *Aided output per frequency* input (row 4) + gain (row 3) = output (row 5)
Row 6: *Threshold of discomfort* at each frequency.

The area between the aided output (row 5) and the unaided threshold curve (row 1) is the *aided residual hearing*. This is what the child hears with the hearing aid. Ross goes on to explain that from Figure 17.3, we observe that this hearing aid is providing too much gain (55dB) at 1000 Hz but not enough in the higher frequencies. Using the $\frac{1}{3}$ to $\frac{1}{2}$ gain rule (required gain = $\frac{1}{3}$ to $\frac{1}{2}$ hearing threshold; see Chapter 11 p. 164), the gain at 1000 Hz would more appropriately be 25dB (75/3). At 4K Hz and 6K Hz the gain should be increased to bring threshold above the 45dB intensity of speech energy at those frequencies. With the hearing aid fitted as shown, the child has adequate reception of speech components to 2000 Hz but will have trouble detecting F2 in front vowels spoken by women and children. He will hear neither the upper frequency components of /ʃ/ nor the energy in /θ/, /ð/, /s/, or /f/, nor the energy burst in voiceless plosives. By increasing the gain of the hearing aid at 3K (+ 15dB), 4K (+ 35dB), and 6K (+ 55dB) (Figure 17.4), the aided thresholds (line 2) are brought above the level of speech energy level at those frequencies, while still staying below the threshold of discomfort. Ensuring the optimal amplification across the full range of residual hearing is an absolute prerequisite to assessment of speech discrimination recognition and comprehension. It will determine whether the child learns to his capacity.

The traditional diagnostic audiology assessment of children includes, when possible, a measure of auditory speech discrimination. The hearing aid evaluation usually assesses the maximum aided discrimination score for words presented at 50dB in quiet. The test materials used to assess speech discrimination ability in young school-age children usually comprise one or more of the following:

- Phonetically Balanced Kindergarten Word List (PB–K) (Haskins, 1949)
  The list is drawn from the vocabulary of hearing children of kindergarten age. The words are selected to ensure that phonemes occur in the word list with approximately the same frequency as they occur in conversational speech. The test requires that the child repeat the word he hears. Oslen and Matkin (1979) have urged that this list not be used to assess the speech discrimination of children whose receptive language age is less than six years.
- Northwestern University Children's Perception of Speech Word List (NU.-CHIPS) (Katz & Elliott, 1978)
  The complete test comprises four lists of monosyllabic words derived from various combinations of a core list of 50 words. This is a closed set task. Each word is illustrated by a picture; the key word is named, and the child is asked to identify the appropriate picture from a set of four.
- Word Intelligibility by Picture Identification (WIPI) (Ross & Lerman, 1970)
  This closed set picture identification test is comprised of 25 cards, each with six pictures. The child is asked to identify the picture named from among the six alternatives. The words illustrated were selected to be appropriate for hard-of-hearing children aged five years and older and were designated as appropriate for testing deaf children above seven years of age.

The audiologist can help by providing additional information for the aided test condition. This should include

- *A record of the child's response to each word.* The word said by the child should be recorded or a "no response" should be indicated. The audiologist usually

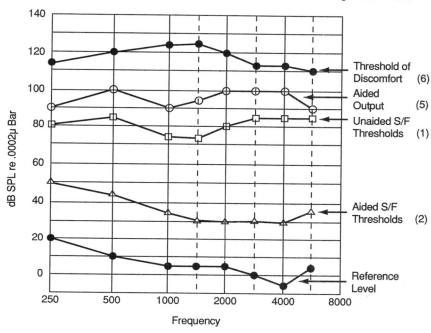

Frequency	250	500	1000	1500	2000	3000	4000	6000
1 Unaided s/f thresholds	80	85	75	75	80	85	85	85
2 Aided s/f thresholds	50	45	35	30	30	30	30	35
3 Gain	30	40	40	45	50	55	55	50
4 Speech input	60	60	50	50	50	45	45	40
5 Aided output		100	90	95	100	100	100	90
6 Threshold of discomfort	115	120	125	125	120	115	115	110

Figure 17.4 Modification of the frequency response plotted in Figure 17.2 to produce a more desirable pattern of amplification. (Ross 1982).

reports only the percentage of words correctly discriminated. Far more useful information can be derived if, as Markides (1978) recommended, the responses are written down by the audiologist for analysis for the percentage of phonemes correctly identified. Given a copy of the child's responses, you can make such an analysis. The results indicate

How much of a word a child correctly discriminated

Which sounds are indiscriminable

Whether sounds not discriminable in one phonetic context are so in another
Patterns of phoneme confusions
This information is valuable in planning auditory discrimination training and
in speech articulation work.

- *A discrimination score based upon an auditory-visual presentation of each word that was incorrectly discriminated by hearing alone.* This provides some indication as to how much benefit the child is deriving from visual cues to the articulation of those sounds that auditorily are not discriminable in certain phonetic contexts.
- *An auditory discrimination score when the test words are presented at a S/N ratio of +5dB using either speech babble or speech spectra noise.* This will provide a very approximate estimate of the percentage of information the child can be expected to derive from the acoustic signal alone when in the classroom. The score, however, must be discounted rather heavily for the other factors that we discussed in Chapter 3. On the other hand, the results do not allow for the child's ability to fill in missing pattern components through closure from linguistic, contextual, and situational constraints.

Supplementing Audiologic Data

You will find it informative to supplement the audiologist's test results by some further testing of your own.

- Ling Five Sound Test (Ling, 1976; Ling & Ling 1978, p. 98)
  This is very informative test that is quick and simple to administer. Five phonemes /a/, /u/, /i/, /s/, and /ʃ/ are presented in isolation using live voice. The sounds are spoken at normal conversational level (50dB HL) at a distance of 3–5 feet, without visible speech cues. The child is asked to indicate each time she hears a sound. As Ling and Ling (1978) explain, audibility of the three vowels indicates that suprasegmental patterns also will be audible, while detection of /ʃ/ indicates F2 of /i/ is audible and that /u/ and /i/ will be discriminable. Once the child's auditory ability is known, the test becomes a reliable and readily available means of checking that the hearing aid is functioning appropriately.
- Glendonald Auditory Screening Procedure (GASP), Phoneme Detection Subtest (Erber, 1982)
  This subtest is very similar to the Ling test but expands the range of phonemes tested. Two further subtests assess word identification and sentence comprehension.
- Pediatric Speech Intelligibility Test 1 (PSI) (Jerger, Lewis, Hawkins, & Jerger, 1980)
  This test is a closed picture identification task with five picture choices. It provides for 20 word discrimination items and 20 sentences. The test items may be administered both in quiet and at various signal-to-noise ratios.

With the exception of the Jerger et al. test, those discussed so far assess speech-sound discrimination in isolation or in monosyllabic words. It has been noted, however, that the Word Intelligibility by Picture Identification (WIPI) test scores, for example, tend to lead to an underestimation of a child's potential for speech discrimination performance in the classroom. Weber and Reddel (1976) in discussing this observation suggest that the task of processing small linguistic units is harder than that of processing larger more meaningful chunks. Certainly there is evidence to support this hypothesis (Sanders, 1971). To accommodate this, the WIPI test was modified by placing the key word in the middle of a sentence. Each sentence was derived from remarks children made when asked about the picture.

The observation that children derive information from surrounding words and from syntax when discriminating test items auditorily emphasizes the symbiotic relationship among various stages of components contributing to speech comprehension. It is clear that while increased discrimination results in greater comprehension of speech, comprehension enhances discrimination. Both, however, are dependent on language-processing capabilities. Thus, before we attempt to assess auditory comprehension, it will be necessary to evaluate linguistic competence.

ASSESSING THE CHILD'S LANGUAGE RESOURCES

I have stressed that the acquisition and use of language must be seen as a process embedded within experience and cognition. At any one time what we say, that is, the choice of words and phrases that our preconscious mind makes available to us, and the manner in which we choose to couch a statement, observation, comment, idea, or reply are influenced by the situation. We choose words and phrases and clothe them in the *paralinguistics* appropriate to the particular circumstance (Bates, 1976). That is to say, we use suprasegmentals, patterns, facial expressions, and gestures to guide our listener to a particular interpretation of our message. Language assessment must encompass all aspects of this process.

We can assess language competence through both a formal and an informal approach. You will need both in your assessment (Moeller, 1985). Formal tests attempt to provide data by constructing very narrow constraints to provoke a particular type of response from a child. Those concerned with assessing language form seek information pertaining to the child's knowledge of the building blocks or structure of language—namely, phonology, morphology, and syntax. They help us determine whether the child can use his knowledge of the value of each of the components to identify or convey meaning linguistically. To use an analogy, unless you know the various strokes in the repertoire of the game of tennis and can use them, you will be unable to play even an elementary game. However, how well you actually function on the court will depend upon your skill in modifying these strokes to accommodate different plays dictated by different circumstances. In communication, this requires a knowledge of how context places constraints on the use of words (semantics) and how context influences the types of utterances we choose (pragmatics).

Formal tests, by design, create contrived language demands. Human communication, however, does not function that way, for it consists of language in action in dynamic circumstances. For this reason formal test results often fail to reflect faithfully the child's true language knowledge and behavior. To overcome this disadvantage, researchers in child language assessment have recommended that we sample the child's use of language as it occurs spontaneously.

Sampling Spontaneous Language

Several samples of spontaneous communication should be recorded. Spontaneity is the essential ingredient in a truly representative sample. A video recording obviously provides the greatest amount of information, for it reveals situational constraints, the use the child makes of them, and her verbal and nonverbal communication skills and use. This, however, may not be possible; you may have to use an audio recording. Use a high-quality recorder and tape, with the microphone positioned to pick up both your speech and the child's. Whichever recording system you use, make a point of repeating exactly any utterance the child makes that may later be difficult to interpret. This will facilitate analysis (Ross, 1982).

The sample is best elicited by involving the child in an activity that stimulates communication. With a young school-age child, this might involve the use of building blocks, toy soldiers, animals, or buildings, or it may involve playing a game. Puppets may depict an event or picture stories may be used. The child is shown a sequence of pictures depicting an event she can appreciate. For example, the sequence might depict a man preparing a meal. While the man works at the counter with his back to the table, his dog enters the kitchen by way of the back door and steals the meat. The man, hearing the noise, turns around, sees the dog, and chases after it down the street. Such sequential event pictures are available commercially and are in many language stimulation kits. The child is then asked to tell you the story with the stimulus available for repetition or reference.

The older child is more likely to enjoy involvement in discussion of a short section of a video film or a cartoon story. He may be asked to begin by describing what took place. This will provide a basis for you to ask about the child's reactions and opinions about why he thought the events occurred, how the characters felt, how he might have felt and reacted, and what the outcome might have been.

Another approach to spontaneous language elicitation is through role playing. This method has been advocated by Ross (1982, p. 93) and developed by Stone (1988) into a complete methodology for assessing and developing conversational competence. This is a variation on the method just described. In role playing the therapist/teacher assigns a role to the child and assumes a role herself, both derived from a scenario communicated visually or verbally to the child. The therapist/teacher explains that she and the child will pretend they are the people and will act out what happened. For example,

"You just came home from school.

You have lost your gym shoes.

Your mother is very angry.

You try to explain it wasn't your fault.

Mother tells you to go back to school to find them.

You want to go out to play with your friends.

Pretend I'm the mother and you are you."

"You are at the dentist's.
He has to put a filling in a tooth.
You are afraid.
You want to know if it will hurt.
You don't want to have the tooth filled.
You want to go home.
I'll be the dentist; you just got up into the chair."

Analyzing the Sample

It first is necessary to gather a large enough sample to provide representative information. There is no general agreement on the number of utterances required for analysis. Most evaluators claim it should be somewhere between 50 and 100 utterances (Kretschmer & Kretschmer, 1978).

Kretschmer and Kretschmer (1978) provide an extensive detailed review of the wide range of analytic procedures suggested in the literature and also suggest a detailed procedure of their own. Obviously the more extensive the analysis the greater is the specificity of prescriptive intervention. Such in-depth analysis, however, requires considerable knowledge of linguistics, psycholinguistics, and child development, as Kretschmer and Kretschmer (1978) point out. The teacher/therapist should aspire to as detailed an analysis as she can provide or as is available through referral to someone well versed in such procedures. The reality of many, if not most, situations is that you will be left to provide the best assessment you can conduct. We will review here just the essential nature of an evaluation. For specific guidance you should refer to the source materials.

Aspects of Linguistic Competence

The aspects of language use that should be examined from the spontaneous language sample include

1. Mean length of utterance
2. Type-token ratio
3. Syntactic complexity
4. Structural complexity score

1. Mean Length of Utterance (MLU). This proves to be a surprisingly powerful measure of language development despite its relative simplicity. It involves counting the number of words or morphemes in each utterance and dividing by the number of utterances. The MLU has been shown to correlate well with other aspects of language development (Shriner, 1969; Brown, 1973). Kretschmer and Kretschmer (1978) state that for children with an MLU of five or less morphemes, "this measure still seems to be the best indicator of language growth" (p. 175).

2. Type-Token Ratio (TTR). This measure is a qualitative assessment of the child's utterances. It measures the relationship between the number of different categories or types of words (nouns, verbs, adjectives, adverbs, etc.) and the total number of words, or "tokens." A modification of the TTR involves determining how many times a particular type of word is used and how many different words or tokens were used in that category. This reflects the richness of vocabulary use (Brannon, 1968; Simmons, 1962).

The findings indicate that the child with impaired hearing exhibits a reduced use of both types and tokens. The effect has been shown to be greatest among severely hearing-impaired children with deficits greater than 75dB ANSI. This group of children was shown to exhibit reduction across all categories of words. Hard-of-hearing children (27–66dB ANSI) by comparison exhibited reductions mainly in the use of pronouns, adverbs, and auxiliaries. By comparison with normal-hearing children's use of 11,400 words, hard-of-hearing children used 5149 words, and severely hearing-impaired children used 4385 words (Brannon, 1968).

3. Syntactic Complexity. The most widely used method of evaluating a spontaneous speech sample for syntactic structure is derived from the Developmental Sentence Types first described by Lee in 1966 and later developed as the Developmental Sentence Types analysis procedure (DST) (Lee, 1974). The procedure requires analysis of a minimum of 100 utterances. These utterances are classified into two categories: (1) presentence types of utterance, that is, those that do not contain a subject and a predicate, and (2) sentences that do possess a subject-verb combination.

Presentences. Lee (1974) classifies the presentence utterances into four developmental patterns, each identifying the most likely linguistic acquisitions in six forms of linguistic function, for example, two-word noun phrases (e.g., "the ball," "Johnny ball," "ball big"), and presentences, containing reference to location or a characteristic (e.g., "Daddy home," "doggie big").

Once 50 true sentences occur in a speech sample, the DSS analysis procedure permits assessment of eight grammatical categories (e.g., primary and secondary verbs, personal pronouns, interrogatives, etc.). Points have been assigned on a weighted basis to the items in each of the eight categories. The weightings derive from the developmental age of occurrence. A total score for each utterance is obtained. The scores for all utterances then are combined and divided by the total number of utterances to provide a mean score. This permits comparison with the norms and percentile scores provided for the procedure. Lee's (1974) developmental sentence analysis procedure allows you to describe and chart the child's use of syntactic structures in spontaneous speech and to determine intervention goals. Kretschmer and Kretschmer (1978), however, caution against its use for establishing a specific set of teaching or training targets (p. 177).

4. Structural Complexity Score (SCS). This is a qualitative measure of the linguistic complexity of the child's utterances. The measure was originated by McCarthy (1930) and later modified by Templin (1957) to provide weighted scores and age norms for six-month intervals from three to six years and in 12-month intervals from six to eight years. Templin's (1957) categories for assignment of values are

Score: 0 Incomplete responses including those that are functionally incomplete
1 Simple sentence with or without phrases
2 Simple sentence with two or more phrases or a compound subject or predicate with a phrase
3 Compound sentence
4 Complex and elaborated sentences

Norms are based on 50 utterances making a maximum score of 200 points.

Another example of a method of evaluating a spontaneous sample of the child's utterances is the Bloom and Lahey (1978) procedure. The authors classify eight stages of progressively increasing linguistic sophistication, ranging from one-word utterances through two- and three-word syntactic structures, connected related utterances, to relative clauses. The transcription first is analyzed to extract all utterances that belong to the same semantic category. For example,

Action designators: "Me go," "Man down," "crash," "the boy broke the window."
Nonexistence: "Car no wheel," "I have no pencil," "There is no milk."
Location: "Boy in school," "Mother went to store."

The sentences in a given category then are compared to a model for that semantic category to determine which components of the model form are present and which are missing. This procedure permits the description of the child's ability to use speech semantically, that is, for the conveyance of meaning, rather than focusing on the correctness of syntactic structure.

These are but two examples of ways in which spontaneous language samples can be analyzed. By far the most comprehensive and detailed procedure is that described by Kretschmer and Kretschmer (1978, pp. 184–210). Their procedure provides information about the semantic content of each utterance, describes the syntactic devices used to convey that meaning, assesses the effectiveness of the child's utterance, and identifies the violations of restricted forms of English (e.g., using adjectives as nouns; "the bad will get me"; or omitting plurality indicators; "Five car"). The authors not only detail the step-by-step analysis, they also provide examples of the analytic procedure results and data summary of elicited samples from a normal and a hearing-impaired adolescent.

Another methods of spontaneous speech analysis has been described by Tyack and Gottsleben (1974).

FORMAL TESTS OF LANGUAGE KNOWLEDGE

As we have seen, the advantage of formal tests lies in their structure. They provide norms against which we can measure a child's linguistic knowledge and performance. Standardized tests, however, are not without flaws. The problem of selecting an appropriate test is one with which you must deal. Kretschmer and Kretschmer (1978, pp. 144–145) have provided eight questions you can ask when determining which test to choose:

1. Does the test objectively measure what it purports to measure?
2. Are the normative data for the test adequate in variety and quantity, and were the standardization samples representative of the children to whom the test will be administered?
3. Is the test reliable?
4. What is the definition of language used in the development of this test?
5. On what aspects of language/communication performance does this particular test focus?
6. Is there evidence of knowledge of contemporary research in child language or linguistics to support the definitions and applications for the test?
7. Do the names and contents of subtests or test components articulate in a logical manner based on the theoretical orientation of the test?
8. Are the justifications for the definitions and selection of test items clear enough, so that a user could generate additional test items or exercises to fit the test model? If so, then the theoretical bases and the test items are consistent with one another. If it is not possible to generate new items, then the reader may not understand the purposes of the task well enough, the theoretical underpinnings of the test may be questionable, or the items in the test may not support the test model.

Guidelines for Administering Formal Tests

We saw that obtaining a representative sample of spontaneous language for analysis requires care to establish the motivation for natural communicative interaction. Formal test administration, which involves standard procedures and scoring, requires even greater care. We must make sure that the child both hears and understands the directions lest his responses be limited by auditory discrimination or by the linguistic complexity of the instructions rather than by his ability to perform the task. The guidelines for formal test administration advise that you

- *Establish a comfortable informal relationship with the child.* Failure to do this not only negatively prejudices a child's performance, but it also deprives you of information that may influence how you administer the test and how you interpret the results.
- *Ensure optimal listening conditions.* Select a test environment with as little noise as possible. Ensure that you will not be disturbed during the test. Hearing aids should have new batteries or they should be tested to ensure they have the required voltage charge. Test each aid by administering the Ling Five Sound Test. If the child has a personal FM system, use it when conducting the evaluation.
- *Ensure optimal lighting to favor speech-reading.* The child should be seated opposite you. You should sit so that your face is well lit. This usually means you should be facing the windows. If you can arrange to sit with your back to a dark surface such as a screen or blackboard, the contrast will further enhance speech-reading.
- *Gain the child's auditory-visual attention.* Make certain you have the child's full auditory-visual attention before giving instructions or identifying a test item to be responded to. Allow the child to look at any objects or pictures to be responded to before you explain the task.
- *Be certain the child understands the directions.* Directions should be worded simply, repeated and rephrased if necessary. Verbal instructions, when not scored as

part of test performance, may be clarified by sign, gesture, or demonstration. Practice items, when not liable to contaminate the actual test results, are very helpful. Be sure the child understands before beginning a test item. Note all modifications on the test record and include them in the assessment report.
- *Recheck incorrect responses at the end of a test unit.* To be sure that a child did not respond incorrectly due to misunderstanding, recheck missed or incorrect responses after completion of the test. This avoids encouraging a child to choose a different response based only on your negative or doubtful acceptance of his first choice.
- *Provide encouragement as needed.* Hearing-impaired children need encouragement and reassurance during test taking. This must relate, however, only to their efforts, not to their responses. Reassure with such statements as "You're doing very well Marjorie." "You really are trying hard." Avoid saying, "That's right" or "Good girl" after correct answers while failing to respond to inappropriate ones.
- *Be sure not to push the child beyond her attention span.* If a child's attention and motivation are flagging, take a break in test administration, recording where in the test such a break was taken. Plan to test over several sessions rather than trying to achieve a complete assessment in one. A record of how long the child was able to pay appropriate attention is important information for intervention planning.

Formal evaluation procedures seek to assess the child's level of receptive and/or expressive language abilities. Receptive assessment involves the use of spoken directions for the child to carry out, for example,

"Give me the airplane and the car.
"Show me that picture of the girl crying."
"Put the baby in the crib" ["behind the mother" or "next to the dog"].

Assessment of expressive abilities requires that the child describe what he/she observes (object relationships: "Where is the baby"; "What happened to the little girl?") and make assumptions ("Why is the little girl crying?" "What will happen when the father comes home?").

Obtaining Responses

Various means exist for obtaining responses.

Imitation. This method is based on the presumption that children will recode into their own expressive language rules what you ask them to repeat. If their rules are deviant, the error will be apparent. If the child has the correct form as part of his language system, he will repeat your sentence correctly. Many researchers have highlighted the potential problems with this method. They include variability in the ability of some children with normal language to imitate (Bloom, Lightbown, & Hood, 1975), the violation of natural pragmatics (Bohannan, 1975; Lund & Duchan, 1983), the possibility that the sentence to be imitated exceeds the child's memory capacity (Lund & Duchan, 1983; Miller & Chapman, 1975) and the question of whether imitation is indeed a natural component of developmental language of hearing-impaired children (Kretschmer & Kretschmer, 1978).

Language Completion. This technique permits you to explore specific kinds of language and conceptual knowledge, for example, plurality rules, tenses, and personal pronouns.

Plurality: This is a car. This is two _____.
This is a knife. This is two _____.
Tenses: John is eating his dinner.
Now he has _____ it.
This morning John _____ breakfast.
Pronouns: That is yours.
I have this book.
This book is _____.

Knowledge of the use of objects or actions can also be assessed:

We stir coffee with _____.
In tennis we hit with a _____.
Birds fly but fish _____.
We drive a car but we _____ a boat.

Demonstration. The child is asked to carry out age-appropriate directions that increase in complexity, for example,

Put the car in the garage and the mother in the house.
Find a red pencil, draw a man on the paper, put the paper in the book.
Open the envelope, find the picture of the city, draw a circle around the large truck, then put the picture back in the book.

It is important to ensure that the child is familiar with the vocabulary used in the instructions; otherwise, it is not possible to determine whether the problem arises from morphological or syntactic deficiency. Care also must be taken to limit clues so that the child must decode the instructions rather than deduce your intentions. For example, if the instruction is to open the *envelope* when no other items could be opened, the measure of language comprehension is reduced.

Picture Identification. This is a widely used test format. It involves identifying a picture named or described by the tester. For example, the test item might be to select a picture of "the bird is flying." This will require that foil items be presented. For the response of the child to represent a valid language/concept decision, it is necessary that all three foil items involve a bird. If two of them involve another animal, the choice can be narrowed to a 50–50 chance on the basis of the word *bird*. In administering picture identification items, care must be taken to allow time for the children to process and respond to the information. It has been shown that performance decreases as the rate of the tester's speech increases (Berry & Erickson, 1973). Special care must be taken with hearing-impaired children whose rate of information processing is known to be slower than that of normal-hearing children.

Just as the results of formal assessment of auditory discrimination are easily contaminated by processing difficulties at the language level, so are language results subject to limitations imposed by difficulty in discriminating what was said. This may result either in a failure of the child to respond or in an inappropriate response due to a misheard word. The child may put the *house* instead of the *mouse* on the toy table.

Difficulty in understanding the instructions or the role he is expected to play in the language interaction may easily distort the results. It is essential to assess the child's understanding of what he is to do. If necessary, reword or rephrase the directions. For children using a total-communication method, you must realize that asking the child to understand directions through hearing only means that he may not respond due to inadequate ability to receive the auditory signal. This does not determine whether he can process the linguistic structure into which the message has been encoded. The same is true in reverse; a child may be able to write or sign the correct response, but may lack the ability to formulate it orally, at least not so that it is intelligible.

Thus you must ask yourself:

- What is it I wish this test or analysis procedure to evaluate for me?
- How will the method of *test presentation* affect the knowledge it will provide?
- How will the method of *response* affect the knowledge it will provide?
- Do I have the manual communication skills necessary to evaluate this child's English language knowledge?

An assessment of oral use of language may be very important to make, but it should not be interpreted as an assessment of English language knowledge.

Formal Language Tests

A bewildering array of commercially available tests and published test procedures confronts you when you need to obtain some quantifiable measure of the child's performance. It is well beyond the scope of this chapter to review all the major tests, even more to recommend specific ones to you. Some tests assess a specific ability; others cover a range of abilities. Consider first the need to assess the child's vocabulary. Some of the more commonly encountered tests of vocabulary designed for use with hearing children are described briefly.

Vocabulary Assessment. The delay in general language development exhibited by hearing-impaired children affects both the quantity and quality of vocabulary at any given age. Keep in mind that the elimination of acoustic information places some words below the level of intensity necessary to create an echoic image. Other words will have only part of the phonemes audible, which distorts the pattern and makes it difficult to discriminate, to restructure, and to store for recall. This is a situation you may identify with by trying to recall foreign names heard over a poor telephone connection. An added factor affecting vocabulary acquisition by the hearing-impaired child is that words that refer to objects or actions are easier to acquire than words that serve a grammatical function, that is, words that are nonreferential. Thus nouns and verbs of action occur in the hearing-impaired child's vocabulary in a far greater proportion than function words such as articles, auxiliaries, adverbs, and pronouns (Brannon, 1968; Brannon & Murray, 1966).

NAME OF TEST	BRIEF DESCRIPTION
Peabody Picture Vocabulary Test, Revised Ed. 1981 (Dunn, 1965)	Test of receptive vocabulary. A closed set picture identification task—test item plus three foils. Progressive difficulty of items. Raw score derived from subtraction of total incorrect responses from a ceiling score. Approximate vocabulary age derived from normative data.
Vocabulary Comprehension Scale (Bangs, 1975)	Qualitative vocabulary test, 61 items. Norms for hearing children 2–6 years of age. Manipulation of toy objects in response to tester's directions. Instructions explore knowledge of pronouns; adjectives, indicating size and quality; prepositions; and comparatives. Record forms sort responses by class and developmental progression.
Test of Word Finding (German, 1966)	Age norms 6.11–12.11 years, grades 1–6. Designed to assess accessibility of child's vocabulary (e.g., word finding). Based on accuracy and speed of response. Six sections: picture naming (nouns), sentence completion, description, picture naming (words), picture naming (categories), and comprehension. Percentile ratings from raw score for comparison with norms.
Expressive One Word Picture Vocabulary Test (Gardner, 1981)	Object naming; items of decreasing familiarity. Scoring may be complicated by a child's poor or unintelligible verbal responses.
Michigan Picture Language Inventory (Lerea, 1958)	Vocabulary subtest assesses receptive and expressive vocabulary picture naming task. Receptive test administered only to items not correct on expressive testing. Norms for ages 3–9.

Syntax Assessment. An essential component in the task of using the language code to establish meaning is the order in which types of words are placed and the rules that govern the relationships among word types, words, and their endings. Effective communication is thus predicated on the ability to use and modify vocabulary according to the rules of syntax and grammar.

Many of the language assessment procedures described in the literature, as well as those commercially available, include components that address the evaluation of syntax and grammar. The most well-known of these is the Northwestern Syntax Screening Test by Lee (1969, 1971).

NAME OF TEST	BRIEF DESCRIPTION
Northwestern Syntax Screening Test (Lee, 1969, 1971)	Provides general picture of syntactic performance rather than specific description of syntactic knowledge. Not to be used as diagnostic tool (Lee, 1971). Receptive section requires identification of two of four items on each of 20 plates. Max score 40. Expressive section comprises 20 plates of two similar pictures (e.g., The baby is sleeping; the baby is not sleeping). Responses must be exactly correct. Norms 3.0 to 7–11 years. Percentile scores provided. Untimed; test items may be repeated.

Multilevel Assessment Tests. Every test of language necessarily involves the child's knowledge at the word level. Levels above this can be assessed only when all vocabulary involved is familiar to the child. As a result, most tests are not designed to evaluate one level alone but include measures of other level functions.

NAME OF TEST	BRIEF DESCRIPTION
Assessment of Children's Language Comprehension (Foster, Giddan, & Stark, 1973)	Vocabulary: 50 items, one- or two-syllable words (nouns, action verbs, adjectives, prepositions). Four picture plates for each item; one is the test word. Syntax: identification of two, three, and four critical elements representing common semantic relationships. Norms 3.0–6.5 years. No percentile rankings, thus indicates strengths and needs rather than linguistic age.
Test of Auditory Comprehension and Language, Revised Ed. (Carrow-Woolfolk, 1985)	Assesses vocabulary, grammatical morphology, and syntax. Picture selection, two foils per test item. Suggested entry norms for each age level 3.0–9.11 years. Norms also grades K–6.
Test of Language Development (Newcomer & Hamill, 1977)	Primary level 4–9 years, intermediate 8.5–13 years. Assesses receptive and expressive language at levels of phonology, morphology, syntax, and semantics. Picture selection required in response to sentence descriptions. Expressive skills

tested by sentence imitation and sentence completion. Grammatical knowledge test includes verb tenses, plurals, comparatives, and possessives. Raw scores converted to standard scores and percentile rank, permitting strengths/ weaknesses to be identified. Sum of subtest scaled scores generates overall language quotient calculation.

Tests of Semantics and Concepts. Among those tests already discussed, the Test of Auditory Comprehension and Language and the Test of Language Development include measures of semantic abilities. Further information on semantic and conceptual knowledge can be obtained from the Basic Language Concepts Test (Engleman, Ross, & Bingham, 1982 and the Boehm Test of Basic Concepts (Boehm, 1971).

NAME OF TEST	BRIEF DESCRIPTION
Basic Language Concepts Test (Engleman, Ross, & Bingham, 1982)	Assessment of comprehension of concepts fundamental to classroom performance. Uses picture stimuli to assess knowledge of such concepts as plurality, negation, and so on. Child selects appropriate item from verbal description. Other tasks include answering questions, recognizing patterns, blending syllables. Age norms 4.0–6.5 years with 6-month categories. Errors scored by type.
Boehm Test of Basic Concepts (Boehm, 1970)	Designed to assess functional adequacy in kindergarten and grade 1. Fifty vocabulary items drawn from classroom topics and instructions include time, space, quantity, and so on.
Houston Test for Language Development, Part I and II (Crabtree, 1958, 1963)	Vocabulary: requires naming or descriptive performance of body parts, gestures. A communicative behavior analysis provides description of language structure and function. Norms 3–6 years. Overall language age calculated.
McCarthy Scales of Children's Abilities (McCarthy, 1972)	Five of six scales cover verbal language. The most useful of these are word knowledge from picture recognition; verbal memory from retelling a story; verbal fluency; a timed subtest from naming words in four categories; opposite analogies. Norms 2.6–8.6 years.

Tests with Norms for Hearing-Impaired or Language-Delayed Children

Each of the previous tests provides normative data that allows you to determine how closely the child's language performance approximates that of her hearing peers of the same age. They allow you to assess the child's language development age as well as provide helpful information about the child's linguistic strengths and weaknesses. They do not provide information specifically related to hearing-impaired children. Kretschmer and Kretschmer (1978) point out that the analysis of the language used by hearing-impaired children is complicated by the discrepancy that often exists between cognitive abilities and knowledge of standard English forms (p. 184). They stress the need for evaluating and understanding the utterances that are deviant rather than simply identifying the presence or absence of standard forms.

Kretschmer Spontaneous Language Analysis Procedure (1978). This is by far the most comprehensive method of evaluating the spoken and/or written language of hearing-impaired children. Based upon several samples taken on different occasions representing several communication situations, the assessment format covers in great detail a full range of language functions. It begins with preverbal behaviors essential to speech, sign language, and communication competence. The system progresses to identification of a variety of syntactic and semantic functions at the one- and two-word level and at the level of single propositions and finally provides for syntactic analysis of complex sentences. At each level specific syntactic and semantic descriptions are provided. In addition, the analysis system provides for an assessment of communication behaviors. Such speech acts as asking for information, making a request, promising to do something, as well as a number of pragmatic communication strategies such as initiating and ending conversation and changing topic are identified. To permit identification and description of restricted language forms used by hearing-impaired children, 11 types of such violations are described for classification. These include violations of semantics, omission of nodes in a sentence frame (e.g., omission of conjunctions, verbs, or sentence subject), errors of word order, and omission of verb selection.

The use of the analysis system is demonstrated by two samples that are analyzed and summarized.

The Grammatical Analysis of Elicited Language (GAEL) (Moog & Geers, 1979). Three levels of the test are provided. These are the Pre-Sentence Level (GAEL-P), standardized on hearing-impaired children aged 3–6; the Simple Sentence Level (GAEL-S), with norms for hearing-impaired children 5–9 years and normal-hearing children 2.6–5 years; and finally, the Complex Sentence Level (GAEL-C), with norms for hearing-impaired children 8–12 years and 3–6 years for hearing children.

The test evaluates receptive and expressive language using imitation and prompted responses as the two methods of assessment. Because the imitation and prompting technique allows you to know what the child is attempting to say, the test is particularly appropriate for those children whose speech may make it difficult to analyze a spontaneous utterances sample accurately. The GAEL is designed to permit a grammatical analysis of the child's language structure knowledge and thus to describe grammatical categories requiring repair. Scoring procedures do not provide for semantic or pragmatic language skills to be credited, though the authors encourage you to examine the responses obtained for insight into these abilities. The test is a long one. The GAEL-S requires a total of 2½ hours to administer and score. It does provide, however, a very detailed and complete assessment of grammatical knowledge.

The Teacher Assessment of Grammatical Structures (TAGS) (Moog & Kozak, 1983). This evaluation tool is recommended for use with the GAEL test. The rating forms parallel the three assessment levels of the GAEL (TAGS-P, S, and C) with essentially the same age norms. Horizontally the record form provides six developmental levels for TAGS S and C, suggesting a sequence of grammatical teaching structures for each of six grammatical categories (nouns, pronouns, verb inflections, secondary verbs, conjunctions, and questions) that are listed horizontally on the form, thus providing a visual profile of the child's use of grammatical structures.

The Rhode Island Test of Language Structures (RITLS) (Engen & Engen, 1983). This test also has been standardized for use with hearing-impaired subjects. It uses a variety of simple and complex forms to assess receptive language comprehension. The child is asked to point to the picture that the statement describes. The results permit an analysis of syntactic knowledge with norms for hearing-impaired children and young adults 3.0–20.0 years.

The Test of Syntactic Ability (Quigley, Steincamp, Power, & Jones, 1978). This test was standardized on hearing-impaired children and young adults ages 8–18. It assesses the subject's knowledge of a wide range of different syntactic functions and grammatical knowledge. The reading and writing forms of expression are utilized to assess the subject across 20 subareas with a total of 1400 items. Like the GAEL test, it is very extensive and takes a long time to administer, approximately an hour per subtest. However, a 120-item screening test is available as an alternative.

Two other tests designed for use in assessing the knowledge and use of basic grammatical structures by hearing-impaired children are the *Test of Receptive Language Ability (TERLA)* and the *Test of Expressive Language Ability* (TEXLA), both developed by Bunch (1978). The *TERLA,* which provides norms for hearing-impaired children ages 6–12 and for hearing children in grade 1, requires that the child have a basic reading ability. This is necessary because the task for the child is to select the picture that best illustrates a written word or phrase. The grammatical structures assessed cover plural nouns, pronouns, adjectives (comparatives, superlatives, and descriptives), prepositions, and verb tenses.

The TEXLA is the expressive counterpart covering the same language structures as the TERLA, with the child providing a written response. The age norms are for hearing-impaired children 7–12 years and for hearing children at grade 1 level.

PRAGMATIC LANGUAGE ABILITIES

Pragmatics is about the various influences that determine how we use and interpret language. Muma has described it as "a set of sociolinguistic rules one knows and uses in determining who says what, to whom, how, why, when and in what situations" (Muma, 1978, p. 137). Lund and Duchan (1988) stress that the overriding determinant in communication is that it makes sense, that what is heard or said is in accord with the totality of the circumstances at the time and with the speaker/listener's interpretation of what is going on, in other words, what it is all about. The prime contributor to sense making is the event itself. Lund and Duchan point out that the event for a given individual is "the participant's conceptualization of the kind of interaction he or she is having" (1988, p. 49).

Interpersonal transactions and social communication are governed by rules for various events. Each interaction with another person is a miniceremony that will vary in the degrees of freedom accorded to each participant. These vary from the ones that govern your presentation to the Queen of England at Buckingham Palace or to the president of the United States at the White House to those that operate when you ask a friend to go to a movie with you. For these interactions to occur smoothly, we need to be aware of what is expected of us. Even Queen Elizabeth was somewhat at a loss when she awoke in the middle of the night at the Palace to find a male intruder sitting on the end of her bed. The event was not governed by the rules of a formal presentation at Court; the intruder merely wanted to chat. It says much for the Queen's sense of the event that chat they did, for some 20 minutes before she was able to feel comfortable about ringing for attention. How we perceive an event greatly influences how we act. According to news reports the Queen did not perceive herself to be in danger; she sensed that the young man really did wish to chat with her. Her reactions, therefore, were appropriate to that expectation, modified somewhat, no doubt, by the fact that she did not share his desire to chat. Consider how the sense of the event modifies your behavior in the following situations:

- Employment interview
- Protest before a student committee
- Confession to a priest/minister/rabbi
- Bridal shower or stag party
- Football game
- Religious ceremony
- "Roasting" of a colleague

When we do not have an adequate sense of the event, we feel apprehensive and fearful of behaving in a manner that will embarrass us, or if we have our parents or Uncle Joe with us, that they will embarrass us:

"I almost died when my mother said . . . ,"
"I did not know where to put my face when Uncle Joe . . . "

When we examine the nature of the constraints imposed by the type of event, we find that they consist of

- *Physical setting:* This includes where the event takes place, the number of people present, how they are dressed, what they are doing, what the furnishings are, what equipment or other objects are to be seen.
- *Action patterns or "scripts:"* These constitute the sequential occurrences that characterize such formal or everyday routines as getting ready for school, arriving in school, going on a picnic, getting a library book, playing tennis, or attending a weekly religious service or a baseball game.

Communication/Discourse Events

Each communication event fits into a certain "frame" that characterizes the type of discourse (Lund & Duchan, 1988). The frame characteristics that differentiate the following types of discourse greatly influence our communication behavior:

informing	requesting	protesting
instructing	debating	pleading
disagreeing	arguing	chastising

Discourse Topic. Each communication event refers to something: the topic frame, the types of things we may talk about within that topic frame, the ordering of what we say, and the vocabulary we use. We derive the topic from the physical context, from actions, and from what already has occurred. I frequently irritate my wife by making a statement or asking a question without providing any topic frame, out of the blue, so to speak:

"Where did you say she was going?"
"Who?"
"Mary"
"Mary who?"
"You know who I mean."
"I certainly don't, I haven't any idea what you're talking about."
"Oh never mind, you never understand me."

Discourse Rules. I, like many hearing-impaired children, obviously need to pay attention to the rules for introducing, maintaining, changing, and ending topics. Conversational communication is analogous to a game, for it too has its phases just as games have kickoffs, serves, sets, or quarters. Consider the major plays or *regulators* in the communication game.

Initiating Strategies. These open the communication in a manner appropriate to the social relationship of the partners. To a person in authority, one might begin "Good morning. I have an appointment with you." With a friend or acquaintance, such informal greetings as "Hi—how are you doing?" or even, "What gives?" will serve as openers. When we need to divert someone's attention to us or we are not sure if he/she is too busy to talk, we modify the initiator:

"Excuse me. Can you tell me where . . ."
"Am I interrupting?"
"Are you busy?"
"Do you have a moment?"
"Is this an inconvenient time?"

Once a conversation is initiated, it must be maintained. For this to occur there must be mutual participation which requires turn taking.

Turn Taking. Conversational rules allow the two parties to interact about the topic. This requires that the parties take turns. There is little that is more frustrating in conversation than "not being able to get a word in edgeways" because one's partner or a group member "monopolizes the conversation." We communicate our willingness to allow the speaker to continue to hold the floor by facial expressions that convey appropriate reactions, nods and utterances, (uh-huh, hmm) whistles of surprise, and verbal comments such as "really," "you're kidding," "good heavens," "I thought that was what happened," "I know." Turns are signaled by the speaker's dropping the pitch of the voice, pausing, asking a question, and concentrating his gaze on the listener. If the speaker fails to allow the exchange of roles with his listener at appropriate points, the listener may signal a desire for a turn or may intercept the conversation. She may interrupt with a statement or question:

"But I thought . . ."
"Excuse me, but how did you do that?"
"Oh I know how you felt. John said that to me once and . . ."

The bouncing of the conversation between or among participants is an important factor in maintaining it. The ability to maintain a conversation relates to turn taking but involves more than the mechanics of give and take.

Maintenance Strategies. A conversation, which by definition involves turn taking, is moved forward and developed by various strategies employed by the participants. Maintenance is achieved by

- *Acknowledging what a speaker says:* "My sister and I are going on a cycle trip."—"Oh that's great"; or "John said he couldn't make it."—"Oh I'm sorry."
- *Requesting further information:* "I was so embarrassed, I spilled the soup all over her dress."—"Oh my goodness, what did you do?"; "We went to the movies with David's parents."—"Oh, how did that work out?"
- *Commenting on what has been said:* "It was such a disappointment."—"I know how you must have felt"; "Mark was at the party."—"He's gorgeous isn't he"; or "We rented the movie, *ET*."—"Oh that movie was great."
- *Answering a question:* "Did you go on the school ski trip?"—"Oh yes we had a wonderful time"; "Did you get to talk with Jane?"—"No, I don't think she was there. I heard she was sick."

At some point the conversational interaction will become exhausted or it will be necessary for one of the participants to leave. As one might expect, we have developed rituals for achieving this.

Closing Strategies. You surely will remember conversations over the telephone or face to face that you had great difficulty bringing to a close. Some people seem not to recognize or to override the rules for terminating conversations. We can close conversations with such devices as

"Well I suppose I'd better get some work done."

"Goodness look at the time."

"Listen, call me sometime when I can really talk."

"I really must be going."

"Listen it's been really nice seeing you but . . ."

"Look we really must get together."

"Is that everything?"

It probably is apparent to you already that assessing a child's knowledge of and ability to use the rules of discourse is not a simple task. Yet in the hearing-impaired child these abilities, which are essential to ease of communication within the hearing world, most commonly are deficient. Therefore, it is necessary to gain as clear a profile as possible of the child's needs for learning or strengthening the various pragmatic strategies common to conversational and other communicative events.

Assessing Pragmatic Knowledge

Pragmatics, as we have seen, arise from the embodiment of a communicative event within a specific situational context, which operates on both receptive and expressive communication. Pragmatic knowledge enables the speaker-listener to behave linguistically in a manner appropriate to the particular sociolinguistic rules operative at the stage of communication reached in a given set of circumstances. These rules change from minute to minute in accord with the context and interpersonal interactions of the communicative event. For this reason it has not proven possible to formalize a test protocol or to develop standardized tests that assess the body of knowledge we identify by pragmatic behaviors. Two structured procedures have been described in the literature (Blagden & McConnell, 1983; Simon, 1984a, 1984b).

Blagden and McConnell (1983) developed the *Interpersonal Language Skills Assessment* procedure for children 8–14 years old. The procedure establishes a game playing situation involving the child to be assessed and several friends. This requirement is relatively easy to meet in the school environment, rather more difficult in the clinic setting. A "score sheet" guides the teacher/therapist in recording the observed child's utterances under a range of functional categories. Thus the communication of the child is analyzed for correct and incorrect incidences of, for example, observed requests, commands, criticisms, information given, advice imparted, and so on. This procedure, though structured by the activity, does not comprise a test. It meets the requirement of a normal communication situation that creates the need to use functional language forms representative of this age range.

Simon (1984a, 1984b) has described procedures for assessing pragmatic competence. She developed guidelines in a published procedure entitled *Evaluating Communicative Competence*. She has used items from other published tests to assess both receptive and expressive pragmatic language competencies. Simon supplements these with loosely structured communication situations such as story telling, recognizing semantic absurdities, and role playing. Once again, this is a set of controlled communication demands rather than a test.

Both Blagden and McConnell and Simon have attempted to provide control and a repeatable structure for exploring a child's functional knowledge of pragmatics. This approach is a refinement of the less structured procedures used more generally. For this, two methods of assessment have been recommended. The first is to obtain information from observation of the child's communicative behaviors in class (Lund & Duchan, 1988; Ripich & Spinelli, 1985). The second is to analyze a sample of the child's communicative utterances in a discourse situation (Kretschmer & Kretschmer, 1978; Lund & Duchan, 1988; Miller, 1981; Stone, 1988).

Naturally, the occasion to demonstrate even some of the listed behaviors in a class period will be limited. Thus, a single observation will not suffice; several observations will need to be made at different times. Even then, not all the child's abilities will have been assessed. Therefore, a more controlled assessment method must accompany classroom observation. This method is the discourse sample analysis.

Analysis of Discourse Sample

We have discussed already the techniques for obtaining a language sample (p. 344). Stone (1988) stresses the importance of ensuring the quality of the audio or video recording made for this purpose. For video recording both teacher and child should be on camera. If an audio recording is used, it is helpful to note any gestures used either by teacher or child. I suggest that you will find the enactment of miniscenarios as the most productive method of generating a representative sample. The scenario, you will recall, is a situation in which two persons play roles. The situation and the roles are described to the child who then is asked to pretend to be one of the participants as the teacher/therapist and the child act out the scene. By controlling the scenario you can ensure that you collect samples of the child's knowledge and ability to apply the major pragmatic functions appropriate to conversation. Stone offers the following guidelines for ensuring this:

> The scenarios should call for the student to initiate and end conversation with a variety of role play partners of different social status and age (e.g., parents, adults, children).
>
> The scenarios should call for the student to use comments and requests to introduce topics.

The scenarios should be carried out so that the student will need to request clarification.

The scenarios should contain opportunity for the student to use each of the extended turns.

The scenarios should contain opportunity for several single turn exchanges. (Stone, 1988, p. 41)

The communication sample obtained from the scenario first must be transcribed orthographically from audio- or videotape. Lund and Duchan (1988) recommend that in transcribing the conversation, the basic unit for analysis should be the clause. To facilitate this, each clause should be transcribed on a separate line and numbered in the transcript. Stone (1988) provides 29 very specific questions to ask in analyzing the sample. These questions address the aspects of:

Structure: Does the child have a repertoire of initiating routines?
Are the ending routines appropriate to the age and status of the conversational partner?

Function: Does the child maintain topics?
Are requests for clarification specific?

Form: For the child producing three-word and longer utterances, what levels of syntactic and morphologic usage are present?

A recording form is designed to facilitate sample analyses. Stone (1988) also provides an example of a completed conversational competence evaluation assessment including identification of strengths and weaknesses in each of the structure, function, and form categories. A sample scenario from Stone's text is provided in Table 17.1. Lund and Duchan (1988) provide detailed guidelines for identifying the type of discourse as narrative, event description, conversation, or lesson. They proceed to show how to analyze the sample for "referencing abilities," that is, the ability of the speaker to inform the listener as to what specifically she is talking about (referring to), whether it be object, person, action, or event. They also provide a means of analyzing "focus and perspective," that is, the ability to use language that highlights the central topic and to take a point of view (perspective), as well as being sensitive to the listener's perspective.

Because of hearing and possible speech-language deviances, an aspect of pragmatics that is of particular importance to the hearing-impaired child is that concerned with communication breakdowns and the strategies adopted by the child and partner to repair the breakdown. Possible repair options include repeating what was just said, emphasizing key words or phrases, changing the language in which the message was couched, and providing additional clarifying information. It is obvious that breakdowns in communication acts will occur frequently for the hearing-impaired child. The causes of the breakdowns we have seen lie in reduced acoustic information due to the hearing problem which is aggravated by noise and reverberations, reduced language skills and at the expressive stage, poor language formulation and impaired speech. These factors cause the breakdown, but lack of pragmatic skills means that the child is not sophisticated in dealing with it. The situation is further aggravated by the hearing partner who, not understanding the child's needs, commonly uses repair strategies that

TABLE 17.1 Conversational evaluation scenario (Stone 1988)

Scenario Six—Description	Comments on Scenario Six—Description
T: "This time let's pretend that you are walking to school and you see someone stealing a bike. So you call the police and tell them what happened. I'll be the policeman."	
C1: "O.K."	C1: Acknowledged understanding of scenario.
T: "Let's start."	
C2: (Pretending to walk to school.) Says to herself, "Oh no! Steal the bike. (Pretends to find phone booth and make a call.)	C2: Commented on action. Inappropriate verb tense.
T: "Hello. Police Department."	
C3: "This is D. I need help. The boy stole the bike."	C3: Initiated appropriately. Twice used "the" to introduce new information.
T: "What did it look like?"	
C4: "It blue, a blue seat and brake."	C4: Answered request for information. Provided almost adequate description. Included distinctive features. Omitted "with". Omitted verb.
T: "What did the boy look like?"	
C5: "A blue jacket and brown hair with blue eyes and red stripe shirt and brown pants. That's it."	C5: Answered request for information. Provided unorganized description. Used "with" phrase. Alternated clothing and physical features. Conjoined using "and."
T: "Thank you for calling. We will try to find the boy and the bike."	
C6: "You're welcome."	C6: Ended appropriately.

(continued)

perpetuate the original communication impedance. Duchan (1988), in reviewing literature on the repair strategies used by hearing-impaired children, found that they approximated the techniques of their hearing peers. They tend to repeat what they said in exactly the same form (Donnelly & Brackett, 1982; Givens & Greenfield, 1982). The incidence of revising the utterance was shown to be significantly low. In an earlier study by Erber and Greer (1973), reviewed by Duchan, it was found that "emphasis" was the most common repair strategy used by teachers when talking with a hearing-impaired child. The second most common repair strategy used was to repeat what they had just said. Neither strategy adds any more information or restructures difficult language forms to facilitate comprehension. Thus, in assessing the child's use of pragmatics, attention should be paid to the strategies employed to repair breakdowns in communication.

It will be apparent from this discussion that pragmatic assessment is complex and time-consuming, yet it is perhaps social communication deficiencies that impact most heavily on the normal development of hear-

TABLE 17.1 Conversational evaluation scenario (Stone 1988) *(continued)*

Scenario Seven—Conversation	Comments on Scenario Seven—Conversation
T: "Now I will pretend to be your mom and you be yourself. You go over to your friend Rachel's house and she has some new puppies. You would like to have one. So you come home and ask your mom if you can have one. O.K.?"	
C1: "O.K." (Walks to door and pretends to come in). "Mom."	C1: Acknowledged understanding of scenario. Initiated appropriately.
T: (As mom) "What?"	
C2: "I saw Rachel have puppy. Rachel have four puppy. Can I take one?"	C2: Commented. Attempted to conjoin but omitted connector. Used incorrect form of verb. Commented. Used incorrect form of verb. Omitted plural marker. Requested information. Included auxiliary.
T: "Will you take care of it?"	
C3: "I take care of puppy."	C3: Answered request for information. Omitted tense marker. Used noun instead of pronoun.
T: "Mmmm."	
C4: "Feed the dog and make for a doghouse."	C4: Expanded answer to request for information. Omitted subject. Omitted tense marker. Confused verb phrase.
T: "Well, I don't know."	
C5: "I feed him dog food. Brush hair and put bow on."	C5: Acknowledged comment. Omitted tense marker. Omitted subject.
T: "O.K. You can."	
C6: "Oh, thank you. I will call Rachel."	C6: Acknowledged comment. Commented. Included tense marker.

ing-impaired children (Prutting, 1982). This is particularly true for the large number of hearing-impaired children for whom mainstream placement in normal schools has become the norm. For this reason you should do everything possible to increase your understanding of the nature and role of pragmatics in communication, especially as it applies to the hearing-impaired child.

The formal and informal assessment means we have considered so far can provide valuable information about the child's linguistic strengths and weaknesses. They can be supplemented by your own informal procedures.

INFORMAL ASSESSMENT

Informal evaluation can provide insight into the extent to which a child is able to draw upon situational, contextual, and linguistic context to achieve closure. It also allows you to approximate some of the communication demands that will occur in the classroom. The information that you may find helpful includes the child's ability to

- Follow oral directions when the language is familiar
- Capitalize on visual constraints
- Receive orally presented information

You also will want to determine how these abilities are affected by the variables we discussed earlier—namely, distance, background noise, and degree of constraints.

Ability to Follow Directions

In assessing the child's ability to follow directions, you should replicate the type of requests he would experience in the classroom. First review critical vocabulary. In the following instruction given to a third-grade class, the concept of odd and even numbers would be checked before giving the direction:

"Take out your blue reader. Open it to page 172. I want you to do exercise number four. Answer only the even-numbered questions. Stop when you reach 20."

Questions:

- Did the child select the reading book?
- Did he turn to the correct page?
- Which exercise is he prepared to do?
- Which questions will he answer?
- How many will he do?

For a child in ninth grade, one might use an arithmetic assignment:

"You should solve problems 8 through 14 omitting number 12. Remember to work out everything in the brackets first and show all your working. When you finish, check your answers against the answer key on page 144."

Questions:

- Which problems should the child do?
- Will he answer all the questions from 8 through 14?
- Which will he omit?
- Which part of the problem will he solve first?
- Can he just write down his answer in his book?
- What will he do when he has completed all the problems?
- On which page is the answer key?

Remember that the underlined questionable vocabulary such as omit in the previous example must be reviewed first. The directions should be given without visual cues. They should be repeated with visual communication cues if the child fails to understand the directions.

Give the instructions from what would be a teaching distance, usually some 10 to 15 feet from an optimal seating position in the front row. You can introduce background noise by using a tape recording of speech babble set at a loudness that is audible to you but is not noticeably disturbing.

Ability to Receive Information Orally and to Use Visual Cues

These abilities may be informally assessed together. The material again should be taken from the child's texts. You might choose, for example, a section on European social geography. The child is presented with a map of western Europe. She listens while you present a short paragraph of information using an auditory-visual mode:

"The Netherlands is one of the smallest countries in Europe. It also is called Holland and is one of the Low Countries. It has borders with Germany on the east and Belgium on the south. Its remaining borders are with the North Sea. Much of the country is below sea level, protected by dikes. The Hague is the capital but Amsterdam is the largest city."

Repeat the information to allow the child to remember it. Next, ask her what she can tell you about the Netherlands. Now write a list of key words on the blackboard.

Netherlands	sea level
Low Countries	dikes (check for familiarity)
borders	protected
capital city	

Repeat the information to determine how well the child is making use of the visual information. Finally, turning to the map, ask the child to answer the following questions:

Which two countries border Holland?
Which sea borders on the Netherlands?
Show me Holland's North Sea coastline.
Point to Holland's largest city.
Is Amsterdam the capital?
What is the capital of Holland?
Why is Holland one of the Low Countries?
What keeps out the North Sea?

You can develop specific assessment tasks and materials to better assist you in understanding the difficulties the child encounters and how she functions in school situations.

A thorough language assessment of a child clearly represents a major undertaking. It is, moreover, but one component in the complete evaluation process. You will need to keep in mind the fact that initially, your goal will be to screen areas of language to determine where more intensive evaluation is appropriate. You certainly can begin intervention before all facets of language ability have been assessed since you will continue collecting and refining evaluation data over the complete period of work with the child.

ASSESSING THE CHILD'S SPEECH PRODUCTION

Speech articulation probably is the aspect of assessment with which you will be likely to feel most comfortable. Many of the problems of voice and articulation experienced by hearing-impaired children also are found in hearing children with speech defects, though the cause is different. The degree of speech impairment will be influenced markedly by the age of onset of hearing impairment, the severity of the deficit, when intervention began, when amplification was fitted, and the quality of aided hearing. Severely and profoundly hearing-impaired children, unlike their hearing peers, frequently experience considerable difficulty with the control and quality of their own voice. Because of the difficulty in monitoring their own voice auditorily, children with this degree of hearing deficit tend to speak too loudly (Penn, 1955) or, conversely, too softly (Calvert & Silverman, 1975), with reduced modulation of loudness in spontaneous speech (Hood & Dixon, 1969). They tend also to experience problems in the production of vowels—diphthongizing, neutralizing them to a schwa /ə/, or nasalizing them. The production of the diphthongs themselves also is likely to be distorted.

The same factors of severity, pattern and quality of aided residual hearing, and age at which amplification was provided and intervention begun affect consonant production. Consonant errors among deaf children are most commonly shown to be

- Incorrect voicing, in which a voiceless consonant is voiced or a voiced consonant fails to be vocalized
- Omission of consonants, singly and in blends
- Distortion
- Nasalization

Consonant errors, in addition to being affected by their reduced audibility, are influenced by visibility—those that are less visible are the ones most often not acquired (Geffner & Freeman, 1980).

Evaluation

The procedure for evaluation of voice and speech production in the preschool child with impaired hearing, as recommended by Ling (1976) and described in Chapter 15, increases in value for use with the older child. For analysis of voice quality and control in speech communication, and for phonologic assessment, you can use the spontaneous speech sample recorded for your analysis of the child's language skills. The multiple uses for this tape emphasize the importance of ensuring that a truly representative spontaneous speech sample is obtained under good acoustic conditions using quality instrumentation.

Two other methods of judging voice and suprasegmental encoding have been described by Stark and Levitt (1974) and Subtelny, Orlando, and Whitehead (1981).

Stark and Levitt (1974) developed the *Prosodic Feature Production Test*, which is a tool for measuring contour, stress, and use of pause. Four sentences, each three to five syllables in length, are judged by experienced listeners according to whether they are a statement or question or exhibit a specified pause and a particular stress pattern. The rating points categorize the degree of intelligibility. In a similar approach, Subtelny et al. (1981) produced training tapes that provide the rater with a set of standards for the prosodic characteristics of hearing-impaired children. The recorded sample of the child's speech is matched to the appropriate standard provided by the taped examples.

Vowel and Dipthong Production

Ling's (1976) criteria for assessing vowel/diphthong production, which we discussed earlier, are

- Maintenance of quality for three seconds
- Ability to repeat at a three per second rate at three voice intensity levels
- Ability to alternate any two vowels
- Ability to vary pitch over eight semitones while maintaining quality

Performance is recorded on the score sheet as "S" indicating correct in a single pitch, "R" for repeated pitches, "A" for alternated pitches, and "P" for variable pitches. Ling further assesses each as being produced consistently ($\sqrt{}$), inconsistently ($+$), or not al all ($-$). The same scoring system is used for consonant evaluation.

Although Ling offers one of the few methods for evaluating vowel production, assessment of consonant articulation can be made using a variety of tests designed for hearing children. These include McDonald's (1964) *Deep Test of Articulation*. This is a particularly useful tool as it seeks to assess sounds in various phonetic contexts that require the ability to coarticulate sounds. Coarticulation contributes to speech intelligibility since it generates the acoustic transitions so important for speech discrimination. In this test, the child is asked to name pictures without pausing between them. In this way each sound can be paired with any other that it can precede or follow. The test is a very long one. This limitation is acknowledged by the author who provides a shortened version to cover the speech sounds most commonly misarticulated by hearing children. McDonald further recommends using the test to deep test those sounds identified as misarticulated in the recorded spontaneous speech.

Two other researchers, Kenny and Prather, also provide a test based upon recognition of the importance of coarticulatory skills in speech intelligibility. Their test, *The Coarticulation Assessment in Meaningful Language* (Kenny & Prather, 1984), is further discussed in an article by the same authors (Kenny & Prather, 1986).

The Goldman-Fristoe Test of Articulation (Goldman & Fristoe, 1969) is a widely used test for assessing speech articulation. It has been enhanced in its usefulness with the hearing-impaired population by a modification made by Geffner and Freeman (1980). They eliminated a number of the test items with which profoundly hearing-impaired children might be unfamiliar, replacing them with items more likely to be known to them. This change recognized the caution Ross (1982) made regarding speech articulation assessment of hearing-impaired children:

> One must ensure that it is the children's expressive status which is being evaluated, and not their ability or inability to understand what is required of them (naming pictures when the word is not in their lexicon for example).

Ling's (1976) assessment of articulation was developed specifically for the hearing-impaired child. We discussed the outline of Ling's method in Chapter 15. The procedure tests each consonant in single and repeated syllables using the vowels /u/, /a/, and /i/ and assesses the child's ability to alternate consonants in syllables such as ba-ma ba-ma ba-ma. Where appropriate, consonants are assessed in the initial, medial, and final positions. A complete range of word-initial blends (e.g., /sma smi smu/, /θra θri θru/) and word-final blends (e.g., /ɪfs/, /isn/, / æps/, /emblz/, /itnz/) is tested.

The procedure appears impractically long; however, as Ling points out, one rarely has cause to test all levels of sophistication except as the child makes progress over a period of intervention. One enters the testing at a point at which the child can articulate the items and stops when a ceiling is reached:

> If the teacher is familiar with the child's speech, and hence with what tasks he is likely to accomplish (and she should be if she is teaching subskills systematically day by day), then the evaluation can be completed in 20 minutes. (Ling, 1976, p. 151)

Ling recommends reevaluation of phonetic articulation at intervals of no less than three months, since the charting of progress is important to ensuring that normal developmental progression dictates teaching order. The goal of speech articulation training is increased intelligibility. Therefore, you will want to determine whether gains are being made as measured by that functional criterion.

Assessment of Speech Intelligibility

A major consideration in the assessment of intelligibility is that it involves both the speaker's production and the listener's perception. Even deviant speech patterns are rule governed. Thus a listener, exposed over a period of time to consistent patterns of deviant articulation, becomes familiar with its rules. Then, with varying degrees of success, the listener recodes the deviant rules to approximate normal articulation with a resulting improvement in intelligibility unrelated to the speaker's articulation. This process is apparent in a study by Markides (1970a) of 58 hearing-impaired children aged seven to nine. A comparison of their intelligibility to their teachers and to naive listeners evidenced a 31 percent word intelligibility to teachers but only a 19 percent word intelligibility to naive listeners.

The problem of judging speech intelligibility is further compounded by the fact that auditory discrimination of words and comprehension of spoken language involve different speech perceptual processing strategies. When a word is placed in a sentence, dependence on the acoustic information about the test word is decreased markedly as we draw upon linguistic constraint information. The acoustics of the word are diminished yet further in importance as the sentence is placed in context.

The relationship between the intelligibility of elicited words and spontaneous speech grows closer as the severity of the speech deviance increases. Children with very poor speech, primarily those with severe to profound hearing deficits, produce conversational speech that is sufficiently distorted as to preclude the listener from utilizing the linguistic and contextual information. This information usually also is deviant in the severely to profoundly hearing-impaired child. You will need, therefore, to obtain baseline and reassessment data for both speech articulation and for speech comprehension. The latter measure will reflect the interaction of articulation and language. Thus it will require a measure of the intelligibility of the child's identifying pictured items, repeating preselected sentences, and generating continuous speech. You also must recognize the limits of the validity of your own judgments of speech intelligibility and should use naive listeners as judges if you wish to quantify improvement more objectively.

A number of evaluation scales and tests are available for assessing intelligibility, including,

> Larr and Stockwell (1959), a speech intelligibility test
> Magner (1970), speech intelligibility test for deaf children
> Markides (1970b), rating scales of speech intelligibility
> Monsen (1982), speech intelligibility evaluation test
> Seewald (1981), test of speech production intelligibility

Ling (1976) cautions us against placing a great deal of value on tests of intelligibility that use meaningful material to assess speech skills except when the child has advanced language abilities. He points out that early speech production tends to evidence distortions originating from syntactic or morphologic incompetence rather than from articulatory difficulty. He maintains that even a valid measure of intelligibility, if available, would be of doubtful usefulness to planning speech training, stressing that

> Economy demands that the measures we use for this purpose are simple to administer, reliable, quick and easy to score even without the help of judges, and structured to reveal not general deficits but particular faults for which specific step-by-step remedial work can be planned. (Ling, 1976, p. 137)

Once more we see that assessing the communication skills of children with impaired hearing is a complex process. It is wise to use a great deal of caution in using results even when carefully obtained. Perhaps the overriding determinants of what you do will be, as Ling suggests, economy of time and effort and the effective utility of the results obtained.

READING AND WRITING AS COMMUNICATION MEDIA

We seldom, if ever, stop to contemplate what in fact we are doing when we read a book. Asked to write one, or a thesis or term paper, we become more aware of the complexity of the task. In reading we may find occasionally that we are unfamiliar with words used by the writer. Our difficulties may begin at the level of pronunciation. How does one say *quinquagenarian*, *chthonic,* or *mesembryanthemum?* However, learning the correct articulation does not mean that we can read, even though reading begins with the acquisition of skills, one of which is knowing the correspondence between written letters, articulation patterns, and the resultant sounds. So now we can pronounce a word, but what does it mean? What is a *solecism?* What are *pursy little faces, hieractic poses,* or *contumelious attitudes?* We look up the unfamiliar words in the dictionary. Are we now easily able to generate sentences in which each word is used correctly?

Even when a hearing-impaired child can pronounce and knows the meaning of every word in a sentence, he still may not be able to derive meaning from the sentence he can "read." In such a case, although he is saying familiar words, he is unable to synthesize them syntactically. Achieving this requires an understanding of the interrelated meanings and functions of the words. The meaning of a word often is further modified by the context in which it occurs. Consider the following uses of the word *engaged:*

John and Mary just became engaged.
I'm sorry, Dr. Jackson is engaged at the moment.
We have engaged a lawyer.
Gradually release the clutch to engage the gears.
The Queen engaged the intruder in conversation.
The patrol engaged the enemy.
Elizabeth is engaged in dramatics.

Truax (1978) states categorically that

No one can assume that helping a child with a hearing loss learn to read can be done without understanding language—how it functions, how it develops, how the various modes interrelate, and how language relates to the reading process. (p. 303)

Reading ability is a reflection of receptive language competence. It is related inextricably to

- The child's experience
- Understanding what was experienced
- Linguistic coding of experience at all levels of language from morphology to semantics
- Linguistic sophistication
- Phonetic skills
- Speech articulation skills

Each of these categories falls fully within the area of competence of the speech-language pathologist. Other aspects of reading acquisition are within the professional competencies of the classroom teacher, special education teacher or reading specialist. They include methods of teaching reading, remedial reading techniques, and the development of appropriate reading strategies for informational reading, functional reading, and recreational reading. I am not suggesting that it is your role to assume these responsibilities. What I am stressing is that a successful intervention program depends upon a transdisciplinary model. Such a model assigns to each person the primary responsibility for her own area of professional expertise. For you that is cognition, language, and speech. However, beyond this it requires that you coordinate your efforts with those of other teachers/therapists in such a way that each of you contributes your particular expertise and reinforces the contributions of the others.

Written Language

My university students often complain that I critique their written work for spelling, syntax, and grammar and that I take these into consideration when determining a grade. My belief is that how you express yourself reflects how you understand what you are attempting to communicate. Written language is not identical to spoken language; it has rules and formulae of its own. However, these are nuances of the medium—they do not change the fundamental fact that written language is a twin of spoken language, if not an identical twin.

It has been shown that the self-generated written language of severely hearing-impaired children is replete with examples of the deficient language abilities from which it derives. Kretschmer and Kretschmer (1978) point out, however, that written compositions cannot provide a complete understanding of the child's linguistic competencies because compounding factors such as carelessness, poor proofreading, or visual or motor problems may inhibit the use of written expression. These authors also refer to Wilbur's (1977) claim that the written expression of deaf subjects reflects not only the influence of the deafness but also that of a methodology of teaching. Wilbur suggests that the children are taught to write in a sentence-by-sentence manner, uncharacteristic of the form in which we express ideas in speech. If this is so, it stresses the need to include self-generated written expression in a holistic model of communication intervention. To do so reinforces newly encountered vocabulary, actualizes in visual imagery patterns of phonemic and word relationships, transforms thoughts into an enduring observable form, and provides an effective medium for feedback and self-correction. To the extent that we can enhance experience and cognitive linguistic knowledge, we can enhance reading ability. To the extent that reading ability is increased so is access to knowledge of the world through printed language. The ability then to express that knowledge in written form completes the spiral of learning one seeks from holistic teaching of linguistic communication.

Assessment of reading ability is an area in which regular and special education teachers receive instruction seldom included in the curricula of speech-language pathologists. Therefore, the actual reading assessment should be left to the teacher. However, unless the teacher is a certified teacher of the hearing impaired and deaf, your input into assessment will be important, since it will be necessary to accommodate the limitations imposed on test procedures by the hearing deficit. Furthermore, your input will help to differentiate the problems with reading from those rooted in the language deficit itself. This is a differentiation frequently not made (Smith, 1975).

ASSESSING THE CHILD'S SOCIOEMOTIONAL RESOURCES

Socioemotional Adjustment

If there were to be one criterion by which the effectiveness of a program of intervention for hearing-impaired children might best be assessed, it would be the child's personal adjustment. It is the impact of the communication/learning handicap on the child's sense of self-worth and well-being that most seriously limits the quality of his life. Everything we do, from hearing aid fitting to speech training, is geared toward the goal of making the individual feel greater self-respect and self-confidence.

The presence of a communication handicap in an otherwise normal child should be expected to give rise to frustration. Van Riper and Emerick (1990) identify the major components of the emotional aspect of a communication disorder as frustration, penalty, anxiety, guilt, and hostility. *Frustration* arises because the basic need to interact easily with others is impeded. The need to express feelings, ideas, and desires and to share experiences is thwarted. To exacerbate the situation, ineffective communication is unacceptable in our society; it draws attention to itself. It identifies the child as different, which often results in stigmatization as the *penalty* we impose on those thus characterized. Fear of failure during required or voluntary attempts to communicate frequently gives rise to *anxiety*. The child lives in a state of apprehension. Not only does he know the penalty that will be imposed upon him by others if he fails, but he judges himself and finds himself lacking. Disabled persons often feel that the penalty imposed upon them is deserved. After all, they are different; they are unable to communicate and participate like others. Recognition of their inadequacy leads to feelings of *guilt*. They are ashamed, often believing they have done something for which the disability is a punishment. These feelings must be dealt with by the child. Lacking understanding of why this is all happening, he protects himself either by withdrawal, probably the most common defense, or by *hostility*. Withdrawal from threat of penalizing situations, self-isolation, is self-destructive and is a way to seek to atone for the guilt. It reduces the anxiety at the expense of self-respect and is often accompanied by apathy and unhappiness. Hostility, by contrast, seeks to resolve the situation by externalizing the guilt and frustration. By verbal or physical hostility we seek to punish others for the hurt we feel.

A number of deviant personality characteristics have been attributed to the hearing-impaired population, including neurosis, introversion, aggression, emotional immaturity, egocentricity, and so on (Altschuler, 1962; Levine, 1956; Meadow & Schlesinger, 1971; Stewart, 1971). Hearing-impaired children have been reported to be significantly less emotionally well adjusted than their hearing peers (Fisher, 1966; Goetzinger, Harrison, & Baer, 1964; Reich, Hambleton, & Houldin, 1977). However, the conclusion one reaches from reviewing the results of studies that have used formal tests of personality, even when administered by persons qualified in their use, is that they are less than helpful. The results obtained are inconclusive, sometimes conflicting. Because of language deficiencies and resultant conceptual limitations, along with communication difficulties during testing, poor knowledge of social expectations and behaviors, and poor social problem resolution strategies, test findings may well be misleading. In any case, lacking appropriate training, the teacher/therapist should not be administering, far less interpreting and using, results of such tests.

Perhaps the most helpful way to consider the emotional behaviors of hearing-impaired children is to assume that they represent the child's best attempt to deal with an abnormal experience. They are the mechanisms that any normal individual will adopt when threatened (Freedman & Doob, 1968). In fact, Yuker and Black (1979) showed that we "normals" exhibit the same stress anxiety and adopt withdrawal-linked behaviors in the presence of disabled persons. Thus the reactions of the disabled person must be considered warranted as an attempt at self-protection. You may judge their behavior to be undesirable and ineffective, but it is understandable.

Your role in counseling will be particularly important because it will acknowledge the normality of the reactions to the handicap. Occasionally a child, particularly in the teenage years, may find the stress too great to manage. The behavior may reach a level of severity that you consider to be destructive to the child's well-being, to be acting as a major barrier to her progress with you and in class. Whenever you suspect the child's needs will exceed what intervention support and rehabilitation can provide, you should consider making a referral for psychological consultation. You should consult with the parents and teacher, explaining what you are concerned about and what you observe. You should explain how the child's behavior is restricting progress and make clear your need for input and guidance from a professional qualified to assess a child's need for special counseling support. Ask the teacher and parents whether they observe similar problems and whether they share your feeling that it would be helpful to seek the guidance of a professional counselor. Your own observations of the child, and those of parents and teachers, should address behaviors that suggest unusual levels of shyness, withdrawal from classmates and activities, apathy, denial of any problems, anger, hostility, and spitefulness. The child who appears unmotivated to accept help, who appears not to care about improving, or who is resistant to genuine offers of support needs more help than you alone can provide. Unfortunately, when a child's attitude or behavior leads her to reject the assistance we offer, we become frustrated. It is easy to take personal affront when our help is rejected and to label the child as lazy, uncooperative, having a bad attitude. We may adopt a "take it or leave it" attitude when, in fact, the child is showing very clearly that she is unable to accept help because of the strength of her negative feelings.

Most children will manage the emotional stresses of being hearing impaired at least well enough not to revert persistently to negative defensive behaviors. However, their needs may go unnoticed unless you provide opportunities for them to share their feelings with you. Confiding in others is not easy for anyone until a sufficient level of trust has been established. It will be some time before you will be able to approach a discussion of feelings with the child. In the early period of your contacts, you will need to depend on behavioral observations, made by you, the teacher, and parents, to identify undue socioemotional difficulties. Later, as trust between you and the child develops, you will feel comfortable in a more direct approach to the topic. This can occur through raising the question in discussion:

So how are things going in school?

O.K. I suppose.

That sounds like it's not so easy.

Well no, I have a tough time some days.

Is that because of the school work?

Well yeah, that and other things.

I can imagine it must be hard for you to keep up with the work; it's hard enough when you can hear okay. What are the things that make it difficult?

Well sometimes the other kids give me a hard time.

You mean they pick on you?

Yeah, they can be pretty mean sometimes.

For younger children you might wish to direct the discussion somewhat more, asking questions about friends in school and at home, activities, feelings about how other children treat them, how they feel about their hearing loss and about themselves, whether they are teased, liked, popular, and so on. You might wish to work together on seeing which of a series of statements best describes how they feel about situations. These may be grouped into choices as in Table 17.2 or you may prefer to randomize the statements and rate each as true or not true as to disability and handicap. Observation of behavior by you and others, augmented by what the child can share about her experiences and feelings, will provide an adequate basis from which to offer emotional support. That support should never be a separate unit in our intervention program. It will represent rather an extension of the climate of trust and respect that we build with these children. Counseling will be interwoven with the other support services we provide within our holistic model.

In other areas of evaluation, we have looked to standardized tests to provide us with quantifiable data and norms for various age-related abilities. We have rejected this approach to understanding the emotional status of a child on the grounds that the validity of such tests is questionable and because we are not qualified to administer and interpret them. Your need is twofold, first to be alert to indications that the child needs specialized counseling intervention and second, to assist the child in dealing with normal emotional reactions.

OBSERVING THE CHILD IN THE CLASSROOM

Observation of the child in school by you and/or by a parent can provide a helpful description of the child's communicative/learning behavior in the classroom setting. Ideally the observation should be made by a parent of

TABLE 17.2 Socioemotional adjustment guide

I enjoy school.	School's O.K.	I don't like school.
I have good friends in school.	I wish I had more friends.	I don't have good friends.
I have a best friend.	I sort of have a best friend.	There's no one who really is my friend.
Other children/students like me.	I get along O.K.	Other children/students don't really like me.
I have good friends after school.	Sometimes I do things with friends.	I don't see anyone after school.
We often play in each other's houses.*	Sometimes I play at a friend's house.	I never go to a friend's house.
I get to sleep over a lot.*	Sometimes I get to sleep over.	I never go to sleep-overs.
Other children/students are nice to me.	Other children/students are O.K.	Other children/students are mean to me.
I like to be with other children/students.	I only like to be with some children/students.	I like to be by myself.
I never get lonely.	Sometimes I'm lonely.	I like to be by myself.
I am never teased about my hearing problem.	Sometimes I get teased about my hearing problem.	They make fun of me.
My hearing problem is not important to other children/students.	If I didn't have a hearing problem, they would like me better.	They don't like me because of my hearing problem.
My speech is not a problem.	Sometimes I get teased about my speech.	I don't like to speak because the others can't understand me.
I get to do a lot of things after school.	I don't do much after school.	I get bored at home.
I do a lot of things with my friends.	I don't have anyone to do things with.	Mostly I do things with my parents.
I don't mind wearing my hearing aids.	My hearing aids are such a pain.	I hate having to wear hearing aids.

* Suitable only for primary graders.

another hearing-impaired child rather than the child's own parent(s). Try to pair parents to exchange this service. This arrangement greatly enhances the objectivity of the observation and provides both of the observers with an opportunity to share their educational concerns. It is still highly desirable for parents to observe their own child in school, but the greatest benefit occurs when they can do so with the knowledge of what someone else perceived. A comparison of the two observations can then be made by you and the parents, allowing discussion of any differences observed, the possible reason for those differences (e.g., the awareness by the child of his own mother/father in the room), and the significance of behaviors observed. Combined with test results, this discussion provides a comprehensive basis upon which you and the parent together can identify needs and decide upon intervention goals. This approach educates the parent about the child's problem and the rationale for your intervention plan. Most important, it invites the parent into a partnership, fosters cooperation, and maximizes the resources available for management.

Guidelines for Observation

A single visit to a classroom often proves misleading. If at all possible, several visits of about a half hour each should be made on different days. The visits should sample the different subjects studied with an emphasis on language-based subjects. Much less would be gained from observing the child in gym or art than in English or social studies. Observation must be directed to be of value. Therefore, you should prepare for a visit by reviewing the criteria for observation in order to know what to look for. The following checklist guides the process of observing and recording general observations.

Classroom Observations

Physical environment
Room size:
  large   average   small
Acoustics:
  reverberant/echoes   sound well absorbed
Average noise level:
  high   acceptable   low
Structures:
  floors:
    hard   carpeted
  ceilings:
    hard   sound tiled
  walls:
    hard   mainly blackboards
  windows:
    old sash   modern double glazed
  ventilation:
    forced air   radiators
  air conditioning:
    yes   no
Seating:
  row   small groups   other
Child's seat:
  front   center   rear
Teacher:
  male   female
  Primary teaching position:
    left   center   right   other
    front   center   rear
  Use of blackboard/visual aids:
    frequent   sometimes   little
  Writes up key words:
    usually   sometimes   seldom
  Teacher's voice:
    strong   adequate   soft

Classroom Observations (*continued*)

Clarity of speech:
  clear   sometimes hard to understand
Rate of speaking:
  rapid   normal   slow
Interaction with class:
  frequent   some   little
Encourages questions:
  often   sometimes   seldom
Keeps children involved:
  greatly   somewhat   little
Checks on children's understanding:
  often   sometimes   seldom
Progresses through lesson:
  rapidly   normally   slowly
Children seem to follow:
  easily   with difficulty
Children are attentive:
  very   mostly   not very

Child's behavior:
  Appears to be attentive:
    mostly   sometimes   seldom
  Asks questions:
    frequently   sometimes   seldom
  Participates in discussion:
    frequently   sometimes   seldom
  Appears to understand:
    frequently   sometimes   seldom

Teacher/child interaction:
  Teacher stands close to child when teaching   yes   no
  Teacher encourages child to contribute   yes   no
  Teacher rephrases and simplifies questions   yes   no
  Teacher checks child's understanding   yes   no
  Teacher asks child questions   yes   no
  Teacher tends to ignore child   yes   no
  Teacher works individually with child   yes   no
  Teacher uses FM unit *consistently*   yes   no   n/a

Overall impression:

In a similar approach Ross (1982, pp. 104–5), under each of seven categories, lists four or five questions to ask about the child's behavior in class. The seven categories include the

- Participation of the child in classroom discussions
- Interactions between the child and his teacher
- Adaptation of the teacher's classroom style
- Interactions between the child and his classmates
- Child's strategies for learning and processing content material
- Use of an FM trainer by the teacher and child
- Source level and location of speech and noise sources relative to the child

In an attempt to profile the child's classroom participation, Ripich and Spinelli (1985) have provided a systematic procedure for screening discourse ability from classroom observations. They use a rating scale to assess the child's level of communication participation. The behaviors rated cover attentiveness, number of questions asked, participation in classroom discourse, and appropriateness of communications.

A speech-language pathologist or a special education teacher could refine this procedure to provide a record of the types of conversational competencies observed. These would include imitation of communicative interaction, maintenance of the interaction, and appropriate exit strategies. Particular abilities observed should be noted. These include evidence of the use of appropriate forms to make requests, answer questions, ask for explanations, express needs and opinions, give directions, recount events, describe pictures or happenings, and explain ideas.

The advantage of classroom observation is that the information gathered is from real rather than contrived communication events. As such it focuses on the child's ability to meet the actual demands placed upon him and to see if he conforms to the classrooms rules (Duchan, 1988). Classroom observation, therefore, can provide a helpful general profile and can alert the teacher/speech-language pathologist to gaps between the child's knowledge and his application of that knowledge in the classroom. The disadvantage lies in the fact that such an uncontrolled method fails to ensure that a complete picture of the child's language proficiency will be obtained.

REPORTING FINDINGS

We have now completed our review of the many areas of need arising from the discrepancy that exists between demands placed upon the hearing-impaired child and his ability to meet them. The task that you confront may seem monumental. With so much to determine you may wonder how you can hope to complete the assessment. Remember, however, that assessment is a cooperative process involving the input of several specialists as well as the parents. If you are an audiologist, your major roles are to measure residual hearing and its usefulness and to optimize its potential use through the fitting and monitoring of hearing aids. Beyond this, you will have a major role to play in providing to parents and the professionals working with the child the information they will need in order to plan and conduct effective management procedures. Your expertise lies in the ways amplification can be used to facilitate learning, in predicting the effect of different environmental acoustics on the amount of auditory information the child might be expected to receive, and in working with the team when problems arise concerning the child's use of audition. Your help in deciding how much emphasis should be placed on auditory training and on speech-reading will be appreciated. You can guide the teacher/therapist in how to integrate auditory training into a holistic intervention model, advise on the use of the personal hearing aids and FM amplification units in class and in therapy, and make predictions concerning which speech sounds may and may not readily be taught through aided hearing. Your ultimate goal will be to help teachers and other professionals better understand the nature and practicalimplications of the child's hearing impairment and to give them confidence in their use of amplification for education.

A summary report accompanying an unaided and aided audiogram, with unaided and aided speech discrimination and comprehension results, will help guide the therapist and speech-language pathologist. The following report on Elizabeth illustrates how your findings may be communicated in a practical form.

Elizabeth

Elizabeth has a moderate, permanent hearing impairment in both ears. She is able to hear the low tones of speech and noise quite well. Thus she is aware of things going on around her, including people speaking. However, her difficulty hearing middle- and high-pitched tones makes it very hard for her to comprehend speech without a hearing aid. Without the aid she hears conversational speech at a just-audible level; a very loud voice would be necessary to make speech comfortably loud.

Elizabeth now has two hearing aids. With these aids she hears speech at a comfortable listening level. She is able to discriminate most of what she hears without needing to watch the speaker. However, you should know that:

1. In a noisy situation when others are talking, Elizabeth's discrimination by hearing alone drops to 65 percent. She misses over a quarter of what is said.
2. When Elizabeth is 15 feet from the speaker she hears clearly only a little over half of what is said. At this distance in noise, she barely understands speech.
3. Even with the aid, Elizabeth has difficulty hearing high-pitched speech sounds such as s, z, f, v, sh, ch, t. The s and sh are noticeably defective in her speech because she does not hear them well.
4. Elizabeth compensates well for her hearing impairment by watching the speaker. When she can clearly see the speaker she scores 100 percent on a word-discrimination task in quiet, 88 percent in noise, and 78 percent in noise at 15 feet.
5. Because of her long-standing hearing impairment Elizabeth's language level is 1½ years below her age. This makes understanding what she hears more difficult. Complex sentences, new vocabulary, unfamiliar concepts, even in good listening/watching conditions, cause Elizabeth to appear confused, to be afraid to volunteer a response, or to guess wildly. When she misunderstands you will need to determine whether it is becuase she has not heard or does not understand what has been asked.

Elizabeth will understand you best when she is
1. Within 4 feet of you
2. Able to see your face clearly
3. Familiar with the language and topic
4. In a place with a low noise level

She will have difficulty understanding
1. Group conversations
2. Speakers whom she cannot see
3. Tape recordings
4. Television when she cannot see the speaker
5. New material presented orally

As a speech-language pathologist or teacher of hearing-impaired children, your summary focuses on receptive and expressive use of communication. You will wish to summarize the child's language performance from vocabulary to semantics and to include a statement regarding her pragmatic skills. The child's familiarity with the particular academic vocabulary and pragmatic language of the classroom should be noted.

Performance in reading as measured by a reading teacher along with a summary of the child's written language expression should be described in terms of the demonstrated language deficiencies.

Auditory discrimination with hearing aids should have been a facet of communication included in the audiologist's report. Your report should note the child's use of audition in communication along with a description of the child's ability to capitalize on visual and contextual cues to meaning. Your focus should be on your findings concerning auditory and auditory-visual comprehension of familiar language material. The results of your speech articulation assessment at the phonetic and phonologic level should be summarized to focus on the types of problems identified rather than on difficulties with particular sounds. General speech intelligibility may be commented on. Finally, you should comment on your impression of the child's general sense of well-being. Note the ease with which she related to you during assessment, her attitude to the tasks, and her reaction to difficulty. Any observations by the classroom teacher concerning her participation and behavior in class may be included.

SUMMARY

- Assessment of the classroom demands on a child requires evaluating the environment, the required knowledge, the method and complexity of teaching, and the expected reading level.
- An evaluation needs to be made for each classroom the student encounters during the day.
- Assessment of the student's resources include
  - Aided residual hearing
  - Linguistic knowledge
  - Pragmatic competence
  - Speech production
  - Auditory-visual processing skills
  - Linguistic competence
  - Classroom behavior
  - Socioemotional adjustment
- A comparison of the classroom demands and the student's resources identifies strengths and weaknesses, and indicates needs.
- Assessment of the maximum to be expected from aided residual hearing indicates the needs for special classroom amplification systems and the emphasis to be placed on the visual modality as an information resource.
- When testing it is essential to ensure that
  Listening and viewing conditions are optimal.
  The child feels secure.
  You have his attention.
  Directions are understood.
  The child is encouraged but not pressured.
  You recheck incorrect responses.
- The conclusions you draw from test results standardized on children with normal hearing and those with norms for children with impaired hearing should be differentiated.

- Test results need to be supplemented by structured classroom observations of
  - Classroom environment
  - Teacher behavior
  - Teacher/child interaction
  - Seating placement
  - Child behavior
  - Child participation
- Speech should be analyzed in detail to document
  - Vocal control
  - Vowel production
  - Phonetic and phonologic skills
  - Coarticulatory skills
  - Rapid articulation of syllables
  - Intelligibility
- Socioemotional assessment should be informal. Careful observation, sensitive exploration of the child's feelings, and anecdotal reports from parents and teachers should guide general impressions.

Conclusion

Evaluation of the school-age child requires that you assess the demands the child must meet, the environments in which they arise, and the present resources with which the child can accommodate those demands. It will be necessary to account for the various learning situations in the child's school day. In assessing the child's present resources, particular attention is focused on performance with aided residual hearing, use of supplementary visual skills, language and speech competence, and general socioemotional adjustment. Your testing procedures must accommodate difficulties in hearing and comprehending instructions. Your selection of tests should be guided by whether you wish to compare the child to his normal hearing peers or to other hearing-impaired children. Finally, general conclusions should not be reached without obtaining information about how the child functions communicatively in the classroom, and how he adjusts to and deals with difficulties encountered there.

18

Management of the School-Age Child

You have completed your initial assessment of a school-age child. The reports from other professionals have been received and you are now confronted with the task of providing intervention support. Before we address how to go about doing this, it will be helpful to consider the general nature of a communication rehabilitation program for school-age children with impaired hearing. You will find it reassuring to have a global understanding of the task.

It is important to realize that the hearing disability and the hearing handicap are not synonymous. In virtually every case that we are asked to help, it has been determined that nothing more can be done to ameliorate the disability; it is the handicap that we must endeavor to reduce. The handicap has its roots in reduced auditory information, but in the school-age child this has resulted in a complex overlay of reduced auditory experience, the effects of reduced linguistic competence, reduced cognitive knowledge, and as a result, retarded learning. Quite commonly these deficits have in turn spawned problems in socioemotional development. Certainly we will wish to make every effort to increase the child's ability to make better use of whatever extrinsic sources of information are available, and we will endeavor to optimize the circumstances relevant to the reception of information potentially available from those sources. In addition, however, we will have as a major goal the enrichment of intrinsic resources and the skills relevant to their strategic use. Ideally we wish to increase the ratio of dependence on intrinsic to extrinsic resources. Our role, therefore, is to manage circumstances and facilitate change through learning. Let us examine the steps we can take to achieve that.

EFFECTING CHANGE IN THE CLASSROOM

Establishing Action Priorities

I refer to *action priorities* rather than to *need priorities* because actions are governed by both recognized needs and availability of resources to provide for them. For example, a child fitted with a monaural hearing aid may have, as a major priority, a need for a second hearing aid. You may know, however, that neither state nor private resources are available to pay for one. In such a case, although the need remains high, its immediate priority on your list of actions realistically must drop, even though you do not give up your efforts to obtain funding. Another example is a child who clearly needs the support of a resource room teacher to enable her to continue effective mainstream placement. Absence of such a resource within practical reach of the school district precludes immediate effective action. This necessitates that the need be redefined.

To establish your action priorities, you have to consider those needs that both urgently require attention and can be met by immediate action. For example, the child who is experiencing emotional adjustment difficulties in class to a degree that labels her as a problem and prevents her from making academic progress presents a need for immediate psychological referral. Similarly, a child whose hearing aid is not working needs immediate audiological attention.

For many children the situation will be relatively well under control—no particular need will be especially demanding. These are the children who require a program of support across various areas of communication and learning rather than emergency intervention in one or two. Nevertheless, you will wish to monitor how well the child is meeting academic and social demands to ensure that your broad intervention plan is flexible enough to adjust to changing circumstances. To determine priorities for this group of children, you will be guided by your assessment results. The paradigm you should keep in mind is

- Identify the problem
- Define the demands
- Describe the needs
- Modify the situation
- Provide additional resources

Changing the Environment

Your goal is to optimize, as far as possible, the classroom conditions for communication and for learning. When you exert a positive change in class, you reduce the child's learning difficulties throughout the school day, or at least for the time spent in that room. Accept that in each situation there are limits to what you can achieve. These limits are financial and lie also in the degree to which the child and other persons involved are willing to cooperate.

It is from the rehabilitative diagnostic results that we identify the child's needs. Our overall goal is to reduce impedance to communication and learning through effecting a change. The possibilities for achieving this lie on two fronts:

- The child's relationship to the learning environment
- The communication resources and behaviors of the child

Informational Support to the Classroom Teacher. Flexer, Wray, and Ireland (1990) have drawn attention to the fact that the overwhelming majority of hearing-impaired children are mainstreamed. Ross (1982, p. 35) showed academic retardation among this population even with monaural hearing deficits of as little as 14dB in the better ear. He found an average of 9 to 12 months retardation in language comprehension and paragraph meaning and 12 months in vocabulary. In the 15–25dB hearing deficit category, the delay increased to over a year. An increase of an extra year's delay occurred for each additional 10dB of impairment up to a plateau of three years. This finding confirmed earlier observations by Kodman (1963), Quigley and Thomure (1968), and Hine (1970). Yet half the teachers in Ross's study did not believe the hearing impairment had anything to do with the academic delay, a finding also reported by Bess (1985). Martin, Bernstein, Daly, and Cody (1988) found not only that regular classroom teachers had little or no knowledge of hearing impairment and its educational implications, but that they frequently even were unaware that a child in the class was wearing hearing aids. The fault lies not with the teachers. Ringaleben and Price (1981) reported that a survey of regular classroom teachers revealed that 54 percent had received no inservice training on how to help handicapped children in their classes.

It is patently clear that we must provide these teachers with the information they need if we are to maximize the hearing-impaired child's potential for learning in the mainstream placement. This must be done supportively, not authoritatively. We must inform so we can discuss shared concerns. Do not tell teachers what they must do. Rather, help them understand the problems, identify the needs, and explore with them possible strategies and solutions.

Flexer et al. state that information "needs to 'begin at the beginning' by promoting an understanding of hearing and hearing loss" (1990, p. 18). Fitch (1982) describes an inservice workshop by the speech-language pathologist on the hearing-impaired child intended for teachers. It utilizes the System O.N.E. Kit (Bitter & Johnson, 1974), which contains 11 sections. These include introduction and orientation, planning for the child, classroom management, parent involvement, communication skills, peer interaction, academic skills, Individuals with Disabilities Act (IDEA) Public Law 94-142 and review. Another set of materials for inservice training was published by Nober (1975). Organized workshops may be very effective but are often difficult to arrange. More commonly, and often more effectively, you will rely upon ongoing personal consultations with the teacher as I will illustrate later. In general, the main information the teacher needs to know is that

- Hearing-impaired children hear speech less loudly and less clearly than normal-hearing children even when hearing aids are worn. No child hears normally with hearing aids.
- Audibility guarantees neither intelligibility nor comprehension.
- Some sounds, words, and phrases will be clear, others not.
- Listening and understanding for these children are unusually demanding and exhausting, which is why attention wanders.
- The child will not understand until close attention is paid.
- Seeing the speaker often is essential to understanding.
- Noise and increased distance from the speaker may make speech unintelligible.
- Hearing impairment causes language, reading, and academic retardation.
- New or difficult material will be unusually hard to learn without special help.
- Without functioning hearing aids, learning may be impossible.

Every teacher who is asked to use an FM system *must* receive considerate, uncomplicated, practical inservice training in its use and care. I refer you to Ross (1982, pp. 161–177) for such a practical learning unit.

Teacher guidelines of the type developed by Gildstone (1973) and Walsvik (1966) for what to do and what not to do to help the mainstreamed hearing-impaired child, in my opinion, overload a teacher with a lot of often ill-considered demands. I believe you will be far more successful, and far better received, if you individualize your counseling of teachers and address the specific needs of a particular child, as we will discuss later. Above all do not overwhelm the teacher with demands and expectations likely to cause him/her to feel insecure.

Classroom Seating Changes. Consider whether the child's seating position can be improved to shorten the teacher-child distance, to improve directionality, and to optimize visual processing of speech and written material.

From the classroom profile of Jessica, whom we discussed in the previous chapter (p. 333), we see that she has optimal seating for hearing her teacher but has difficulty hearing her classmates' questions and comments. This latter difficulty cannot be managed by changing her seating but must depend upon other modifications we will discuss. Anthony (p. 331) also has optimal seating in social studies class but is seated inappropriately in English and chemistry classes. The ideal action would be to move him to the front in English and to the left-hand end of a middle bench in chemistry, placing him next to the blackboards. However, while Jessica might accept a seating change without comment, Anthony enjoys sitting in the back of the English class among his friends. This class, you will recall, is taught by an inexperienced and rather ineffective teacher. There is a lot of talking, giggling, and distracting behavior going on. This leads one to wonder how much learning occurs in the class in general and how much Anthony would gain from a seating change, particularly since it would mean singling him out for the move and separating him from his friends. Social acceptance is very important in the teenage years; it is a factor one must consider seriously when intervention might place it in jeopardy. It is unlikely that the gain expected from a seating change in this class would outweight the social cost. The situation in chemistry class is different. Placement involves teams rather than individuals, a placement change would be expected to have definite advantage. Anthony will appreciate any facilitation of learning chemistry and Mr. Davis appears to be a reasonable person. You first would discuss with Anthony the need for reseating his group. Then inquire about the possibility of such a change in a meeting with Mr. Davis. Ask also about the possibility of assigning Anthony to a more cohesive group of pupils, preferably as part of a larger reshuffle that it might be reasonable to make at the end of a particular curriculum unit. You will recall that Jessica, who also works in a group situation in social studies, derives considerable support from other members of her team. The effect upon learning that comes from placing a less emotionally and academically secure child in among children who work well together often can be greater than all our one-on-one rehabilitation efforts (Kidder, 1989). Whenever you include a consideration of a seating change in a discussion with a teacher, you should explain the acoustic problem the child experiences and describe the move as part of a complete support program. When help is sought, rather than change demanded, most teachers are very accommodating.

Jessica's seating placement left unresolved the problem of her not hearing contributions made by classmates. You may recall (p. 333) that Anthony reported that in mathematics his teacher commonly repeated questions and comments by the students, greatly facilitating Anthony's ability to follow the class. Such a suggestion to Mrs. Burwick, with appropriate explanation of the problem, most likely will be received favorably. However, it would be wise to explore the possibility of a personal FM amplification system for Jessica. Her young age makes its acceptance much easier, and it will prove particularly valuable when she begins to have different teachers for different subjects. Anthony, by contrast, might have a difficult time accepting the use of such a unit, which might make him feel more different than do his personal hearing aids, which he feels are not very conspicuous and, most important, are accepted by his friends. He has but another year in high school, perhaps rather late to first consider an FM unit. Your responsibility remains, however, to explore options and to educate the hearing-impaired student about the hearing impairment and its management. You also wish to encourage Anthony to take responsibility for his own future. For this reason, I recommend that you review with him the needs that are not met in school and explain what FM is and outline how it functions and what it can do. Recognizing that Anthony hopes to go to college, I would stress that in college, classes will be much larger, with as many as 400 students in some of them. At the same time, the subject matter will be more difficult. Explain that FM can relieve much of this problem and suggest that high school might be an excellent place to learn, with support, how to really put state of the art technology to work.

Other Strategies for Reducing Learning Impedance

Consider some further strategies you might choose to use in reducing the impedance to learning experienced by Jessica and Anthony. We concluded that for Anthony a change in seating probably would prove of very little gain in Miss Lee's English class. The difficulty encountered with the subject might, however, be reduced if Anthony were less dependent on the oral information presented in class. The need is to identify other sources from which knowledge about the subject matter, *Julius Caesar*, for example, might be gained. There are study guides, such as *Cliffs Notes, Coles Notes,* and *Monarch Notes*; there are books that retell Shakespeare as stories for somewhat younger students, and there are audiotapes and video films of the plays. Knowing what the story is about, with insights into the twists and turns of the plot, will make the play more intelligible. Furthermore, Anthony will no longer have the same difficulty extracting meaning from obtuse language. He would gain extra help from some study strategies with which you can familiarize him, for example, writing characters' names, roles, and relationships on 3×5 inch cards, summarizing events in each act, and so on. This information then can serve as the basis for a communication training session with you. It provides material for specialized vocabulary, syntactic knowledge, spontaneous discussion, auditory and visual communication upgrading, role playing, and reading and writing.

There are two other impedance barriers to classroom communication that we left unresolved for Jessica. The first was the difficulty she has in spelling. Of course you will plan to use classroom spelling lists as material for your sessions with her, expanding those words for meaning, using them for syntactic exercises, and giving auditory-visual training with them. However, you first will want to seek to modify the situation in class. You might achieve this by explaining the difficulty to Mrs. Burwick, describing your support plans, and identifying Jessica's needs during spelling tests. Words in isolation are particularly vulnerable to loss of acoustic information due to poor acoustics and increased dependency on the speech signal. Thus Jessica, more than other students, needs to see the word spoken, to hear it from the closest distance possible, to hear it more than once, and to hear it in context. We would explain to the teacher that it would help greatly if she could stand close to Jessica when giving the test, in a position where Jessica can see her face clearly, if she could ensure that Jessica is ready for the word, and if she could first state the word, for example, *emigrate* and then place it in a sentence, "The Pilgrims decided to *emigrate* to America," and then restate the word, "Spell *emigrate*."

Jessica also needs help with video film instruction. This is a difficult situation that is resistant to resolution. If an FM unit is used, the microphone-transmitter should be placed very close to the set. It may be possible for Mrs. Burwick to provide the parents and you with a copy of a synopsis of content for review prior to the showing of the video. Probably the most practical step would be to look to other sources for the same content.

Note Taking. A problem encountered by Anthony and by many hearing-impaired students in high school is being unable to take adequate notes.

Two factors underlie this difficulty. The first is that few of these students can comprehend speech easily without the aid of visual cues. Thus, looking down to write notes shuts off the source of information for those notes. This is the same problem encountered when a teacher expects the students to follow his explanation while carefully studying in the textbook the formula, figure, map or illustration being explained. The second factor is that reduced language abilities make extremely difficult the complex task of hearing what is said, decoding the message, restating it in one's own cognitive-linguistic form, and writing it down. These students can benefit from the use of an assigned note taker. Care must be taken in seeking the assistance of another student in the class. The following steps should be taken:

- Discuss with Anthony the need for adequate notes for studying and preparing for exams.
- Discuss the classes in which this is presenting a problem.
- Discuss the solution of having access to another student's notes.
- Identify a student who takes effective notes, whose handwriting is legible, whose vocabulary is not exceptional, and who would be willing to assist in this way.
- Explain the need to the potential note taker, then have Anthony and the note taker discuss the procedure with you. Notes may be taken on special paper placed in a notebook, which obviates the messiness of carbon paper, or they may be photocopied in the school office.

Sometimes it helps to have teachers tape record a lesson for subsequent review with the notes. This requires appropriate placement of a high-quality cassette recorder and tape.

Tutoring. It may be appropriate to arrange for tutoring in critical subjects in which a student experiences difficulties. This may be provided by a resource teacher. In some cases volunteer services from students in upper grades or even a local college may be available. In such a case some guidance in how to tutor should be provided. It helps greatly if the subject teacher identifies the information to be covered. Both preview of vocabulary and concepts in approaching curriculum and review of material not understood should be considered.

What I have tried to do in this section is to illustrate that intervention in the classroom calls for highly individualized strategies based on the paradigm identified earlier:

- Identify the problem
- Define the demands
- Describe the needs
- Modify the situation
- Provide additional resources

I stress again that this calls for a cooperative approach with the classroom teacher. You appeal to the teacher to help you understand her perception of the student's difficulties and for information that will help you to explore options with the teacher. The goal is to facilitate the student's classroom learning. The extent to which this is possible also will facilitate the teacher's task.

Having effected the possible changes in the classroom in order to minimize the impedance to learning, we now must consider the student as an important resource. We must examine how we can upgrade his own potential for communication and learning.

ENRICHING RESOURCES WITHIN THE CHILD

We considered one by one the several areas of development that need to be included in a diagnostic evaluation of a child's communication function. Unfortunately, it will be necessary for us to examine, in the same sequential manner, ways in which we can increase the communication abilities of the student. I say, unfortunately, because sequential discussion of intervention procedures suggests that one devotes a lesson on a given day to a particular aspect of communication upgrading and on another day to another aspect. "Today we are going to work on auditory training and speech-reading" or "Today's the day we work on speech," and so on. Such a model is inefficient and ineffective, based as it is upon the assumption that such aspects of communication function independently. I have emphasized throughout our discussion that all components in communication are intimately interrelated, so that changes in any one impact upon all others. I also have stressed that all the components must fit together as a functioning whole. Thus, when we provide a program to upgrade communication, one of our aims will be to balance abilities, to move them all along in concert. Truax (1978) has stated this very clearly:

> For a child with a language deficiency of any kind it would seem appropriate to provide an integrated communication curriculum. Within the framework of such a curriculum a child's development would be charted in all areas. His individualized program would reflect his needs in all modes of communication. Activities designed to foster aural-oral language development and usage could be related to activities emphasizing reading development and usage. Learning to express ideas in drama or through creative and expository writing could grow out of reading experiences. If a child's language program in communication areas such as writing and spelling, reading, and speech and auditory training is not coordinated and not based on an overall language acquisition and development plan, then the child may spend much valuable time in fragmented learning experiences, which in some instances might be counterproductive to educational progress. (p. 294)

The model of intervention you should keep in mind is one that

- Recognizes all areas of need
- Is sensitive to priority needs
- Monitors changing needs
- Is flexible
- Accommodates the acknowledged interdependence of component functions
- Seeks to generalize improvements across all aspects of receptive and expressive communication

The areas of communication that should be included in a supportive intervention model are

1. Information counseling
2. Understanding the hearing impairment and use of personal hearing aids and FM units
3. Auditory and visual communication upgrading
4. Language knowledge and use enrichment
5. Speech intelligibility improvement
6. Reading, writing, and communication
7. Adjustment counseling

I wish to stress again that this list does not imply a sequential order in which enrichment is provided. On different days at different times in the child's school career some components will require special emphasis. This is what makes the criteria of monitoring changing needs and flexibility so important. However, most of your sessions will be devoted to working intensively on an ability for a short time, then integrating it with the whole, moving everything along together. With this concept clearly in mind, we now can consider intervention procedures.

1. Information Counseling

It is unfortunate that few young people with impaired hearing know much at all about the very condition that causes most of their difficulties. A 20-year-old totally oral university student with a severe congenital hearing impairment asked with serious concern, "I know this may sound like a stupid question, but am I deaf or hard-of-hearing?" A high school student asked, "Why do I have to wear aids behind my ears when I see in magazines advertisements for hearing aids that are invisible?" An eight year old still wondered when she would not need to wear her aids anymore, while another asked, "Well if I've got a hearing loss how come I can hear people talk?" These examples reflect a failure of us professionals to prepare school-age children for management of their own problems. It derives from the concept of providing "rehabilitation therapy" rather than perceiving our role as one of educating the child to deal with problems he will encounter throughout his life. Even adult clients say to me, "Oh, no one ever gave me a copy of my test results or explained what they mean."

Educating the child about the hearing impairment, about its effects and how to minimize those effects, should be a continuing component of an intervention program throughout the school years. By the time the young person leaves high school, either for postsecondary education or for employment, she should understand the nature of the problem and have gained confidence in the ability to manage its effects.

2. Understanding the Hearing Impairment

It is not easy to present complex information simply. Neither the young person nor the adult needs to know everything you know about hearing impairment and its management. You must present only the basics and must do so quite simply. The hearing-impaired student deserves to understand his hearing problem and its effects. He needs this understanding in order to cooperate fully in the measures you and he will take to maximize his ability to function in communication-learning situations and social environments. Do not forget that this young person soon will be entering college or the adult work world where the support team available in school does not exist. Our intervention strategies should serve to ameliorate present difficulties. However, they also should be used to help the student learn to solve problems he ultimately will have to resolve alone. Information counseling should be an ongoing component of intervention, not confined to a short explanation given by the audiologist or teacher/therapist during a session with the student. It should serve to help the student to

- Understand how his hearing is different
- Realize and accept it will not improve
- Learn the type, severity, and shape of the hearing impairment
- Understand what the hearing impairment does to speech perception
- Understand how hearing aids make more speech audible
- Know the conditions that provide the best and poorest listening
- Know how to use and care for the hearing aids
- Understand thoroughly how to use the FM unit correctly, including what the teacher needs to know

This information is not inclusive. As you encourage the student to think about the hearing difficulty objectively, as a problem to be managed, other needs for information and understanding will arise. Obviously, what a first-grade child needs to know is different from what a twelfth-grade student needs to know. The core topics remain constant; however, the level of sophistication of knowledge needed increases, and additional topics arise that must be dealt with. Do not lecture the student; set out instead to learn the information together. Encourage the keeping of a notebook or folder in which a record is kept of what was learned, for example, hints given; problems with solutions noted; and illustrations and brochures about hearing, hearing deficiency, and hearing aids; and helpful tips. It is essential that you avoid a professional approach to imparting this information. For example, the audiogram can be explained quite simply thus:

Here is a chart of your hearing. We call it an <u>audiogram</u>.*

You remember you pressed the button, raised your hand each time you just heard a sound?

Let's learn how to read this chart. Across the top here, these numbers 125, 250 to 8000 tell use the <u>pitch</u> of the sound, a low buzz like this [make a low-pitched sound] is at this end, a high whistle or squeak is up here. We call all these pitches <u>frequency</u>.

Will a tone near 4000 frequency be high or low pitch? Make a sound like that? Good. How about 250 frequency? Great.

O.K. Now, the numbers down the side tell us how strong the sound is. We measure this in numbers called <u>decibels</u>, like we measure milk in pints. The larger the number the louder the sound.

---

* All underlined words should be checked for familiarity and emphasized when used. Note where possible new vocabulary is paired with a familiar term that subsequently is omitted.

When you took the hearing test, the audiologist was measuring how loud she had to make the sound, how far down these numbers, these decibels, she had to go before you just heard it.

So, here is your chart. What do we call it? It's an audiogram. There are circles and crosses. The circles are your right ear, the crosses your left. Forget the other stuff (bc/responses, masked responses, etc.). Now we can read your audiogram.

What does it tell us? Well, here is where people who have no hearing problem hear—those faint tones [draw a line across at 20dB Hz]. So you can see first that you have a problem in both ears. Which is the right ear?—Good, circles—and left ear? Crosses. Your left ear is a bit better than your right. When you look at the frequency (pitch) numbers, the ones at the top, you can see you hear the low frequencies (pitches). Can you show where you hear low pitches? Right—you hear these low frequencies better than these high frequencies. Now, let's just go over what I told you.

In the notebook, place a copy of just the a/c audiogram and the notes.

A hearing chart is called an audiogram.

It shows when you just hear a faint sound.

Numbers at the top are pitches, low to high. They are called frequencies.

Numbers down the side are measures of loudness called decibels. The bigger the number the louder the sound.

Circles are my right ear, crosses my left.

The circle, under a pitch/frequency number at the top, by a loudness/decibel number at the side, shows how loud the sound had to be before I could just faintly hear it.

If I had normal hearing the circles and crosses would be above the 20 decibel line.

Both my ears have a problem.

My left ear is a little better than my right.

I hear low frequency sounds better than high frequency ones.

The teacher probably would find a copy of this synopsis helpful. This information would take a while for the student to digest. There is no hurry; review it briefly several times every third session or so. Ask questions about the audiogram. The information then can be woven into vocabulary and semantic knowledge. For example, the word *frequency* needs to be understood in general terms.

Frequency: number of times something happens. We could talk about the frequency of homework, visits to your class, visits to the dentist.

Frequent: we would learn how to use the adjective, "He was a frequent visitor." "She was a frequent winner."

Frequently: we would learn to qualify verbs. "He missed school frequently." "She frequently interrupted." "We frequently missed the school bus."

To frequent: to be at often, to go to many times, to hang out. "Teenagers like to frequent the mall." "He frequented the video game places."

I would use words such as *pitch* to illustrate multiple meanings:

Pitch: the sound of a note; a black, sticky substance for making roads and roofs *watertight.*

A pitch: a throw—"He made a good pitch to the batter."

To pitch: to throw something such as a ball in baseball; to rock as in a boat or in sleep, to "pitch and turn."

To pitch in: to help.

I would use these examples for auditory-visual communication material. Everything learned has to fit into all levels of communication processing. When the student seems to understand the audiogram, I would ask for a short written explanation entitled, "My Hearing Impairment."

Hearing for speech can be taught (not just explained once), in a similar manner.

Let's talk about why your hearing problem makes it hard for you to hear speech. First you need to know about speech. When I say a sound /u/ or /a/ or /d/ or a word or sentence, what you hear is a mixture of a lot of frequencies, or pitches which make a particular pattern of, for example, the sound /sh/ or the word /tie/. Think of baking a cake. First you need ingredients. A lot of cakes use many of the same ingredients, for example, flour, milk, sugar, but some cakes are special because they have one special ingredient—fruit, chocolate, banana. Next, you need a recipe which tells you how much of each ingredient you need—1 lb. flour, two eggs, etc. Finally, the recipe tells you how to put the ingredients together—first sift the flour then add sugar and mix well.

Speech is like this. Each speech sound or word has a recipe. Each has certain frequency ingredients in a certain measure (strength/intensity) and in a certain order (pattern). When they are all present in the right amounts and correct order, you hear a clear speech sound just as you ended up with an excellent cake. But when hearing impairment takes out some of those frequencies or even reduces their loudness, it's the same as not following the cake recipe. Just as the cake gets soggy or dry, so does speech get mushy, fuzzy, unclear. sometimes your hearing impairment takes out a very important ingredient, one that makes the sound special. That's like leaving the currants out of a currant cake. The result is you can't tell the difference between a currant cake and a plain cake. So you may not hear any difference between /sh/ and /s/ because the ingredient (feature) which makes them different can't be heard. 'Shy' and 'sigh' might sound exactly the same. Now let's look at which sounds you don't hear or get mixed up.

I would go on to show which words were not discriminated correctly, which sounds in those words were not heard, and which sounds were confused. We would look at the audiogram to illustrate why some of them were not heard, for example, hearing above 2000 Hz means /s/ not audible, or problems distinguishing between /e/ and /ɛ/ occur because the high frequency ingredient F2 must be audible. The same exploration can be made with the student of important information regarding amplification.

Maximizing Use of Amplification. Maximal use of the hearing aid and classroom amplification systems requires acceptance of these instruments by the child and a willingness to wear them based on an understanding of them. The child needs to know

What the hearing aid is
What difference it makes (aided hearing, aided speech discrimination)
How to take care of the hearing aids by checking mold for wax, reporting discomfort, checking tubing flexibility and discoloration, using a battery tester, having new batteries available, and knowing when it is reasonable to turn off or take off the aids
What the FM receiver is, how it works, and what the settings (M, M-FM, FM) mean

It is also important to devote special attention to educating the student in how to maximize auditory-visual reception. Thus she needs to understand in lay terms the practical effects of noise and reverberation, distance from the person talking, directionality, advantageous seating, and appropriate lighting.

The student needs to understand these factors, know how they affect ability to hear, and know what actions to take in order to account for them. This information cannot be explained just once. It and its applications should be discussed and reviewed frequently.

Every word I have underlined may be used in language and communication enrichment, so one is never neglecting the broad front while attacking a particular need. The extent to which you use and generalize specific vocabulary will depend upon the language age of the child. The opportunities to develop general vocabulary from specific vocabulary abound. Consider for example, some of the words I have underlined:

Watertight In addition to the literal meaning you could expand to include: a watertight case in court or a watertight excuse or argument—we must be sure the plan is watertight.

Mixture We used a mixture of colors. The city has a mixture of races.

Recipe If you do what you say, it's a recipe for disaster. So do you have a recipe for what we can do?

Measure Measure the carpet.
He took his measure [summed him up].
She took an umbrella for good measure.
He took measures to stop the plan from being carried out.
His contribution was beyond measure.
She failed to measure up to my expectations.
My suit was made to measure.
He measured his words.

No matter which aspect you are focusing on, you can branch out to encompass other needs, providing listening-watching training, auditory discrimination training, and speech articulation training. Words defined are placed in various needed syntactic structures; the student is asked to read sentences illustrating their different uses and assigned exercises to write sentences illustrating meaning. Sessions never need be boring because they are relevant and varied. We will adopt the same approach to upgrading language abilities.

3. Auditory and Visual Communication Upgrading.

Our model does not accommodate a separate activity identified as auditory-visual training, far less one that addresses auditory and visual cue processing separately. The final goal we seek to achieve through educational guidance and training in receptive communication skills is comprehension. If you understand what is said to you, the level of your performance in subskills is irrelevant to this goal. On the other hand, as a component of the process leading to spoken language comprehension, the acoustic, and to a lesser extent the visual, speech signal is important. Therefore, to understand how auditory and visual constraint information can be incorporated best into communication training, you need to recall our earlier discussion of the role of constraints, probabilities, predictions, serial versus parallel processing, and bottom up versus top down processing (see Chapter 8). To review those concepts briefly as they apply to the question in hand, I will remind you that communication occurs in a context of place, people, behaviors, and the preceding discussion, if any. The listener sizes up the situation, that is, uses these broad constraints to compute what probably is going on and/or, in communication terms, what topics are likely to be addressed. This, in turn, permits predictions to be made as to what will be said. This is the expectancy stage of the Solley and Murphy model (p. 78). Remember the prediction is of content, of topics. It further is governed by the constraints imposed by the speaker's knowledge of pragmatics as it applies to the situation. For example, you would have little difficulty matching the following scenarios with the questions that follow:

Scenario 1: A restaurant: dinner is over but the diners are still talking freely. The waiter approaches a diner from her left . . .
Scenario 2: Street scene: A pedestrian, piece of paper in hand, stops a passerby.
Scenario 3: Pizza parlor: At the counter after the customer has ordered a medium pizza.
  a. "What do you want on it?"
  b. "Excuse me. Could you tell me where the Motor Vehicle Bureau is?"
  c. "More coffee Madam?"

Having identified the situation and its associated communication probabilities, content constrains vocabulary, making it easy for you to match the following related words and phrases to the appropriate scenarios:

decaffeinated   pepperoni
license   to go
about 15 minutes   black or with milk
                       renew

Your need for the spoken message, for its acoustic and visual pattern, is now relatively small. In fact, all you need is to confirm your prediction (trial and check). On the other hand, if you are on the phone and you need to record the name of a person introduced as Mr. Papadimitrios, you are going to depend very highly on the acoustic speech signal. In the earlier scenarios you were processing top down, synthetically; in the recording of an unfamiliar name you process bottom up, analytically, and will continue to do so until you are able to reply immediately, "Ah Mr. Papadimitrios, how are you?" without any hesitation over the now-familiar name, a process we call *recognition*. At this stage you process top down.

What these examples illustrate is that cognition and spoken language in communication logically cannot be viewed as independent functions. For this reason it is impossible to think of auditory and visual communication training as addressing processing skills that can be worked on independently from the student's cognitive and linguistic needs. There is, however, one exception—working at the phonetic level of speech articulation. This task, as Ling (1976) emphasizes, is nonlinguistic, unrelated to meaning. We will pursue this point when we consider speech training.

It might appear, therefore, that there is little or no role for auditory and visual training; however, this is not so. In fact Ross (1986), addressing auditory training for hearing-impaired children who use hearing in complement with vision, says, "For these children at this stage, auditory training cannot only be a certain period set aside for that purpose; it must permeate the entire school day" (p. 446).

It is apparent that we must understand auditory training in a context different from what used to be called *ear training*. You can exercise and train eyes because they depend upon muscular action, but you cannot train ears. What we train is the auditory cortex by means of the efferent neural pathways, which affect how stimuli received are processed. As I explained earlier, how and what we perceive depend upon how we process information. For the brain to make a prediction, the predicted word or phrase must exist in memory. The image may be an acoustic one, as when you talk in your head, recall a conversation, or hear people talking in dreams. The image also may be motor kinesthetic, as when you silently mouth your thoughts. These relate to the acoustic and motor theories I spoke of earlier.

I wish to emphasize again that there is no justification for auditory and visual training as an end in itself. These are tools not products. The training is cognitive linguistic. We train the brain to recognize and make use of information available in the auditory and visual channels to identify patterns.

Auditory-Visual Training Vocabulary. The first goal of auditory-visual training, therefore, is to ensure that an optimal auditory and visual image is acquired for all new word or phrase patterns.

When confronted with an unfamiliar word pattern, for example *chthonic*, you need to hear it spoken in order to know how to say it. You then speak it several times in order to map the auditory image clearly in the brain and to establish its equivalent motor-articulatory-kinesthetic image; /eɔnɪk/eɔnɪk/. When doing this you often need to have the word said for you several times before you internalize a sufficiently detailed auditory image to allow you to try to make the sound pattern. Try, for example, the name of a local highway, Scajaquada, or even Poughkeepsie. To learn how to pronounce these names you must first hear them. Once learned the word is familiar when heard again; it can be recognized with only minimal cues, just enough to evoke the familiar pattern of the whole. The word now will tolerate considerable distortion while still remaining identifiable.

When working on unfamiliar vocabulary or phrases, use this same model:

- Explain the meaning, given several examples in context (*language cognition*).
- Next, ask the student to listen intently to the sound of the word or phrase repeated five times with a pause between each presentation. This should be done without the student watching (*auditory imaging*).
- Repeat the words five more times while the student watches you say it (*auditory-visual imaging*).
- Have the student say the word several times. If the pronunciation is not correct, model the correct words. Teach correct articulation only when the prob-

lem is compatible with your speech correction curriculum (*motor-articulatory-kinesthetic imaging*).
- Place the word in several simple sentences and repeat each sentence slowly and clearly twice (*contextual imaging*).
- Compare and contrast the word with any similar sounding word. For example, *County-Country*, repeating the pair several times (*discriminatory imaging*).
- Work on the spelling of the word. Request that the student use the word in a sentence. Write the sentence down (*orthographic imaging*).

The new word then should be added to a vocabulary list comprised of recently acquired words. These should be written in a notebook in groups of six. At each session the two latest groups are used for auditory-visual discrimination, for spelling, and for sentence construction. A third group, comprised of words drawn from previous groups, can be used for review. Present the word first in a sentence:

"The Indians were the original <u>inhabitants</u> of North America."

"Say <u>inhabitants</u>."

"Can you make another sentence using the word <u>inhabitants</u>? Try using it to describe people who live in an apartment building."

"The <u>inhabitants</u> of the apartment building had to leave because it caught fire." "Good. You also could say, the <u>inhabitants</u> of the apartments were <u>evacuated</u>. There's a new word—listen, evacuated, evacuated. The <u>inhabitants</u> were <u>evacuated</u>."

All words should arise from the student's vocabulary needs.

Presentations should be made using the best available amplification. When using a hand microphone, the child should speak into it directly when listening to his own speech productions.

Auditory-Visual Training for Comprehension. The manner in which we listen is determined by the purpose for which we listen. That is to say, we process speech differently for different purposes. This processing includes the level of attention we devote to the speaker, the levels of memory used to process the signal (echoic, short term, long term), and the size of the unit processed. Listening for comprehension demands that the student process fairly large chunks for meaning, focusing on key words and phrases in the message. Your activities must reward correct predictions, even approximations of meaning, while ignoring discrimination of parts. To achieve this, activities must emphasize *utilization* of information. The student must be required to *respond* to what he hears. Word discrimination, multiple-choice answers, and repetition of what is heard are inappropriate responses for this purpose. Boothroyd (1978), in a discussion of this language approach to auditory management of hearing-impaired children, described his own experience:

> Everything had to do with comprehension and communication. We did not use discrimination tasks or multiple choice responses. The children's reactions were interesting. They were all children whom we felt ought to be doing better auditorily than they were. They hated training at first, but later came to enjoy it, and they succeeded. When we tested their performance using both analytic discrimination tests and global comprehension tests we didn't get any im-

provement in discrimination. The improvement was in the perception of words in sentences and not in isolated words. (p. 327)

Training for auditory-visual comprehension, therefore, should be an ongoing component of your academic-language-communication and learning support model. The purpose is to modify how the student listens for meaning. This is more linguistically then auditorily determined.

The student's academic content, draw from a textbook or class topic, provides the material. The following sequence outlines the steps:

Add key words and phrases from the unit to new vocabulary already learned, checking to ensure meanings are understood.

Read or present a subsection of the unit. The length will depend upon the student's ability; it might be three or four sentences, or a paragraph

Working with the student, begin to extract from memory general concepts. These may be identified by such questions as

T: *"What is this paragraph about?"*
S: *"Foods."*
T: *"Yes what does it tell you about foods?"*
S: *"I can't remember."*
T: *"Listen again to the sentence, there are four major food groups—there are four major food groups."*
S: *"That there are four groups."*
T: *"Good—there are four major groups."* [check meaning of major]
  "Listen, I will name some foods, you tell me which major group they belong to, butter, milk, cream, eggs.
  Which group? No?
  O.K. Let's review the four groups. Listen, the four groups are meats, dairy products, vegetables and fruit, cereals."

Then review the categories of proteins, fats, carbohydrates, sugars, and so on.

When comprehension has been ensured, read the unit over again before progressing to the next. Then for auditory or auditory-visual training, place key vocabulary in sentences that require a response.

"Name a food in the vegetable group."
"Is an egg a meat product or a dairy product?"
"What does milk give the body?"
"Doughnuts contain mostly _____."

Predictions can be encouraged by techniques such as forced choice. Write the choices on the board:

"Tell me which word I say—Breads and cereals provide <u>carbohydrates—carbohydrates</u>."

	dairy products	meats and fish
choices	fats	<u>carbohydrates</u>
	vegetables	proteins

Put up a word, for example, chicken or energy. Then tell the student you will say something about it but that she has to provide the missing word.

Chicken is a good food because it gives our body _____.

We get quick energy when we eat _____.

If a word is not correctly identified, put several words on the board including the answer, then repeat the question.

It is important to keep in mind that the purpose of this lesson must be communication enrichment, not auditory training and speech-reading. These skills are practiced as part of the whole process of receiving and processing spoken language for the purpose of learning. Remember also that your purpose is to support language growth in accord with classroom demands, not to teach academic content. It also is to teach communication strategies as a means of compensating for the hearing deficit. I see no place for intensive general listening-watching drills. Focused intensive listening is of value when pursued for a very specific purpose. For example, if the student is having difficulty discriminating between two similar words, take the following steps:

- Ensure that the meaning of the words is clearly differentiated.
- Place the words in sentences that indicate the meaning.
- Listen carefully to each of the words presented separately several times immediately after you say it in the sentence.
- Present one of the words three times, then the other three times.
- Present the two words in pairs for comparison.
- Test to see if discrimination has been achieved.
- Generate sentences that omit the key word. Ask the child to deduce from the context which word should be used.

Most confusions can be resolved linguistically. You should question, however, whether the discrimination difficulty occurs only in certain consonant-vowel, consonant-vowel-consonant, or vowel-consonant combinations. If this is the case very intensive short sessions (1–2 minutes) spent listening to those combinations might enhance discrimination. Fry (1978) has explained that when a child cannot hear the acoustic cues to a speech sound, he may learn to use the second formant transition cue to identify it. That is, the child predicts the inaudible sound from its foreshadowing by its coarticulatory influence on the audible preceding sounds.

As with everything else you do, the ultimate determinant will be time, relevance, and efficiency. You must determine how your limited time with the child may be invested for maximum return. We will return to a discussion of auditory training when we discuss phonetic level speech training. I leave the topic at this point by quoting four of a number of conclusions Ling (1978, p. 210) reached about auditory training.

1. Auditory training may be considered as a series of structured, progressively ordered exercises in the detection, discrimination, identification, and comprehension of speech.
2. Auditory training should be closely related to cognitive and linguistic growth and to motor speech development.
3. Auditory training should be geared toward meeting the needs of individual children. Because cognitive, linguistic, and speech skills vary from one child to another and as hearing impairment may range from slight to total deafness, the notion of an "auditory training syllabus" that could be applicable to all hearing-impaired children is untenable.

4. Auditory training is distinct from auditory experience. Auditory experience, exposure to an abundance of meaningful speech and sound, may be sufficient for one child to master spoken language skills, but insufficient for another. Auditory training should be provided prescriptively as a supplement when particular auditory skills cannot be acquired simply through auditory experience (Ling, 1978, p. 210).

4. Language Knowledge and Use Enrichment

Language lies at the core of the hearing-impaired child's success or failure in school because the learning experience is embedded within it. Laughton and Hasenstab (1986) state that

> school equals language use, whether the task involves listening to reading, speaking or writing language. Through awareness of school language, a child is expected to function independently in the use of receptive language (listening, reading) and expressive language (speaking, writing) by the fourth grade in order to support learning in the content subjects (e.g., the language of math or history books). (p. 9)

During the preschool years our emphasis was on the teaching of language. We used naturally occurring situations and we contrived circumstances to foster a need for verbal communication so we could provide appropriate language for the child to learn. Language, we decided, must be learned; it cannot be taught. Our task was to optimize the learning opportunities through molding experience and participation in the language. By the time the child enters the primary grades, she not only must be able to learn through language, she must be able to contemplate it. *Metalinguistics*, as this process is called, involves analyzing and talking about language, that is, knowing how it works (Menyuk, 1976). It is to this self-awareness of how to make language function better for her that our efforts with the student will be directed. This does not mean that we provide the student with an intensive course on linguistics, but that we lead her to an awareness of the processes involved. When you self-correct the linguistic form of something you have said, or wonder whether you should say "him and me" or "he and I," you are using linguistic awareness without necessarily knowing the linguistic rule.

Consider first these guidelines for language enrichment:

- Language enrichment should address both expressive and receptive forms.
- All aspects of language from phonology to pragmatics should be addressed.
- Interaction of language aspects should be demonstrated.
- Current language needs should direct lesson goals.
- New language content and structures should be founded on experience.
- New language content and form should be linked to old knowledge.
- Emphasis must be on language use. The student must learn how to understand and to generate language rules.

When you work with the student, your perception of your task will determine your approach. It should be to enrich learning through improved communication competence. When we discussed auditory-visual training, we linked it to vocabulary syntax and semantics. Similarly when you work on language vocabulary, form, and structure or on pragmatics and conversation, you will ensure that the auditory-visual patterns are well learned. You also will deal with the spoken and written forms of what is learned.

Enriching Vocabulary. The possession of an extensive vocabulary is of little use unless it has contextual meaning and can be used in sentence frames. You could learn every word in the dictionary yet lack the understanding of how the words can be used in communication. Thus words must be learned contextually within the framework of the student's syntactic and experiential knowledge. In this way the other words and the syntax of the sentence contribute to the semantic value of the new word, providing the broadest possible understanding of its meaning. To achieve this the base meaning of the word needs to be highlighted, generalizing from the specific context to broader frames of reference. Other forms of the word derived from the same root should be explored and placed in context. Finally you should discuss words that commonly occur in the same topical context as the key word or phrase. For example, if the word *settlers* occurs in a social studies text you would

EXPLAIN THE WORD

Settlers (noun): people who move to a new country or to another part of the country to develop new land, build new communities (homes, churches, stores, schools). It is a word we use about people in history.

USE IN EXISTING CONTEXT

The early settlers in America were Pilgrims from England. The settlers had to get all their tools and equipment from England. The lives of the Pilgrim settlers were hard.

TEACH DERIVATIVES

To settle (verb): to set up a colony or community, to place firmly, to alight, to cease to move and come to rest (to settle down), to put things in order.

USE IN CONTEXT

The Pilgrims *settled* in the northeastern part of North America.
They *settled* their disagreements with the Indians.

USE IN DIFFERENT CONTEXTS

My family finally *settled* in Oregon.
We are very *settled* here.
The butterfly *settled* on the flower.
The campers *settled* down for the night.
The victim *settled* his lawsuit out of court.
He *settled* his affairs with the store.
O.K. then, its all *settled*.
I want to *settle* the bill.
Let me *settle* up with you.
I wouldn't *settle* for less.

EXPLAIN THE WORD

Settlement (noun): the community built by the settlers.
A settling up. What people agree to accept.

USE IN CONTEXT

The new communities the Pilgrims built were called *settlements*.
Today there are religious *settlements* in Pennsylvania called Amish *settlements*.
The Pilgrims reached a *settlement* of their differences with England.

OTHER RELATED VOCABULARY

Emigrant, emigrate, immigrant, immigrate
Community (in all its applications)
Pioneer(s), inhabitants

Such vocabulary enrichment is highly relevant to the student's needs, creating an opportunity to expand cognitive knowledge. Auditory and visual communication training is given as the words are used in context. The words are written up by the student on the board or on a pad, read by the student, and discriminated auditorily and visually. The response to auditory presentation should be written to ensure correct spelling of the words presented in context, as I explained in the previous section.

The vocabulary needs of the child are primarily subject specific, since it is academic content and classroom activities that are creating the demand. The student should be encouraged to identify all words in textbooks, handouts, and laboratory experiment instructions with which he is unfamiliar. It helps for you or the teacher to spot check understanding of key vocabulary. Be alert also for uncertainties about the vocabulary of instructions and directions (see discussion of the Boehm Test of Basic Concepts [Chapter 17, p. 354] and the assessment of the student's ability to follow directions [Chapter 17, p. 365]). Do not assume an understanding of such words and phrases as

alternate, omit, except, compare, place in order, that fit,
group, fill in, compose, complete, underline, the exercise,
following, word down, word across, even numbered, every other

The demands of each subject need to be considered, including art, music, sports, industrial arts, and driver education. You cannot meet every need, but if you are to address the most demanding, it will be necessary to monitor them all in cooperation with classroom teachers.

In addition to subject-specific needs, the need for enrichment of general vocabulary knowledge is present for most hearing-impaired children throughout their school years. This cannot be achieved by creating lists of words to be learned. The way to enrich general vocabulary is to create situations that give rise to such words. This can be achieved best by

- Extending the meanings of subject-specific vocabulary to more general usage.
- Raising topical social issues to which the student can relate. These could include the school plays, a class outing, clubs, hobbies, organizations, sporting activities, the orchestra or chorus, little league, the junior prom, dating, college, or work plans.
- Developing conversational scenarios that can be constructed around such familiar experiences as asking someone to a prom, going out on a date, and interviewing for a summer job or with younger students, inviting someone to a birthday party or sleep-over and meeting new friends at boy or girl scout meetings.

The need for vocabulary must arise from contextually cued experiences. Words are the material of communication. They must be used in meaningful situations to be comprehended. They must link to related words and thus to related experiences. This link either *expands* a conceptual category:

> *Cow*—expands to cattle and refers also to female elephants, buffalo, moose, and whales

or *contracts* a conceptual category:

> *Cattle*—contracts to cow, heifer, bull, bullock, steer.
> *Cow*—contracts to heifer
> *Bull*—contracts to bullock or steer

Sometimes it is essential to differentiate between meanings of words in similar categories, for example, between cow and heifer, bull and steer.

Vocabulary alone does not make language. Meanings lie not just within the building materials but in the design, as illustrated by the sentence

> Grew puritans corn first the

Enrichment of syntax, therefore, should dovetail with the other language enrichment approaches rather than being concentrated on teaching students the basic patterns of English sentence structure (Laughton & Hasenstab, 1986). The specific structures that you select to teach or correct will be drawn from the diagnostic assessment of syntax we discussed in the previous chapter. Your task now is to use the vocabulary and semantics of academic content and context to illustrate and provide meaningful structures to be acquired. Take, for example, the student who exhibits incorrect use of the gerund (a verbal noun that also has verbal properties). For example, a student says

> The coastline was very rocky.
> The Pilgrims *avoided to land* there.

She is failing to follow the verb with the gerund, *landing.*

> The Pilgrims avoided landing there.

Explain that certain verbs (check that the student understands that verbs are words of actions or happenings) take the *-ing* form, never *to.* Generate examples related to the topic.

> The Pilgrims *avoided landing* on the rocks.
> *not* The Pilgrims avoided to land on the rocks.

> They *enjoyed resting* after the awful journey.
> *not* They enjoyed to rest after the awful journey.

> The early settlers *kept moving* west.
> *not* The early settlers kept to move west.

Generalize to other examples:

> I *practice playing* the piano.
> *not* I practice to play the piano.

I will *suggest going* to the zoo.
not I will suggest to go to the zoo.

She *imagined running* in the Olympics.
not She imagined to run in the Olympics.

It would be absurd to assume that you could teach this form for every verb to which it applies (admit, appreciate, miss, mind, postpone, prefer, etc.). The goal is to establish a strong linguistic model for this structure in the student's mind. By establishing such a model and by drawing attention to it when it occurs in spoken and written language, we increase the chances of its being noticed when attention is not drawn to it. Eventually, a process of adaptation to the norm in appropriate circumstances will occur.

Another example of teaching such a model might involve the difference between active and passive voice, or the form of the verb.

Check that the student understands subjects (Who? or What?), verbs (Did what or Experienced what?), and objects (To whom or Because of whom?). Explain that in the *active* form there is action or experience by the subject. The subject does something to someone or something.
Illustrate active voice:
The Pilgrims put up tents.
The Indians attacked the settlers.
John forgot his homework.
Mary raised her hand.
Explain that in the passive form the subject has something happen to him/her or it. The subject does not act.
The tents *were put up*.
The settlers *were attacked*.
John's homework *was forgotten*.
Mary's hand *was raised*.

Practice in the use of the new form should be incorporated into *receptive processing* (listening only, listening and watching, reading) and into *expressive processing* (speaking and writing the sentences). For example, for auditory training you can put on the board sentences in active and passive voice. The student is asked to listen carefully to one of the first pair. She must select the one you said and decide whether it is active or passive. If it is not discriminable auditorily, the sentence should be repeated with visual cues. For spelling, practice sentences of both kinds can be dictated without and with visual speech cues. Similarly sentences can be read from a list with decisions being made as to their active or passive nature.

A helpful guide to the types of language problems experienced by hearing-impaired persons is *Better English Usage—A Guide for the Deaf* by Greenberg and Withers (1965). This text gives examples in aspects of language usage most commonly in error in the communication of congenitally hearing-impaired persons.

In each stage of language we have discussed, I have stressed the importance of context. Situational and contextual constraints, as we have seen, play an important role both in perceiving the message being received and in encoding messages to enhance their ease of comprehension by others. This use of constraints culminates in the processes of pragmatics and conversation, which will constitute the final components in our discussion of enhancement of language use.

Enriching Pragmatic and Conversational Skills. You may recall the quote I drew from Lund and Duchan who said that pragmatics involves "the participant's conceptualization of the kind of interaction he or she is having" (1988, p. 49). This ability to perceive and interpret the nature of a situation, the roles of the people in it, and one's own place in the situation is a prerequisite to appropriate, as opposed to structurally correct, linguistic behavior. Activities chosen to enhance pragmatic skills seek to increase this awareness. The three types of constraints we wish the student to be more aware of are (1) the physical setting, (2) the action patterns or scripts, and (3) discourse events.

1. *Physical Setting.* The student should be able to sum up the environmental situation and recognize people in context and the probable roles they play. To do this we must encourage the student to make predictions and form hypotheses based upon probabilities. We must encourage predictions concerning which transactions are most probable, which are most unlikely. This knowledge will facilitate identification of the discourse topic, since it permits a rank ordering of probabilities that in turn influences the linguistic set.

2. *Action Patterns/Scripts.* To read these the student needs to know the ritual associated with the physical environment and the likely transactions to occur within it. This reading further constrains probabilities by associating probable behaviors and discourse topics with the environment and the people within it.

3. *Discourse Events.* The pragmatic knowledge that steers discourse commonly is deficient in students with congenitally and prelinguistically acquired hearing impairment. This knowledge permits the participants in discourse to track conversational exchanges and to interpret the underlying intent of the linguistic message, referred to as *illocutionary force* (Searle, 1975). For example, when mother says,

"You're not going to walk all over my carpet in those dirty boots?," she knows the answer and expects action, not a verbal response.
"I'm hungry" usually has the hidden intent of "I would like to eat."
"Do you think that's a good idea?" means "I don't think that's a good idea."

These speech acts are further clarified by presumptions or *presuppositions* we make about what our listener already knows. "Jane isn't coming" presupposes that you know Jane. Pragmatic assumptions such as "Take out your reading book" depend on knowledge that there is but one reading book, while the semantic presupposition "Last time we read chapter six; I want you to read the next two chapters" makes the command dependent on carrying forward semantic information from the first statement.

Enrichment in understanding of these functions in discourse and conversation requires that we develop activities that generate occurrences of such communication behaviors. Consider now the types of activities that will foster this.

Physical Environment. To enhance the student's ability to read the probable informational constraints of environment, you could use photos or illustrations of various settings as the constraining information. For each setting ask the student to identify the people usually encountered in that setting and what they usually do. Such pictures might illustrate a(an)

fast food outlet	physics/chemistry lab
post office counter	gymnasium
dentist's office	industrial arts classroom
department store	swimming pool

The student is asked to identify where he is from each environment, and to identify people he expects to find there:

clerk
swimming instructor
dentist
teacher
salesperson

These names can be given auditorily or auditorily-visually (auditory-visual training) or written on cards (reading) and can be placed in sentences using constructions appropriate to the student's syntactic needs. They also can be used for phonologic speech practice.

Typical situational scenarios might be

We wait in the waiting room.
We look at the magazines.
A lady in a white coat tells us to come in.
We sit in the big chair.
The lady puts a white bib around our necks.
Another lady or man comes.
We open our mouth.

We go in the car.
We park the car.
We go up to a counter.
We look up at a list of things.
A girl asks us a question.
She talks into a microphone.
We wait.
The girl gives us a bag.
We give her money.
We go to a table.

Again, all aspects of communication training can be incorporated.

Discourse Events. The ultimate goal of all language enrichment is to facilitate communication exchanges. Discourse, either dyadic or small group, demands the functional use of the language abilities we have been discussing. It also creates the need to become familiar and comfortable with the use of the formal rules of conversation.

We are so used to *teaching* handicapped children and adults that we often control the communication-learning event throughout the session. Yet you will agree that we all learn best through involvement in a task, since experience makes knowledge functional. When this philosophy is applied to communication, it demands that we serve as facilitators and models for the student, in a partnership relationship rather than as instructor and student. Therefore, as far as possible, control should lie with the student. It is important to move with her comments or contributions rather than insist she provide the response we require, or even that she stay within our lesson plan. This requires that we allow the student to use her language to explore ideas or experiences within a roughly defined topic. Our purpose must be to use the techniques we know to facilitate her formulation, organization, and expression of those ideas through conversation. You will not achieve this immediately for it requires a different mental set from the teaching model most of us were trained to use. It requires a commitment to the belief that the knowledge to be acquired can be learned best through participation.

Developing Conversational Skills. The conversational framework developed by Stone and described in his 1988 text lends itself perfectly to your needs for a model by which to increase the student's conversational resources. Stone's framework includes

- Structure: rules for managing the conversation, namely initiating, turn taking, and ending
- Function: sharing of thoughts, ideas, and feelings achieved through commenting on what has been said, requesting information, acknowledging, and replying to what is said
- Form: created by semantic, syntactic, and morphologic constructions

Stone tabulates the relationship among these three components as shown in Table 18.1.

Using the Scenario Model. Stone uses the scenario as the basis for enrichment of structure, function, and form through dialogue or conversation. Scenarios are described as

role playing situations which contain appropriate dialogue. They are planned by the teacher and presented to the child in such a way that a realistic conversation takes place between teacher and child. (Stone, 1988, p. 28)

TABLE 18.1 Conversational framework

Structure	Function	Form
• Initiation	• Topic Introduction Requests Comments	• Semantics
		• Syntax
• Turn Taking	• Topic Maintenance Answers Acknowledgements Requests Comments	• Morphology
• Ending		

The goal of the scenario is to provide an opportunity to demonstrate and allow the student to model and practice a particular aspect of conversation. To achieve this, Stone identifies five essential elements of the conversational scenario:

- The student must be familiar with the situational topic. It is only possible to converse in a meaningful way about situations or topics with which one has some familiarity. Familiarity should further be refined by the requirement of relevance.
- The student understands the situation before you begin.
- The scenario generates a demand for the targeted skill.
- You do not tell the child what to say, though you model a correct form of what he has said.
- The situation and conversation come to a logical completion.

Topics for Scenarios. Our philosophy throughout has been to take an integrated holistic approach to providing communicative-learning enrichment. Thus topics for discussion should be drawn from school-related situations, both academic and nonacademic, and from the student's social needs. Conversational scenarios may be very simple with limited vocabulary and basic syntactic structures. A topic for an early primary-grade child might be a homework assignment not handed in. The goal is for David to practice

- Opening a discourse
- Maintaining a topic
- Requesting information

First describe the scenario:

You: *"David do you remember last week you told me your teacher was cross because you did not do your homework?"*
David: *"Yes."*
You: *"Let's pretend that I am your teacher and you have forgotten your homework again. This time you did it, but you forgot to bring it. You were late this morning and almost missed the school bus. O.K. I'm the teacher and you're you. Do you understand?"*
David: *"Yes."*
You: *"Who am I?"*
David: *"The teacher."*
You: *"Right, and who are you?"*
David: *"Me."*
You: *"Yes, let's begin."* (as teacher) *"David, you haven't given me your homework yet."*
David: *"I forget."* (incorrect tense)
You: (as teacher) *"You forgot? You forgot last week too."* [correct tense modeled]
David: *"No."*
You: (as teacher) *"No what?"* [expansion requested]
David: *"I have it—home."* [preposition omitted]
You: (as teacher) *"You left it at home. You left your homework at home?"* [preposition emphasized]
David: *"Yes, at home."* [corrected preposition] *"I late. School bus."*
You: (as teacher) *"You were late for the bus."* [corrected verb] *"You forgot your homework. You left it at home."*
David: *"Yes, I forgot."* [David corrects verb]
You: (as teacher) *"You did your homework but you forgot it because you were late. How will you remember it tomorrow?"*

David: *"Don't know."*
You: *(as teacher) "Will you put it in your bag?"*
David: *"Yes, in my bag, tonight."*
You: *(as teacher) "Good, you'll remember to put your homework in your bag tonight." (as therapist) "That's good David; now let's change places. You pretend to be the teacher; I will be David."*

Note that during the scenario you presented a model of the teacher's role and you modeled for David the conversational structures with which he had difficulty. Emphasis was placed upon missing parts of speech and on correcting tenses. By reversing the roles David now gets to observe the role he just played and to experience the teacher's role and perspective. At this point, since the scenario has now been established, more attention can be paid to structure. Each time the student uses a clearly defective or inappropriate structure you stop the conversation in order to reverse roles. You actually change seats to help keep roles separate. This permits you to model the correct structure within the actual conversational transaction. It provides for experiential learning rather than academic instruction. Once modeled you resume your original role for a replay. Observe how this works. David, you will remember, has now assumed the teacher's role.

David: *(as teacher) "Where your homework David?"*
You: *"Change seats with me, I'll be the teacher."*
You: *(as teacher) "Where is your homework David?"*
You: *"Change again. You are the teacher."*
David: *(as teacher) "Where is your homework David?"*
You: *(as David) "It's at home."*
David: *(as teacher) "Why home?"*
You: *(as David) "I forgot it. I was late for the school bus."*
David: *(as teacher) "OK." (This response is inappropriate so you model one that is more logical.)*
You: *"Change again—I'm the teacher."*
You: *(as teacher) "Oh you forgot it. Bring it tomorrow. Don't forget."*
You: *"Change again; now you are the teacher, David."*
David: *(as teacher) "Oh you forget it."*
    [change]
You: *(as David) "Oh you forgot it."*
    [change]
David: *"Oh you forgot it. Tomorrow bring it."*
You: *(as David) "I'll put it in my bag tonight."*
David: *(as teacher) "Good. OK."*
You: *"Good David, you did that well."*

Conversational scenarios can be selected and structured to emphasize the modeling and use of initiating conversation, introducing new topics, requesting information or offering opinions. A series of short scenarios may be selected to rehearse turn taking and topic maintenance or may emphasize ways of terminating a communication transaction.

The same techniques are effective with older students with whom the conversational model may be used to review academic subject matter taught in class. At the same time experience with the use of vocabulary and syntax is provided and an opportunity for self-monitoring of quality speech is created in context. For example, the topic may have been a basic introduction to magnetism and electricity. Key vocabulary first has been reviewed for meaning, for audiovisual recognition, and for spoken and written expression. The vocabulary list included:

Magnet	Attract
Poles	Repel
Polarity	Magnetic field
Alternating	Lines of force
Filings	

You will have reviewed the vocabulary in the context of physics, but you also will have generalized the meaning of such terms as

Attraction: "She felt an attraction for John"; "The concert was a real attraction; everyone wanted to go"; "Coming attractions at the movies were listed."

Attractive: "She was a very attractive girl."

To attract: "He attracted the teacher's attention."

Magnetism: "He had a certain magnetism; everyone was attracted to him."

Magnet: "The concert was a real magnet; it attracted everyone."

To magnetize: "The speaker magnetized the audience. You could feel the electricity."

To file: "The teacher told the students to file their notes in the binder."

Filing: "Mary was filing her nails."

Filings: "The nail filings made a mess."

The topic for discussion will be an experiment that Margaret conducted. In the experiment she did two things. First she took two magnets and observed that depending upon which ends she chose, the magnets either *attracted* each other, snapping together, or they *repelled* each other, illustrating polarity. You may depict this visually by diagram to remind Margaret.

$$S \rightarrow \leftarrow N \qquad \leftarrow N \qquad N \rightarrow \qquad \leftarrow S \qquad S \rightarrow$$

Next she sprinkled iron filings on a sheet of paper and held it over a magnet. She saw how the iron filings formed a pattern illustrating the *lines of magnetic force.* The words and simple diagrams to remind Margaret of the experiment are on the blackboard or in a note pad. You will not talk together about the experiment. The goal is for Margaret to

Initiate conversation using appropriate routines
Provide a complete setting for what is to be recounted
Explain fully facts not known to the listener
Develop the conversation in a logical sequence

You: *"Margaret, you asked if we could go over that physics lab project you did. Pretend that I know nothing about it. You want to tell me what you did. Remember the way we do this is when what you say needs improvement we change places, I say it for you, then we change back. Do you remember how we do this?"*

Margaret: *"Yes."*

You: *"OK, why don't you begin."*

Margaret: *"We used magnets."*

You: *"Let's change on that because I do not know anything about your physics class."* [change]

You: *(as Margaret) "In physics class we did a lab experiment."*
or
"Our physics lab experiment was really fun."
or
"I have to tell you what we did in physics lab."
[change]
Margaret: *"We had fun in physics lab."*
You: *"Oh—what did you do?"*
Margaret: *"They push each other but then they pulled."*
You: *"I don't understand—let's change."*
You: *(as Margaret): "We did an experiment. We put two magnets together."*
[change]
Margaret: *"We did experiment. We put the magnets together."*
You: *"What happened?"*
Margaret: *"They pulled and pushed."*
You: *"I'm not sure I understand. Let's change."*
You: *(as Margaret) "When we put the same ends, the same poles together, they pushed apart—they repelled. When we put different poles together, they pulled together—they attracted."*
[change]
Margaret: *"The same ends, I mean poles, pushed away. The different ends pulled together, attract."*
You: *"Did you do anything else?"*
Margaret: *"Yes, iron on paper."*
[change]
You: *(as Margaret) "Yes. We did an experiment with iron filings. We put them on a piece of paper."*
Margaret: *"We put iron filings on piece paper."*
You: *"Then what did you do?"*
Margaret: *"When magnet under the paper the iron made pattern."*
[change]
You: *(as Margaret) "We put a magnet under the piece of paper. The magnet made the filings move. They made a pattern."*

So the discourse continues. Conversational discourse is a useful technique for reinforcing vocabulary, for helping the student to conceptualize experience linguistically, and for enhancing her capacity to participate effectively as a communicator. It provides a learning model that intergrates the several aspects of spoken communication in a realistic and meaningful manner. Phonologic speech production is among the components that can be given attention during the conversation, though phonetic level production will still need separate instruction.

5. Speech Intelligibility Improvement

It is unrealistic to assume that a primary- or even secondary-level student can benefit from a whole session devoted only to speech teaching and improvement. Furthermore, it is a rare student whose hearing impairment creates no more than a need for speech training. Thus, speech intelligibility improvement effort also must be part of an integrated management program related most closely to vocabulary, spelling, and reading. The Ling method of teaching speech, which I outlined in Chapter 15, will prove practical and, I believe, efficient for use with students in primary and secondary schools. Your assessment data will have identified the baseline phonetic level performance of the student in voice production and control, vowel and dipthong production, and consonant production. This data identifies consonant-vowel, vowel-consonant, and vowel-consonant-vowel combinations that must yet be acquired or raised to automaticity. You can use this information to select the particular voice and/or articulation behaviors to be targeted for intervention.

The analysis of the spontaneous spoken language sample will provide details of which sounds at the phonologic level are used correctly either intermittently or consistently. By comparing the phonetic assessment data with the phonological data, you will be able to identify sounds that can be produced but are not being used phonologically. You have, therefore, the information you require (1) to select one or two targets to teach at the phonetic level and (2) to identify sounds to be reinforced or introduced at the phonologic level.

Phonetic Level. The teaching strategies for this level have been specified sound-by-sound in the Ling (1976) text. Having identified one or two targets to be achieved, you will need to plan each intervention session to include several brief interludes of two or three minutes to be devoted to intensive phonetic level speech teaching. You naturally will incorporate auditory and visual awareness of the speech-sound patterns into the teaching of the speech sounds. Remember to protect phonetic integrity from the phonologic contamination of habitual speech patterns of already acquired words. Do not be tempted to use words or pictures at this level of instruction. Work intensively and fast during each minisession. Ensure that newly acquired articulation patterns can be produced in the full range of phonetic contexts and that they are practiced to the level of automaticity.

Phonologic Level. At the phonologic level, you will have identified sounds that are used correctly in some phonetic contexts but not in others and some that are used correctly but not consistently in a given context. You will drop back to the phonetic level to teach the production of sounds in contexts in which they are not used phonologically and will practice to automaticity those intermittently used. Sounds newly raised to automaticity will be introduced into words in context. You will need to gain the cooperation of teachers and parents to expect correct articulation in the spoken language and oral reading of those sounds that the student can produce to the level of automaticity. Reinforcement of the correct articulation of these sounds in communication can be achieved by acknowledging their appropriate use, by modeling, and often by simply drawing the student's attention to the word in question. This reinforcement needs to be provided at appropriate times in the classroom and at home. Activities such as learning or reviewing vocabulary words, learning to discriminate and spell new words, and learning syntactic structures and discourse role playing all present opportunities by which phonologic speech improvement can be integrated into a holistic model of intervention. Reading aloud also lends itself well to this end and provides an additional rationale for incorporating reading into your intervention program.

6. Reading, Writing, and Communication

Teaching reading skills to hearing-impaired children, as I pointed out in the previous chapter, requires an expertise that is not part of the qualifications of a speech-language pathologist or audiologist. Thus our role is to use the reading skills the child has acquired in class or with the remedial reading specialist to reinforce all levels of language knowledge from vocabulary to semantics. Reading can be used to enhance conceptualization through language, to broaden conceptual knowledge, and to provide a controlled structure for phonologic speech monitoring. Reading aloud helps the student become aware of individual word units within speech and focuses his articulation of them, and it generates a need for appropriate use of suprasegmentals, focusing attention on syntactic structure. It thus provides a valuable tool for integrating most of the language components we have discussed.

The reading of information presented or reviewed in your sessions should constitute the last stage of each activity. It should serve as a reinforcement to all other stages. Thus if we are reviewing key vocabulary for a lesson, reading the words will culminate the sequence of listen, watch, discriminate, say, explain, and place in a sentence. When this sequence has been completed, the student reads the key words and sentences in the list presented in random order. Finally she writes them from dictation. A lesson or experiment that you have reviewed with a student, establishing what occurred, what information was presented, in what order, with what result, or to what conclusion, can be read from the text to determine comprehension of the written information. The student might then, as an assignment, describe the content in her own words.

In a discourse activity, a summary of the scenario to be enacted may be written on a card. Once you have explained the roles, the student can be asked to read the description of the scenario. Likewise, reading will be a primary component in reviewing grade level survival knowledge for specific subjects. For example, in understanding the instructions pertaining to solving a quadratic equation or calculating the cubic area of a box, the student must comprehend the printed explanation. Consider written expression as a tool with which the student can discover her own needs in the use of verbal expression and organization of thoughts. Short written assignments read aloud to you or in a small-group situation provide a means of monitoring and thus providing for language needs.

Although written English does not mirror spoken language exactly, it is dependent upon linguistic competence in all aspects of language. We cannot afford to neglect this form of communication in our effort to upgrade the communicative-learning abilities of the hearing-impaired student. Finally, we must acknowledge that coordination of our written language planning with the work of the classroom teacher and reading specialist is essential. Although we each have a different contribution to make, we need to ensure cooperative supportive assistance to the student. We should not, for example, be setting quite separate vocabulary learning assignments, as occurred with one 13-year-old hearing-impaired student. He ended up with three times the number of vocabulary words his hearing peers had to learn because he had separate lists from his classroom teacher, itinerant teacher, and speech-language pathologist.

Receptive and expressive language skills constitute the primary means of knowledge acquisition in secondary and postsecondary education. Since both are extensions of listening and speaking, accommodating them within our holistic model is unavoidable. For older children, the use of the written language form also may provide a valuable vehicle for expressing, exploring, and discussing feelings related to being hearing impaired. The need to address the socioemotional cost of hearing impairment constitutes the final component in our consideration of intervention strategies for the school-age child and young adult.

7. Adjustment Counseling

Of all the areas of need created by a communication difficulty, it is the need for support in resolving feelings and problems of interpersonal relationships that beginning teacher/therapists and audiologists feel the least competent to address. This situation cannot be resolved by referring all hearing-impaired students to a psychologist to ensure that their socioemotional needs are adequately provided for. Perhaps more important is the fact that almost all of the feelings and experiences that are troubling these young people are quite understandable in light of the handicap with which they must deal. Their reactions to the difficult situations they encounter usually are justifiable even though not satisfactory. What you are asked to provide, therefore, is a relationship in which these understandable emotional feelings and interpersonal difficulties are safe to express and explore. You are asked to encourage a sharing of difficulties and to provide empathy, acceptance, and a genuine interest in understanding those experiences and feelings. This model demands that you focus on providing support rather than directive counseling. Management of the socioemotional needs of the student is based on the application of the model we have used throughout our discussions.

Describe the Problem. In the previous chapter we considered ways in which we can explore informally the socioemotional status of the student in school. You will have learned from the class teacher(s) how well the student manages the stresses that arise from the learning demands of the classroom. The teacher will have profiled the student's behavior in terms of attitude to work, level of frustration, reaction to frustration, relationships with classmates, and so on. You also will have discussed with the student's parents their feelings about how well their child is coping with the effects of hearing impairment. They will have profiled his relationships at home, how he reacts to frustrations, and how often his verbal or perhaps physical expressions of anger or his withdrawal behaviors, prove difficult to understand. The parents will have expressed their concerns and anxieties about this aspect of their son's problem, and they will have responded to questions about his social activities and friends and how he spends his free time. You may even have been successful in exploring with teacher(s) and parents how they react to the student's expression of frustration at being different.

Finally over a number of sessions, during which you will be working with the student to better meet a range of communication-learning demands, you gradually will learn how he feels about the situation in which he finds himself. At this point, having a fairly clear picture of the student's difficulties, you will turn to available resources to attempt to begin to effect change.

Resources. Resources consist of

- Teacher(s) willing to explore modification in demands and management procedures to reduce stress in class
- Parents who are prepared to attempt to explore alternate ways of handling frustrating situations at home
- Siblings who may be influential in contributing to changing relationships
- Peers, particularly special girl or boy friends whose influence with older students usually is particularly strong
- Other students with hearing impairments or even other physical disabilities who will have credibility in discussions of feelings and how to react in difficult situations
- Leaders of extracurricular activities that may be of interest to the student
- Counselor/psychologist who may be used as a consultant to provide you with reassurance or direction with difficult situations and for referral of the student if you feel that is necessary
- The student himself, whose usefulness as a resource could prove equal to or more important than all others

Plan a Strategy for Intervention. Your first goal should be to endeavor to effect a more supportive environment for the student. This involves discussing the situation with the counselor/psychologist and teachers to share ideas concerning ways to reduce the pressures felt by the student. This usually is achieved as a result of a better understanding of the situations that cause frustration and a better appreciation of the relationship of the student's attitudes and behaviors to the communication/learning handicap. Identification of specific situations in which unproductive or unacceptable attitudes and behaviors are manifest facilitates analysis of how these were managed, how the student reacted, and how management techniques might be modified to be more effective. Discussion needs to focus on goals for socioemotional growth. You will recall we explored this approach when we discussed behavior management with the preschool child (Chapter 15, p. 301).

Socioemotional goals for a particular student, Amy, might be to

Increase her willingness to participate in class
Reduce the amount of stress she experiences over homework assignments
Reduce the self-negation she experiences when her efforts are not successful

For Michael, who response to these difficulties is different, short-term goals might be to

Reduce his need for constant attention from teachers and classmates
Increase his self-confidence in assuming responsibility
Increase his ability to participate in group tasks

For each goal a strategy needs to be identified. This requires that the present management support techniques be examined and possible other approaches explored. The following discussion might take place to deal with Amy's problems:

You: *"How do you handle Amy's unwillingness to participate in class now?"*

Teacher: *"Well, I used to put some pressure on her but that usually ended up with her in tears which meant she withdrew totally from the lesson. Now I just never call on her; in fact, I tend to avoid eye contact with her."*

Counselor/Psychologist: *"Where does she sit in class?"*

Teacher: *"About two-thirds of the way back."*

You: *"Would it help to move her more forward? Not to the front, but closer."*

Teacher: *"It might make me give her more attention."*

Counselor/Psychologist: *"You would have to do it as part of a more general seat adjustment."*

Teacher: *"Yes, but that won't be enough."*

You: *"Perhaps if we took Amy into our confidence, explained how we want to help her and plan a strategy together it might work. What I am thinking of is that she and I really prepare for an upcoming lesson; work out with you two or three topic areas you could ask her about. We could role play them so she would feel more confident after rehearsal, and you could bring her into the class participation."*

Teacher: *"It might work."*

Counselor/Psychologist: *"You would need to treat her just like any of the other kids in the discussion—not make a big deal over her participation, moving on easily whether she responds or not."*

Teacher: *"I'm willing to try."*

What you are endeavoring to bring about little by little is a change in the experience the student has in specific situations in which failure, frustration, and stress are experienced. For Amy, coordination of efforts on homework may be fruitful in reducing stress—perhaps a lighter load would represent a more realistic challenge. Other possible interventions include the support of a resource teacher; a senior-student coach for difficult subjects; and advanced assignment notice to you, the teacher/therapist, allowing for preview of topics.

It should be apparent that socioemotional needs are inextricably interwoven with the student's personal resources, with the situations she encounters, and with the demands arising from them. Counseling is, therefore, an integrated component of general management. Just as we must work in close cooperation with school personnel interacting with the student, so must we work together with parents to the extent that they are willing and able to cooperate. Once again, we need to discuss their perceptions of, and feelings about, their child's social and emotional behavior. We need to listen to their concerns, to identify specific examples of problems, and to examine together how the parents handle them. Goals should be explored and agreed upon and strategies identified and discussed. We must be particularly careful only to inquire and suggest, never to reject parents' suggestions or tell them what they must do or how they should handle situations. Our goal is to effect change in the parents' perception of their child's needs through greater insight into the child's frustrations. We seek to explore with them strategies that may reduce the stress they and their child experience in conflict situations. For example, we might enlist their participation in a management strategy to reduce Michael's need for constant attention.

You: *"I wanted a chance to talk with you about Michael. His teacher, counselor, and I have been discussing ways of building his confidence. I know his counselor mentioned to you earlier that he is very demanding of attention in class and that sometimes this can be disruptive of a lesson."*

Parent: *"Yes, he's like that a lot at home; he jokes around a lot, silly like. I get very annoyed with him sometimes."*

You: *"We've talked about this here at school and we have decided that it might help if we give Michael more responsibility. His biology teacher, Mr. Daniels, has agreed to give Michael some responsibilities in the lab; Miss Davis, his English teacher, plans to encourage him to become directly involved in the stage work for the school play. Michael's been hovering on the fringe of that, so I think he will be pleased to have a real role. Also, the librarian, Mrs. Eaton, has a project she plans to ask his help with. We wonder if you think such an approach might work at home."*

Parent: *"Well, we never really thought of Michael as responsible; we are forever nagging him to get his chores done."*

You: *"Are there things he might enjoy doing if he were given the responsibility?"*

Parent: *"He's always on about getting a job after school. The man at the garden shop said he could use a boy like Michael, but we think his schoolwork is more important."*

You: *"Perhaps he could work Friday after school and on Saturday, that would still give him time for school work."*

Michael did get a job along the guidelines suggested. His parents agreed to support his efforts and to give him full responsibility for being at work on time and for taking care of homework. He responded responsibly to the special assignments at school, particularly to involvement in the school play. The general reports from his teachers indicated a noticeable improvement in Michael's behavior, including more cooperation and less attention-getting behaviors. Michael is also one of a small group of regular and special students involved in a social studies project pertaining to how minority and disabled students are treated in school. The topic suggested to the teacher by one of the counselors covers everything from accessibility to prejudice. The group meets weekly with the counselor who has agreed to help with the project. Michael feels somewhat of an authority in this group; he has taken the task quite seriously. He also has proven quite sensitive to the other students with special needs.

Amy and Michael illustrate how the socioemotional needs of students are interactive with the other needs arising from the demands of school. In addition to these academically related demands, the student experiences all the normal emotions associated with growing up. The impairment of hearing only makes more complex any questions about personal identity, sexuality, relations with the opposite sex, career opportunities and directions, and the drug culture. Each of these issues contributes to answering the question, "Who am I?" (Cohen, 1978). The need for an answer to this question becomes acute as the child moves into the adolescent years.

SPECIAL CONSIDERATIONS FOR THE POSTPRIMARY STUDENT

The adolescent years in western society are notable for the adjustment demands they make on the individual. The child must move from the relative stability and protection of childhood through a period of intense biological, psychological, and social change to the independence and responsibility of adulthood. The extent of the upheaval varies from child to child as a result of a complex of interacting factors. These include the child's personality, previous level of academic and social success, the attitudes and support of the family, whether one or both parents are closely involved with the child, the ages of brothers and sisters, and the cultural mores of the peer group. The hearing-impaired child will be subject to these influences as well as to additional factors arising from the hearing impairment. It is important to remember, however, that each child is different, and no general description can be written to accommodate the personal experiences of every child. You will encounter the same range of difficulties and reactions among hearing-impaired students in the postprimary years as are apparent among hearing students.

Defining the Problems

The special needs that may arise for young hearing-impaired persons in the postprimary school years occur in several categories. They relate to the need for the students to define themselves and to develop the self-confidence necessary to handle the increasing independence they must assume on the way to adulthood. The maturing students also will need to deal with more sophisticated social relationships with peers. As they move through junior high and senior high school, they will have to accommodate increasing academic demands, and ultimately, they will have to face the question of career choice.

We ended our consideration of the needs of the primary school child by discussing the need for counseling. This need increases when the child moves into the adolescent years. At this time the child must find an answer to the question "Who am I?" This answer will be sought in relation to the child's aspirations for the kind of person he hopes to be, in the expectations of the parents and peers, in the child's social success, and in his academic achievement. At this stage of life, the potential for a personal metamorphosis exists, as is evidenced by the unpredictable changes we frequently observe in hearing children. Although adolescence is a period of upheaval, often turbulent, it is also a period of great potential, a period of optimism. As a person whose training and experience makes you sensitive to the special difficulties associated with hearing impairment, you will be viewed by the hearing-impaired student differently from other normal-hearing adults. You know about the handicap and are sympathetic toward the person who suffers it. When this is recognized, the young handicapped person will usually categorize you among the group of family and close friends to whom Goffman (1963) refers as "the wise." This acceptance of you provides the potential for frank, open discussion of the feelings and anxieties, hopes and despairs that the young adolescent will experience. Your uncritical acceptance of these confidences will create a neutral climate that will encourage the hearing-impaired adolescent to explore his feelings. It will encourage him to verbalize the fear of not being accepted, to express any doubts about self-worth, to externalize anger about the way others treat him. It will permit the student to express aspirations and to explore how realistic they are, to assess assets, and to identify and test what he perceives to be personal limitations.

It is important, therefore, that in your early contacts with the postprimary student you define your role in the broadest terms. Explain that you hope to provide a support in whatever form it is likely to be effective. Establish a cooperative interaction rather than a teacher-child relationship. Explain that you will adopt a problem-solving approach.

The student, with your encouragement, will attempt to identify and define trouble areas as carefully as possible. Together you will explore and test ways of reducing problems. Make it clear that your goal is to help the student to learn how to define and resolve difficulties, and to assume responsibilities that in the primary school were assumed by others. Depending on the needs of the child, much of your time may be spent discussing such expressed opinions as

> Most of the kids don't have much time for me because I don't hear everything they say.
> I'm afraid to tell the other kids that I'm hearing impaired. They don't know I wear an aid.
> I'm always afraid to speak up in class in case I didn't understand. I'm afraid I'll make a fool of myself.
> There's this cute boy who my friend says likes me, but I'm afraid to talk to him because when he finds out I'm hard-of-hearing, he won't want anything to do with me.
> I've stopped wearing my aid to school because I'm embarrassed by it.
> Kids call me deaf. Am I deaf or hard-of-hearing?
> I'd like to try out for cheerleading, but I don't' think my speech is good enough.
> The teachers never call on me to give oral reports because my speech embarrasses everyone.

You cannot, and should not, in any way minimize the significance of the feelings expressed. Your role is to accept what the student says and to help explore the feelings more carefully, to try to describe them more specifically, to consider the situation that gave rise to those feelings or perceptions and to discuss their implications, and to investigate ways of dealing with the difficulties.

You may find it helpful to stimulate self-exploration of feelings and attitudes by using inventories that help to structure the students' thinking about themselves. Libbey (1978) developed an inventory to identify the attitudes of hearing-impaired adolescents in mainstream situations. This inventory contains information about how a student reacts to the types of situations encountered in school and provides a means of comparing the responses of an individual student with those reported by other hearing-impaired students in similar situations. Alpiner (1987) developed a scale of communication function that is heavily weighted in terms of the client's attitudes about the effects of the hearing impairment on her own ability to communicate and of the attitudes of others toward her. Although the Denver Scale developed by Alpiner was designed for us with adults who have acquired hearing losses, the judicious selection of appropriate items, the modification of others, and the addition of some items specific to the age group we are discussing will provide you with a useful inventory to help the student explore self-perceptions.

An increase in self-confidence can only arise from a better understanding of oneself. The insight gained then permits one to control the degree of risk taking so that the risk is assumable and the consequences of failure are manageable. Each situation that represents a threat to the student's sense of security must first be examined and understood and then approached with a management strategy with which the student feels comfortable.

The limitations the student perceives will be those that

1. Jeopardize relationships with peers, including participation in peer-group social activities
2. Limit developing relationships with members of the opposite sex
3. Affect acceptance by teachers
4. Limit academic achievement

Your plan of intervention must grow out of an understanding of the way the student perceives the difficulties encountered in these areas. The student's perceptions are always legitimate in terms of selection and interpretation of the evidence. Your task is to work with the student to determine whether there is evidence that has not been taken into consideration and whether the existing evidence can be interpreted differently. To the extent that the student's perceptions arise from objective evidence, both of you together should attempt to modify either the situation that gives rise to the difficulty, or the strategy the student is using to deal with it. When insufficient concrete evidence is available to justify the student's feelings, then you need to discuss other feelings that are contributing to the perception of the problem, and other ways of viewing the difficulty. Let us now examine some possible areas of difficulty that may result from any of the categories we have already identified.

Peer Relationships and Social Experiences

In the early adolescent years, there is a very strong desire not to deviate in any way from what the group determines is acceptable. This is clearly seen in the vagaries of teenage fashions, which suddenly label a certain type of shoe or brand of jeans as prerequisite to acceptance—the criterion by which crazes are determined. Not only is there a desire on the part of the individual teenager to conform, there also appears to be an almost malevolent determination to root out differences among one's peers. This is behavior to which every teenager is prone. The difference may be as obtrusive as wearing a dress when slacks are identified as the uniform of the event, or as subtle as having eyebrows that meet above the nose. A hearing aid that is visible is obtrusive. Its identification by a peer who comments upon it negatively frequently results in a rejection of the aid that has been worn unprotestingly for years. This rejection must not be met with entreaties to wear it, or threats of the dire consequence if it is not worn. Rather the feelings about it must be accepted and discussed. The normal teasing behavior must be talked about. It can be counteracted by the student's understanding the nature of the hearing impairment and the use of amplification, accepting the need for the aid, and examining the limitations she will experience communicating with friends without it. If through informational and adjustment counseling you can restore the student's self-dignity, she will probably feel able to minimize the significance of the teasing and by so doing may indirectly contribute to its reduction.

A more serious threat to the student's relationship to hearing classmates will arise if she experiences difficulty in using the telephone. In junior high school the telephone begins to be a major means of social contact as well as a way of cooperating on homework assignments. It may be essential to consider whether the hearing-impaired student can benefit from a hearing aid with a telecoil amplification circuit on the aid or, if she has one, whether its use is understood. It may be important to explore commercially available modifications, which are designed to improve the ability of a hearing-impaired person to use the telephone. Parents should encourage a child who simply cannot communicate over the phone to invite a friend to do homework at the house and to have friends over just to keep up with school gossip.

Participation in extracurricular activities in school and within the community should also be encouraged and facilitated. Talk with the student about the types of activities he wishes to pursue. Discuss what such activities demand, whether the student feels the hearing impairment is preventing participation, and if so, in what ways. Explore ways of overcoming perceived problems. Suggest that you both discuss the situation with a hearing student club or activity member, a club advisor, or activity leader. The hearing-impaired student's reluctance to participate in peer-related activities often lies in a lack of understanding of the demands of the situation. The group leader often has an incorrect perception of what the hearing-impaired student can handle and does not know how to limit difficulties. Both parties need support and help in working together to ensure that the hearing-impaired student has a satisfactory experience. Most handicapped persons are subjected to the limited expectancies nonhandicapped persons have encouraged them to accept. Their limited aspirations are often a reflection of others' perceptions of them. It is up to you to help change that situation. It is likely that hearing-impaired girls will experience fewer acceptance difficulties than boys, because boys in general are under heavy social pressure not to manifest weakness. A hearing impairment may be considered as an imperfection resulting in negative feedback from the group.

Acceptance by the peer group will be greatly influenced by the image the young people project of themselves. Hearing-impaired students must be able to counteract the assumption that their handicap generalizes to all areas of competence. They must be encouraged to explore their abilities in as many areas as possible, never assuming limits until they have tested them. You must help them express how they feel about themselves and their abilities and must provide support in their experiments to expand their experiences. You will need to work with their parents, who will be the major source of stability and encouragement even though these are not easy years for them. It is not easy for parents to avoid being overprotective toward hearing-impaired children out of concern for their physical and emotional well-being. It is important to recognize this as a normal reaction, but it can be tempered by the parents' evaluating the assets and competencies of their teenage sons or daughters. They must understand the importance of encouraging peer relationships and of being sympathetic to appeals from their sons or daughters for the material prerequisites to serious participation in group social activities, whether this be shorts and sneakers for the track team, skis to join the ski club, or financial support to permit participation in an overnight school trip.

It may not be possible for parents to finance the more expensive activities. It is necessary, however, for the children to realize that the parents would like them to participate but that money rather than lack of confidence is the deciding factor. When support can be given, it should be in proportion to the students' commitments. Parents should not feel that they can compensate for their children's handicaps by giving them everything they ask for.

Relationships with the Opposite Sex

Relationships with the opposite sex are difficult for most preteen and teenage students. They will be somewhat more difficult for hearing-impaired students. These students' concepts of self will determine how they think others will receive them. Helping the students to decide what makes a person attractive to others and to identify the characteristics they value most will permit them to better evaluate their own attributes. You can consider the criteria of physical appearance, dress, styles, personal grooming, interests, general behavior, attitudes and behavior to others, choice of friends, willingness to participate in group activities, willingness to reach out to others, and ability to handle disappointment. Discuss how they rate themselves in these categories. Consideration of each student as a whole person is important if you are to counteract the tendency to make a self-evaluation exclusively on the basis of the hearing impairment.

Assessing the effectiveness of communication skills and sociolinguistic competencies may motivate greater concern for improvement of auditory and visual speech-recognition abilities, speech articulation, voice quality, and modulation and linguistic competence, particularly in terms of current teenage usage. The quality of a student's present hearing aid, the possibility of changing the aid to add a telephone circuit, automatic volume control, or directional microphone may need to be discussed along with the possible advantages and disadvantages of binaural aids.

You should talk about ways of getting to know members of the opposite sex in a social context, of currently acceptable ways of inviting a girl/ boy to a school dance, to a party, or to a movie. How and when to raise the issue of the hearing impairment is often a problem faced by a teenager who begins to relate to members of the opposite sex. "If I talk about it, will they be embarrassed?" "Should I tell him/her the first time we go out if he/she does not know? If so, how?"

In a mainstream situation in which several hearing-impaired students attend the same school, a small group discussion of these topics may prove possible and valuable. It may also be helpful to invite hearing friends to one or two sessions.

If you can serve as a resource person with whom a student can raise problem issues and discuss feelings as they occur, you have the potential for contributing to the student's adjustment to the reality of the significance of the hearing impairment rather than to an unacceptable perception of it.

Acceptance by Teachers

During the primary school years we tend to show considerable concern for helping the classroom teacher understand the needs of the hearing-impaired child. Unfortunately we do not usually extend such counsel in the postsecondary grades. One of the reasons is that instead of a single teacher, the student must relate to several teachers of different subjects. As more students with hearing handicaps are mainstreamed, inservice training becomes increasingly necessary. At least at the beginning of each school year, the staff should consider the special needs of the handicapped students. There should be discussion concerning how these can realistically be provided for. Handicapped students should receive counseling from a person who has an in-depth appreciation of the functional effects of impaired hearing. Such counseling information should be shared with the teachers. Realistically, at present, the most likely route to success is for the itinerant or resource teacher or the therapist/teacher to work closely with a school guidance counselor selected for her interest, sensitivity, and willingness to work with the hearing-impaired students. The counselor may then use you as a resource, just as the classroom teacher uses the counselor. It is highly valuable for those who serve the hearing-impaired child to meet at the end of each school semester to assess the student's progress, to identify difficulties experienced by both student and teachers, and to coordinate intervention approaches.

It is equally important that junior and senior high schools encourage the student to participate in planning for his own needs. The ultimate goal is the preparation of a student with sufficient knowledge and self-confidence to pursue career training commensurate with abilities and interests. The older the student, the more essential it is that he should be involved in a cooperative program of problem identification, definition, and solution. If the student is to gain acceptance by teachers, then those teachers must have an understanding of the impact of the hearing impairment on the student's ability to learn in class, and they must have guidance and support in making reasonable adjustments necessary to accommodate the student. This will mainly involve attempting to accommodate special needs and to minimize those factors that the student perceives as limiting academic performance.

Academic Limitations

As for the primary school child, a comprehensive evaluation should be made of the older student's communicative learning abilities. These should be compared to a profile of the learning demands the student will encounter in each of the classes he takes. These demands should be assessed in terms of

- The subjects involved
- The course requirements
- The environment in which the class is taught
- The method of teaching

Special note should be made of the level of language complexity represented by the textbooks in the various subjects, the nature of the homework assignments, the size of the class, whether the class is taught in a room, laboratory, or auditorium. Note also whether independent or group projects are assigned and what the student is expected to do in order to complete these assignments.

From such an assessment you should be able to identify the student's primary needs for support.

Additional supportive help may include audiologic referrals for improving present amplification and recommendations concerning possible use of an FM system; provision of academic tutoring, either by the regular extra-help sessions given by teacher, itinerant-teacher service, or if appropriate, private arrangement; special note-taking privileges or the substitution of alternate means of fulfilling course requirements.

The need profile also will allow you to determine how you can best serve the student. While one may need intensive help in the expressive use of language, another may primarily need speech and voice improvement, or help in resolving feelings of frustration arising from particular communication situations.

A high school student finally will need help in career guidance. This should be the role of the guidance counselor. However, since school counselors are not trained to know the effects of hearing impairment on the student's potential for higher education or on the potential for pursuing a particular course of employment training, your input will be very valuable. You will have an understanding of the student's communication and learning abilities, and of the effects of various listening environments and communication situations upon the ability to understand speech. The guidance counselor will be aware of the many career opportunities and what each demands of its applicants. Increasingly the counselor will be familiar with the types of support services available in colleges and of the role of vocational rehabilitation services. Together with the student and parents, you and the guidance counselor should be able to identify realistic opportunities that neither underestimate nor overestimate the student's potentials. The counselor should outline the procedures for pursuing those opportunities.

Adjusting your services to the changing needs of the maturing student through adolescence and young adulthood represents a management approach. This is as challenging and rewarding for you as it is meaningful and effective for the student and the parents.

In concluding, I would refer back to the fact that, in general, beginning teachers and speech-language pathologists feel apprehensive about providing "counseling." What I have tried to show is that by conceptualizing counseling differently, by seeing it as a continuation of your role as a sympathetic facilitator, the justification for the apprehension dissipates considerably. I have described the secondary counseling task, as opposed to the primary role played by the psychologist or trained counselor, as one of a relationship in which all significant parties play a problem-solving role. Emotions have cause and effect. They arise from perceptions and result in behaviors. Both perceptions and behavior are modifiable through changes in demands and resources, and through insight into the problems encountered. Counseling, as described here, requires practical management of situational elements and a different perspective for the viewing of demands and resources. As we perceive so we react. Each of us contributing to reducing the impact of hearing impairment, whether we be the student, the parents, the teacher, or a helping professional, needs the broadest possible perspective. This we achieve through sharing, which is what counseling is all about.

SUMMARY

- Intervention begins by maximizing the support to the classroom teacher.
- The teacher needs to understand the nature and cause of the child's communication difficulties in class:
- The teacher needs constructive suggestions about how to reduce the learning difficulties for the child.
- Suggestions must derive from an understanding of the situation the teacher must function in, thus suggestions must be practical and capable of being followed without stress on the teacher.
- Use should be made of note takers and tutors where appropriate and available.
- Enriching the child's resources requires a holistic approach.

- All areas of function should be addressed, all needs prioritorized, and strategies integrated.
- Intervention strategies should be flexible to accommodate changing needs.
- The child needs to be educated to understand the nature of the hearing impairment and its effects on understanding speech.
- Understanding of amplification encourages acceptance and correct use of hearing aids and special amplifying systems.
- Auditory and visual communication training should be incorporated with language and cognition training. The emphasis primarily should be on comprehension.
- Language enrichment should relate to academic content.
- New subject-specific vocabulary and phrases should be generalized to nonspecific contexts whenever possible.
- Pragmatic and conversational skills are best improved through actual communication interactions.
- Speech articulation and vocal control need to be taught without language stimuli.
- Reading and writing as communication skills related to understanding of instructions and enriching language should be integrated into a holistic management plan.
- Provision of socioemotional support involves utilization of the support of significant others.
- An analytic approach to socioemotional problems facilitates a management solution based on modifying contributing factors and behavioral strategies.
- Postprimary students should be encouraged to participate in planning intervention goals and methods.
- Practical approaches to problem analysis and modification should predominate.
- The socioemotional needs of teenage students should be treated seriously.

Conclusion

The difficulties and needs experienced by the school-age child are complex and interrelated. In addressing these needs we must seek to modify the classroom environment and the behavior of significant persons in that environment. We strive to do this through understanding the teachers' need to communicate more easily with the student. This requires a mutual understanding of classroom demands and the nature of the students' difficulties in meeting them. Cooperative approaches to problem identification and resolution are likely to prove practical and acceptable.

Our special task is to upgrade the students' resources. To achieve this we first maximize the effectiveness of personal and classroom amplification devices. Then we focus on enrichment of cognitive linguistic competence in academic subjects, and on the practical use of language in class. Communication skills are upgraded through speech improvement and conversational discourse training. The socioemotional difficulties arising from or exacerbated by the communication difficulties and by the perception of difference require an ongoing counseling relationship built on sensitivity, acceptance, and trust.

19

Assessment of Hearing Handicap in the Hearing-Impaired Adult

Working with the hearing-impaired adult lacks the immediate dramatic appeal of working with the young child. Unfortunately it is commonly felt that the adjustment the adult must make is not a great one. After all, it is reasoned, he already has the communication abilities we often must work so diligently to develop in the child. The needs of the adult tend to be seen as adjusting to the use of amplification and acquiring some speech-reading skills. This view is supported by the fact that many hearing-impaired persons, once fitted with a hearing aid, are able to compensate for their hearing handicap. They become satisfied hearing aid users who need no more than periodic attention to their hearing aid by a dispensing audiologist.

Realistically it is probably true that the majority of hearing-impaired adults, when carefully fitted with appropriate amplification, are able to adapt successfully to its use with only minimal guidance. Certainly when approached, few hearing-impaired adults express an interest in a program of aural rehabilitation (Rossi & Harford, 1968).

et al. (1976) sought to identify the reasons underlying clients' rough on recommendations for aural rehabilitation. Of viewed, 66 percent gave lack of motivation as the reason herapy. The second two most frequently occurring rea- awareness of the service and its value (approximately 25 eduling difficulties (approximately 25 percent). Audiologists apparently are failing to convince clients of the value of effective rehabilitation management. Oyer et al. (1976) interpret their data as suggesting that audiologists themselves may be unconvinced of the value of such programs and thus devote little time to demonstrating their worth.

These findings are over 15 years old, but more recent research has not shown that the situation today is significantly different. There appears to be a discrepancy between hearing-impaired persons' assessments of their needs and those of the audiologist, even when aural rehabilitation is recommended. This was evidenced by the client's lack of motivation to accept a recommendation that they enroll in a program of aural rehabilitation.

Motivation is an internally derived drive—it can be stimulated from without but it cannot be imposed. As audiologists and speech-language therapists, we must not assume that our goal is to ensure that once fitted with a hearing aid(s), the adult client will wish to begin a course of aural rehabilitation. Such a philosophy is incompatible with the model of cooperative management stressed throughout our discussions. To gain a clear picture of our responsibility to the client, we need to examine the process by which the client will accept or decline our suggestions, as well as the factors that contribute to that decision.

RECOGNIZING AND ACKNOWLEDGING THE HEARING DIFFICULTY

In the overwhelming number of cases, the appearance of hearing impairment in the adult is insidious, slow, and progressive. Moreover, for most of us it represents part of the aging process. Because we see it as yet another symptom of growing old, we decline to recognize it for as long as we can. In my own experience I found myself progressively prouder of my annual audiogram indicating thresholds of less than 10dB across the frequency range—that is, until the results indicated a significant drop at 8000 Hz and a moderate decline at 6000 Hz. I refused to believe the change and insisted on a retest: "I'm not old enough to have a hearing loss." So often I hear a client seek the same reassurance: "I don't need a hearing aid yet, do I Doc?," or "I don't have enough of a loss to need an aid, do I?" as though the ultimate criterion for using a hearing aid is the audiogram.

Unable to face our own mortality and the progressive physiologic and psychological processes associated with it, we adopt strategies to delay our recognition of the symptoms of aging and the stigma we feel they carry. We do so even when the symptoms occur relatively early in our middle years.

The first strategy most of us adopt to deal with our suspicions is *denial*. We simply refuse to acknowledge the problem. "Perhaps it's your hearing" we suggest when we accuse father of not listening. "There's nothing wrong with my hearing," he protests, flatly denying the possibility both to others and to himself. Denial usually is supported by *rationalization*. This occurs in two ways. We provide evidence that we do not have a problem: "If I had a hearing problem, I'd have trouble on the phone and I don't" or "I don't have a problem hearing you now; it's just when you all talk at once."

The second device is to *attribute the problem to the speaker*:

"Well the priest just mumbles; everyone in church says he's hard to hear."
"How do you expect me to understand when you talk with your mouth full?"
"It's his accent; I have real trouble with his accent."

For a time, members of the family simply accept the communication difficulties experienced in just a few situations. It avoids upsetting father. However, as the months pass the problem grows and communication situations begin to be increasingly difficult for everyone. A nonverbalized acknowledgment of the problem by the person with the hearing difficulty begins to be evidenced by the strategy of *retrenchment*.

Retrenchment is based upon the acknowledged inability to cope with certain communication situations. These commonly are group situations, dinner table conversations, noisy environments, and movies and theaters. The insecurity felt by the hearing-impaired person in these situations, or the lack of enjoyment derived from them, causes the person to withdraw from them. The individual shrinks his lifestyle to one that he can handle. By avoiding the situations he avoids the stress. The person pulls back to a position of safety, but at a cost. This too may be rationalized: "I don't care for the movies they make these days—I can watch them on video. Anyway, who wants to go out in the winter" or "I guess I never really got along with Joe and Mary; Joe always annoyed me with his boasting about his job—I don't miss seeing them." Throughout this period family members, even friends, become increasingly aware that mother, father, or spouse does not hear adequately. With increasing frequency, they experience being misheard, not being replied to, or receiving an inappropriate answer to a question. Spouses in particular find their social lives shrinking along with that of their partner. Finally the price of retrenchment, along with family pressure, usually effects a grudging acknowledgment by the sufferer of the hearing difficulty and of the need for help. Consultation is then sought.

The process of acknowledging the hearing impairment that I have described is quite common. I need to stress, however, that not everyone reacts to the problem that way. Some persons gradually begin to notice that in certain situations they are not catching what people are saying, that listening is becoming quite tiring, and that they are having to ask people to repeat what they said. Once they suspect it is their hearing, they seek consultation and are enthusiastic about rectifying the problem. That amplification might well be of help to them may come as a surprise, because the general assumption is that you have to have quite a loss before you can be helped by a hearing aid. However, once informed about the benefits of amplification, even for a mild or moderate loss, they are ready to try a hearing aid and are quite receptive to a binaural fitting when recommended.

These two patterns of psychological reactions to suspicions of a problem illustrate the individuality of the management needs we will encounter. Each adult comes to us with a particular set of attitudes, feelings, and emotional resources along with a range of complex situational factors. Together these account for the situation in which the person finds herself, as well as the way in which she is managing her problem when we see her. No matter how well or how poorly she is adapting, we must recognize that for any given individual, the way she is functioning represents the best she can achieve alone. Unless resources are modified or supplemented, the situation is only likely to deteriorate.

Whether the individual comes to us willingly or reluctantly, the decision to seek help is based on the recognition that

- Communication abilities are no longer adequate to permit the client to meet the demands encountered.
- The psychological cost of meeting daily demands is judged to be too high.
- The present level of communication abilities, though adequate for current demands, is recognized to limit the adult in the pursuit of advancement.

Given that perceived needs are specific to each person, only an individually tailored approach is likely to be effective.

The element of cost effectiveness of your intervention efforts is crucial when working with adults. A client's willingness to participate in a rehabilitation management program usually is determined by her perception of the value of anticipated gain for the cost and inconvenience. Cost must be measured in terms of

- Total fees paid
- The price and cost of operating and maintaining the hearing aid(s)
- Income lost by absence from the workplace
- Cosmetic considerations
- The psychological adjustment

Inconveniences are perceived as

Using and keeping the hearing aid in working order
The need to rearrange schedules and to accommodate the rehabilitation sessions
The inconvenience of traveling to and from the center
The total time involved

Motivation to seek help must be based, therefore, on a (an)

- Acknowledgment of the need for help and willingness to accept it
- A clear understanding of those needs
- Understanding of the methods for meeting needs
- Acceptable cost in terms of money, time, and inconvenience
- Definite and acceptable time frame for the intervention program
- Clear understanding of expected benefits
- Set of realistic and meaningful goals
- Acceptable schedule of appointments

The client will use this information to determine whether the financial, time, and the psychological costs are justified by the anticipated benefits. To minimize these costs, our intervention plan should

- Address specific needs
- Order need priorities
- Provide a clear practical plan that addresses individual circumstances
- Be designed in separate units that terminate after a predetermined number of sessions

A cooperative working relationship with the client and significant family members is essential. The client and family should be encouraged to participate in all stages of evaluation, intervention planning, decision making, and progress assessment. You should not make decisions for the client in anything but technical matters pertaining to amplification. It even is wise to be very sparing with advice since your role is to provide maximum information and to help the client make the decisions, not to recommend one solution over another.

The participation of significant family members, particularly a spouse, or increasingly a partner who, though not a family member, has a close relationship with the client, is very important. We need to remember that communication requires two or more people. Thus if one partner experiences a communication problem so does the other. In fact the impact of a person's hearing handicap on a partner or close family member may be so severe as to disrupt the relationship. Whenever possible a spouse, partner, son or daughter, or son/daughter-in-law should participate in the informational counseling and diagnostic processes. We should try also to involve them in management planning. We certainly will need their help in modifying the communication conditions in the home. The assessment and management plan you will pursue together follows the model we have adopted throughout our discussions. The stages include:

- *Problem definition*: a careful assessment of all factors that have a direct bearing on the communication difficulties experienced by the client and significant others
- *Need assessment*: identification of the needs of the client and significant others that must be provided for if a significant improvement in their daily lives is to be effected
- *Establishment of goals*: the formulation and acceptance of a set of goals that will be achieved within the agreed time frame of the rehabilitation unit
- *Determination of intervention strategies*: the formulation of specific methods by which the identified goals will be achieved
- *Implementation of intervention strategies*: the application of the specific management strategies selected as appropriate
- *Evaluation*: the monitoring of progress and assessment of the effectiveness of intervention strategies

ASSESSMENT OF AMPLIFICATION NEEDS

Assessment of the client's amplification needs constitutes the initial stage of the rehabilitative management process for any person with impaired hearing. Amplification comprises the single most effective resource for reducing hearing handicap for the overwhelming majority of individuals. Determining the client's needs and prescribing appropriate hearing aids are the responsibility of the audiologist. It is important for those of you who have this role to be very aware of the fact that a successful hearing aid fitting requires attention to more than the acoustic needs of the patient. Although the function of the impaired ear remains the primary determinant in the selection of amplification specifications, it is by no means the sole factor in determining the successful use of hearing aids. It has been demonstrated that for many persons with impaired hearing, the subjective assessment of the degree of handicap experienced correlates poorly with the objective measures of the severity of the disability (Brainerd & Frankel, 1985). Thus, in assessing the need for amplification you should include careful consideration of the other factors that will influence your assessment of the probable benefit that the hearing aid(s) will provide. Such factors include the:

- Client's real acceptance of the need for amplification
- Cosmetic acceptability of the type of aid(s) recommended
- Physical health of the client
- Client's ability to insert and remove the hearing aid(s) and to adjust the controls
- Financial ability to purchase and operate the aid(s)
- Demands placed upon the client for auditory-oral communication at work and in social situations
- Types of environments in which the client must function

Hearing aid fitting and dispensing involve a great deal of counseling. You cannot assume that the presence of a client in your office means that he has either accepted the reality of the impairment or is now willing to wear a hearing aid, to say nothing of both. Even the purchase of the aid(s) does not ensure their optimal use. Often the client who has decided reluctantly that he will have to wear a hearing aid also has decided that it has to be "one of those tiny ones that goes in your ear so no one can see it." Unfortunately, a canal aid may be quite inappropriate for this person. By contrast, as I explained earlier, another client will wear anything you recommend "so long as it gives me the best help I can get." Assessment of the degree of acceptance by the client of the hearing impairment and the need to use a hearing aid(s), as well as the degree of willingness to do so, will influence your management plan.

If the hearing aid(s) are to be judged by the client to be truly beneficial, they must be seen to be providing the amount of benefit that you realistically counseled the client to expect in the varying situations he encounters. They also must be augmented by the communication strategies you will have developed with the client to deal with difficult listening environments. You can encourage realistic expectations only when you know both the client's performance with the aid(s) in the audiometric booth and the situations and environments in which he must function. Both will vary with each client.

Profiling Communication Difficulties

The customary sequence of assisting persons who experience hearing difficulties begins with audiologic assessment followed by otologic examination. The recommendation for hearing aid evaluation then comes from the otologist. In other instances the medical clearance, which in some states is a requirement unless waived in writing by the client, is given by a family physician. The client may then go to a certified audiologist who dispenses hearing aid(s) or to a hearing aid dealer.

audiologic assessment → otologic examination

To conduct a hearing aid evaluation and fitting with an understanding of the client's needs, I require background information concerning the particular demands for auditory communication that the client has difficulty satisfying. I need information about difficult situations encountered in specific environments at work, at home, and in social activities. This information helps me to select the most appropriate amplification specifications. It also provides the basis for counseling the client concerning realistic expectations for the hearing aid and the possible need for further rehabilitative management. Usually I obtain the essential information during an informal exploration of the problems with the client. In my discussion with the client I ask when the hearing difficulty was first noticed, what was experienced, and whether the difficulty has become greater over the past few years. I inquire if the client has "a better ear" and whether she has ever worn a hearing aid. I ask the client and family member(s) to help me to understand the nature of the communication difficulty and the circumstances in which it occurs. I ask about types of communication situations at work that present difficulty and I explore home and social situations. These include hearing radio and television news and entertainment; using the telephone; talking at dinner; entertaining guests in the house and garden; traveling in the car; attending a place of worship, cinema theater, or concert; attending meetings or clubs; pursuing a hobby; and so on. I also ask the client and family member to help me understand what it feels like to have these difficulties, encouraging them to speak of the stress, anxiety, apprehension, and embarrassment associated with communication insecurity. Finally, I ask how the client feels about wearing hearing aids.

Usually an informal exploration of the problem provides me with the information I need. Sometimes, however, a more structured case history is considered helpful.

The Structured Profile of Difficulties

The primary determinant of a detailed profile is cost effectiveness because services must be paid for and should be included only when they are likely to provide a significant benefit. To obtain more detailed information, one turns to published measures, profiles, and scales.

A structured assessment tool requires time to administer, score, and interpret. The self-administered tool has the advantage of obviating your need to administer the questionnaire. However, this type of instrument needs to be used with caution. Even when the client is completing the assessment on his own time, the length of the task may affect the care taken to read and answer the questions. Furthermore, on questions relating to function, there is no way to be sure that the answers given represent reality, that they are not distorted by the client's inability to acknowledge that reality.

The power of wish fulfillment was recently emphasized for me when I completed a dietary profile as part of a wellness program. To the question, "How many cookies do you typically eat in a week?," I confidently and quite sincerely answered, "Two or three." My wife, checking the questionnaire, was astounded. "I can't believe this about the cookies," she exclaimed. "Two or three a week! You regularly have three or four every evening with your coffee." She was correct; "but," I protested, "I don't eat dessert."

Answers also may be invalid if the question is misinterpreted by the client, or if it does not quite apply. There is the further problem that the assessment tool may be too limited, ask too few questions, and thus fail to profile accurately the client's difficulties. Finally, since no normative data are provided for any of the available tools, the results obtained should be accepted as advisory only.

In selecting an assessment tool or tools for profiling the client's needs, you should seek to cover the situations and environments that comprise the particular client's world. You may choose to use the complete list of items or to select only appropriate sections or questions. This is acceptable since the inventories have not been normed. In some cases it may be advisable to complete the selected sections together with the client. In this way the questions serve as probes to the area being explored. In any case it always is advisable to review and discuss the answers with the client rather than simply accepting the raw or indexed scores.

An extensive profiling of the hearing handicap experienced by the client sometimes is undertaken by the audiologist fitting the hearing aid(s). More commonly, however, it is carried out by a speech-language therapist who undertakes a rehabilitative intervention program with the client. The results obtained are used to develop an individualized intervention plan.

Published Hearing Handicap Assessment Tools

A number of scales and indexes are available that were designed to profile and assess the severity of the handicap created by the hearing deficit. The very first of these was the Social Adequacy Index (SAI) published by Davis in 1948. Its importance is its recognition that a hearing handicap could not be assessed simply from a pure tone audiogram or as a percentage loss. The SAI is based on the subject's ability to process speech rather than to detect pure tones. It combines the measure of intensity at which speech begins to be useful, the *speech reception threshold* (SRT), with the measure of residual discrimination provided by the percentage of phonetically balanced words *incorrectly identified*, that is to say, the percentage loss. The intersection of these two measures on a numerical chart provides a number that constitutes a social adequacy score for that relationship of SRT to percentage discrimination loss. This is then compared to a social adequacy *threshold* score, which represents the value designated as normal function. The intent of the SAI is excellent; unfortunately, it is not without flaws. Davis himself states that it lacks effectiveness because the phonetically balanced (PB) word list recording used in establishing the figures was insufficiently standardized. Newby (1964) identifies a further limitation, which is that our current W22 PB word lists are a modified version of the lists used to compute the SAI figures and thus cannot be assumed to provide completely compatible measures. Finally, as Alpiner (1987) emphasizes, the reliance on quantified data fails to allow for differences in individual behavioral characteristics. To this observation I would add that the SAI score obtained reflects the unrealistic environment of the sound room. In no way does it allow for the varied environments and situations in which the individual must be socially adequate, nor does it attempt to assess comprehension of connected discourse.

Despite these reservations, or perhaps bearing them in mind, the SAI can be a helpful and simple baseline tool for assessing the relative impact on predicted social adequacy of such changes as the wearing of a hearing aid, the addition of visual cues to word presentation, or the varying of signal-to-noise ratios.

Subsequent to the Social Adequacy Index, attempts to assess hearing handicap moved away from computation based on quantified measures of hearing. Researchers approached hearing handicap, as compared to hearing deficiency, from the subjective view of the hearing-impaired person. The assumption is made that a hearing handicap is that degree of deficiency a person perceives himself to have in meeting the communication demands encountered in his daily life. Such an approach aims to permit the individual to generate an individualized picture of difficult situations as he perceives them. The descriptive profile then provides a basis for a problem reduction approach to management.

The Hearing Handicap Scale. The first descriptive inventory, The Hearing Handicap Scale, was published by High, Fairbanks, and Glorig in 1964. The inventory has two forms, A and B, each comprising 20 questions surveying a variety of communication demands and situations. It was designed to be self-administered by the hearing-impaired person who responds by indicating the frequency of difficulty on a five-point scale from "almost always" to "almost never." Sample questions taken from the test are

Q2. Can you carry on a telephone conversation without difficulty?
Q7. Can you understand a person when you are seated beside him and cannot see his face?
Q15. Can you follow the conversation when you are at a large dinner table or in a meeting with a small group?
Q17. If you are seated under the balcony of a theater, can you hear well enough to follow what is going on?

The scale presents a rather narrow homogeneous range of items sampling only one aspect of communication (Giolas, 1970). No questions relate to problems encountered in the workplace, nor are the client's attitude or feelings about the hearing handicap addressed. The scale was designed to explore the effects of the hearing impairment on communication; no method for quantifying results was provided. Schow and Tannahill (1977) have attempted to provide a means of categorizing the Hearing Handicap Scale scores and classifying clients into one of three degrees of hearing handicap: nonhandicap, slight handicap, and severe handicap. The value of quantifying the results lies in the baseline score that can be used to assess the results of the intervention procedures we adopt in our attempt to reduce the communication handicap.

It is not clear to what use categorization by severity of handicap might be put. This same difficulty exists with the computation of percentage hearing loss, except for medical-legal purposes. Neither categorization serves as functional use since the primary purpose of our efforts is to document areas of difficulty, to describe them, and to develop strategies for reducing the communication impedance. Such individualized measures cannot be based on a general category of severity of handicap.

Hearing Measurement Scale. The Hearing Measurement Scale (Noble & Atherley, 1970) explores a much wider range of factors contributing to hearing handicap. It covers seven areas:

- Speech and hearing
- Acuity for nonspeech sounds
- Localization
- Reaction to the handicap
- Speech distortion
- Tinnitus
- Personal opinion of the hearing loss

Examples of questions from this scale follow.

SPEECH AND HEARING (11 ITEMS)

Q1. Do you ever have difficulty hearing in the conversation when you're with one other person when you're at home?

Q5. Do you have difficulty hearing conversation at work?

Q11. Do you ever have difficulty hearing what's said in a film?

ACUITY FOR NONSPEECH SOUNDS (8 ITEMS)

Q13. Can you hear it when someone rings the doorbell or knocks on the door?

Q18. Can you hear the tap running when you turn it on?

LOCALIZATION (7 ITEMS)

Q21. If you're with a group of people and someone you can't see starts to speak, would you be able to tell where that person was sitting?

Q20. Outside do you always move out of the way of something coming up from behind, for instance a car, a trolley or someone walking faster?

REACTION TO THE HANDICAP (7 ITEMS)

Q27. Do you think you are more irritable than other people or less so?

Q32. Do you ever get bothered or upset if you are unable to follow a conversation?

SPEECH DISTORTION (3 ITEMS)

Q34. Do you find that people fail to speak clearly?

Q35. What about speakers on TV or radio? Do they fail to speak clearly?

TINNITUS (8 ITEMS)

Q37. Do you ever get noise in your ears or in your head?

Q39. Does it upset you?

PERSONAL OPINION OF THE HEARING LOSS (9 ITEMS)

Q40. Do you think your hearing is normal?

Q42. Does any difficulty with your hearing restrict your social or personal life?

Although originally designed to be administered by a professional in an interview format, a self-administered version has been made available (Noble, 1979). In the interview format the session is taped and scored by two clinicians. Although this procedure may be essential in industrial hearing loss assessment for which the scale was designed (assessment of industrial workers usually involves compensation payments), it would be a prohibitively expensive procedure in the rehabilitative management model we are addressing.

Denver Scale of Communication Function. This scale, developed by Alpiner, Chevrette, Glascoe, Metz, and Olsen (1974) is unlike the two already reviewed in that it seeks to measure attitudes of hearing-impaired subjects rather than to identify problem situations. Twenty-five statements are made covering four areas: family, self, social-vocational, and communication. The statements encourage the person to reflect on how she perceives her reactions and those of others to the problems created by the hearing difficulty. The statements also explore the person's feelings about being hearing impaired and the effects it has had. In responding the person is asked to agree or disagree on a five-point scale from "strongly disagree" to "strongly agree." Examples of questions follow:

Q1. The members of my family are annoyed with my loss of hearing. (family)
Q5. I am not an "outgoing" person because I have a hearing loss. (self)
Q14. I do not enjoy my job as much as I did before I began to lose my hearing. (social-vocational)
Q19. Conversations in a noisy room prevent me from attempting to communicate with others. (social-vocational)
Q22. I feel threatened by many communication situations due to difficulty hearing. (communication).

McCarthy-Alpiner Scale of Hearing Handicap. Another scale similar to the Denver Scale is the one developed by McCarthy and Alpiner (1980). It, too, seeks to assess the effects of the hearing impairment on psychological, social, and vocational functioning. Thirty-four statements are presented, including nine relative to adjustment, five to social activities, and ten to vocational activities. The person is asked to rate each statement on a five-point scale indicating whether it is true (1) always, (2) usually, (3) sometimes, (4) rarely, (5) never. Examples of questions include the following:

Q4. I feel negative about life in general because of my hearing loss. (psychological)
Q11. I tend to avoid people because of my hearing loss. (psychological)
Q22. I enjoy social situations with considerable conversation. (social)
Q27. My co-workers know what it is like to have a hearing loss. (vocational)
Q33. I try to hide my hearing loss from my employer. (vocational)

McCarthy and Alpiner (1987) reported on an interesting study designed to test the validity of their scale. A second form was devised that differed from the first only in that the statements were expressed in the third person. The original scale then was administered to the client and the revised scale was completed quite independently by a close family member. The results revealed a low level of agreement between the responses given by the hearing-handicapped person and those given by the family member. This appears to document what those of us in practice observe so often—namely, there is a significant gap between the hearing-impaired person's perceptions of the problems and the perceptions the family has of those difficulties and how they are being handled. Throughout the text I have emphasized that communication difficulty, by definition, involves both the sender and receiver. A hearing disability handicaps both the hearing-impaired person and his family. Unfortunately clinical observations and the findings of McCarthy and Alpiner illustrate that neither party sees their common problem in the same way. This in essence means there are two problems rather than one. A primary goal in management, therefore, must be to fuse the two images into one. Our counseling model accepts the perceptions of both parties as valid but seeks closure through expanding the sensitivity of each party to the other's views and needs. Only through a cooperative approach to problem definition and resolution can we hope to effect significant improvement in the situations experienced by both the client and members of the family.

Quantified Denver Scale. The Denver Scale of Communication Function subsequently was modified by Schow and Nerbonne (1980) to permit quantification of the results. The subjects were separated into three hearing categories, 0–15dB HL, 16–26dB HL, and 27–40dB HL, based on the unaided pure tone average of the better ear. The Quantified Denver Scale scores obtained by subjects in the three groups averaged respectively 6.5 percent, 21.3 percent, and 37 percent. This evidences the increased hearing handicap occurring with increased hearing thresholds. As I explained earlier, quantification provides a score against which to measure the impact of a hearing aid fitting and of subsequent intervention strategies.

The Hearing Performance Inventory Revised Form. This self-administered inventory developed originally by Giolas, Owens, Lamb, Schubert in 1979 was published in revised form by Lamb, Owens, and Schubert and again in 1983. The revised form comprises a lengthy scale of 90 items that explore six categories: (1) understanding speech, (2) intensity, (3) response to auditory failure, (4) social, (5) personal, and (6) occupational. The 90 items represent the refinement by item analysis of an original 158 items. The responses are recorded on a scale of 1–5 from "practically always" to "almost never." Examples of questions include

1. Can you understand what a woman is saying on the telephone when her voice is loud enough for you?

   You are at a party or gathering of less than ten people and the room is fairly quiet. Can you understand what a friend or family member is saying to you when his/her voice is loud enough for you, but you cannot see his/her face?

2. When an announcement is given over a public address system in a bus station or airport, is it loud enough for you to hear?

   When others are listening to speech on the television or radio, is it loud enough for you?

3. You are talking with a friend or family member. When you miss something that was said, do you pretend you misunderstood?

You are having dinner with five or six friends. When you miss something important that was said, do you ask the person talking to repeat it?

4. Does your hearing problem discourage you from going to the movies?
   Does your hearing problem discourage you from attending lectures?

5. Does your hearing problem lower your self-confidence?
   Do you feel that others cannot understand what it is to have a hearing problem?

6. Does your hearing problem interfere with helping or instructing others on the job?
   You are talking with a co-worker at work. When you miss something important that was said, do you ask for it to be repeated?

All questions are classified by category in a key that enables you to sort the responses back into the original six categories. Questions in the "understanding speech" category can be separated according to the "with vision" and "without vision" criteria.

Self-Assessment of Communication. The most recent scale to be published is the Self-Assessment of Communication Scale by Schow and Nerbonne (1982). This scale was designed as a screening tool for hearing-impaired adults, including the elderly. Six broad descriptions cover a variety of communication situations to be rated for frequency of occurrence. In addition, two questions pertain to feelings and two to the behavior of others. The five-point ratings are (1) almost never or never, (2) occasionally, about ¼ time, (3) about half the time, (4) frequently, about ¾ time, and (5) practically always or always. Sample questions include:

Q1. Do you experience communication difficulties in situations when speaking with one other person? (For example, at home, at work, in a social situation, with a waitress, a store clerk, with a spouse, boss, etc.)

Q7. Do you feel that any difficulty with your hearing limits or hampers your personal or social life?

Q9. Do others leave you out of conversations or become annoyed because of your hearing?

To calculate a percentage score, the values of the individual ratings first are added. The formula, percent = (2 × total raw score) − 20 multiplied by 1.25 is then used. Schow and Nerbonne provided a modified version of this scale to permit the same evaluations to be completed by a family member or significant other person. They have identified this as the *Significant Other Assessment of Communication Scale*. Its function is the same as that discussed for the modified version of the Denver Scale of Communication Function.

For none of the scales and inventories have I provided a complete list of questions. If you feel it appropriate to administer a full scale, it is important that you work from the source publication. The developers of a scale accompany its publication with information about its development and standardization together with instructions for its use and interpretation. It is unwise simply to ignore the author's guidelines. However, I do include in the appendix to this chapter a copy of a scale that I developed.

Profiles for Communicative Performance. These three scales (see chapter appendix) are intended to serve as examples of nonstandardized inventories that can apply to specific populations and lifestyles. Only communication difficulty is addressed; the scales do not allow for assessment of a person's feelings or the attitudes of others. A significant difference has been introduced into the method of scoring. I believe that the impact of a hearing handicap in any given communication situation is a function of three important factors: (1) the importance of the communication situation, (2) the degree of difficulty, and (3) the frequency with which that situation occurs. The importance of the situation usually is the most critical factor for the hearing-impaired person. An upcoming employment interview, a meeting with the boss, a wedding ceremony, and a particular celebration dinner may warrant great concern by the hearing-impaired person even though they may be infrequent occurrences. Missing the punchline in a TV sitcom, though it occurs frequently, may not be considered terribly significant by the same person. By contrast, however, to an invalid elderly person, TV may be of great importance. These three factors are rated separately in my *Communication Profiles*. For each question, the degree of difficulty is rated on a four-point scale from $+2$ (little or no difficulty) to -2 (great difficulty). The frequency of occurrence is rated from 1 (seldom) to 3 (very often), while importance of the situation is rated 1 (relatively little) to 3 (highly important). By multiplying the results one obtains a score indicating the impact of the handicap for each situation. The magnitude of the scores provides an overall measure of impact by category. Two examples of scoring follow.

OCCUPATIONAL ENVIRONMENT

Q4a. If I have to take notes by dictation in a fairly quiet room, I have

$\boxed{+2}$	$+1$	$\widehat{-1}$	-2
little or no difficulty	some difficulty (but not a lot)	a fair amount of difficulty (quite a lot)	great difficulty in understanding

Q4b. This happens

1	$\boxed{2}$	$\widehat{3}$
seldom	often	very often

Q4c. The importance of this situation is

1	$\boxed{2}$	$\widehat{3}$
not very important	fairly important	highly important

The first example □ "Little or no difficulty": $\widehat{+2}$ multiplied by "Often" $\widehat{+2}$ and by "Fairly important" $\widehat{+2}$ yields a score of $+8$.

If, however, the person has indicated having "a fair amount of difficulty" $\widehat{-1}$ "very often," $\widehat{3} \times$ in this highly important situation $\widehat{3}$, the score becomes

−9. The lower the positive number, the less the interactive impact; the higher the negative number, the greater the impact.

A Review of the Use of Scales

It seems necessary and appropriate at this point to review our discussion of hearing-handicap assessment tools. We will do so by posing a series of questions.

What Is the Purpose of These Scales? Hearing-handicap assessment scales are intended primarily to provide information about the impact of the hearing disability of the client's ability to communicate effectively.

Do They Assess a Range of Communication Circumstances? Scales and inventories usually try to assess communication handicap in the home, at work, and in social settings. Some scales assess only difficulty of communication; some include feelings and behavioral reactions associated with the hearing impairment.

Are the Scales Self-Assessment Tools? Almost all scales can be used either as self-assessment tools or they may be administered by the clinician. Some scales have been modified to provide a second form to be administered to a significant other person.

What Is the Purpose of the Significant Other Person Evaluation? It provides helpful information about discrepancies between how the hearing handicap is perceived by the hearing-impaired person and by family members that must be addressed and resolved through counseling.

Which Is the Best Scale to Use? There is no best scale. Only by examining the full version of each together with the author's comments can you decide which to select to meet your particular needs.

What Criteria Should I Use When Assessing Scales? First, the scale should meet your needs, either to screen quickly or to provide comprehensive information. You should consider the number of items and thus the length of time required to complete the scale in relation to the client's availability and the time you need to read and evaluate responses and, if appropriate, to administer the scale yourself. The scale selected should provide some way to quantify the results if you need baseline data for comparison of pre- and postintervention measures.

Are There Concerns Regarding These Scales? The reservations about the scales include that we cannot be sure that the client's responses truly reflect the degree of difficulty or feelings actually experienced since we have no measure of internal validity. Even though two of the scales provide a comparative form for completion by a significant other person, one study designed to assess level of agreement found very poor correlations (Alpiner, 1987). Thus, the question of whose perception was valid remains unanswered. The fact that not all scales cover all factors contributing to hearing handicap justifies concern that important problem areas may not be revealed. Finally, though intended to facilitate rehabilitative management, no guidelines are provided concerning how the results can be used in planning an intervention program nor is there data about pre- and post-rehabilitation scores.

Should I Plan to Use Such Scales? The scales should be seen as a means of generating data. Care should be taken in how you interpret and use the results. Some scales are needlessly long, asking such specific questions as, "Can you understand if someone speaks to you while you are chewing crisp foods such as potato chips or celery?" "Can you hear night sounds such as distant trains, bells, dogs barking, trucks passing and so forth?" Other scales generate relatively little information. We do not know whether there is an optimal number of questions nor is there evidence to show the relative value of any particular question for any particular client. Despite these reservations the various scales have made us aware of the need to obtain information concerning the handicap imposed by the interaction of the hearing impairment and the communication demands encountered by the client. You must decide how best to assess this.

How Can I Make That Decision? The determining factors in selecting an approach to profiling should be (1) extent of need, (2) usefulness, and (3) time, cost, and inconvenience.

1. The Extent of the Need. Since sensorineural hearing disability is not reversible, amplification cannot restore normal listening conditions. It will help to reduce, by varying degrees, the handicap of the hearing deficiency, but it invariably falls short of eliminating all communication difficulties. The extent of the hearing handicap remaining after hearing aid fitting and a period of adjustment to amplification varies from client to client. The severity and configuration of the residual hearing and the degree of speech distortion interact with the client's attitude and personality, the acoustic conditions under which communication takes place and the variable cost of not understanding. With most clients you, the audiologist, will be able to gain the relative information concerning specific communication difficulties through an efficient initial hearing aid evaluation interview. The purpose of such an interview is to guide the client in a description of the types of communication difficulties that are causing concern, where they arise, and what the effects of those problems are. You should ask about communication at home, work, and social situations and about attitudes and feelings. The presence of a significant other person allows you to ask how the client's difficulties affect them both. Much can be learned by sensitive observation of how each person reacts to the other's perceptions and needs arising from communication difficulties. The client should be counseled appropriately concerning what to expect from the hearing aids. A set of realistic expectations for improved communication in specific problem situations should be established. After an appropriate trial period, you and the client will be able to explore and discuss the remaining hearing handicap. If this is significantly serious, a decision best reached by the client, an in-depth analysis of problem situations, current communication strategies, and negative feelings will be appropriate. At this point the use of an inventory or scale may be advisable.

2. *Usefulness.* There is little point in administering a tool unless it provides useful information. Useful, for our purpose, might better be termed *useable*. Whether the information can be used will depend upon its relevance for each client. The problem with administering a long scale is that many of the questions may have marginal relevance and detract the client from carefully responding to those that are important. Thus in proceeding to a more in-depth evaluation than provided by the initial interview, you may wish to be selective in the questions asked or descriptions provided. It is possible to develop a pool of useful profile items on a computer disk. This makes it possible for various combinations to be put together to increase their appropriateness for a given client. The questions you might ask an office worker might be very different from those appropriate for a factory worker or an airline pilot. You must ask yourself what you will do with the client's responses when you have them. How will they influence your management strategies? If you cannot say, in all honesty, that the profile developed from the scale played a significant part in planning rehabilitative management, that it really made a difference, then its use cannot be justified.

3. *Time, Cost, and Inconvenience.* We are being made increasingly aware of the rising cost of health care and related services. Unfortunately, our services for hearing aid evaluation and dispensing, and for providing rehabilitative management, rarely are covered by health insurance policies. For persons living on fixed incomes, as an increasing percentage of our clients are, the combined cost of the hearing aid(s) purchase and maintenance, the rehabilitation management fees, and travel to and from the center may be prohibitive. It is a sad fact that expenses on our health, except for serious problems, are considered postponable. Indeed, hearing is less important than food and shelter when finances are strained.

Thus, financial cost must be a consideration. The administration, scoring, and interpretation of a lengthy questionnaire can take as much as an hour to complete. Since services must be charged for, this represents an unsubsidized fee of around $60 at the time of writing. You must decide whether you, in fact, obtain $60 worth of valuable useable information and whether this is the most profitable way for the client to invest what usually are limited funds. As I pointed out earlier, for an employed client time often translates as lost income, raising the cost even higher. Inconvenience may also be a major factor in a client's ability to participate in rehabilitation. For retired clients, particularly those who live alone, arranging for transportation frequently is difficult. For many persons it creates dependence upon a family member or friend, a dependence that the client feels guilty about. Not liking to ask for favors, the independent retired citizen often forgoes the service you offer.

I cannot stress too strongly that in the real world, where services become increasingly more expensive, you will not have the luxury afforded by the university clinic setting. That clinic is subsidized to permit you to spend a lot of time with a client in order to learn. Important though this is, it fails to teach fiscal accountability. Maximum effectiveness of your rehabilitative management program must be contained within maximum cost effectiveness. This can be achieved only through maximizing efficiency. You must ensure that all services are fully warranted.

THE AUDIOLOGIST'S ROLE IN MANAGEMENT

As an audiologist you have several functions to provide in the rehabilitative management plan:

- Providing primary education of the client concerning the nature of the hearing impairment and its effects.
- Explaining realistically what can be expected from amplification and what its limitations are.
- Selecting the most appropriate amplification to optimize the potential use of residual hearing. This includes the fitting of the hearing aid(s) and the recommendation of such assistive listening devices as are helpful and acceptable to the client.
- Providing counseling and instruction in the use and care of amplification devices.

These constitute the accepted components of a hearing aid evaluation, fitting, and dispensing service. In addition, the audiologist must determine, with the client, whether further rehabilitative management would be helpful in further minimizing the hearing handicap. Rehabilitation may be provided by the audiologist or, as more commonly occurs, by a speech-language therapist. In either case, existing audiologic findings can be supplemented with useable information. This constitutes another function, namely to provide additional information concerning auditory processing.

In Chapter 10, we discussed the audiologic test information you will need and how you can read those test results. At this point, we will review and expand that discussion with specific reference to the supplementary rehabilitation assessment.

SUPPLEMENTING STANDARD AUDIOLOGIC TEST RESULTS

The standard battery of tests for hearing assessment and hearing aid evaluation will include (1) the audiogram, (2) the speech reception threshold (SRT), and (3) word discrimination scores obtained under headphones and aided in a free field. For hearing aid assessment, we extend this battery to include the most comfortable listening level (MCL). In addition you may find an aided real-ear measurement printout or perhaps an aided audiogram helpful. The additional information needed should include

- An aided audiogram if real-ear measurement printout is not available.
- A list of phonetically balanced words missed or incorrectly identified in the aided condition together with the subject's response to each word missed. This permits a subsequent phonetic analysis of errors.
- For subjects with mild deficits in the low and mid frequencies and steeply

falling thresholds above 1000 Hz, unaided and aided discrimination scores on the California Consonant Test (Owens & Schubert, 1977) are helpful.

The California Consonant Test consists of 100 multiple-choice items in sets of four words. Each word differs from the other three by only one phoneme. The phonemes were selected as difficult for subjects with high frequency hearing deficits and because of a high rate of confusion with two or three other phonemes. The variable phoneme occurs in the initial position (36 sets) and in the final position (64 sets). The subject is asked to check the word she hears spoken. The sensitivity of the test to high frequency discrimination problems has been demonstrated by Schwartz and Surr (1979). Examples of the items follow:

1	Back	2	Rice	3	Seen	4	Bail
	Batch		Dice		Seed		Tale
	Bag		Nice		Seal		Sale
	Bath		Lice		Seat		Dale

Since spoken language comprehension depends heavily on knowledge of linguistic probabilities, it is helpful to supplement word discrimination information with a measure of discrimination that better approximates conversational speech. The Central Institute for the Deaf (CID) Everyday Speech Sentences (Davis & Silverman, 1970) provides a useful test for this purpose. It comprises 100 sentences representing the vocabulary, syntax, and form of everyday English including colloquial speech. The words are divided into 10 lists of 10 sentences each. Sample sentences include the following:

A2. How do you feel about changing the time when we begin work?
B8. Don't try to get out of it this time!
C4. That's right.
D1. It's a real dark night so watch your driving.
E9. Time's up.
F2. My brother's in town for a short while on business.
G2. See you later.
H1. Believe me!
I2. I like those big red apples we always get in the fall.
J5. Weeds are spoiling the yard.

Another test involving sentences is the Speech Perception in Noise (SPIN) test (Kalikow, Stevens, & Elliott, 1977). This test consists of several lists comprising 50 sentences each. The last word in each list is the test item. The listener is asked to repeat only the last word. The placing of the test word in a sentence moves the perceptual task away from dependence upon purely acoustic information and toward utilization of linguistic knowledge to predict the word. This is far more representative of how we process speech than is isolated word discrimination (see Figure 9-2). To further reflect linguistic effects, the sentences were constructed so that the constraints operating on the final word vary its predictability from high to low. Equivalency among the lists was increased by a revision carried out by Bilger, Rzcez, Kowski, Neutzel, and Rabinowitz (1979). Each 50-sentence list consists of an equal number of high and low predictability items in a random order. Each sentence is keyed for high or low predictability. Examples of high and low probability of the test word as determined by contextual cues follow.

HIGH PREDICTABILITY
Crocodiles live in a muddy *swamp*.
They played a game of cat and *mouse*.
The steamship left on a *cruise*.
We saw a flock of wild *geese*.

LOW PREDICTABILITY
The old man discussed the *dive*.
Miss Black knew about the *doll*.
Nancy had considered the *sleeves*.
The old man thinks about the *mast*.
He hopes Tom asks about the *bar*.

The results of the test administered in an aided condition, in quiet, and in a sound field at 50dB HL provide information about the ability of the listener to discriminate the test words on the basis of audition, and about his ability to capitalize on linguistic constraints. When the scores on the high and low predictability sentences show a large difference (e.g., 40–50 percent), one can assume that effective use is being made of linguistic constraints. When scores on both sentence types are depressed by about the same amount, a need for work on utilizing linguistic cues to supplement poor auditory discrimination would appear to have potential benefits. The test further allows for an assessment of how noise interferes with the client's discrimination. A practice run is provided using a few sentences that will not be included among the test items. These are presented against a background of speech babble at a favorable S/N ratio of + 10dB (i.e., S60/N50). Once accustomed to the interference, the S/N ratio is lowered to + 5dB and then to 0dB.

When the supplementary information previously discussed is not included in the case report of a client referred to you, the speech-language pathologist, every effort should be made to have such an evaluation completed by the audiologist. After all, the reason for the referral is that the client needs some very individualized intervention procedures. We need to foster acceptance of the fact that a careful rehabilitative diagnostic evaluation is as necessary as the initial hearing-impairment diagnostic battery. If for some reason such an assessment by an audiologist is not possible, you should generate as much of the information yourself as you can. Try to work in a quiet environment and administer the aided speech discrimination tests at normal conversational voice level at a distance of approximately four feet from the client. Conceal your mouth from the client but do not hold the cover close to your lips lest you block and distort the sound.

Assessment and Use of Supplementary Visual Cues

The comprehension of low redundancy speech information, as we have seen, can be enhanced considerably by the addition of visual cues. It is helpful to know, therefore, the extent to which a client already capitalizes on this additional source of information.

In my earlier text (Sanders, 1982), I made a point of not separating vision from audition in the communication training of hearing-impaired children and adults. I stated:

> Except for a person with little or no useable residual hearing visual communication training is inseparable from auditory training. To consider it as a separate aspect of communication requiring separate training is to ignore the indisputable finding that audiovisual speech processing is superior to auditory or visual processing alone under degraded listening conditions. (p. 436)

I supported this statement by reference to Binnie and Alpiner's (1969) study of the effectiveness of lip-reading training. They provided nine one-hour weekly lessons to 10 hearing-impaired adults who had had no previous lip-reading instruction. Half the subjects were trained by the Jena analytic method and half by the Nitche synthetic method. A third group of five hearing-impaired adults received no instruction whatsoever. At the end of the experiment a comparison was made of the pre- and postinstruction scores on the Utley silent-film word and sentence test, and on an individual phoneme-recognition test. Statistical analysis showed no significant difference between pre- and posttest conditions for any of the three groups. The subjects who had received lip-reading training proved no better at recognizing the test items than those who had received no training.

Alpiner (1978) also examined the pre- and posttherapy speech-reading test scores of 100 clients who had received eight one-hour per week therapy sessions that included speech-reading and auditory training, communication training, and counseling. Eighty-nine of the clients reported better communication ability after therapy, yet there was no significant change in their speech-reading test scores. O'Neill and Oyer (1973) have pointed out that even though aural rehabilitation centers upon speech-reading and auditory training, we have no body of research findings to provide evidence of its effectiveness or lack of it. Thus in Alpiner's (1978) words: "We find ourselves utilizing techniques which have no supportive documentation for their success" (p. 4).

In a subsequent publication Alpiner (1987, p. 61) states:

> Our own experience in utilizing lipreading tests under a visual only condition continues to show no outstanding improvement in lipreading ability when comparing pre-service scores. Further there does not appear to be any valid relationship between scores on lipreading tests and success in communication ability.

These findings place the hearing therapist in a dilemma, for it is hard to justify asking a client to pay for a therapy for which we have no demonstrable evidence of success. If anything, the little evidence we do have suggests its ineffectiveness. Why, then, do we persist in providing auditory and visual communication training? Should we continue to include this type of instruction as part of our rehabilitation program for adults? If so, how much time should be spent on such training? These are difficult questions to answer because we lack objective evidence upon which to base decisions. Once again you are forced to use your own judgment in each individual case.

From our discussion we have seen that communication involves the ability to predict the meaning the speaker wishes to convey. We do this by using information inherent within patterns of nonverbal and verbal cues that the speaker transmits. These cues have informational value when correctly decoded. The greatest information is encoded into the acoustic cues of speech. These acoustic patterns are equivalent to linguistic patterns, which, in turn, identify semantic and cognitive values—that is, meanings and concepts. Speech articulation, the means by which we generate the acoustic pattern, is visible to varying degrees. Thus, what we can observe of speech articulation is directly correlated with the acoustic pattern being produced. This makes the visible cues to speech potentially informative. However, at the level of individual phonemes, the visible articulatory information is insufficient to permit identification of each speech sound. Moreover the visual revealing characteristics of speech sounds, like their acoustic correlates, vary with coarticulation. Thus it seems reasonable to assume that visible speech cues, like acoustic cues, are processed in syllable-sized or larger chunks.

We have discussed the fact that we are capable of processing speech at several levels, ranging from listening to the actual sounds (phonetic) to listening only to extract the meaning (semantic). In normal communication we listen for meaning. This is necessitated in part by the rate at which the speech signal is generated. The rate of transmission precludes auditory or visual analysis of individual sound units, so that we must scan for patterns that can be accommodated by syntactic structures. In conversation we listen linguistically rather than acoustically. For this reason our perception of speech is heavily influenced by what we know about the language rules governing the speaker.

Finally, we know that communication does not take place in a vacuum. The study of the pragmatics of language has shown how the choice of topics for communication, the ways in which we introduce and terminate discussion of a topic, as well as the manner in which conversations are developed are all rule bound. Communication takes place in context. Context is determined by content and by the relation of content to previous content. Simultaneous to broadcasting verbal information, the speaker frequently encodes nonverbal cues in the form of gestures. These may be deliberately encoded to clarify the spoken message or they may occur naturally as part of the situation. These visual cues potentially constrain the listener in predicting what is being said.

We know from the study of normal communication that for the reasons just identified, speech involves a high level of redundancy. We know that as the acoustic signal is progressively degraded, the normal listener begins to draw more and more upon that redundancy. As the auditory signal deteriorates, normal-hearing subjects increasingly use visual cues to help retain the ability to process the linguistic pattern. Of particular relevance to this discussion is the unequivocal evidence that on tasks involving recognition of spoken language samples, both normal and hearing-impaired adult subjects score higher when auditory and visual cues to speech are simultaneously available. The bimodal processing of information appears to be integrative rather than additive, resulting in a better definition of the linguistic pattern on the basis of the sensory cues.

PRECEPTS BASIC TO AUDITORY-VISUAL PROCESSING

From this discussion we can identify a number of precepts basic to a rationale for providing auditory and visual communication training, rather than for teaching speech-reading as a separate skill.

1. Speech communication involves the identification of cognitive values.
2. These cognitive values are tapped by use of the language code.
3. In normal communication the system attempts to process units in chunks as large as possible.
4. Comprehension occurs as a result of reconstructing language patterns.
5. Providing meaning can be correctly attributed to a pattern. The actual components of the pattern are not relevant and have probably not been paid attention to or processed.
6. In communication, information already understood will facilitate the processing of new, related information. The greatest dependency on the details of the auditory-visual speech pattern occurs, therefore, when the topic has yet to be identified.
7. The acoustic signal is the primary vehicle for speech information. It far exceeds the visual-speech signal as a source of speech information for all but the severely hearing impaired.
8. Speech comprehension through the recognition of individual speech sounds by their visible characteristics is not possible due to factors discussed earlier.
9. The available visible aspects of articulation can, in many instances, serve to increase the total amount of linguistic constraints upon which prediction of message content is made.
10. Because visible speech articulation is part of spoken language, it is subject to the same factors discussed in items 1 to 5.
11. If the visual intelligibility of speech is low, and visual constraints are integrated with auditory constraints under conditions of acoustic degradation, the overall level of information exceeds that available in either modality alone.
12. Visual and auditory cues are computed by an interactive, not an additive, formula.

Assessment of the Contribution of Vision to Speech Comprehension

Given the preceding precepts, we can state that we are not interested in how well a client scores on visual cues alone since we wish the person always to make maximum use of whatever hearing remains. Assessment thus aims to determine how much better a client discriminates and comprehends speech when visual cues are added to auditory ones than when she must depend upon auditory cues alone.

With the criterion of cost effectiveness in mind, we can gain much of this information by extending the speech discrimination and perception testing to include a recheck with visual cues of each item incorrectly identified by hearing alone. This obviates the need to repeat all the items since

TABLE 19.1

Clients Name				
Date		Test condition		
Aided Free Field		(A) Auditory only		
Signal level (50 dB HL)		(B) Auditory-visual		

Test		Signal-to-Noise levels		
		50/30	50/45	50/50
		1	2	3
Northwestern University	A	74	54	40
Words (NUWT)	B	92	78	72
California consonant Test	A	62	44	36
(CCT)	B	78	58	48
Speech Perception in Noise	Redundancy:	Low High	Low High	Low High
Test (SPIN)	A	54 84	30 64	16 50
	B	66 88	40 80	28 72
CID Everyday Speech	A	80	65	45
Sentences (CID)	B	90	85	75

those correctly discriminated auditorily would have enhanced redundancy with added visual cues. For those incorrectly heard we ascertain whether vision provides sufficient additional constraints to the acoustic constraints to raise the total information above the threshold of comprehension under the conditions of the test. To the auditory-only score we add the items correctly identified under the auditory-visual recheck condition information. The results permit you to gain insight into the extent to which the client is capitalizing on visual cues and on linguistic constraints.

In the example in Table 19.1 (1B) you can see that this person when wearing hearing aids scores 92 percent (NUW test) word discrimination when listening and watching the speaker saying the words in quiet (30dB) in normal conversational voice (50dB HL). In this condition the scores are high for all tests except the low-redundancy words on the SPIN test. When deprived of visual cues under the same condition (Column 1A) discrimination falls by 10–15 percent. However in unfavorable conditions (Column 3. S/N = 50/50) the auditory only scores drop to around 45 percent. The higher scores on the SPIN test high redundancy and the CID test suggest that use is being made of linguistic constraints when they are available.

Thus this client, as expected, experiences difficulty processing speech in low S/N ratios. However, she compensates quite well by using visual and linguistic cues.

During your early sessions with this client, you may wish to take assessment one step further by making a subjective assessment of her ə' to follow conversational speech and to understand a short anecdote. This assessment should be conducted at normal conversational level at a distance of four feet. You should evaluate comprehension by hearing alone and then by hearing with vision. Both conditions can be made against a competing speech babble tape at a low level and at a level you would judge to be distracting for you but not disruptive.

The information obtained for the conditions and materials discussed should prove helpful in identifying the client's needs and in guiding you in planning intervention strategies.

SUMMARY

- Acknowledgment of a hearing impairment is a frequent barrier to an adult's seeking help.
- Reluctance to acknowledge the cause of difficulties encountered leads to rationalization and retrenchment.
- A decision to contract for help is based on the client's perception of cost and inconvenience related to a variety of areas.
- Our program outline must address specifically the cost in each area. Emphasis is on demonstrating the projected benefits from rehabilitation.
- Assessment should detail specific difficulties and the situations in which they arise. It also should determine the priorities for intervention planning.
- The use of formal or informal profiles helps to identify specific situations and tasks that present difficulty. Profiles also tap into difficulties in dealing with feelings about the handicap.
- Hearing-handicap scales should be used judiciously with concern for need, usefulness, and cost.
- Provision of optimal amplification is the primary concern.
- The audiologist can provide comprehensive information concerning aided residual hearing potential or limitations.
- Determination of the contribution of vision to auditory comprehension of speech should be part of the assessment.

Conclusion

It is essential to recognize that impairment of hearing inevitably requires the hearing-impaired person to acknowledge an inability to continue to function normally. Such a recognition calls forth a range of reactions all of which seek to preserve the image of self as normal. This phenomenon must be acknowledged by a management program and accommodated within both the assessment and intervention plan. The concerns of each client derive from a lifestyle peculiar to that client. Thus the thrust of assessment must be to determine the ways in which the hearing deficiency imposes on all facets of the person's life. The assessment task is to identify areas in which difficulties arise. To this end, use of formally structured profiles or a more informal interview approach will permit the identification, detailing, and significance of a range of problem situations. Emotional and behavioral reactions also can be identified in this way. However, one always must bear in mind cost effectiveness of assessment procedures. Together the audiologist and speech-language pathologist should chart the client's performance with the hearing aids in everyday circumstances. A practical assessment process that documents difficulties in direct relation to daily demands and expectations provides a sound basis for effective rehabilitative management.

Appendix 19.A
PROFILE QUESTIONNAIRE FOR RATING COMMUNICATIVE PERFORMANCE IN A HOME ENVIRONMENT

1. a) In my living room, when I can see the speaker's face, I have:

+2	+1	−1	−2
little or no difficulty in understanding	some difficulty (but not a lot)	a fair amount of difficulty (quite a lot)	great difficulty in understanding

b) This happens:

1	2	3
seldom	often	very often

c) The importance of this is:

1	2	3
of relatively little importance	fairly important	highly important

2. a) If I am talking with a person in my living room or family room while the television, radio, or record player is on, I have:

+2	+1	−1	−2
little or no difficulty in understanding	some difficulty (but not a lot)	a fair amount of difficulty (quite a lot)	great difficulty in understanding

b) This happens:

1	2	3
seldom	often	very often

c) The importance of this is:

1	2	3
of relatively little importance	fairly important	highly important

3. a) In a quiet room in my house, if I cannot see the speaker's face, I have:

+2	+1	−1	−2
little or no difficulty in understanding	some difficulty (but not a lot)	a fair amount of difficulty (quite a lot)	great difficulty in understanding

453

b) This happens:

1	2	3
seldom	often	very often

c) The importance of this is:

1	2	3
of relatively little importance	fairly important	highly important

4. a) If someone in my house speaks to me from another room on the same floor, I experience:

+2	+1	−1	−2
little or no difficulty in understanding	some difficulty (but not a lot)	a fair amount of difficulty (quite a lot)	great difficulty in understanding

b) This happens:

1	2	3
seldom	often	very often

c) The importance of this is:

1	2	3
of relatively little importance	fairly important	highly important

5. a) If someone calls me from upstairs when I am downstairs, or from the window when I am in the garden, I will experience:

+2	+1	−1	−2
little or no difficulty in understanding	some difficulty (but not a lot)	a fair amount of difficulty (quite a lot)	great difficulty in understanding

b) This happens:

1	2	3
seldom	often	very often

c) The importance of this is:

1	2	3
of relatively little importance	fairly important	highly important

6. a) Understanding people at the dinner table gives me:

$+2$	$+1$	-1	-2
little or no difficulty in understanding	some difficulty (but not a lot)	a fair amount of difficulty (quite a lot)	great difficulty in understanding

b) This happens:

1	2	3
seldom	often	very often

c) The importance of this is:

1	2	3
of relatively little importance	fairly important	highly important

7. a) When I sit talking with friends in a quiet room, I have:

$+2$	$+1$	-1	-2
little or no difficulty in understanding	some difficulty (but not a lot)	a fair amount of difficulty (quite a lot)	great difficulty in understanding

b) This happens:

1	2	3
seldom	often	very often

c) The importance of this is:

1	2	3
of relatively little importance	fairly important	highly important

8. a) Listening to the radio or record player or watching TV gives me:

$+2$	$+1$	-1	-2
little or no difficulty in understanding	some difficulty (but not a lot)	a fair amount of difficulty (quite a lot)	great difficulty in understanding

b) This happens:

1	2	3
seldom	often	very often

c) The importance of this is:

1	2	3
of relatively little importance	fairly important	highly important

9. a) When I use the phone at home, I have:

$+2$	$+1$	-1	-2
little or no difficulty in understanding	some difficulty (but not a lot)	a fair amount of difficulty (quite a lot)	great difficulty in understanding

b) This happens:

1	2	3
seldom	often	very often

c) The importance of this is:

1	2	3
of relatively little importance	fairly important	highly important

Appendix 19.B
PROFILE QUESTIONNAIRE FOR RATING
COMMUNICATIVE PERFORMANCE IN AN OCCUPATIONAL
ENVIRONMENT

1. a) In talking with someone in the room where I work, I have:

+2	+1	−1	−2
little or no difficulty in understanding	some difficulty (but not a lot)	a fair amount of difficulty (quite a lot)	great difficulty in understanding

b) This happens:

1	2	3
seldom	often	very often

c) The importance of this is:

1	2	3
of relatively little importance	fairly important	highly important

2. a) When I am in a room at work where there is noise, I have:

+2	+1	−1	−2
little or no difficulty in understanding	some difficulty (but not a lot)	a fair amount of difficulty (quite a lot)	great difficulty in understanding

b) This happens:

1	2	3
seldom	often	very often

c) The importance of this is:

1	2	3
of relatively little importance	fairly important	highly important

3. a) When I am at a meeting with a small group of people, around a table in a fairly quiet room, I have:

+2	+1	−1	−2
little or no difficulty in understanding	some difficulty (but not a lot)	a fair amount of difficulty (quite a lot)	great difficulty in understanding

b) This happens:

1	2	3
seldom	often	very often

c) The importance of this is:

1	2	3
of relatively little importance	fairly important	highly important

4. a) If I have to take notes by dictation in a fairly quiet room, I have:

$+2$	$+1$	-1	-2
little or no difficulty in understanding	some difficulty (but not a lot)	a fair amount of difficulty (quite a lot)	great difficulty in understanding

b) This happens:

1	2	3
seldom	often	very often

c) The importance of this is:

1	2	3
of relatively little importance	fairly important	highly important

5. a) If I have to take notes at a meeting, I have:

$+2$	$+1$	-1	-2
little or no difficulty in understanding	some difficulty (but not a lot)	a fair amount of difficulty (quite a lot)	great difficulty in understanding

b) This happens:

1	2	3
seldom	often	very often

c) The importance of this is:

1	2	3
of relatively little importance	fairly important	highly important

6. a) If I have to use the phone at work, I have:

$+2$	$+1$	-1	-2
little or no difficulty in understanding	some difficulty (but not a lot)	a fair amount of difficulty (quite a lot)	great difficulty in understanding

b) This happens:

1	2	3
seldom	often	very often

c) The importance of this is:

1	2	3
of relatively little importance	fairly important	highly important

Appendix 19.C
PROFILE QUESTIONNAIRE FOR RATING
COMMUNICATIVE PERFORMANCE IN A SOCIAL
ENVIRONMENT

1. a) If I am entertaining a group of friends, understanding someone against the background of others talking gives me:

$+2$	$+1$	-1	-2
little or no difficulty in understanding	some difficulty (but not a lot)	a fair amount of difficulty (quite a lot)	great difficulty in understanding

b) This happens:

1	2	3
seldom	often	very often

c) The importance of this is:

1	2	3
of relatively little importance	fairly important	highly important

2. a) If I am playing cards, understanding my partner gives me:

$+2$	$+1$	-1	-2
little or no difficulty in understanding	some difficulty (but not a lot)	a fair amount of difficulty (quite a lot)	great difficulty in understanding

b) This happens:

1	2	3
seldom	often	very often

c) The importance of this is:

1	2	3
of relatively little importance	fairly important	highly important

3. a) When I am at the theater or the movies, I have:

$+2$	$+1$	-1	-2
little or no difficulty in understanding	some difficulty (but not a lot)	a fair amount of difficulty (quite a lot)	great difficulty in understanding

b) This happens:

1	2	3
seldom	often	very often

c) The importance of this is:

1	2	3
of relatively little importance	fairly important	highly important

4. a) In church, when the minister gives the sermon, I have:

$+2$	$+1$	-1	-2
little or no difficulty in understanding	some difficulty (but not a lot)	a fair amount of difficulty (quite a lot)	great difficulty in understanding

b) This happens:

1	2	3
seldom	often	very often

c) The importance of this is:

1	2	3
of relatively little importance	fairly important	highly important

5. a) In following the conversation when I eat out, I have:

$+2$	$+1$	-1	-2
little or no difficulty in understanding	some difficulty (but not a lot)	a fair amount of difficulty (quite a lot)	great difficulty in understanding

b) This happens:

1	2	3
seldom	often	very often

c) The importance of this is:

1	2	3
of relatively little importance	fairly important	highly important

6. a) In the car, I find that understanding what people are saying gives me:

$+2$	$+1$	-1	-2
little or no difficulty in understanding	some difficulty (but not a lot)	a fair amount of difficulty (quite a lot)	great difficulty in understanding

b) This happens:

1	2	3
seldom	often	very often

c) The importance of this is:

1	2	3
of relatively little importance	fairly important	highly important

7. a) When I am outside talking with someone, I have:

+2	+1	−1	−2
little or no difficulty in understanding	some difficulty (but not a lot)	a fair amount of difficulty (quite a lot)	great difficulty in understanding

b) This happens:

1	2	3
seldom	often	very often

c) The importance of this is:

1	2	3
of relatively little importance	fairly important	highly important

20

Rehabilitative Management of Hearing Handicap in the Adult

In general, the rehabilitative management needs of the adult are considerably less extensive than those of the child, but they are more individualized because adults' language and cognition abilities usually are intact, and there is less emphasis on the use of residual hearing for learning. On the other hand, the types of communication demands a client must meet, and the situations in which they arise, are as varied as their occupations and private lifestyles. Thus the need for an individualized intervention plan for an adult is great. It is comprised of five stages:

1. Collection, summarization, and interpretation of findings
2. Identification of needs
3. Statement of goals
4. Determination of methods for goal attainment
5. Evaluation of progress

COLLECTION, SUMMARIZATION, AND INTERPRETATION OF FINDINGS

Our first task is to pull together the information we have gathered and to record it in a manner that allows us to see it as a whole. One way of doing this is suggested by Table 20.1. Such a summary facilitates our interpretation of the findings and allows others to become familiar with the records very

TABLE 20.1

Name: J. Iles   Date: Occupation: Personnel Manager
                                            Hearing aid model

History Summary:
Slow progressive loss over 15 years. Wore single postauricular aid 4 years ago, unsatisfactorily: has learned to get by. Now feels his work threatened.

Problems Reported:
Group meetings and large lecture presentations at work. Understanding wife in car, eating in restaurants, dinner parties. Uncomfortable about aids, self-conscious, others insensitive.

Audiogram

SRT: 50
Unaided discrimination at 50dBHL
PB N/A: NU 56%: CCT 44%

SRT: 35
Aided results at 50dBHL
Discrimination:
PB N/A: NU 88%: CCT 76%
SPIN S/N 50 = 56% 50 = 72%
              55   40

Aid + Vis
PB N/A: NU 92%: CCT 84%

CID N/A
SPIN
  S/N

  50/55 = 68%
  50/40 = 80%

Key: Unaided freefield = F   Aided: AR = right,   AL = left
                                           AB = binaural

General impression: The aids provide considerable benefit. The speech area is encompassed. Discrimination improvement marked but noise remains a problem. Even aided plus vision leaves gaps (68%) at S/N +5dB. Visual cues not well capitalized on. Reluctant to consider wearing hearing aids.

General goals: To foster acceptance of the hearing aids through an understanding of their capabilities and limitations. To analyze communication difficulties and seek strategies to reduce them to help Mr. Iles come to terms with his hearing impairment.

quickly. The process of pulling the available information together encourages us to think of the interactive implications of test scores. It also makes clear whether it would be helpful to provide any further data. When we have the data assembled, consider what we can deduce from it. In the case presented in Table 20.1, it is appropriate to note that

Mr. Iles is a business man.
He encounters different acoustic environments and different situations.
Distance, noise, and numbers of people present listening difficulties.
Similar problems are encountered at home and socially.

- He has not come to terms with his hearing handicap.
- He is sensitive about wearing the hearing aids.
- He wore a single hearing aid four years ago without success.
- He has been "getting by."
- He feels his career is in jeopardy.

Looking at the test results we note that

- The unaided hearing is no longer adequate to permit "getting by."
- Aided hearing brings sensitivity within normal speech intensity boundaries.
- Aided discrimination in quiet approximates normal.
- A frequently encountered S/N condition of $+5dB$ reduces auditory discrimination to only 56 percent.
- Noise is a major problem for Mr. Iles.
- Vision appears not to contribute as much to discrimination in noise as might be expected (56 percent improves to 68 percent).

Now look at the observations you have made in order to identify needs.

IDENTIFICATION OF NEEDS

Mr. Iles demonstrates a number of different needs. These are

1. Acknowledgment and acceptance of his difficulties
2. An understanding of the nature of his hearing problem and its relation to his hearing handicap
3. A set of realistic expectations for amplification
4. Honest information about the limitations of amplification in reducing problems
5. Help in coming to terms with his need to wear hearing aids
6. An understanding of how to obtain maximum benefits from the hearing aids
7. Development of confidence in his hearing aids
8. Help to objectify his fear of losing his job as a result of his hearing handicap
9. Strategies for dealing with problem communication in work and social situations
10. Help in improving his use of visual cues to communication

I would be frank in my relationship with Mr. Iles and discuss the 10 needs I perceive and ask him if they are valid and whether he can improve upon the list. As I drew up the list, I was thinking about the problem developmentally. Because all problems cannot be addressed at once, it will be necessary to identify those needs that are most pressing and most easily addressed.

Under the first criterion, "most pressing," I would expect the most critical needs to be 3, 4, 6, and 7—that is, to develop realistic expectations for amplification and to obtain maximum benefit from it. Strategies for communication problem management, 9, also will be a primary need. Under the criterion of "most easily addressed needs," I would identify 1 and 2.

STATEMENT OF GOALS

Goals are derived from need priorities. They must be stated clearly and be judged by you and the client as realistic and attainable. For Mr. Iles, restated primary needs provide the specific goals:

- That he be able to explain the nature of hearing deficit and the types of listening problems it creates
- That he be able to apply problem-solving strategies to minimize communication difficulties
- That he be able to describe the degree of benefit he should expect to get from his hearing aids in the situations he encounters, and that he be able to identify the limits of amplification
- That he will feel at ease in describing and exploring his difficulties in the management sessions

These represent our initial goals. They set the agenda for our first meeting or two. Subsequent long-term goals will meet the remaining needs:

- That he will explore the subjective and objective evidence pertaining to his fear of loss of employment and will develop ways of addressing these issues
- That he will express and resolve the negative effects of his feelings about having impaired hearing
- That he will achieve confidence in the value of amplification and a positive attitude toward its use
- That he will make better use of visual cues to speech

Correlating, analyzing, and interpreting test results, along with identifying needs and establishing goals, take time and effort. They are, however, essential functions because they focus your intervention efforts. Time invested initially is recouped through the relevance and effectiveness of your resultant management planning. Such a systematic approach, adopted in a climate of acceptance, builds confidence in the process, both the client's confidence and your own. You will know what you are planning, you will have justification for it, and you are assured of its relevance.

Having established goals, you need to identify the means by which they will be achieved.

DETERMINATION OF METHODS FOR GOAL ATTAINMENT AND EVALUATION OF PROGRESS

As with every other stage, choosing intervention methods and evaluating progress are cooperative processes. You need to work with the client and, whenever possible, with a significant other person. It is wise to avoid an open-ended management plan even when a client's needs are extensive. An individual always is better motivated when there is an end to a commitment in sight; it offers a possibility of achievement. If you limit your plan to six sessions or less, you sharpen goal selection and definition and focus your efforts more effectively. A limited number of sessions ensures that you will define your plans realistically and economically, addressing priority needs first. At the end of the unit you will evaluate progress and decide together whether another unit is appropriate. The second unit will have new or revised goals and probably modified strategies for their achievement. This process fosters self-confidence and independence in the client. It offers the opportunity to reduce gradually the amount of support provided in a given time frame. Thus the client who does not wish to make a heavy commitment can negotiate an acceptable unit size while the client who might grow dependent on your support can be moved through progressive stages of reduced appointments per unit until she is placed on a periodic check-up list.

In planning how to achieve the goals the client has accepted as relevant, you will have both general and specific procedures to follow. First we will examine the general approaches to reducing hearing handicap, then we will consider how to address a set of specific needs.

General Procedures

There are three methods of effecting change in the degree of handicap a hearing-impaired client experiences:

1. Education
2. Adjustment counseling
3. Experimental learning

1. Education. Handicap reduction through education occurs when information provided effects a change in the person's understanding of a problem, the significance of a problem, or of possible ways to reduce it. Such change cannot be effected simply by telling the client what you think he should know. As Luterman (1990) has pointed out:

> Unfortunately, most diagnostic interactions are information based and prescriptive in quality; the professional tells or "advises" the client what to do, and the client becomes a passive participant in the rehabilitation program by just following the doctor's orders. (p. 35)

To be educational information must

- Address a need for specific knowledge
- Be provided at a time when the client needs it
- Be presented in an amount, manner, and rate compatible with the person's ability to absorb it
- Be interacted with by the person, that is to say, used for rethinking a topic, situation, or emotion
- Effect change in perceptions, feelings, or behavior

We must make sure, therefore, that we and the client identify information needs together and that we discuss the information we provide. The client may not know initially what information she needs, but neither do we, though we can make general predictions. Our role at first is to find out from our client what is understood, experienced, perceived, or felt. Then together we need to establish goals for knowledge and understanding. Once this has been achieved, we become the resource for providing the appropriate information. Clients commonly have a need for extra information about the following general topics:

Type of Hearing Impairment.

- *Confirmation that there is indeed no cure for the type of loss they have.* Clients often still nurture the thought that perhaps someone knows of an ear specialist who has a special cure for hearing loss. For example, they often inquire about cochlear implant surgery. The need here is to be restored to normal, to eliminate the handicap. This is a healthy desire providing it does not delay or prevent rehabilitation.
- *Information about the chance of losing residual hearing.* The person may have forgotten the answer or may have been afraid to ask this question of the otolaryngologist. The most common need behind the question is for reassurance that she will not "go deaf."
- *How severe the hearing impairment is.* The request often is made to know the percentage loss, which really tells nothing useful. What is usually needed is reassurance that she is not "deaf" or sometimes confirmation that she really has a severe impairment that explains the communication difficulties.

Hearing Aid(s).

- *Need for information about the hearing aid, its use, and maintenance.* Often a person is overwhelmed when the audiologist explains the care and use of the hearing aid. A client frequently will say, "I feel so stupid" when expressing difficulty in inserting the aid or earmold, knowing how to set the volume control, or replacing a battery. The need often derives from a feeling of inadequacy or apprehension. A client may apologize for not being able to manage, saying, "I'm so clumsy" or "I never can make anything work." It also may evidence a struggle between the need to wear the hearing aid(s) and a resentment at having to do so, with the resultant feelings of frustration and anger.
- *A need to know about other makes or models of hearing aids.* Clients will ask why they were not fitted with "one of those little ones you can't see" or one manufactured by X company that "my cousin swears by." Clients sometimes were persuaded to accept the audiologist's recommendation with reluctance. They remain unsure of their decision and need more information or perhaps just reassurance.

Assistive Listening Devices.

- *A need to know if there is anything else to improve hearing.* This need is most likely experienced by a client who leads a varied business and social life in which communication demands are encountered in a variety of situations and acoustic conditions. It evidences the fact that the client still encounters difficulty in certain situations. It is a need for extra practical support. Information about such extra help should cover all forms of assistive listening devices that the client considers relevant to the range of circumstances with which he must deal.

Legal Rights. Our commitment is to the management of hearing handicap. Although this focuses primarily on communication, we must recognize that a hearing disability, along with other disabilities, results in the handicapping of the adult in more ways than their own ability to hear or speak. Society has added to the burden of the disabled by discriminating against them in various ways. Congress has placed limits on such discriminations against disabled children by legally defining their rights. The same action has now been taken to protect disabled adults. The Americans with Disabilities Act (Public Law 101-336), passed by Congress in 1990, extends to the disabled adult the protection against discrimination in the private sector previously afforded to women, persons from minority groups, and the elderly. The law covers a wide range of well-defined rights that can be enforced by the federal government. For individuals with communication disabilities, the law provides the right to communication unimpeded by barriers. This applies to the person's workplace, to public and private service operations, to public accommodations, and to telecommunication services. The list of environments and services included under "public accommodations" is extensive. It includes shops, department stores, restaurants and bars, hotels and motels; all places of entertainment from movie houses to stadiums; offices of doctors, health care professionals, lawyers, other professionals, beauticians, and hairdressers; and even laundromats. Almost no public place of service is excluded, from the college classroom to the bowling alley.

The ramifications of this act for hearing-impaired adults are enormous. It means that employers and all who provide a service to the general public are called upon to ensure that communication environments do not handicap unreasonably the hearing-impaired person. Thus the provision of assistive listening and alerting devices, of interpreters and of information in written form, can now be demanded. All telephone locations must provide for the needs of a hearing-impaired adult, including the use of telecommunication devices (TDD) and telecommunication relay services for the person who has a profound hearing impairment (see Chapter 12).

Finally, the act prohibits discrimination against qualified disabled persons during the hiring process. Their right to "reasonable accommodation" of their disability during the hiring process, and in all facets of their work experience, is protected under law. They must, in other words, be provided the same access rights as their nondisabled co-workers at no additional cost to them.

As audiologists, speech-language pathologists, and teachers of hearing-impaired people, we must serve as advocates for those with whom we work. We must be knowledgeable of the legal rights of the disabled person, be prepared to advise them of such rights as part of the counseling process, and be willing to support them in their effort to have those rights enforced. Our concern must not be simply for the hearing impairment but for the person who is hearing impaired and for the family of that person.

2. Adjustment Counseling. From our discussion of a number of types of information most commonly needed by the person with impaired hearing, I hope you will appreciate that there is no clear separation between the need for information and the need for counseling support. A great deal of the information we seek, perhaps most of it, arises from concern, anxiety, or even fear of the unknown. Our feelings about our disability and all its ramifications are a major part of our handicap. Interactive counseling thus constitutes a powerful method for reducing the hearing handicap. In Chapter 13 we examined the general principles of interactive counseling. I stressed that it involves the nurturing of a dynamic relationship between you and the client. For the most part counseling is woven throughout all our interactions with the client. It involves being sensitive to or willing to explore the feelings and concerns that lie beneath the verbal messages (Webster, 1977). As I have endeavored to show, a demonstrated or expressed need for information that appears on the surface to be intellectual very frequently has an underlying emotional motivation. In some instances the emotional need may be primary. Interactive counseling does not justify your making this assumption, but it requires that you be sensitive to its possibility and that you check it out. Often the client herself is unaware of the specific underlying anxiety that has become part of a general worry about the whole problem of the hearing impairment and all its actual and potential ramifications. Interactive counseling, as the occasion arises, seeks to identify the single strands of the tangled problem and to unravel them over a period of time. Fortunately, as with a tangled skein of wool, unraveling one piece tends to loosen others.

In Chapter 14 p. 236 we reviewed the types of requests persons make. We discussed Webster's (1977) guidelines for categorizing questions. As a reminder, these included requests for facts, opinions, clarification, and discussion. We must endeavor to identify the nature of the expressed need if we are to respond appropriately. Counseling seeks to facilitate a change in the client's attitudes, feelings, and behavior as they relate to the hearing impairment. The changes made become possible when the client acknowledges a need for change, is able to resolve or accommodate the attitudinal and emotional resistance to the change, and finds acceptable the change and the means by which it will be achieved. I stress that both the decision to accept a change and the means by which it can be made must be the client's, made without pressure. Our role is to help the client reach that decision, not to make it for her.

It is not uncommon for a client who is trying to deal with the impact of a hearing impairment to raise aspects of the problem that we feel uncomfortable dealing with. The idea of counseling is in itself a somewhat intimidating one for many audiologists and speech-language pathologists. Even those of us who have been involved with counseling still feel insecure in many situations. Charles Van Riper (1979), one of the foundation stones of speech pathology, responded to a student clinician's expressed intense apprehension about working with her first client by telling her:

> I, who had worked with speech handicapped individuals for so many years, still felt inadequate whenever a new client was confronted for the first time. . . . Any clinician who feels absolutely confident or competent at such a time is probably insensitive, egocentric, or stupid. (Van Riper, 1979, p. 74)

This initial feeling of inadequacy usually passes as you develop a relationship with the client. However, I encounter these feelings again from time to time even when I know a client. In fact the greater the client's confidence in me as a sensitive person, the more likely is it that he will share with me intimate concerns that may make me feel uncomfortable. Some years ago I had a woman in her mid-years talk with my counseling class. She was severely hard-of-hearing and wore binaural hearing aids. This woman was herself a rehabilitation counselor. My class expected to be given professional guidance in the techniques of counseling. I had told my colleague to feel free to address any issue she felt particularly important for them to consider. She chose to discuss the impact of hearing impairment on a person's sexual life. She spoke about her own experiences and generalized them to the larger population of hearing-impaired persons. It was interesting to observe my students' reactions. They felt very uncomfortable and expressed the opinion that this was not a topic they should be expected to deal with. My guest insisted that her problem was not with her sexuality but with the impact her hearing impairment had on her ability to communicate in intimate relationships. Psychologists, she said, do not know very much about hearing impairment, hearing aids, acoustic feedback, or visual communication. She insisted she did not need sexual counseling—she needed aural rehabilitation. Several months later the December 1987 issue of the journal *ASHA* devoted nine pages to four articles discussing sexuality in communicative disorders, one of which was titled "Romance, Sexuality and Hearing Loss" (Reiter, 1987).

Hearing impairment affects sexual communication between partners. If this handicap is ignored, it may severely affect the relationship. Monat Halle (1987) advocates that speech-language pathologists accept responsibility for serving as counselors and sexuality educators:

> Because of our technical training and expertise in communication speech-language pathologists can assume special roles in enhancing social interaction. One of these is the role of facilitator when social interaction or sexuality issues are discussed in a group or with a client. (pp. 35–36)

I chose sexuality as an example of a counseling need we often ignore or treat as insignificant, as, for example, when we answer with an immediate "Yes" the question, "Should I take my aid(s) off when I go to bed?" We should reply that the answer depends upon the client's need to communicate with a spouse or partner in that situation. Sexuality is not the only area in which the hearing aid becomes a part of the larger need. One lady I saw for a hearing aid evaluation showed a high level of resistance to accepting her need for one hearing aid, and I was recommending that she consider wearing two. My client was discourteous to the receptionist who warned me not to expect an easy fitting. The woman spoke to me abruptly, advising me that her appointment was at three o'clock but that it now was eight minutes past the hour (she had inquired at three o'clock whether I was ready for her) and that she had other important things to attend to. Already this woman had told me a lot about her situation. I listened to her calmly, realizing that though I was the recipient of her feelings I was not the cause.

I explained why I was running a little late. I told her my previous client needed a little more time than I had expected and that I intended to provide the same personal attention to her. After some discussion of her amplification needs during which her attitude changed only a little, I decided I needed a broader understanding of this woman's attitude. In a sympathetic tone of voice I said:

I get the feeling you are having a particularly difficult time. I know you find the idea of the hearing aids difficult to come to terms with, but I suspect that's not the whole problem. It seems that perhaps it really is the idea of being hearing impaired rather than just the hearing aids that you cannot face. Perhaps it would help to talk about why you feel so angry at everything and everyone.

I thought I had identified the real justification for her attitude, so I was not surprised when she burst into tears. It was several minutes before she composed herself. I simply handed her a box of tissues and waited. When she was ready to talk, I learned that my perception of her problem was still too narrow. She explained:

Oh, it's not just the hearing aids or my hearing loss, though they do bother me. It's everything, it's my life. I'm lonely, I'm overweight, I'm getting old. I don't look good, now I have to wear these things because I'm deaf. Why would anyone ever be interested in me? I'm sorry, I shouldn't take my problems out on you people.

Once again here is evidence that for many the hearing impairment is but a part of a larger handicap. This woman perceived her handicap primarily to be one of appearance and age. Her problem was loneliness, a condition exacerbated by her moderate hearing impairment. The hearing aids were for her "the last straw"; like her weight, they stigmatized her. What should you do? Should you reassure her that her weight is not 'that bad," that fat people are likeable, that we all get old, that lots of people wear hearing aids, and that you're sure she will meet someone? Hardly an empathetic response. Should you ignore these other problems and get back to discuss the hearing aids? Should you refer this client to a psychologist? Should you acknowledge her feelings, accept that things can be very difficult at times, and suggest that it might help to spend the session talking about these feelings and how the hearing impairment fits into the picture? Should you discuss possible ways for your client to address each of these problems including, of course, the need for amplification.

I pursued the latter course. We devoted two consultations to talking about the whole situation, about the feelings she had been bottling up, sharing with no one, about being hearing impaired. We discussed action on several fronts, Weight Watchers for physical appearance along with a fitness program at the YMCA, attendance at meetings of the local Self-Help for the Hard of Hearing chapter, and volunteer opportunities to focus concerns away from herself. We talked about hair styles and hearing aids, about beauticians and manicurists, and about a new wardrobe as a motivation and a reward for successful weight control.

What is it that makes us so reluctant to accept such responsibility for counseling in general and most particularly for consideration of aspects of the client's life that are not obviously related to speech and hearing rehabilitation? The most immediate cause of the attitude of speech and hearing professionals rests in lack of training. McCarthy, Culpepper, and Lucks (1987) and Stone and Olswang (1989) recognize this deficiency in counseling training but look beyond it to more fundamental causes of the discomfort and uncertainty we feel about our role as counselors. Stone and Olswang suggest that a major but neglected barrier to the provision of counseling by most of us is that of professional boundaries. They cite the Merriam-Webster Dictionary (1974) definition of boundary as "[Things] that mark or fix a limit." Audiologists and speech-language pathologists, they state, "have for the most part been working with 'blurry boundaries.' " This, they claim, is the fundamental cause of our anxiety and insecurity about counseling responsibilities. In their excellent examination of barriers to effective counseling Stone and Olswang lay out a set of very helpful and practical guidelines to a better appreciation of valid boundaries. These are fairly flexible criteria to accommodate different professional experiences and work settings. Two aspects of the counseling relationship are considered by the authors—namely, focus (content) and style (dynamics). *Focus* involves "what you talk about" (p. 28). Within the acceptable content boundary are included "feelings, attitudes, information or problems directly related to the communication disorder and treatment process." Such topics as marital problems, depression, and major financial difficulties would fall outside the boundary and call for referral to an appropriate support service. The authors explain that boundary problems are identified not because they arise in one particular session but because they begin to detract progressively from the major task of communication handicap reduction.

Style is defined by Stone and Olswang (1989) as "how the clinician and client interact, share power, and assume responsibility" (p. 29). They strongly support Luterman's (1984) model of the counseling relationship, which empowers the client while maintaining mutual respect. When the dynamics of the relationship lead to client dependency, when the client evidences marked swings in behavior or emotions, or when your relationship with the client becomes unsatisfactory or causes you to feel uneasy and insecure, then there is evidence that the boundary has been crossed. Failure to make progress in problem solving, entrenched fear of change, and regression instead of progression also indicate that boundaries have been exceeded, placing the need within the territorial competence of another type of professional.

The Stone and Olswang article goes on to point out that we, the audiologist or speech-language pathologist, are equal partners in the dynamics. Our own needs and feelings may interact with those of the client, often in a selfish manner. We may encourage dependence to bolster our sense of self-worth or even to feel the power that comes with control. We may adopt the clients' pain and suffering and experience their feelings, or we may worry so much about clients' feelings that we must resolve their problems for them. We may be angry because they are not striving for what we believe they or their child have the potential to achieve.

In matters pertaining to sexuality, we run up against our own personal barriers. These may cause us to avoid or suppress the expression of need for guidance pertaining to the sexual implications for the hearing handicap. In today's liberal environment such topics may be expected to occur more frequently, particularly in support groups. Neither our criteria for what is appropriate nor our personal feelings should discourage a client or spouse from raising such sensitive issues. The fact that these concerns are expressed is evidence of trust. Such trust may be received and honored. A need expressed must be addressed. We must be prepared to listen, to acknowledge the legitimacy of the concern, and to assist the client in locating a professional trained to deal with issues that we feel fall outside our boundary.

As professionals in a helping profession, we cannot avoid the counseling responsibility. A hearing handicap creates communication problems with which we have been trained to deal. It also creates confusion about identity and personal values, disrupts personal relationships, and creates a feeling of insecurity and apprehension about the future. Hearing handicap aggravates other personal concerns and generally erodes self-confidence. These problems in turn create a need to share the burden with someone who is able to empathize and who has the ability to guide the client.

Counseling for Progressive and Sudden Onset Deafness. An acute need for interactive counseling support occurs when the loss of hearing progresses fairly rapidly or when it is traumatic. The loss may be familial or may result from an accident, illness, vascular lesion, or chemotherapy involving ototoxic drugs, or its cause may remain unknown. The rate of progression of the impairment will determine the pressure on the client for rapid adaptation. Slow progressive hearing loss allows the person to spend more time in each of the stages involved in denying, acknowledging, protesting, and finally adapting. Time for this client is a luxury; it makes the process of coming to terms with the changing reality somewhat easier. What is not easy is the terror that the concept of *deafness* evokes. The client feels he has seen the future and it is intolerable.

For the person with a sudden onset of irreversible deafness, the impact is immediate. She suddenly has been transported into a world of silence. In a matter of days all lines of auditory input are blocked, and communication is seriously impaired. Her relationship with her loved ones and friends is disrupted, made abnormal, as is their relationship with her. She no longer has confidence that she can drive, take care of her young children, or even go shopping, since she cannot understand what shop assistants say. Her ability to continue working may be seriously in doubt and with it the whole question of the ability of the family to manage without her paycheck. Most forms of entertainment are denied her (e.g., radio, television, movies, theater, music) as is the comfort of a religious service or the challenge of a sermon. Serious depression is a very real threat for this client who suddenly becomes extremely dependent (Lieberth, 1986).

Neither the person who is "going deaf" and sees the inevitability of silence nor the person who already is in that world knows how to cope. Their families do not know how to behave or manage either. This is a situation that frequently calls for a different form of counseling than most of us are qualified to provide. If the client is in a state of depression, she and her family will not benefit from rehabilitative management counseling until the depression lifts and she can afford to direct her attention to understanding the implications of the hearing impairment and how to minimize the handicap. Stone and Olswang (1989) contrast educational supportive counseling with psychotherapy, which is essential to the management of depression. The latter, they point out, encourages the exploration of unconscious material, having as its goal the provision of new emotional experiences and enhancement of sensitivity to emotion: "It aims to alter a person's or family's basic way of relating and functioning" (p. 28). This clearly falls outside our competence boundary. Thus we must make an appropriate medical-psychological referral. However, psychotherapy will not address the communication needs of the client; it will not seek to lessen the hearing handicap or help the client to investigate the serious anxieties that arise form the practical problems to be confronted. These concerns reflect very real problems—the feelings are normal and justified. They are within the client's ability to address constructively given appropriate education and support counseling. This responsibility lies well within our area of competence.

Progressive hearing impairment demands that the client look into the future. Its advance is inexorable; we can ignore it, but ultimately, we must come face to face with it. The alternative to denial is to prepare for the loss of hearing to the extent that we can anticipate what it will bring. The future for people with a progressive hearing impairment is frightening. They and their family see a progressive erosion of their relationship and of their means of deriving pleasure from life. Their very existence may be perceived to be in jeopardy as a result of possible loss of financial income. The potential loss of employment due to the communication barrier means loss of a role and identify, self-confidence, and self-respect. Thus, for man or woman, the justifiable fears are of loneliness, dependency, and loss of self-respect.

Luterman (1984, p. 38) explains that almost all anxiety stems from awareness of separation and that all change is a loneliness experience. This he defines as existential loneliness, an experience we all go through. To this fundamental loneliness now is added the realization that because of the increasing hearing loss, we will be more and more isolated from others. Luterman says:

> As a practicing audiologist it became apparent to me that the underlying terror of progressive hearing loss experienced by the clients was the feeling of being cut off and isolated. The major means by which we alleviate our interpersonal loneliness is verbal communication, and when that is defective we become very disturbed. (1984, p. 40)

Anxiety loneliness results from being cut off from others. To assuage our fears we seek the support of others and

> We try to merge with another to avoid dealing with our existential loneliness (and also responsibility). This love is the romantic kind (I will die if you leave me), and does not allow for growth. It fosters a mutually dependent relationship in which there is no growth. (Luterman, 1984, p. 39).

We must be extremely cautious in our reactions to progressive or sudden deafness. Although acceptance of the seriousness of the situation is important, we must avoid accepting responsibility for dealing with the problem. Dependence is a serious threat to a client in this situation because he sees no hope. Life often has become meaningless. Don Juan, in Castanada's (1972) *Journey to Ixtlan*, a novel I highly recommend, which is much quoted by Luterman, says:

> When you feel as you always do, that everything is going wrong and you're about to be annihilated, turn to your death and ask if that is so. Your death will tell you that you're wrong; that nothing really matters outside its touch. Your death will tell you, "I haven't touched you yet." (Castanada, 1972, p. 34)

If life appears meaningless, the urgent need is to give it a meaning. Once the acute sense of loss begins to subside, the person needs to become involved in a problem-solving task.

The first stage of problem solving involves providing the client and loved ones with encouragement to express the feelings they are experiencing, to verbalize the unspeakable. Until these fears are externalized, they cannot be reduced through action. It is very important to treat the problem as a family problem, since those close to the person who experiences a sudden loss of hearing also experience considerable anxiety and apprehension. As with any serious disability, both the victim and family become handicapped; that is to say, both experience significant limitations on their existing lifestyle—they even may feel they have lost control of their lives. Rehabilitative counseling will involve modifying family perceptions and behaviors to minimize the degree of handicap experienced by all members. This includes children in the family who will feel equally threatened by being shut off from a parent who, in addition to the communication difficulties, reasonably may be expected to be overwhelmed emotionally and possibly functionally. The children, therefore, also may experience feelings of isolation and loneliness and may fear that the same thing may happen to the other parent or perhaps to themselves. They may perceive their future to be in jeopardy due to the handicap of the parent. Children often experience guilt in such circumstances in the belief that this is some sort of punishment for their behavior, a fear that somehow they may have caused it. At the same time a child may feel and act resentful and angry at the parent for letting this happen. The confused feelings of children in the family add to the total problem and must be recognized as part of the solution. We must do everything we can to protect family unity. We must remember constantly what Luterman stresses:

> Clinicians must come to realize that the people we deal with are part of a system and that we cannot treat one element (the person with the communication disorder) without some attention to the entire system (the family). (1984, p. 160)

Our reaction to the situation must be especially neutral. Above all it is important to avoid expressing great sympathy or trying to minimize the pain. What the family needs more than anything else at this time is hope. They need to know that you see a meaningful resolution of the difficulties, that there are resources to draw upon in the community, and that they themselves also have resources. They need not feel alone since you will be able to help them deal with the impossible. An understanding yet very professional manner will lead to confidence. While accepting the seriousness of the trauma and legitimizing the feelings associated with it, you must make quite clear that the client and family cannot afford self-pity. Self-pity represents a focus on the past, on the notion of fairness and unfairness, and it magnifies the negatives of the situation. When we feel sorry for ourself, we feel we have been unfairly singled out. We concentrate on our inadequacies; we feel helpless. Castanada's Don Juan addresses this feeling:

> "You feel like a leaf at the mercy of the wind don't you?" he finally said, staring at me. That was exactly the way I felt. He seemed to empathize with me. . . . "Since the day you were born, one way or another someone has been doing something to you," he said. "That's correct," I said.
> "And they have been doing something to you against your will."
> "True."
> "And by now, you're helpless, like a leaf in the wind."
> "That's correct. That's the way it is." I said that the circumstances of my life had sometimes been devastating. He listened attentively but I could not figure out whether he was just being agreeable or genuinely concerned until I noticed that he was trying to hide a smile.
> "No matter how much you like to feel sorry for yourself you have to change that," he said in a soft tone. "It doesn't jibe with the life of a warrior. . . . It is no use being sad and complain and feel justified in doing so believing that someone is always doing something to us. Nobody is doing anything to anybody." (Castanada, 1972, pp. 109–110)

Self-pity effects no positive change in circumstances; more important, it puts off action. Self-pity "doesn't jibe with power" says Castanada and power is what the client must assume if he is to take control of the situation and dictate a positive change. Point out that problems compound if left unaddressed, while power, by contrast, builds strengths.

Although the philosophical and psychological issues are at first primary, they only prepare us for change. Progress is measured by concrete evidence of problem reduction. For this type of hearing loss as for our clients in general we must identify the most pressing needs, which may include

> Ensuring optimal use of any residual hearing
> Exploring alternate family communication modes and strategies
> Obtaining a TTY system for telephone communication and a telephone answering machine
> Dealing with the practical needs relative to employment
> Consulting the motor vehicle department regarding the driving license
> Consulting the insurance agent concerning automobile coverage
> Identifying needs for assistive alerting devices in the home

We also need to determine the structure of a program of management and communication training that will include

> Retention of normal speech and enhancement of visual information processing skills

The teaching of essential signs to the whole family
Teaching strategies for difficult situations
Enrichment of social life, which may include obtaining captioned TV; subscribing to magazines; pursuing a new activity; taking up a sport or hobby; joining a class involving practical instruction, such as indoor gardening, bonsai, pottery, or weaving; joining a self-help group or association for the hearing impaired; or offering to talk with students in training about being deafened. All these may offer both interest and insight to the client. Devoting time to volunteer work, particularly for others with special needs, is an excellent therapy for self-pity and loneliness.
The maintenance of normal voice and speech

The education and counseling for the client and the family of the hearing-impaired person must underpin all our management and training efforts. This holds true whether the impairment is mild or profound, stable or progressive. A client who regains a sense of optimism for the future, who sees that her life need not be restricted in the way she believed, will be motivated to effect change. That change must be reflected in tangible ways. Education provides insight and understanding of the problems to be resolved; support counseling helps to bring about the self-knowledge, attitude, and motivation prerequisite to change. It is the final component of a management trio, namely, experimentation, that explores, implements, and evaluates practical ways to improve functional behavior.

3. Experimental Learning. Experimentation is the process by which you apply appropriately selected resources to address a clearly defined need. It is based upon predictions that a particular strategy will effect positive change in one or more of the factors contributing to functional communication impedance. The impediments to communication lie with the client, with significant persons within the client's family, in factors in work and social settings, and within the physical environment. The means by which the effects of these impediments can be reduced are

1. Technological assistance
2. Environmental modification
3. Modification of communication behavior of significant others
4. Modification of communication strategies used by the client
5. Upgrading of information-processing skills of the client.

We will consider each of these in the order listed since they represent a progression from management strategies that, if feasible, can be implemented quickly to those that will require a longer investment of time.

1. Technological Assistance. The provision of technological assistance is your responsibility as audiologist. You have the expertise necessary for this. However, effective management requires a transdisciplinary model. In such a model we each assume a primary area of responsibility based upon our own training and role definition. We also accept, under the guidance of other professionals, a secondary cooperative responsibility for related areas. This responsibility means that you and the speech-language pathologist must work cooperatively to understand what has been done for the client, what effects those procedures have achieved, and what deficiencies remain.

Equally it requires that you, the speech-language pathologist, provide the audiologist with your observations of the client's present level of function and self-reported abilities and difficulties. You should discuss the communication problems that remain in everyday life situations to ensure that every possible form of technical assistance has been explored.

The universal form of technical assistance is, of course, the personal hearing aid. This, however, does not accommodate all demands for speech comprehension in all situations. This is why rehabilitative management is necessary. When the client who has a realistic understanding of what can be expected of the hearing aid still has difficulty in certain situations or environments, it is essential to determine that nothing further can be done technologically to reduce the communication impedance. If a profile questionnaire has been completed, you will have identified specific communication difficulties. You now must obtain from the client very specific information about the nature of each problem, when and where it occurs, what type of communication activity it is, and how it presently is handled. The problems described should activate an exploration of whether there might be further technological assistance that might prove effective. The factors that need to be considered are

- Binaural amplification unless contraindicated
- Type of output limiting (i.e., peak clipping or compression amplification)
- Upper frequency limits of the hearing aid
- Use of special earmold technology for further signal enhancement
- Possible extra benefits from special fittings (e.g., automatic signal processing [ASP], digital hearing aids, CROS, BICROS)
- Use of special assistive listening and alerting devices

Identify the problem and describe it as carefully as possible, then ask a series of questions about the present fitting and about possible additional technological support. Discuss these with the audiologist. Problems encountered usually center on speech in noise, at a distance, in very quiet settings, in group discussions, at large meetings, in poor acoustics, and on the TV or VCR.

As an example of the questions to ask, consider the following complaint:

Problem: Considerable discrimination problems in competing noise when wearing the hearing aid(s).

Question: Does the aid have compression amplification? Since no signal is lost with compression amplification, it provides more acoustic information than peak clipping, thus reducing signal distortion. Compression amplification also maintains a constant signal-to-noise ratio, which peak clipping does not.

Question: Is it possible that automatic signal processing (ASP) hearing aids or digital hearing aids might help suppress the noise factor?

Question: Is the client wearing binaural hearing aids? We know that signal and noise sources can be spacially separated only when different information is received about them at each ear.

Question: Is the problem significant enough to warrant the use of an assistive device? For persons who must meet professional demands, special or modified amplification systems such as the use of FM microphone pickup units matched to a wearable hearing aid may be considered. For couples who find communicating difficult while traveling by car, plane, train, or bus, a direct audio input microphone to the hearing aid may prove effective. A portable personal FM unit would be equally effective in these situations without the limitations of a microphone cord. Such a system could thus be used by cyclists and walkers and is often used by non–hearing-impaired motorcyclists.

Technological assistance may eliminate, or reduce to acceptable levels, the client's communication problem. Technology, however, always is limited by the processing capability of the damaged cochlea. It also is limited by the willingness of the client to use it. Thus other approaches to handicap reduction frequently are necessary. The next strategy on our list is attempting to modify the environment.

  2. *Environmental Modification.* This is a method of reducing hearing handicap that requires that you be very realistic about the cost of modification. The most effective method of modification of the acoustic environment—namely, technological means, already has been discussed. Beyond this, the amount of environmental modification that is financially realistic and cost effective will depend on the individual client's needs, fiscal resources, and ability to dictate changes. Environmental modifications will seek to

  Reduce reverberation
  Reduce noise
  Shorten speaker-listener distance
  Maximize favorable lighting

In the home, or where possible in the work setting, reverberation may be reduced by lowering ceiling height and by using acoustic ceiling tiles. Extending heavy window drapes beyond the window frame to cover wall space and extending drapes several inches from the wall reduce low frequency reverberation (Nabelek & Nabelek, 1985). Drapes are particularly important when rooms have large picture windows that use plate glass.

  To reduce noise levels, attention should be given to mechanical noise-producing sources that might benefit from replacement or servicing. Noise level should be a prime consideration in the purchasing of air conditioners, fans, space heaters, dishwashers, and all other noise-producing home appliances. Turning off the radio, television, or record player will greatly facilitate communication by reducing the signal-to-noise ratio as will closing doors or windows to reduce outside noise. When purchasing a car, attention should be paid to how quiet the interior is while driving. Air conditioning dramatically reduces wind noise while driving; its use is desirable even when outside temperatures may be moderate. Carpeting in home and office should be wall-to-wall if possible and should have thick underpadding as well as an open weave for maximum effect. Carpet also serves to limit reverberation of high frequency sounds (Nabelek & Nabelek, 1985). Shortening the listener-speaker distance is effective because it increases signal-to-noise ratio. The action should aim to move the listener well within the critical distance (see Chapter 3). In home and office attention should be paid to the arrangement of furniture to provide favorable areas for conversation. At the same time care should be taken to provide seating so the hearing-impaired person can elect to sit with her back to the source of natural light. Good artificial light should be provided with particular attention to seating areas.

I wish to emphasize the importance of being realistic and practical when discussing modifications in the physical environment with the client. Changes that may be possible for a business executive or a partner in a law firm may be totally unrealistic for a bank teller or school teacher. Similarly if a couple is planning to renovate their home, structural changes may be possible; the same changes may be impractical for persons in a well-established home environment, in an apartment, or on a limited income.

Once the physical environment has been favorably modified as far as possible, our effort to reduce communication impedance will be focused on modifying the communication behavior of significant others in the client's life.

3. Modification of Communication Behavior of Significant Others. The most successful method of persuading any one of us to modify our behavior is to convince us that to do so is in our own best interest and that it will improve our situation. This is the most advisable approach to take with family members of the hearing-impaired person. Remember that although the client has the disability, the family shares much of the handicap with him. We have discussed how hearing impairment causes the person to experience a sense of being isolated from others and creates frustration that can lead to anger or withdrawal, particularly in conversational interactions. We saw also that it leads to difficulties in remembering what was said or requested because of information overload, signal distortion, and reduced auditory attention to what is going on. Each of these difficulties directly impacts on the partner in the communication interaction. How members of the family react to the effects of the hearing impairment on their ability to communicate will either increase or decrease the ease of communication. When it is difficult for wife and husband to communicate with each other, or for the children to be understood easily when they speak to a parent, the hearing partner becomes annoyed, irritated, and impatient. Unable to appreciate the invisible disability, or unable to accept it, the hearing partner blames the hearing-impaired person, accusing him of not paying attention, of not listening, or of not being interested in what she has to say:

You seem not to care anymore. You shut yourself off in the newspaper (in your stamp collection, in your gardening, etc.), and you're just not interested in the kids. You could manage, you just don't make the effort. "What's the point of telling Dad, he never pays attention anyway," they complain.

These statements often are made even after amplification has been provided, usually due to the misconception that the hearing aid restores hearing to normal. As the frustration builds for all involved, patterns of social interaction change negatively, increasing the effects of the handicap even further.

Our goal is to provide support for all involved and to bring about a modification of communication interaction in ways that minimize the handicap. To achieve this you, the hearing-impaired person, and the family need to consider the needs of the family and how family members can help. We can do this

- Through sympathetic listening to the concerns of the hearing members of family and acknowledging how difficult and demanding the situation is for them
- Through explaining why these breakdowns occur, familiarizing them with the causative elements
- By having the family carefully document and describe the specific situations in which difficulty arises in order to better understand the factors involved
- Through explaining that there are strategies they can use to reduce the difficulties they are experiencing and thus the frustration
- By considering together specific strategies for minimizing the difficulties

Empathetic listening: The family needs us to acknowledge and legitimize the problems they experience as a result of a loved one's hearing handicap. They need to feel that their frustrations and their reactions are quite understandable, but they also need to realize that it is the situation they really are angry at rather than their hearing-impaired family member. This acceptance of their feelings and the acknowledgment of their needs will do much to enhance their willingness to contribute to change. Family members seldom are fully aware of their contribution to the communication difficulties. They tend to see the problem, and therefore the solution, as lying with the hearing-impaired person.

Identifying and explaining breakdowns: To be able to experiment with new patterns of communicative behavior, the family must understand the factors that contribute to communication problems. This is best achieved by explaining, quite simply and concisely, what hearing loss does to sound patterns. You need to explain that even more important than the loss of the loudness of speech, which alone makes listening difficult, the person suffers from distortion of sound, a problem helped only a little by the hearing aid(s). Explain that for those of us with normal hearing, the signal is comfortably loud and quite clear. We receive far more information in the speech signal than we need under most circumstances. This is analogous to having an excellent income and a healthy balance in a savings account. For the hearing-impaired person, the same speech signal is not loud enough and is very distorted. This often is the case even with the hearing aids. This person can just about make ends meet and has no savings. Savings, in a monetary context, are a cushion against unexpected financial demands that cannot be accommodated by the checking account. Without them a person may find certain periods of the year, such as holiday times when fiscal demands are high, hard to get through. Similarly, for the hearing-impaired person, the demands upon hearing resources often exceed what she can accommodate. As a result she either fails to respond (she has no informational savings on which to draw) or she avoids such situations.

Documenting and describing difficult situations: The family needs to be encouraged to be sensitive and alert to those situations that make listening difficult. By now you are familiar with these. They are

- Competing speech on radio or TV
- Speech at a distance
- Soft speech
- High-pitched voices
- Rapid conversation
- Multiple speakers
- Being addressed before one's attention is captured
- Topic changes
- Unfamiliarity with the topic
- Noisy environments
- Reverberant rooms
- Wind noise when outside
- Poor lighting or glare
- Visual distractions
- Inability to see the speaker

The family may find such a list to be quite helpful to them in identifying the particular situations in which problems occur. In addition to identifying the situations, the family needs to learn to analyze them and to identify how they currently are managing them. Once this has been achieved, the next step is to explore acceptable alternative ways of managing those situations.

Deciding upon strategies to reduce difficulties: Consider carefully how to bring about change. The temptation is simply to give the family a long list of do's and don'ts about how to behave when talking to or with the person with the hearing difficulty. This may save time but it achieves little. You will find it far more effective to help the family to understand why a particular communication situation proves problematic, what the requirements for effective communication are under those circumstances, and how those requirements might be achieved. *The goal is to teach the family how to think about problems and their resolution*. This is an educational training task rather than an informative one. Select one or two of the situations and go over with the family the problem created and their way of handling it. Then analyze the situation in terms of the reasons the person has difficulty. These we just listed. Then explore with the family, do not just tell them, what the person's hearing/seeing needs are in that situation. Finally ask for suggestions as to how these may be met. I again remind you that the goal is to teach the family how to perceive, understand, and use these problem-solving procedures.

Some possible options for communication strategies include

- Make a point of talking only after the person's attention has been alerted.
- Move closer to the person to whom you are speaking.
- Face the listener when speaking.
- Provide topic identification words before talking about the topic.
- Speak only when in the same room.
- Do not expect to compete with the TV or radio; they make communication very difficult.
- Alert a person to a topic change with a key content phrase.

The family members should be encouraged to see communication breakdowns as a challenge to identify effective repair strategies. You should work with them to select one or two problem situations to work on changing. Set a realistic goal, such as "I will use the new approach at least half the time." Ask the hearing-impaired person to agree to make a point of acknowledging the problem reduction each time it is achieved. This builds a reinforcement into the behavior modification and establishes shared acceptance of responsibility, a partnership. The same partnership will be needed in the modification of the communication behaviors of the hearing-impaired person.

4. Modification of Communication Behaviors Used by the Client. The procedure to accomplish this goal follows closely those we already have discussed. You help the client identify and describe the problem situations, then you help him analyze how he reacts and manages the difficulty. Review with him the factors contributing to the problem, consider options for change, and follow through with the most practical of them. Among the available options are to

- Advise the speaker of your hearing impairment, thus increasing her understanding of your difficulty.
- Move close to the speaker.
- Change your seat to reduce distance, to optimize favorable lighting conditions, and to enhance visibility of the speaker.
- Ask for clarification when you are not sure you have understood.
- Repeat the speaker's message saying, "Let me see if I have understood your plan/intention/wish, and so on."
- Acknowledge you lost the topic of conversation when it changed, thus initiating an update or orientation.
- Ask for names, difficult instructions, and figures to be written down.
- Review the main points of the discussion/plan/findings with the speaker or with a colleague at the end of a meeting.
- Ask for written confirmation.
- Use a fax message rather than the telephone when possible.
- Take a note taker or a quality cassette recorder to important meetings.

There will be many other available options in specific situations. You and the client will identify these through creative thinking. As with the family members, you should identify one or two specific situations, review new communication strategies for those situations, set a goal for improvement and then assess the resulting improvement in dealing with those specific difficulties. These conscious behavioral management approaches are practical and easy to understand and can be implemented almost at once. Modifying the way in which the brain processes communication behavior is a more complex and less easily qualifiable task. Upgrading information-processing skills is the final component of our rehabilitative management model.

5. Upgrading of Information-Processing Skills of the Client. I have emphasized throughout our discussion how important it is to keep cost effectiveness in mind when planning the management strategy. It is important to provide no more intervention than is necessary to achieve a level as close as possible to the client's pre–hearing loss status. For most clients the management strategies we have discussed will prove sufficient to achieve their goals. For a few, supplementary intervention to upgrade communication skills will be necessary. For these persons cost may be a crucial issue. Thus you must aim to reeducate the client so that she can modify her own perceptual processing strategies rather than provide her with extensive training. I deliberately avoid adopting the more commonly used term, *auditory and visual communication training*, since I consider such training to be *the tool* we use to upgrade comprehension, not the process itself. I discussed this philosophy in the previous chapter (p. 395).

I have explained in this text a model of speech comprehension that attributes the greatest role to the cognitive-linguistic system. The process of generating semantic hypotheses based on linguistic probabilities at each level, from the phonemic level up, draws upon the acoustic signal only to the extent that raw data is necessary. This process, I explained, is further constrained by visual cues, both speech and nonspeech, and by situational and contextual knowledge. Using this model to design an approach to upgrading the client's ability to process information provides the following goals:

- To increase the ability to make predictions about the probabilities of what might be said given the topic and situational and/or contextual constraints
- To increase ability to make predictions concerning possible message evolution based on awareness of linguistic constraints
- To increase the amount of information the client is able to extract from the acoustic parameters of the speech signal
- To increase the amount of information the client is able to extract from the visual parameters of the speech signal.
- To heighten awareness of nonspeech visual cues

In addition to these receptive processing abilities, we should recognize that communication involves active participation even when one is in the primary role of listener. As I pointed out earlier, even when we are listening passively we still are sending messages concerning how we are reacting to the communication event. When we listen actively we seek to participate in the development of the conversation. We interrupt to slow down the communication when the information rate is too high, to ensure we understand precise meanings when the message has high significance, to identify to whom or to what the message refers when the antecedent is uncertain, or to establish where or when an event occurred when that information is unclear. We do this without demanding our turn as speaker. Such strategies of control aimed at ensuring comprehension should be understood and used by the hearing-impaired person to minimize communication breakdown. Those strategies comprise skills in communication management that increase information-processing effectiveness. As indicated by Nett, Doefler, and Matthews (1960) as cited by Giolas (1982), these skills are sadly lacking among hearing-impaired adults.

THE INTERVENTION PROCESS

The client must have a clear understanding of the goals I have listed and the purpose of each activity should be understood. The goal is to educate, not simply to train. To familiarize the client with the process of making predictions, it helps to begin by reversing the process. Take a simple object and together list all the constraints it generates.

The pencil I am observing

- Is long, about 6 inches, and thin
- Has six sides
- Has smooth sides
- Is light brown in color
- Has words on one side only
- Comes to a point at one end
- Has a black substance at the point
- Has a round metal holder attached around the wood at the opposite end
- Has a fairly soft substance in the metal holder
- Is light in weight
- It leaves marks when the pointed end is lightly pressed on paper
- Removes these marks when the opposite end is rubbed across them

Do this with several objects until the person has the concept of constraints. Next put before him a group of four or five objects. Then provide constraints, one at a time, asking him to identify the object as soon as he knows what it is.

- It is round.
- It appears to be made of metal and glass.
- It has a band attached to it.
- It has numbers on it from 1–12.
- It has three pointers on it.
- One pointer can be seen to move quite quickly around the numbers.

When this can be done for a small group of objects, increase the number of foils; then finally do the same with no visible constraints.

Situational constraints can be reviewed by placing before the client four pictures illustrating four situations, or four cards naming the situations. The client is instructed to watch and listen as you read slowly a list of words and phrases relevant to one of the situations which he must identify.

THE SITUATIONS

Drawing money from a bank   Mailing a letter at the post office
Dining in a fancy restaurant   Checking into a hotel

THE WORDS

register, overnight, expensive,
sheets, far to go, delivery, air
mail, special issue, stamps

Similar word lists can be generated for a variety of situations.

Contextual constraints can be reviewed using the principle of the Speech Perception in Noise test we reviewed earlier (p. 446). This test, you may recall, uses sentences with varying amounts of constraining information operating on the test word. The predictability of that word varied from high to low. In upgrading information-processing skills based on the use of contextual constraints, start by having the client complete the missing parts of sentences of high predictability.

We dined at a very fancy _____.
The _____ misunderstood the order.
The head _____ apologized for the misunderstanding.
He offered us a complementary _____.
We decided to leave only a _____.

When the client can do this, give only the topic, then ask a question about that topic:

FOOTBALL (assuming this is a client's interest)

Who is the quarterback for the Dallas Cowboys?
When does a team go for a field goal?
How many points do you get for a touchdown?

If this proves too difficult, write all key vocabulary words on the board or on a piece of paper. Put them in groups of three so that you can make the task easier by identifying the key word "field goal" as being in list number three or four, or more easily, in list three.

Once the client has the concept of constraints and how they operate, exercises should derive from his own work-related situations and vocabulary and phrases from hobbies and interests. For example, a teller at a bank might need to discriminate the following words and phrases:

Deposit	Pay in
Withdrawal	Take out
Coupon	Federal tax
Interest	Short term/current rate
Bond	Tax free/municipal
Savings	Short term
Account	A special account
Sign/signature	Safety deposit
Loan securities	Home improvement
Deduct	Certificate of deposit/C.D.

Each client can be asked to generate such a list of words and phrases as part of learning about constraints. The list can be used later for communication training activities. Thus you do not have to know which words and phrases are important in the client's environment, the client is encouraged to think in terms of constraints and probabilities, and you save time and expense through this cooperative approach.

Providing Upgrading Communication Activities

We have seen that in speech communication, the ears and the eyes provide the higher levels of the brain with information. Each modality modifies the interpretation of the information provided by the other. The result is a prediction or perception of meaning, based upon the principle of *best-fit*. Thus, bisensory processing of information is superior to unisensory, emphasizing that we should separate the two during practice only rarely and only for very specific purposes. From the evaluation data, you will be aware of the degree of difficulty the client experiences in speech, comprehension, and the conditions under which this occurs. Your challenge is to provide equivalent difficulty in the upgrade activities. The profile identifies the situations, while the assessment of auditory discrimination for words (Northwestern List, California Consonant test, or PB words) suggests to what extent audition will need to be supplemented by visual cues for fine discrimination. The CID Everyday Speech Sentences gives some guidance in how much potential improvement may lie in better utilization of linguistic constraints, while speech tests under three noise conditions will provide evidence of how much environmental noise affects the client's comprehension. All of this we reviewed in the previous chapter. Given this information, you must decide the type of conditions that need to be created for the upgrade activities. There is little to be gained by conducting activities that already are within the competencies of the client.

We have discussed at some length the parameters that contribute to information redundancy, namely,

- High signal-to-noise ratio
- Intensity and fidelity of the acoustic signal
- Knowledge of topic (cognitive constraints)
- Situational constraints
- Familiarity with vocabulary (linguistic constraints)
- Developmental structure of ideas (contextual constraints)
- Simplicity of sentence structure (syntactic constraints)
- Visible speech constraints

The absence of these conditions constitutes the detractors to message decoding, restructuring, and interpretation. It is these detractors that we manipulate in our attempt to upgrade the client's resistance to them. Depending on the client's assessment findings, we will emphasize one or more of the deficient parameters of effective communication. Consider first the techniques for decision making regarding prediction of vocabulary and topics of conversation based upon baseball and the cost of living.

BASEBALL GAME	COST OF LIVING
Did you catch the game on TV last night? I missed the beginning. Wow, the Dodgers were really in good form. I couldn't believe those two home runs in a row. And those weren't easy balls.	It seems like every time I go shopping things have gone up again. I can't believe the price of clothes. It's outrageous what they want for a simple cotton dress. I've bought hardly anything this summer.

This relates to the goal of increasing the client's active listening skills.

Changes in Topic. Using the same two topics, repeat a conversation but, at a particular point, make a statement or ask a question related to the second topic. Ask the client to utilize an acceptable strategy for interrupting the conversation to reenter the topic flow:

"I'm sorry I lost you—are you referring to _____?"
"I think I misunderstood. Are you speaking about _____?"

A second level of processing involves utilizing situational constraints to make predictions.

Situational Constraints. Two situations familiar to the client are identified, for example, waiting in line to buy movie tickets and waiting to board an airplane that is late. Have the client generate the relevant vocabulary and phrases as we discussed when we reviewed situational constraints (p. 100). Ensure that you both have a copy of the list, or write it on a blackboard if available. Ask the client to imagine she is in one of these two situations. Open and develop a conversation as though you were sitting/standing next to her. Difficult words and phrases should be isolated for several presentations in a concentrated listening-only mode, then in a watching-only mode with presentation at minimal voice level, finally in a listening and watching together mode. I suggest six repetitions under each condition. For example, begin by repeating the question, "Are you waiting for the 7:10 showing?" a couple of times at a slower than normal rate, then resume normal conversational rate. Situational constraints also can be imposed by using photographs, pictures, news articles, short printed anecdotes, cartoons, or even videotapes. Whichever stimulus you use, it will serve as the basis of your conversational activity. Since functional communication is the goal, I stress the importance of avoiding activities that require repetition of what you say. The aim is to increase comprehension and appropriate response, not to teach the client how to take dictation. Strive for normal communication behavior. Repeat the activity with the second topic.

Increase Use of Auditory-Visual Constraints by Reducing Developmental Construction. In the activities we have considered, the ability to predict has been influenced by the constraints imposed by logical progressive development of ideas. You can increase the listener's dependency on auditory-visual information by putting up a list of numbered sentences or phrases in either one or two topics. The content and vocabulary of the sentences are now familiar. Ask the client to identify by number, not by repetition, statements or questions. These are in topic context but out of sequential order.

The previous activities, which should not be belabored, are presented in quiet. When a client is able to perform acceptably well in quiet, you can then introduce the noise distractor.

Increasing Noise Interference Tolerance

It is not possible to re-create in the therapy environment the varied acoustic conditions encountered by each client in his daily activities. Therefore you first should make every effort possible to marshal technological resources, utilize environmental modification, and upgrade your client's communication strategies in an attempt to combat and compensate for noise and reverberation effects on speech comprehension. These techniques are likely to contribute most to the reduction of the negative effects of poor acoustics. Beyond this, your expectations for the benefits to be expected from listening practice in noise, except for new hearing aid users, should be guarded at best. The function of introducing noise as a background to the upgrade exercises we have discussed is (1) to require the person to draw more heavily on the redundancy in the message signal (auditory and visual and linguistic) and (2) to resort to the use of more active communication control strategies. The goal is to increase the client's ability to fill in (i.e., predict) more of the figure in an attempt to increase the perceptual figure-to-background ratio, since training will not change the actual acoustic S/N ratio. Ideally we would like to increase the client's use of prediction to the point at which a decrease from a highly favorable $+24$dB to a realistic $+6$dB and finally to a very unfavorable 0dB can be tolerated. An S/N of 0dB, however, probably will prove impossible to manage for most subjects who, therefore, will need to adopt other strategies for dealing with such situations. The experience, however, at least may persuade the person to seek technological support modes previously not considered favorably.

Signal-to-noise ratios are difficult to reproduce closely in a non–test booth situation, which is a further limitation for most rehabilitation management settings. The best you can hope to do is to have an audiologist calibrate a speech babble tape in a cassette player. This should be done so that when the volume control on the cassette player is in a particular position, the measure intensity at a preselected distance, for example, a six-foot radius from a listener, can be shown to be xdB greater than normal conversational voice level. The problem is that as the noise level increases, the Lombard reflex will act automatically to increase a live voice presentation by a compensatory amount (see Chapter 3, p. 33). This means you would need a second cassette with prerecorded messages. This method, however, denies the hearing-impaired person the visual constraints he would expect to turn to for information. Thus the best you can expect to achieve is to use a single noise competition source set at a level you determine to be minimally distracting, distracting, or highly distracting. I would use this procedure very judiciously in a normal therapy setting. If it is possible, you might decide to conduct a session in the coffee shop in your building or in the McDonald's across the road. In such an environment, noise and reverberation are as the client is likely to have to experience them. For the most part, education about the effects of noise and reverberation and how to control compensatory variables to maximum effect probably will achieve the greatest improvement in communication performance in poor acoustics. Practical actions are likely to prove the most effective means of coping with noise. Such actions might be included in the following advice:

- Choose a booth in a coffee shop.
- Do not sit at a counter, which has a higher noise level due to greater activity and proximity to the kitchen and service doors.

- Sit near a window but with your back to it.
- If possible, sit opposite rather than beside people.
- If possible, put people on the side of your better hearing.
- If there is significant noise from the cafeteria, try turning off the hearing aid on the opposite side to a partner sitting next to you in the booth to see if comprehension is improved.

You can problem solve management of poor acoustics as we discussed under modification of the client's behaviors. (p. 484)

A similar approach to the one here described has been developed by Garstecki (1981). His method manipulates message content by progressively decreasing the redundancy, the competing noise by type and S/N ratio, and the amount and type of auditory and visual cues. Eleven levels increase the amount of redundancy above a baseline and decrease it seven levels below. The baseline condition consists of unrelated sentences presented at 0dB S/N against a multispeaker background of speech babble without visual cues. The contributing variables are altered programmatically at each level during the therapy sequence. It does, however, require audiologic equipment and a sound-isolated booth to conduct the program.

To this point I have emphasized a holistic practical management model of intervention that has ignored auditory and visual skill training, taking instead an integrated cognitive problem-solving approach. There is, however, a small role for auditory and visual recognition of individual speech sounds.

Auditory and Visual Speech-Sound Training

Some speech perception failures cannot be resolved by capitalizing on nonacoustic redundancy. Some clients will evidence on analytical speech discrimination tests that there is consistent confusion between two sounds or among sounds in a given category. They may be well aware that those sounds are difficult to discriminate. For these persons you should begin by examining the phonemic analysis of errors made on speech discrimination tests. The California Consonant test is particularly helpful in this respect since it identifies choices among phoneme options. Also helpful in providing for assessment of consonant discrimination and confusions are the Nonsense Syllable Test (Levitt & Resnick, 1978) and the test developed by Edgerton and Danhauer (1979). If you do not have adequate information concerning the types of phonemic errors made during testing, you will need to use the test materials to generate the information. You will find the Larson Sound Test (Larson, 1950) helpful in generalizing the information (Table 20.2). Try to establish whether discrimination failure of a sound or group of sounds involves all phonetic contexts or whether the confusion occurs only in certain vowel-consonant combinations. If the latter is the case, you may assume it in those contexts in which the sound is reliably discriminable. This occurs because transition to or from the adjacent sound either moves the consonant in question into the audible range or colors the adjacent sound sufficiently to make its prediction possible. If you find no phonetic context in which a sound is dependably identified, it is reasonable to presume that

TABLE 20.2 Larson recorded test (after Larson, 1950)

Name: _____

Date: _____

Score: (Errors)

With Aid _____ (_____)

Without Aid _____

Directions to be given the listener: "Draw a line through the words that are pronounced to you from each box."

Box 1	f and ch	Box 2	b and m	Box 3	l and z	Box 4	l and n	Box 5	d and n	m and l
few	chew	lip	loan	lame	zip	dot	name	mine	not	line
fin	chin	loan	dale	light	zone	die	night	mast	nigh	last
filed	child	dale	mail	loan	daze	deed	known	moan	need	loan
calf	catch	mail	hail	pail	maze	ode	pain	name	own	nail
four	chore	hail		rail	haze	did	rain	home	din	hole

Box 6	b and m	Box 7	l and v	Box 8	l and v	Box 9	k and g	Box 10	p and b	m and v
bill	mill	lane	vane	coal	pin	goal	mice	bin	vice
boast	most	lie	vie	came	pie	game	ham	by	have
bake	make	lace	vase	coat	pole	goat	glum	bowl	glove
robe	roam	lull	love	luck	cap	lug	mine	cab	vine
tab	tam	rail	rave	rack	rope	rag	mile	robe	vile

Box 11	n and v	Box 12		Box 13	sh and f	Box 14	f and k	Box 15	f and b	s and sh
nice	vice	show	shore	fit	foe	fun	kit	lease	bun	leash
nurse	verse	shore	shade	four	fore	fig	core	sew	big	show
nine	vine	shade	cash	find	fade	cuff	kind	sigh	cub	shy
loans	loaves	cash	leash	cliff	calf	calf	click	sip	cab	ship
lean	leave	leash		laugh	leaf	graph	lack	save	grab	shave

492

Box 16 — p and f

pour	four
pile	file
par	far
cap	calf
cup	cuff

Box 17 — s and z

ice	eyes
seal	zeal
bus	buzz
lice	lies
juice	Jews

Box 18 — v and f

five	fife
vase	face
leave	leaf
view	few
loaves	loafs

Box 19 — ch and sh

chop	shop
chair	share
watch	wash
catch	cash
cheap	sheep

Box 20 — b and d

bid	did
big	dig
buy	die
rob	rod
robe	rode

Box 21 — d and g

doe	go
date	gate
drove	grove
bud	bug
dad	gag

Box 22 — t and p

tail	pail
cat	cap
cut	cup
tar	par
toll	pole

Box 23 — f and s

fine	sign
flat	slat
cuff	cuss
knife	nice
lift	list

Box 24 — b and v

bet	vet
dub	dove
base	vase
bigger	vigor
robe	rove

Box 25 — v and z

live	lies
have	has
rave	raise
view	zoo
wives	wise

Box 26 — th and f

thin	fin
thirst	first
three	free
thought	fought
thrill	frill

Box 27 — t and th

tie	thigh
tin	thin
trill	thrill
mitt	myth
pat	path

Box 28 — k and t

kick	tick
kite	tight
code	toad
shirk	shirt
park	part

Box 29 — k and p

pike	pipe
car	par
crock	crop
cry	pry
coal	pole

Box 30 — m and n

mine	nine
mew	knew
time	tine
dime	dine
dumb	done

Box 31 — Word endings

store	stores	stored
will	wills	willed
start	starts	started
cough	coughs	coughed
cap	caps	capped

Box 32 — th and s

thumb	sum
truth	truce
path	pass
thing	sing
thank	sank

Box 33 — th and v

than	van
thy	vie
that	vat
thine	vine
loathes	loaves

auditory training will not make discrimination possible. In that case attention must be focused on visual cues to phoneme identification in nonlinguistic contexts. When two sounds are both audible, but not reliably differentiated, intensive listening to repeated contrasts of the two in a variety of nonlinguistic phonetic contexts may evidence increased accuracy of discrimination in certain contexts. Intensive listening means listening with one's whole attention for a brief period of time. It facilitates far more detailed analytic processing of acoustic information than in any other listening state. Present the sounds separately first:

$$\int a - \int a - \int a \cdot t\int a - t\int a - t\int a$$

Then alternate them:

$$\int a - t\int a - \int a - t\int a - \int a - t\int a$$

Only when the client has listened intently to several presentations should you ask her to differentiate between the sounds when presented, first in a series:

$$\int a \int a \int a$$

then in isolation:

$$\int a.$$

All three positions, consonant-vowel, vowel-consonant-vowel, and vowel-consonant should be practiced. Phonemes that cannot be discriminated between auditorily should be presented with visual cues. To emphasize visible speech constraints, the client should turn off her aid(s). You now can continue to use normal voice when repeating the previous activity but this time with your face clearly visible. Do not emphasize the articulation in any way. Turn the aids back on and repeat with both auditory and visual cues.

When targeted phonemes can be differentiated in nonsense syllables, move to word discrimination involving those pairs, for example,

Ship	Chip
Skip	Chip
Skip	Ship
Chose	Shows

Finally place the words back into the context of low redundancy sentences.

The ship was large.
The dog chose well.

Group Activities

It often is most convenient for a client to arrange for individual sessions for intervention management. Certainly a personally tailored intensive program of counseling and strategy planning usually proves most convenient, particularly for the working client. Individualized intervention also is likely to produce the fastest results, thus proving to be time efficient. There are, however, advantages to group activity. It is important to realize that one does not preclude involvement in the other. A judicious mix of individualized and group experiences may prove optimal for some individuals. Once again I wish to emphasize that this is an individual decision to be made with each client.

The advantages to be derived from groups have been identified by Oyer (1966), Binnie (1977), Giolas (1982), and McCarthy and Culpepper (1987). They include

- The realization that their problem is not unique to them
- The experience of interaction, information, and support from persons with a similar handicap
- The positive competitive challenge offered by the group
- A normal interactive communication situation in which to practice communication management/strategies

Inclusion in a group also can do much to help a person deal with the sense of social isolation and loneliness. To be effective a group must have a degree of homogeneity. A group cannot be put together simply by identifying a certain number of hearing-impaired individuals. When a person agrees to participate in a group, he must be justified in assuming that he will have things in common with the other members of the group beyond the fact of the hearing impairment. The types of demands made upon members of the group by their work, the type of social life they pursue, and their interests and hobbies will to some extent be related to age, education, and socioeconomic level. These are factors to be taken into account when forming a group. An equivalent degree of hearing loss will ensure that the group members experience similar severity of communication difficulty (Hardick, 1977). Giolas (1982), addressing this factor, recommends that groups be composed of people who can be shown to have similar communication problems on the basis of a handicap profile. He points out that there are no well-established criteria for composing a group of hearing-impaired persons. You must use common sense and good judgment. It might prove counterproductive, for example, to include a young businesswoman in a group composed of retired persons.

Rationale for Group Experience. It is helpful to take a practical approach to deciding whether you should offer group services once you have a compatible population who might be served in this way. There are a number of economic and logistical reasons to support group services. Consider some of the most important advantages:

- Service delivery is maximal since you can accommodate up to 12 persons at one time. My experience with groups indicates that eight to nine people are an optimal number for discussion and activities. A group of less than six is difficult to run effectively given that there are likely to be absentees.
- A group is economical for the audiologist, speech pathologist, or teacher, since several people are served simultaneously. However, as Webster (1977) points out, this never should be the primary reason for forming a group.
- Cost of service to the client can be reduced in proportion to the size of the group. Remember, however, that while this is true for clients needing only a short-term group experience, longer periods may drive the cost up to what would have been the expense for individualized sessions. The latter may be

assumed to effect progress more rapidly because it is individually tailored to meet a client's needs.

- The group provides an excellent transitional setting for practicing in an evaluative environment those skills learned in individual sessions.
- In particular, it provides an opportunity for practice and evaluation in conversational activities, in experimenting with choice of seating, and in listening to presentations.
- It provides a forum for clients to present problem situations encountered in their daily environments for problem solving along the lines we have discussed.
- It provides an accepting climate in which to express and explore feelings among others who have to deal with the same disability and its stigma.

Luterman (1984) identifies the curative functions of the group as

- Instillation of hope
- Reaffirming the universality of feelings and perceptions
- Imparting (sharing) of information
- Fostering altruism—helping without loss of self-esteem
- Fostering interpersonal learning
- Providing cohesion and a sense of belonging
- Providing catharsis—growth through expression of feelings

Determining Activities and Function. You must have a clear idea of how you plan to function in relation to the group before it meets, and you must have a clear concept of what the options available to the group will be. Determine the functions of the group on the basis of what you know to be the needs of its members. These will follow closely the needs we have discussed for the individual since individuals make up your group. Among the services/information you can provide to a group are

1. Information about the nature and impact of hearing impairment
2. How to understand hearing impairment and test results
3. Why speech is difficult to understand
4. Why some environments make listening very difficult
5. Hearing aids and what they can and cannot do
6. Other assistive listening devices
7. How to improve listening
8. How vision helps hearing
9. Controlling communication situations
10. Practice in listening and predicting
11. Practice in using visual cues, both speech and nonspeech
12. Practice in communication strategies

A group will provide an opportunity to both understand this information and practice using it.

Further, a group provides an opportunity for

13. Sharing and exploring feelings
14. Sharing of personal management strategies
15. Group problem solving of difficulties raised by individuals

In forming a group or including a new client in a group, you first must determine whether there is a need to present the information listed in numbers 1–6. Often it is most effective when this is provided in individual sessions that allow the information to be illustrated using the client's own hearing problems. The information in numbers 6–9 and its implementation (10–12) are best presented in a group, while the sharing and supporting activities (13–15) only can take place in a group.

The topics and activities I list do not have to be presented sequentially; they can constitute a part of each session. Groups should be formed for a limited number of sessions; six to eight meetings seem to be appropriate. Two-hour sessions, including a half hour of social relaxation, can accommodate all the activities. The social half hour probably is most appreciated as a break, though providing it at the end of a session allows those who wish to leave early. The sessions should be set up as a unit and paid for ahead of time, unless financial stress makes this difficult, in which case a flexible fee schedule can be negotiated. When clients pay in advance, or pay after an introductory session that allows them to determine whether they wish to continue, they make a commitment to themselves and to the group. That commitment is financial, but more important, it is a commitment of their presence as contributors to the group. An outline of an eight-week group program based on two-hour sessions has been provided by Giolas (1982) and reproduced in Giolas (1989). Davis and Hardick (1981) also describe in some detail a ten-week group program.

SUMMARY

- The intervention process requires that various types of assessment data be integrated into a descriptive picture that summarizes the client's present level of function in daily activities.
- Needs should be identified and priorities established.
- Short- and long-term practical goals will be derived from this process.
- Specific strategies for need reduction and goal achievement should be devised with the client. These must be fully acceptable to the client.
- The three components in effecting change are education, adjustment counseling, and experimental learning.
- We must be particularly sensitive to the client's *emotional* needs whenever they can be determined to arise from or relate to communication function.
- Often successful practical actions must await more positive feelings in the client that derive from resolution of emotional issues.
- To be effective we professionals must deal with our own feelings and needs in terms of our relationships with our clients.
- Special adjustment needs are experienced by those with sudden traumatic hearing impairment and those with progressive deterioration of hearing.
- Reduction of communication difficulty in specific situation involves
  - Exploring improved amplification
  - Special listening devices
  - Modifying the environment
  - Counseling significant others
  - Improving client communication skills
- Group sessions afford growth opportunities different from individual sessions, including
  - Reduction of loneliness related to the disability
  - Highly credible information and support
  - Challenge
  - Opportunity to practice communication strategies in an interactive setting

Conclusion

We have examined in this chapter the handicapping effects of hearing impairment on the adult and on those persons most important to him/her. I would remind you that while the cause of the problem is reduced hearing, it is the resulting handicap at which we direct our efforts. That handicap, we saw, comprises a lack of understanding by the person and the family of what is happening, feelings of lack of self-worth with its resulting attempts to excuse noncoping behaviors, and the inability to meet the communication demands of daily living. A program of hearing handicap management must address each of these needs as they impact on the client and significant other persons. It must be a holistic management plan individualized to address special needs. Perhaps most important, it must place the responsibility of communication management on the client and family. Thus the goal is to teach, not to train, to educate both client and family in how to approach the task of solving their own communication problems.

The issues discussed in this chapter will apply to adults of all ages. However, certain factors associated with the normal aging process necessitate that special consideration be given to the needs of the elderly person. This will constitute the final two chapters of our discussion.

21

Special Considerations for the Assessment of the Older Client

In titling this section, I deliberately avoided the term *geriatric* for the same reason that I earlier rejected the use of the term *the hearing impaired* along with the terms *the aphasic, the dysarthric, the stutterer,* and so on. I personally never have met "a geriatric." This is more than a semantic quibble; the term *geriatric* immediately identifies a category into which we place people using the single criterion of age—not maturity, not experience, not wisdom, simply age. In Western society, and most acutely in North American society, age carries with it a stigma (Kite & Johnson, 1988). The emphasis in our society remains focused on youth and beauty. Thus the term *geriatric* evokes many negative connotations (Trapp & Spatz, 1988). These include physical and mental deterioration, reduced cognitive function, reduced responsibility, and, above all, loss of power in society. If you question this view, ask yourself whether the terms *pediatric* and *geriatric* convey the same emotional connotation.

A number of naturally occurring changes in our body are associated with aging; none of them enhances our ability to function. In turn, these changes impact upon our ability to meet all of the demands occurring in our environment. To varying degrees they force us to modify our lifestyle, our activities, the amount of assistance we need, and in more severe cases, the type of accommodation in which we can manage acceptably. Nevertheless, I suggest that we need to consider advancing age to be a privilege. As my 92-year-old father tells me, despite the aches and pains, the decreased mobility, the loss of visual acuity, he finds being 92 years old highly preferable to the alternative. He is fortunate that the changes he has experienced have permitted him, with some minor sacrifices, to meet the demands of the lifestyle he has followed since retirement. The aging process is not always so benevolent. The progressive handicap imposed upon us as we age varies considerably from one person to another. Thus as we grow into the later years of our life, we tend to become more different from each other rather than more alike (McPherson, 1983; Salthouse 1982), a fact that further limits the value of discussing *the geriatric client.* Having emphasized yet again the importance of individualizing our approach to each client, we are ready to consider the special needs we might expect to experience in our later years. Recognize that we are considering these in a general context; different individuals will experience different combinations and degrees of these needs.

We have seen that demands arise from needs. The demands arise from within the individual and from others within his social environment. The need we are concerned with is for communication. This need is related to a range of others, including the need to provide

- Sustenance for bodily functions
- Sensory contact with the environment
- Control over our relationship with the environment and those in it
- Social intercourse
- Emotional expression
- Information
- Entertainment to stimulate the brain

The aging process, to varying degrees, impairs the communication function in the older client. It does so by gradually reducing sensory reception and processing abilities (Kimmel, 1974; Marshall, 1981), linguistic abilities (Light, 1986), cognitive function (Heron & Chown, 1967; Kausler, 1982) and expressive processing (Benjamin, 1988). Even in the healthy older person, a modest reduction in these functions may result in a consequential reduction in the motivation to communicate (Elias & Elias, 1977), in the ability to attend (Rabbitt, 1965), and in memory function (Kausler, 1982; Parkinson, Lindholm, & Inman, 1982). Given this reduction in internal resources, the older person finds processing demands exceed processing capabilities far more quickly than in a younger person (Wright, 1981). This difference is exacerbated by a sensory disability.

AGING FACTORS THAT AFFECT COMMUNICATION

Hearing Deficiency

Progressive hearing deficiency with age is a well-documented fact (National Center for Health Statistics, 1977). Figure 21.1 shows that a normal decrease in hearing thresholds begins to be evident in men in the third decade of life and is significant in the high frequencies by age 40–49, presenting

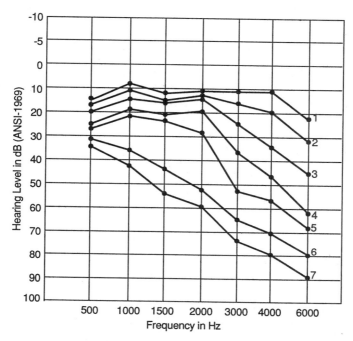

Figure 21.1 Median hearing losses for males ages 10 to 79 (*1*, 10–19; *2*, 20–29; *3*, 30–39; *4*, 40–49; *5*, 50–59; *6*, 60–69; *7*, 70–79). Data are converted to the ANSI-1969 reference from Glorig et al., 1957.

a marked speech reception problem by age 60 (Glorig, Wheeler, Quiggle, Grings, & Summerfield, 1957). In women the deterioration is somewhat slower. For them a significant loss in the speech frequencies (500, 1K, 2K, 4K) does not occur until the 60–69 age range.

The decrease in sensitivity is complicated by the phenomenon of *phonemic regression*. This term characterizes a deterioration of auditory discrimination for speech that exceeds what one normally would attribute to the degree of sensitivity loss evidenced by the pure tone audiogram. Not all older persons with a loss of hearing sensitivity exhibit phonemic regression, but it is a problem commonly encountered among the older population. The discrimination reduction has been shown to affect speech perception at all levels of linguistic structure from nonsense syllables to sentences (Harbert, Young, & Menduke, 1966). Performance reduction has been demonstrated even when hearing thresholds remain within normal limits (Gelfand, Piper, & Silman, 1986). The phenomenon is thought to be due to the cumulative effect of degeneration of both the peripheral and central auditory systems (Grimes, 1991; Konkle, Beasley, & Bess, 1977). Thus the first characteristic that we must recognize about hearing difficulty in the elderly population is the likelihood that even with optimal amplification, the maximum auditory discrimination for speech potential will be limited. As McCarthy (1987) states:

However, despite potential variability in degree and configuration of the hearing loss, reduced speech discrimination ability represents the primary problem associated with aging. (pp. 372–373)

Visual Changes

In Chapter 5 I emphasized the vulnerability of the older person to conditions that reduce visual acuity. It has been demonstrated in addition that visual processing skills deteriorate with age along with other subcortical and cortical functions (Shoop & Binnie, 1979). This represents a further limiting of available information relevant to the spoken message and, thus, a restriction on the available resources with which to compensate for loss of acoustic information. The reduction of visual acuity associated with the normal aging process (Botwinick, 1973; Kimmell, 1974), which for this modality becomes significant in the 40–50 age range (Kimmell, 1974), exerts a demonstrably negative effect on the ability to make use of the visual cues to the spoken message (Fozard, Wolf, Bell, McFarland, & Podolsky, 1977; Hardick, Oyer, & Irion, 1970). This compounds the impact of the hearing impairment on comprehension of the spoken message. In the words of Ryan (1991):

> The cumulative impact of slight changes in both sensory modalities can be substantial because of the tendency to use the complementary sense to compensate for one loss and because of anxiety and social avoidance resulting from the loss of confidence. (p. 90)

Cognitive Linguistic Changes

Language and cognition are the fundamental components of human communication fed primarily by the ear and the eye. Any reduction in the information they receive will reduce communication effectiveness. However, as we have seen, perception is an active rather than a passive process. Cognition and language are highly influential in determining what we attend to auditorily and visually, as well as dictating how information received will be processed. As Kausler states succinctly:

> Cognitive processes direct our attention to specific events present in our environment, enable us to perceive and interpret those events, guide the acquisition of new information about our environment, determine the subsequent memorability of that new information, and find the means of solving problems created by novel environmental demands. Any impairment of cognitive functioning results in the diminished ability to adapt to our physical and social environments. (1988, p. 79)

The literature emphasizes strongly that the assessment of cognitive deterioration as a function of age is fraught with complications. So many factors including research design, evaluation procedures, impact of sensory deficits, health status, medication, and social factors all complicate the assessment of true age changes. Nevertheless, changes in cognition, and to a lesser extent in linguistic processing, do occur. Those that are most relevant to our task of providing assistance in receptive communication are discussed in the following sections.

Rate of Information Processing. We have seen that one of the primary negative effects of impairment of hearing in children and adults is the reduction in the rate at which information can be processed. This reduction arises from the need to depend on closure to compensate for decreased extrinsic redundancy. The aging process, even when normal hearing is present, exacerbates this problem by decreasing the overall rate at which the central nervous system can process sensory information (Salthouse, 1985). The effect is considered to be evident in almost every stage of processing. The impact of this slower processing capability on communication is seen in the reduction that older persons evidence in their ability to discriminate between similar speech patterns (words and sentences) under conditions of noise as compared to younger subjects (Bergman et al., 1976). Such reduced information naturally affects the ease with which older persons can pay and maintain attention.

Attention. We have discussed attention in several places in this text. We considered it as part of the perceptual model proposed by Solley and Murphy (1960), (Chapter 7, p. 78). In that context we saw it as resulting from an active process of editing the flow of information by processing expected patterns in a more complex manner than other stimuli. We saw how it involved maintaining a figure-ground relationship, a process made particularly difficult when the ratio between figure (signal) and ground (noise) is low. We considered also Lawson's (1967) differentiation between nonspecific and specific attention. In our later discussion of the effects of impaired hearing, we saw that inadequate attention has been shown to affect negatively children's ability to learn. We know, therefore, that attention is an important factor in effective communication and cognitive processing, and that it is affected by hearing impairment. Since increasing hearing difficulty is a natural component of aging, it is not surprising to learn that older persons evidence increasing difficulty with attention. Studies have shown that *alertness*, a process we call *vigilance*, which is that constant scanning watchfulness of the sensory systems, is not affected by age (Quilter, Giambra, & Benson, 1983), probably because it is not a task requiring cognitive processing. However, Kirchner (1958) showed that when a memory component is added to a vigilance task, older subjects show a significant decrease in vigilance. For example, when a subject is asked to sort coloured discs depending upon which sound pattern is presented, the colours which each sound represents must be remembered while attention, or vigilance, is devoted to not missing a sound stimulus occurring at different intervals. This suggests that the overall capacity of cortical processing is more limited in elderly persons, who reach overload more quickly than younger adults.

Selective attention, which Lawson refers to as specific attention, a task involving figure-ground separation, suffers far more significantly than vigilance as we grow older. Older persons have been shown to be at a marked disadvantage on tasks requiring the tuning out of irrelevant stimuli (Comalli, Wapner, & Werner, 1962). Kausler (1988) postulates that young adults simply identify nontarget information as irrelevant and suppress it at the periphery (see also Brazier, 1964, noted on p. 79):

> By contrast, elderly adults may have difficulty "turning off" the processing of irrelevant stimuli until it has been completed to the point of identifying them. The net effect would be increased time for elderly adults to reach a reject decision for each irrelevant stimulus. (Kausler, 1988, p. 91)

The end result is that the elderly person cannot keep up with the information flow and may, therefore, appear lost, flustered, or disinterested (i.e., not to be paying attention).

Kausler addresses also the type of attention required to perform two tasks simultaneously, for example, talking while doing something in which both sources of information are relevant. *Divided attention,* as he identifies it, has been shown to deteriorate only for tasks in which the demand of the task is relatively high (Somberg & Salthouse, 1982). For example, you might be pouring a boiling liquid into the narrow neck of a jar, a task that makes divided attention almost impossible, prompting you to say, "Don't talk to me while I'm doing this." Instructions or messages given to an older person, even to a not-so-old person, when that person is engaged in another task demanding specific attention often are not processed into memory.

Learning, Remembering, and Forgetting. We are all quite sure that with increased age comes a deterioration in learning ability and an ever increasing difficulty in remembering. Certainly elderly persons cite memory difficulties as one of the major problems they encounter. The research on memory and recall is complicated by the changes we see occurring in our language processing as we grow older. The findings do support the observation that memory function deteriorates, but it does not affect all types of memory equally and for some types the data are equivocal.

Semantic Memory. This is the store of concepts and the auditory and visual patterns that identify them. It is our reference source for meanings and differences and shades of meaning among the words, the interrelationships of words and auditory and visual word patterns. The research in this area suggests that there is little change with age either in the way semantic memory is organized or how readily we can gain access to its store (Bowles & Poon, 1985; Howard, Lasaga, & McAndrews, 1980).

Short-Term Memory. This you will recall from our discussion (p. 86) is limited in capacity, is linguistic in nature, and allows for rehearsal or reauditorization. Studies of STM in elderly persons evidence a limited decrement of some 10–20 percent across the adult years, the exact amount depending on whether digit series or a list of unrelated words is to be recalled. The experimental research on forgetting, however, has produced no conclusive results relevant to aging effects (Kausler, 1988).

Long-Term Memory. Because of the major linguistic restructuring that occurs between short- and long-term memory (see p. 87), this stage is greatly affected by the cognitive strategies used to enter the information into storage. The encoding strategies involved include the use of semantic values, word and meaning relationships, sophisticated rehearsal techniques coded to semantic values, and contextual keying. Older persons, by virtue of reduced cognitive resources, evidence reduced recall strategies. It has been suggested that this may result from the fact that they use far less complex encoding routines than young adults (Rankin & Collins, 1985). It may be that what they encode are the sound patterns or word patterns of what is said. It is of interest to note, however, that recognition of the item that cannot be remembered evidences about a 10 percent improvement over free recall. This finding suggests that to a limited extent, difficulty of access to what has been stored plays a part in reduced performance (Poon & Fozard, 1978). The problem of long-term memory storage may be complicated further by language processing changes (Light & Caps, 1986).

Changes in Linguistic Abilities. Language comprises two major components, *language competence*, or knowledge of how language works, and *language performance*, our ability to put that knowledge to functional use. The literature tells us that competence is affected hardly at all by aging, while a number of performance abilities have been shown to deteriorate (Ryan, 1991).

Vocabulary and Syntax. Test results (Kausler, 1987) indicate that age effects no change in vocabulary definition (Salthouse, 1988); in fact, there is evidence to suggest that age brings with it some growth in vocabulary (Bowles & Poon, 1985). The Bowles and Poon (1985) study did reveal, however, a marked decrease in the ability to recall the word that identified a definition. This would suggest that expressing ideas through the use of specific vocabulary choice may constitute more of a problem for the older adult than dealing with the vocabulary of others.

Reduced syntactic skills among the older population have been demonstrated. This, however, seems to affect primarily the ability to process complex syntactic structures. Comprehension of simple forms appears to be unaffected (Benjamin, 1988). Benjamin (1988) concludes:

> While older adults demonstrate reduced comprehension for complex syntactical forms in artificial tasks of linguistic ability, the affect [sic] of age-related change in this parameter on daily communication is presumed to be minor. (p. 171)

Discourse Skills. Discourse, or conversational skills, are highly sensitive to the reduction of redundancy from noise and reverberation and from environmental distractions. The result of such interferences is to reduce significantly the amount of extrinsic information, placing increased demands on a cognitive system that has lost some of its capacity for linguistic, contextual, and situational closure. It is not surprising to learn, therefore, that older persons find sentence statements difficult to understand when the linguistic redundancy in the message is low and noise is present (Obler, Nicholas, Albert, & Woodward, 1985). When the linguistic redundancy of the spoken message is high, with resulting high predictability, the difficulty of comprehension was shown to be eliminated for 75 percent of the subjects studied. Ryan (1991), in reviewing the literature on conversational skills among elderly persons, points out that very little information is presently available. She illustrates the influence of memory problems on conversational performance by referring to the findings of three studies (Kausler & Hakami, 1983; Koriat, Ben-Zur, & Scheffer, 1988; Rabbitt, 1981). These identify the main problems as

- Keeping track of who said what in group conversations
- Retaining what was said while actively participating in a conversation
- Remembering what one already had recounted and recalling what was said in a conversation

Let us review now the cognitive linguistic abilities that will change for most of us when we age, though to markedly varying degrees. We know that deterioration of hearing with an associated problem in speech recognition is a natural function of aging. It occurs earlier in men, by about age 60, than in women in whom it occurs about a decade later. Both sensitivity and discrimination are affected. Vision, likewise, becomes less acute but at a much earlier age, being significantly affected by 40–50 years.

The evidence for cognitive changes must be treated with caution because of the many variables that make research difficult. However, there is general agreement that cognitive resources are reduced by progressive age and that slowing of the rate at which information can be processed, rather than a marked reduction in capacity, is the major problem arising with age. Our ability to pay attention as we grow older depends on the nature of the attentional activity. Vigilance remains good, providing the task does not have a memory component, but selective attention has been shown to be affected negatively, probably as a result of inefficient blocking of irrelevant stimuli. Divided attention likewise becomes more difficult with increasing age.

The findings pertaining to changes in memory processing are contaminated by the difficulty in controlling for changes in linguistic skills. Memory appears to be affected but not in all its forms. Short-term memory seems to suffer little from aging, but more significant aging effects have been shown for long-term memory, probably due to reduced skill in the use of sophisticated cognitive encoding strategies by older persons.

Linguistic competence, that is, our knowledge of how language works, resists aging effects. No reduction is seen in vocabulary definition, but word finding ability decreases markedly with age. Complex syntactic forms also present more processing difficulty as we age but are not thought to affect daily communication. In conversational situations the little research available suggests that memory and recall are the primary difficulties. These are affected seriously by poor acoustic conditions.

Health Changes

The realization that one is aging usually is prompted by the mirror. Living with ourselves daily, we are slow to recognize and reluctant to accept the changes occurring in our own bodies, though we have little difficulty in identifying them in others. "He's really showing his age," we say, as though he ought not to, and we are glad that we do not. Eventually, however, we notice the first grey hairs, the first wrinkles and occurrence of age spots on the skin. "Age spots?" I said. "I never knew there were such things."

All systems of the body change as we grow older, some more quickly than others. These intrinsic changes must not be viewed in isolation, for they are affected significantly by such extrinsic factors as diet, lifestyle, occupation, family support systems, stress, medications, smoking, and consumption of alcohol. The effect of the changes is to place increasing demands on the system for adaptation. When the demands exceed the genetic and acquired capacity of the body to adapt, and when supplementary resources are not available, the person becomes vulnerable to sickness and disease. We note, thus, an increasing prevalence of health problems with increasing age. Many of these problems markedly affect the ability of the person to function (Kenney, 1988).

This situation is aggravated by the fact that illness in turn triggers a breakdown of normal social expectancies and demands, with a resultant redefinition of the patient's role, both by himself and by others (Bengston, 1973). As Kenney explains:

> The physiological changes which occur with the passage of years reduce the efficiency of these systems, so that the "world" available for man's activity closes about him. (1988, p. 77)

Yet again it becomes clear that we neither can comprehend the significance and impact of hearing difficulty on a person, nor provide effective intervention, without an appreciation of the complex matrix of factors determining what, for that person, is her life. This realization is even more important than ever when we work with older persons.

The general health status of the older person will influence the amount of personal resources that remain to deal with a hearing problem. She may not have the psychic energy to care about communication, and even less about audiologic assessment, hearing aid use, and rehabilitation management. We will consider this factor in depth when we discuss intervention.

Mobility. Aside from the general health changes occurring with age, reduced mobility resulting from arthritis, poor motor control, and tremors associated with some degenerative conditions must be noted. In general, mobility problems limit the environmental boundaries of the individual and thus the communication situations encountered.

All of the changes we have discussed are associated with the normal aging process. They occur to all of us to various degrees with various rates of onset. Many conditions affect us all; some are confined only to certain individuals. This variability in the time of onset of the changes and in the rate at which they develop emphasizes that we must view each older person as a unique individual. It is helpful for us to have an understanding of what normal aging does to the body and to its systems. However we must avoid, most strenuously, viewing the elderly individuals with whom we work as "a population of geriatrics." These people, well or infirm, are simply further ahead in the life cycle than we are. Reluctant as we may be to face reality, if we live long enough, we too will experience these changes. The model of assessment and management of the needs and resources of the person with impaired hearing, which we have used from preschool to adult years, will serve equally to protect the individuality of the older person.

IMPLICATIONS OF AGE CHANGES FOR ASSESSMENT PROCEDURES

Hearing Deficiency

We know that people 60 years and older are highly likely to have a hearing impairment of sufficient difficulty to impair speech comprehension (Raiford, 1988). We can assume, therefore, that special care must be taken to be sure amplification is provided at all times when talking with the client: when obtaining information, giving directions, and explaining results. Amplification at its simplest can be provided by speech one inch from the ear. This might be appropriate before placing headphones on the client to communicate that you will explain everything through the headphones. In other situations a portable auditory trainer or a personal amplification device, whether hardwire, FM, or infrared, can be used. Whenever possible, arrange seating so that the person can see your face clearly. Our instruction of the older client will be satisfactory only when we accommodate his special needs. By satisfactory I mean that the client feels comfortable in performing what is expected, providing us with reliable and valid responses. Such comfort comes from understanding what is required and having your encouragement and support during testing. To achieve this you need to remember the changing capacities we discussed earlier.

Consider the practical implications of reduced rate of processing. As we grow older, we discover that while our abilities remain intact, we simply cannot function at the same rate. I run four miles very comfortably, but I cannot run them as fast as my daughter. Thus, in seeking information, giving instructions, or presenting test material, we must ensure that we do not exceed the client's intake rate, and we must allow adequate time for the client to process and respond to information (Canestrari, 1963). The rate of processing and responding to information is decreased even further when noise is introduced into the system.

These changes in processing rate need to be accommodated during testing. We need to allow for delayed responses to pure tones. If we assume too quickly that a tone was not heard and proceed to present it at a 5dB higher level, we are likely to confuse the client. The rate of spondee or P.B. word presentation that characterizes taped test materials frequently exceeds an older client's processing rate. As a result she often misses words. Realizing that she cannot cope with the task, she may become very nervous. Live-voice presentation, which allows you to control rate of presentation and to provide frequent reassurance and encouragement, often provides far more representative results than taped materials.

Attention Problems

Once you allow for rate of presentation, listening for the tone is not a difficult task for older persons who have been made to feel comfortable. We know from our review of attention in elderly persons that vigilance, which is the process involved here, is not affected by aging. The time taken to make the response/nonresponse decision, however, may be much longer than normal and must be allowed for. Selective attention also is reduced in efficiency. This you will recall requires tuning out nonrelevant stimuli. Thus speech in noise is a particularly difficult task for older persons. Even masking in the nontest ear often confuses a patient, making accurate assessment of speech discrimination in the test ear difficult (Kasten & Miller, 1982).

It particularly is important to obtain results that relate to the actual communication demands the client encounters each day. This concern will be addressed also when we consider profiling the older client's potential for understanding speech communication. In selecting speech discrimination materials, you will learn most from those that permit the client to call upon internal linguistic and contextual redundancy to compensate for reduced auditory information. The CID Test of Everyday Speech Sentences provides a useful tool that gives the client the opportunity to capitalize on linguistic redundancy. The Speech Perception in Noise Test (Kalikow, Stevens, & Elliott, 1977) similarly provides linguistic constraints providing suppression of the noise is not a factor.

Formal testing can be supplemented by some of the procedures we discussed for use with children. You can assess the client's ability to participate in responding to questions, following directions, and listening to and retelling a short anecdote. Remember, however, that these abilities involve more than auditory discrimination. Abilities prone to normal aging effects, compounded by acoustic information loss, may contribute greatly to the observed performance.

Visual Change Effects

Visual changes need to be assessed in terms of the extent to which reduced auditory information can be supplemented by visual cues to speech. Optimal visual functioning is essential to maximize speech comprehension. Thus we must provide every encouragement to the client, and to significant others, to ensure that the best corrected vision is obtained and that such conditions as glaucoma, macular degeneration of the retina, and cataracts, which occur in this age group, are under opthalmological care and monitoring. During interviewing, testing, and counseling, it will be important to assure optimal lighting conditions and to avoid glare. Self-administered questionnaires and tests that require reading, such as the California Consonant Test, may be impossible for the client with poor vision.

Mobility Limitations

Mobility problems that keep a patient wheelchair-bound make obvious demands for adjustment on our part. Less obvious are the implications of restricted mobility of the arms, wrist, and fingers. The method of test response the client is asked to use must be considered carefully, since buttons and switches may be difficult to manipulate. Special consideration also must be given to the mobility factor when selecting the type of hearing aid to be recommended. The postauricular placement of a hearing aid or the insertion of an in-the-ear or canal aid or an earmold may prove very difficult. I further have noted that older persons often experience difficulty in perceptually imaging the task of inserting a hearing aid or earmold. They cannot direct the movements of the hand(s) relative to the auricle and ear canal. I had such an experience in a science museum when I stood facing a mirror that failed to reverse my image as mirrors usually do. My mind did not know how to direct my body. Small on-off switches, volume controls, and telephone switches on hearing aids can make wearing the aid very frustrating. Equally frustrating may be the task of replacing a battery. In addition to the dexterity needed on account of the small size of ITE and canal hearing aid batteries, the batteries themselves may be barely visible to the person with poor vision. Certain difficulty will be experienced in identifying the positive sign on the battery and the number or notches on the volume control. It may be necessary, therefore, to mark controls and batteries with red nail polish indicating appropriate positions and battery side. Even so, the operation of the hearing aid may prove simply too much for some elderly clients to manage mentally or physically (Weinstein, 1984), necessitating that a significant other person assume that responsibility where feasible.

Attitudinal Problems

Finally, it is necessary to be sensitive to the attitude of the hearing-impaired person toward his handicap and to take steps for its management. Rather than getting simpler as we age, life often seems to grow more complicated, just as our resources to deal with problems decrease. Some healthy persons in their later years function as well as or better than you and I. Others, burdened with worries about spouses, sons, daughters, grandchildren, health problems, and finances, carry a heavy burden. We need to see the attitudes expressed toward the hearing problem and its management within the larger framework of the client's feelings about life in general:

> Older adults who have not reconciled themselves to the aging process, or who have not adjusted to the many upheavals associated with age, like the death of a spouse or friends, forced retirement or frequent illnesses, may be less apt to accept the hearing impairment and the wearing of a hearing aid. (Rollin, 1987, p. 282)

Rollin goes on to explain that such attitudes may arise from a lifestyle that essentially has become fixed. The client resists even positive changes, preferring to cling to the existing status even when it can be improved. Assistance from the outside is seen as interference and is resented. Unless you are prepared to provide or obtain counseling for the client and family, you are unlikely to achieve management goals.

PROFILING THE COMMUNICATION DIFFICULTIES OF THE OLDER CLIENT

The attitudes and feelings of the hearing-impaired older person, the family, and in the case of individuals in long-care residential facilities, the professional staff need to be evaluated. These are important aspects in determining relevant factors. To this end, profiles designed for working adults have been modified to make them applicable for use with an older population of hearing-impaired individuals. Others have been designed specifically for this age group; some of them are specific to residential care environments. The modifications involved

- The elimination of work-related questions
- A recognition that questions that were exclusively family directed need to be expanded to include other persons and the professional staff in long-term care facilities
- Questions exploring the individual's attitude to rehabilitation management
- The assessment of the client's participation in social activities

Recognition is given by the profiles to the difficulty many older individuals have in reading questions and in writing or recording responses. Thus most profile questionnaires are intended to be administered by the audiologist or speech-language pathologist. We will examine the modifications made in existing profiles as well as those profiles specifically designed for use with older persons.

Denver Scale of Communication Function—Modified

You will remember this scale from our earlier discussion of it in its original form, along with its quantified version (Chapter 19, p. 438). The modified form, which was adapted by Kaplan, Feeley, and Brown (1978), has a contracted rating scale of five rather than seven. The client evaluates her agreement or disagreement with the statements, ranging from "definitely agree" through "slightly agree" and "irrelevant" to "slightly" and "definitely disagree." The number of questions has been increased from 25 to 34 to include specific listening situations such as listening to radio or TV at normal volume, talking in a quiet room, playing cards, and hearing intercom announcements.

Hearing Handicap Inventory for the Elderly (HHIE)

Designed by Ventry and Weinstein (1982), the inventory is for use with people living independently or with their children. Intended for assessment of unaided hearing handicap, it explores emotional, social, and situational perceptions. Each of 25 questions is coded and identified as emotional or social. Examples of questions follow.

	YES (4 points)	SOMETIMES (2 points)	NO (0 points)

SOCIAL

Does a hearing loss cause you
to use the phone less often
than you would like?

Does a hearing problem cause
you difficulty when visiting
relatives or neighbors?

EMOTIONAL

Does a hearing problem cause
you to be nervous?

Does a hearing problem cause
you to have arguments with
your family?

Each response is assigned a value of four points for a "yes" response, two for a "sometimes" response, and zero for a "no" or "nonapplicable" response. A maximum of 100 points is thus possible, with higher scores indicating a high level of perceived handicap. One of the few scales that has been standardized, it was found to have high reliability on test-retest. This finding would support the use of the tool as a pre- and post–hearing aid trial period assessment tool, or a pre- and post–management effectiveness measure. A shorter version of the inventory for use as a screening tool (HHIE-S), which involves only 10 questions, five from the social and five from the emotional categories, was found to have high statistical reliability and validity correlations with the longer form. Both forms may be administered by interview or as a written questionnaire.

Communication Assessment Procedure for Seniors (CAPS)

This tool was developed by Alpiner and Baker (1981) for use with persons in residential care. It consists of 35 questions divided into six sections: general communication, group situations, other persons, self-concept, family, and rehabilitation. They explore communication difficulties and behaviors, feelings and perceptions, self-perceptions, and perceptions of the family's feelings and behaviors. Judgments are made on a three-point scale: "always," "sometimes," "never," with a "not applicable" option. Some sample questions follow.

GENERAL COMMUNICATION

Do you talk to people during your meals?
Do you have trouble hearing in certain situations?

GROUP SITUATIONS

Do you ask a person to repeat if you don't understand what he says?
Do you feel isolated from group situations because of your hearing loss?

OTHER PERSONS (FAMILY, FRIENDS, AND STAFF)

Does anyone ever leave you out of conversations because of your hearing problem?
Do others avoid you because of your hearing loss?

SELF-CONCEPT

Would you describe yourself as a relaxed person?
Does your hearing loss make you irritable?

FAMILY

Do they make decisions for you because of your hearing loss?
Does your family understand what it is like to have a hearing loss?

REHABILITATION

Do you need help in overcoming your hearing problems?
Do you wear your hearing aid?

Scale of Communication Adequacy in Daily Situations

This scale was not designed specifically for use with hearing-impaired persons but would appear to address some relevant topics. It is presented by Clark and Witte (1991) in discussing communication management of persons with Alzheimer's disease. This scale also is designed to provide an assessment both from the individual's and from the caregiver's perspective; there are parallel questions in each category. Of the 13 questions in each list, four deal with expressive speech and are inapplicable for our purpose. Of the remaining nine, three deal with communication difficulty, three with communication behavior, two with feelings, and one with perception of family reactions. Responses are scaled on a five-point scale from "almost always" to "almost never."

Nursing Home Hearing Handicap Index

Specifically constructed to profile the communication behavior of a person in a long-term care setting is the Nursing Home Hearing Handicap Index (NHHHI) developed by Schow and Nerbonne (1977). It has two adaptations, one to gather information from the client (the Self Version for Resident) and a mirrored set of questions to obtain comparative assessment by the staff (Staff Version). Each form contains 10 items; each question occurs in both client and staff versions. Of the 10 questions, two pertain to communication difficulties, four to feelings, two to perception of other's feelings or behaviors, and two to communication behaviors. Each item is rated on a five-point scale of frequency from "very often" to "never." The authors report that on analysis, the staff scores were found to reflect the average pure tone loss of the resident more closely than did the resident's perceptions. You may recall that Alpiner and McCarthy (1987) also administered their scale to both the client and a significant other person. In that case it was a family member. They, too, found a significant difference in ratings by the two groups, reflecting different viewpoints of the problems. Both Schow and Nerbonne and Alpiner and McCarthy consider the significant-other assessment responses as more objective. Alpiner stresses, however, that neither perception can be considered the correct one but rather that both represent different insights. We should pay attention to what family and staff reveal to us because they are part of the communication cycle, but we must avoid accepting their perceptions as more valid than those of the hearing-impaired person.

The Denver Scale of Communication Function for Senior Citizens Living in Retirement Centers (DSSC)

This is another modification of the original Denver Scale of Communication Function adapted by Zarnoch and Alpiner (1977). The scale is more specifically focused on the difficulties experienced by older hearing-impaired persons. It adopts a three-step process of exploration. First a general question is asked. For example

Q4. Do you avoid communicating with other people because of your hearing problem?

If the answer is "yes," the profile moves to the second stage, identified as the *probe effect*. Questions in this stage seek to specify the difficulty more narrowly. For example,

Q4. Do you communicate with people during mealtimes?
Do you communicate with your roommate(s)?
Do you communicate during the social activities in the home?
Do you communicate with visiting family or friends?
Do you communicate with the staff?

The final step, which may have more than one stage, is called the *exploration effect*. The questions now seek to explore a specific problem in greater detail. For example,

Q4. Is your roommate capable of communication?
What are the social activities of the home?
Which ones do you attend?

The general areas covered by the test are family, emotional concerns, other persons, general communication, self-concept, group situations, and rehabilitation.

Not normed, the profile is intended to provide a picture of the individual's perceptions of his communication abilities. It is useful for pre- and postmanagement performance comparisons.

SUMMARY

- For the older person it is necessary that we be sensitive to the interactive effects of the aging process *and* the hearing impairment.
- The capacity of the older individual to compensate for information loss without special help is more limited than that of younger persons while the effect is more pervasive.
- It is common for the maximal use of residual hearing among persons in this age group to be limited by poor speech discrimination potential and reduced tolerance for loudness.
- In addition to a reduction in visual acuity, older persons experience reduced visual processing capability with a resultant impact on compensatory speech-reading potential.
- Cognitive changes arising from normal aging processes include reduced selective

attention ability, some short- and long-term memory reduction, and some diminution of word finding.

- The rate at which older persons can process information comfortably is reduced.
- Particular difficulty is experienced in comprehension of conversation when redundancy is low and in tracing the topic in group conversations and even one's own contribution to it.
- *No* evidence of change with age has been documented in semantic memory function, language competence, or syntactic processing.
- Health factors must be considered when working with older persons, since health problems reduce their ability to cope with other difficulties.
- Special adaptation(s) of assessment procedures to accommodate these changes are called for, particularly during hearing assessment and hearing aid evaluations.
- Mobility restrictions of arms and hands and with ambulation need to be considered in relation to hearing aids and assistive devices.
- Sensitivity is needed to older persons' feelings about aging, to the perspective they have on life in general, and to their attitude toward change.
- Modification of profiling to acknowledge specific circumstances and lifestyles as well as limitations in response modes must be considered.

Conclusion

Older people may be expected to be subjected to most of the effects of hearing impairment we have discussed. In addition they must accommodate to normal aging changes and the interactive effect of these two sources of limitations. Therefore, it is essential that in our assessment and management of persons in this age category, we are sensitive to and allow for their special circumstances. In particular, we must present information less quickly and more carefully than normal, since the older person often has difficulty processing rapid low-redundancy messages. Instructions may need to be repeated due to possible memory problems; mobility problems need to be recognized both in test procedures and in selecting amplification devices. Above all, we need to preserve the dignity of these people by respecting their rights to participate actively in planning and decision making and not to have management strategies imposed upon them.

22

Special Considerations in Management of Hearing Handicap in the Older Client

Respect for the client lies at the very core of all effective management models. Two groups of individuals more than any others need our full commitment to this philosophy. These are children and elderly persons. My rejection of the nonmedical use of the term *geriatric* is due primarily to the fact that it strips the older person of his dignity. We younger individuals (note that there is no pejorative term for us!) owe our elders the respect other societies accord them naturally. They are people who either served or had loved ones who served in a world war and in other regional wars. They also worked to permit us to live as we do now. I make this point strongly because its realization fosters a genuine attitude of concern and consideration. Genuineness is crucial. Mawkish sentimentality, overly solicitous behavior toward an elderly person, or a tone and manner of speaking suitable only to an infant disqualify you from affording real help to others. Genuine evidence of your concern and your desire to be of assistance to the client and the family will do much to motivate them. It will encourage them to think and act positively and to assume responsibility for their own welfare.

As we consider guidelines to direct us in our management of resources to meet the needs of our older clients, it is essential that we have a broader frame of reference than hearing impairment and its implications. For this population, hearing impairment is just one variable in the level of handicap imposed as a function of the normal aging process. For a smaller group of people, the aging handicaps will be complicated further by chronic medical ailments and ill health and by the setting in which they reside.

There are two implications for intervention

- The personal needs and resources among individuals will vary greatly as a result of factors other than the hearing loss. This means very sensitive individualized assessment and planning for each person. You will need to take into account the influence of environment, health, mental capacities, emotional status, and psychosocial opportunities.
- Many of these persons will be in the care of family or professional staff. The resultant increased dependence means that to achieve your goals you will have to be successful in working with caregivers as well as with the client.

ADAPTING PROCEDURES

The management model we have followed for other age groups is equally valid for the older client. It affords you the flexibility to adapt your procedures to accommodate special needs. The stages of the model, you should recall, are

- Problem definition
- Need assessment
- Establishment of goals
- Determination of intervention strategies
- Evaluation

To help us consider the special needs of this client age group, we will break the group into three main categories: (1) the working older client, (2) the retired client living independently, and (3) the client in residential care. These are listed in increasing order of client dependence. The progression through the categories represents the increasing need of the client for various types of support personnel and services as she becomes less able to cope with the demands of daily living. That reduced ability to cope alone represents a progressive reduction in the client's control over daily experiences. For those in the third category, the extent of daily living experiences may be curtailed considerably.

The Working Older Client

In the working world we each make a daily contribution to society in return for financial reward and fringe benefits. Power accrues to us by virtue of society's need for our knowledge, expertise, skills, and labor. Our position in the hierarchical structure will determine how many people are dependent upon us and thus the responsibility and power we possess. In this way our roles outside the family are defined clearly for us and are supported by society. Within the family our roles as parent, homemaker, breadwinner, and/or wage earning partner also are defined.

For the working older client, employment roles usually will have remained fairly stable over several years, though they may have diminished somewhat as children have grown up and become independent. The communication situations and demands probably also have remained stable. However, a slow deterioration of hearing will aggravate the normal aging effects that impact on communication and information processing in ways we have discussed. Thus the significance of a hearing impairment, compounded as it is by these other factors, will be greater for the older working individual than for a younger person not experiencing age effects. Of course each person's circumstance is unique, but in general the assumption that hearing impairment jeopardizes the older worker's performance more than that of the younger worker is true. Awareness of this double jeopardy helps us to appreciate the concerns of the older working person. It emphasizes the need to explore fully the ramifications of hearing impairment upon employment of a person who also may be experiencing difficulty in coming to terms with the approach of retirement. With these individuals we must consider not only the hearing needs, but also the communication needs that the age factor alone creates. We will wish to learn what the person's hopes and concerns are for the next few years.

The major special consideration for the working older person lies in counseling. We need to explore the relationship of the aging effects and the implications of the change represented by approaching retirement to the expressed difficulty in communication. A further consideration is the need to involved the spouse in all stages of rehabilitation management. Transition from a full-time working role, with all its social recognition and its responsibilities and challenges, to the circumstance of full-time retirement frequently is difficult even without a handicap. Communication between spouses or partners at this time is at a premium as each works out his/her place in a changed relationship. When that communication is impaired at the surface level by poor hearing and by lack of awareness of the effects of hearing impairment, negative patterns of adaptation are fostered. So, for preretired older persons, our management plan will follow that for the younger working adult. In addition, we will be particularly sensitive to the fact that communication difficulties arising from impaired hearing and age, to varying degrees, may be expected to contribute additional problems. We must be sensitive to the psychological implications of being near the end of one's career and to the prejudices society expresses toward older persons—against prejudices that the older person may feel he warrants (Kalish, 1977). These factors will encourage us to place particular emphasis on the potential help that counseling offers. Finally, we will be certain to involve the person's partner since in these transition years, easy communication will be essential to effective adaptation of both parties.

The Retired Client Living Independently

This person has moved from the working category to the retirement category, a change of considerable magnitude. Cumming and Henry (1961) describe the process as one of disengagement. Withdrawal from the expectations and demands of society imposed by employment must be replaced by other forms of social interaction that permit the individual to maintain a positive self-identity. This may be achieved through the pursuit of hobbies, sports, travel, and expanded social activities. It also may be achieved through involvement in volunteer organizations and civic activities. Almost all the pursuits mentioned bring the individual into social contact with others; many involve the person in an organizational and administrative structure. To cope with the demands associated with such pursuits, a functional level of communication is prerequisite. Therefore, we must be ready to consider as significant limiting factors to effective social communication such effects as, for example, wind noise interfering with communication on a golf course or while working outdoors. We need to treat the problems of hearing the numbers in a Bingo game or of understanding from a distance when serving on a committee or board as being just as important as work-related communication demands.

Recognize that the attitudes of the retired hearing-impaired person toward rehabilitative intervention planning and management may be complicated significantly by attitudes toward self. The usual low spirits, self-pity, and sense of inadequacy we feel when we experience even a temporary limitation of our abilities is much more serious when we see it as a permanent aspect of the life ahead. Thus, age plays a big role in our reaction to disability and handicap, particularly when other disabilities, such as arthritis or diabetes, coexist. We are unlikely to make great progress in reducing the hearing handicap until the person has a positive approach to the larger task of restructuring her life as a retired person. It is not uncommon for the hearing difficulty to be used as a cover for a deeper problem of not having a social world to relate to, of feeling that society no longer values the abilities she has to offer. Alpiner (1979) has stated that if elderly persons believe that "they are at terminal stages in their lives, if they believe that society has relegated them to hasbeens, the hearing aids, counseling, and rehabilitative audiology are of no import in everyday living" (p. 170). It also is important when working with the retired client to pay particular attention to his perception of his problems and his attitudes toward efforts to ameliorate them. You will not understand the person's attitude toward hearing handicap until you can see it within the larger framework of his attitude to the situation in general. Older persons particularly need to have their problems acknowledged and to talk about their feelings in a climate of acceptance. Counseling thus will play an important part in your work with persons in this group.

When we discussed intervention strategies with children, I stressed the importance of respecting the child's need to understand why she is experiencing difficulty and to involve the child in the management process to the limits of her ability. I cautioned against counseling only the parent, particularly in the presence of the child, because of the importance of recognizing the need to foster responsibility for self-help and to communicate your respect for the child and her ability to learn problem-solving techniques. This need again is accentuated in the older client. It grows greater as the person's dependence on others grows, since dependence fosters learned helplessness. Lubinski (1991a) defines *learned helplessness* as occurring "when individuals perceive that events and outcomes are independent of their responses and that further action is fruitless" (p. 144). In many instances we begin to see attitudes and behaviors reflecting reduced acceptance of personal responsibility for communication management when a widow or widower moves in with a son or daughter. We need to attempt to break the pattern of increased dependence by giving responsibility for decisions and actions squarely to both the hearing-impaired person and to the family. We should acknowledge the separate and equally important needs of both. Explain to all concerned that the impact of hearing impairment, with resultant communication difficulty, imposes a handicap on each family member. Each person experiences communication inadequacies that intervention strategies can help minimize. By emphasizing the mutuality of the problem, you stress that each person must assume an active role in problem reduction. Lubinski (1991a) points out that when communication becomes inadequate, older persons "become marginal members within their families, and even more so within the larger social framework" (p. 142). Our goal must be to make increased independence through acceptance of individualized responsibilities a family goal. Increased independence means an expansion of lifestyle and enriched communication experiences.

Retirement lifestyles, as I have pointed out, often include participation in group activities, such as playing cards or golf; doing handicrafts; attending a book or gardening club or a lecture; or going to a theater, or out to dinner, or on a group tour. You, the client, and the spouse or significant other person will need to monitor each situation to identify and follow problem-solving procedures for maximizing communication (see Chapter 20). Group activities involving active strategies for managing communication situations to favor listening conditions, as well as active strategies for controlling conversations to maximize comprehension and to repair breakdowns, can be very effective. Auditory and visual perceptual training activities designed to increase message prediction should center on the vocabulary and language appropriate to the activities and interests of group members. In addition to participating in regular local community activities, retired persons may be interested in becoming actively involved in the lobbying, educational programming, and social activities of the organization Self Help for the Hard of Hearing, or working with a group such as the American Association of Retired Persons.

Retirement should be a positive productive period. Impairment of hearing represents an impediment to the enjoyment of retirement; hearing handicap management seeks, by all methods, to minimize the effect of that impediment.

The Client Living in a Long-Term Care Facility

When the basic demands of daily living exceed an older person's ability to meet them, accommodation in a long-term care facility that provides the required support services becomes necessary. A small number of residents of such facilities have minimal health problems, but the majority suffer varying degrees of physical and mental health difficulties. What they share is a common physical and social environment that differs significantly from that of the private home. Furthermore, health conditions of residents, and loss of independent mobility in the form of private transport, restrict the experiential and social worlds. In a text specifically addressing the interaction of environmental and aging factors, Lawton (1980) concludes that the effects of environment on a person increase as the competence of the individual decreases. Reduction of communication ability definitely reduces competence, even when potential remains unchanged, since independence and social interaction depend upon it. Lubinski (1991b) lists eight functions communication serves for elderly persons.

- Maintenance of self-identity
- Reception and transmission of information of which that pertaining to physical and health needs assumes great importance both to the individual and to medical and related professionals
- Expression of feelings, particularly those arising from their condition
- Provision of sympathy and guidance to others with needs
- Assumption and use of power to influence people and circumstances
- Maintenance of a sense of life's continuity, linking memories with hopes and concerns
- Cognitive stimulation
- Esthetic and cultural stimulation

Our efforts to minimize negative effects on communication will follow the same model we have followed throughout our discussions—namely, to

- Enhance hearing function
- Modify environmental factors
- Modify communication patterns of significant others
- Modify communication strategies of the client

Although these are listed as separate steps, I emphasize that in reality each is part of a greater whole. We will consider here only those aspects that require special consideration for this population.

ENHANCING HEARING FUNCTION IN ALL HEARING-IMPAIRED OLDER PERSONS

Amplification of speech continues to hold the greatest potential for improvement in communication for most persons. When recommending, selecting, and fitting a personal hearing aid(s) to an elderly person, regardless of where they reside, you must afford the same respect for their concern about appearances as for a younger person. I am delighted when an elderly person confesses to a degree of vanity; it says much that is positive about the person's self-image. Unless the client will accept a hearing aid positively, the likelihood of resistance to its use is high. This is particularly true among older persons. Their resistance tends to be heightened by ill health, which often already has brought the person to the limits of his ability to cope, so that amplification seems an additional burden that cannot be borne. Attitudes toward hearing aid use by the older population indicate that a personal hearing aid results in a devaluation of expectations for the wearer even from other elderly individuals (Johnson, Danhauer, & Edwards, 1982). Thus a hearing aid appears to be seen, both by the general public and by older persons, as a negative factor, exacerbating the stigma of age that we already have discussed. Recommending and educating the client about the use of a personal hearing aid(s) must be approached in a realistic but positive manner. A hearing aid(s) or assistive device is not something a client must or should use. It is a device that we feel can reduce some of the difficulties the client has in hearing. We look to it to reduce frustration and to increase the person's ability to participate in and control communication situations and to participate in social activities. Stress that you do not wish to impose the hearing aid but rather than you wish the client to have the opportunity to decide whether amplification can make life easier. Explain that to do this well, you, the client, and significant others will need to work cooperatively and to allow a fair trial before reaching a conclusion.

Older people need special consideration in determining what information to provide and how to present it. The most common barriers to acceptance of amplification are expressed or hidden feelings of inadequacy. The extent of the feelings increases in accord with the general level of learned helplessness. Countering the sense of inadequacy requires appropriate counseling strategies and practical steps. The expressed or presumed feelings need to be acknowledged by the individual. They must be accepted by you as reasonable and normal. Responsibility for helping you to understand them should be given to the client:

"It must seem like quite an undertaking. Help me to understand your concerns so we can see what we can do together about taking care of them."

The concerns expressed often include

I get confused by all the things to remember.

I never can manage instruments.

I'm sure I'll do something wrong/break something.

I'll never get it in my ear; I'm so clumsy.

I'll never be able to see/manage all those little switches.

I'll never get used to it.

Never negate or belittle such statements; each is a valid description of a real concern. Approach each in a logical manner by endeavoring to understand the concern and by adopting a problem-solving strategy:

I think I know how you feel. I get the same feeling about some appliances.

These aids are really quite sturdy. We'll set things up so you'll not risk breaking it. Remember they can be repaired.

I'll go over the instructions many times with you. I don't expect you to do anything first time; most of us don't. I'll write everything down for you and we'll teach your daughter (wife/ roommate/nurse, etc.) how to do things.

We'll work out ways to solve any problems you have manipulating the aid. There really will be only one switch to worry about.

Everything takes time to get used to. Give yourself time; you can handle it.

Weinstein (1991) makes the following recommendations for hearing aid orientation. She is writing about persons suffering from senile dementia. However, I find the recommended steps valid for all older persons and indeed for a lot of younger adults, too. They provide equally helpful guidance for the speech-language pathologist as for the audiologist:

> To maximize rehabilitation efforts, the audiologist should incorporate the following intervention strategies. Instructions should be simple, repetitive, and to the point. The individual's habits and routines should be maintained. Every effort to promote a sense of competence should be made. One should be wary of signs of frustration or agitation. Finally, each accomplishment should be reinforced, pictorial or written memory aids should be adopted and family members should be integral to the sessions. (p. 231)

Particular attention needs to be paid to how information, instructions, assistance are given:

- Provide a brief explanation of what you are going to do.
- Present information in small units.
- Do not go faster than the person's ability to cope comfortably.
- Have the person explain or demonstrate what she understands.
- Review information, directions, activities as frequently as necessary.
- Make maximal use of demonstration and visual aids.
- Show much patience. If an approach does not work, modify it or change to another. If you become frustrated, the individual will feel guilty and will withdraw from the task
- Give honest constructive feedback in a kindly manner.

Personal hearing aids often do not provide the best listening conditions possible in all environments. When residual hearing capacity is severely limited and other patient problems are present, every extra source of information becomes critical. Therefore, assistive listening devices and alerting devices constitute an important potential resource for the older person. For someone living alone they may be critical to preserving independence and an acceptable lifestyle.

Assistive Listening and Alerting Devices

We have discussed the types of devices and their various functions. When considering the special needs of the older person, your concern will be to

> *Increase safety.* This requires that you pay attention to how alerting devices can be made audible for the client when she is not wearing a hearing aid(s). Most particularly you need to ensure that a smoke/fire/burglar alarm, not audible when she is asleep, will waken her.
>
> *Enable a person to know someone is attempting to reach her.* This involves the ability to know that the telephone is ringing or that someone is at the door.
>
> *Maximize home entertainment.* Television, VCR, radio, and cassette players increasingly have become essential to people's leisure enjoyment. They have special psychological importance in counteracting loneliness, a sense of isolation, and boredom among elderly persons with reduced mobility. This is particularly true for the older person living alone. In many long-term care facilities, television unfortunately often is the only form of entertainment constantly available.

Increase participative interaction with others. This addresses the need to exploit assistive devices that permit the hearing-impaired person to interact with others in a manner that minimizes frustration on both parties' parts. This includes TV listening systems that permit the listening level to be acceptable to all, personal FM or infra red systems that permit the person to hear across a room, and telephone amplifiers that allow others to communicate without unacceptable levels of difficulty. Facilitating interaction with others includes paying attention to the use of devices that facilitate listening at church services; at social activities held in church halls, clubs, or senior citizen centers, or in the social activities room in a long-term care facility.

Care and Maintenance of the Hearing Aid(s) and Listening Devices

You must determine to what extent an older person needs assistance in operating and taking care of the hearing aid or ALD. Some older persons are as competent in doing this as you are; they can assume complete responsibility. Others may need limited help, such as cleaning the ear mold or replacing batteries, while some will need a caregiver to assume full responsibility for putting the hearing aid on the client and for all care and maintenance needs. This necessitates that you educate the significant other person.

Modification of the Environment

One of the most thorough discussions of special considerations for the environment of elderly persons is provided by Lubinski (1991b). Although her discussion is directed to the management of patients with dementia, there is very little she discusses that does not have significance for older persons in general. Our consideration of the environment has been focused primarily upon the acoustic and visual components of the physical environment. In addition, we have explored the role of significant other persons who also are part of the environment. Lubinski expands our concept of environment to include the individual himself. She points out that the person contributes to a matrix of influential environmental factors. These contributions in turn act upon other components thus modifying both the environment and its effects. Lubinski defines environment in these words:

> Thus, the "total environment" is comprised of the physical background, the individual, and the relationship of the individual to others. It should be noted that each of these components changes over time and as a consequence of its relationship with other components. (1991b, p. 258)

We will examine how environmental factors that we considered for the working younger adult almost certainly change for the older retired person. We then will discuss the significance of this knowledge for management strategies.

We already have recognized a difference in the physical setting, mobility, daily life experiences, and level of independence that usually exists between the retired older person living with a spouse or alone and the person in a residential care facility.

The elderly person who moves into the home of a son or daughter falls somewhere between these two sets of circumstances. A move away from fully independent living almost always results in a change and usually means a contraction of options for the older person. We need to acknowledge also that when a person moves in with a son or daughter, the reduction in independence is experienced by all parties. The environmental influences that you need to take into account in terms of the communication demands are considered by Lubinski (1991b) under the headings (1) topographic issues, (2) social environment, (3) environmental fit, and (4) caregiver needs and attitudes. Let us consider these in a little more detail.

Topographic Issues and Social Environment. Topography refers to the surface features of space. In our own home we each have a part that is ours, be it a room or part of a room. The remainder of the house is common to all. When you give up your home as your residence to go to college, often you end up with a half or quarter of a dormitory room. When older persons relinquish their home, they invariably experience the same decrease in space. With that reduction in space usually comes a reduction in the freedom for personal pursuits. Within the confines of your own home, you can pursue whatever interests you wish. You may raise plants, do carpentry, pursue dressmaking, collect various items, invite friends, give parties, and so on. As a student or as a parent who has moved in with a child's family, you may have to give up many or most of those pursuits. Similarly your freedom to come and go within the larger space of your community may now be dependent upon transportation provided by others.

The residential care patient frequently experiences a far greater restriction of space, since institutions, whether they are schools, hospitals, or nursing homes, usually have strict regulations governing the availability and use of both private and public space.

In both the family home and the residential home, the older person also experiences a loss of privacy. In the case of the family situation, it is again important to be sensitive to the other members' reduced levels of privacy. Reduced space and reduced control over both private and shared space, together with restricted mobility within the community, will limit social interaction and communication. When a person is restricted in entertaining friends and participating in community events, the need to communicate diminishes. More basic is the reduction in experiences that give rise to things to talk about, even among those within one's daily social milieu. When the need to communicate is limited, the functional need for amplification or for intervention management disappears. Thus topographic and social factors exert a considerable influence on communication motivation.

Environmental Fit. The compatibility of the older person and her environment determines the degree of stimulation it provides. Although stimuli are sensory, their effects are cognitive. Without ongoing stimulation and cognitive function, there will be little need for more than the most basic functional communication. Thus proposals for communication enrichment will have to take into account the environmental fit the client experiences as well as ways to improve that fit. A comfortable fit with the environment will be lost when a move is made from that environment to another (e.g., to live with family or to enter a residential care facility). Fitting a hearing aid(s) may greatly enhance a person's hearing potential, but it will not suffice alone if a comfortable fit with the new environment has yet to be achieved. A similar loss of environmental fit occurs on the death of a spouse or after divorce, when the central source of gratification of communication needs is lost. Thus we need to view the hearing deficit and the communication difficulty with respect to the existing environmental fit.

Caregiver Needs and Attitudes. Those persons in the environment who relate most closely to the individual with impaired hearing will be extremely important in determining the person-environment fit. As Lubinski (1991b) emphasizes, not only must the needs and perceptions of the elderly person be considered but also those of their caregivers (p. 261). Most of the persons we work with will be in good mental and physical health; some will have health problems and/or disabilities; fewer still will have mental and/or emotional problems. Lubinski's observation applies to each of these categories and certainly fits the model of management I have presented. Communication involves interaction; both parties have needs that influence the nature, quality, and effectiveness of the interaction. We have addressed the needs of parents, teachers, and spouses in relating to hearing-impaired persons. Those needs are shared by family members and by professional caregivers. As we each grow older, our level of tolerance for deviance usually tends to decrease. We find we have to expend more effort on most tasks; we acquire aches and pains; and even our hearing acuity diminishes. The spouse of a hearing-impaired person finds communication difficult, frustrating, and irritating. The demands can exceed the spouse's tolerance level and so communication opportunities are neglected by both partners. The same complaint often is experienced by other family members. The staff in a residential center likewise commonly feel overloaded, their patience worn so thin that communication interaction with hearing-impaired residents is kept to a minimum. Residents are spoken to, not talked with. Therefore, there is an acute need for relevant informational counseling to increase the caregiver's understanding of the client's difficulties, and an even greater need for us to understand the needs and attitudes of family and staff.

Effecting Change

Because less than fully independent older persons have limited power to change their environment, and because dependence makes demands on others who have their own needs, we must be very realistic in what we attempt to achieve. Realism does not excuse you from effort; it simply acknowledges reality, sets goals within existing resources, and focuses opportunity. Any change effected will be primarily in the power of the family member or the staff of a residence. The strategy with the greatest chance of proving effective is to approach the caregiver for information. Make him the educated informant whose guidance you need in order to reduce the present difficulties experienced by all. Make clear that in order to help the client you need to attempt to understand the situation in the family/residence facility as well as the needs of the family members/staff as they relate to your client. Try to identify actual communication problem situations together. Establish goals that the family/staff members feel are realistic and explore with those concerned what resources can be available and how they can be used most effectively.

Family and professional caregivers can be expected to be helpful in reducing the problems of the hearing-impaired individual only when they have insight into those problems. Without understanding, suggestions for change lack import. We need to provide the information these persons lack, but we must be sure they understand how to make use of that information. I urge you, therefore, before listing needs, requesting changes, or suggesting strategies, to help the person understand the nature of the difficulty to be addressed and why it is arising. We need to help people conceptualize problem situations before we can expect them to want to follow our advice about how to manage them effectively. Thus,

- Identify problems specific to an individual client.
- Explain why you think they are arising.
- Identify the needs that must be met if the client's problem is to be ameliorated.
- Explore available resources with the family/staff member.
- Identify intervention strategies and changes that are realistic and acceptable.

Special Considerations for Environmental Changes

Whatever changes may be needed, the overriding factor must be cost. As we discussed earlier, cost is defined in terms of finances, time, effect on other activities and responsibilities, and inconvenience. *Your recommendation must be locally achievable at a cost acceptable to all parties.*

Acoustic Environment. I refer you back to our earlier discussion of factors in the environment that degrade the acoustic signal and the techniques for minimizing this negative effect. As in schools, the acoustics in residential care facilities usually are poor (Maurer, 1976). The effects of structural acoustics are further aggravated by lack of sensitivity to the problems created by noise.

In considering the residential care facility, you should conceptualize the acoustic environment within the larger frame of the spatial, visual, and social environment. Indeed, in reality no one of these functions is independent of the other since each affects information processing.

Combatting noise and reverberation is first approached in terms of special amplification systems, both individual and group. Obtaining and putting such technology as loop induction, FM or infrared systems, and portable amplifiers into effective monitored operation in a residential setting always should be a goal; usually it must be a long-term goal. This demands resources not always available. Similarly, the acoustic benefits provided by well-hung drapes, appropriate floor coverings, sound insulation on walls and ceilings, double-glazed windows, double doors, as well as the purchase of low noise generating fans (ceiling fans, for example), air conditioners, and heaters should be stressed to administrators as affording benefits applicable to all residents and to staff. Your goal is to affect future planning, budget proposals, and purchases. More immediately you should survey more easily controlled noise sources. Among these are radios and TVs left on when no one is paying attention to them, and open doors to the kitchen, laundry room, or staff lounge. The trundling of equipment through social areas, frequent use of the personal address (PA) system for less than essential messages, use of a PA system that is difficult to understand even with good hearing, use of bell systems for alerting staff members to the fact that they are needed—all can be controlled given administrative and staff concern. In one-to-one or small-group contacts, endeavor to have staff realize the importance of the use of the client's hearing aid(s) or ALD. Help staff understand that reducing speaker-listener distance rather than raising the voice level greatly increases discrimination and comprehension while reducing stress on the staff member.

The Visual Environment. In Chapter 5 we discussed the various factors that limit visual information relevant to communication. We examined also ways in which those negative factors may be combatted. Those suggestions apply equally to the visual needs of the older client. Indeed the needs of the older person for optimal reception of visual stimuli are increased by the effects of aging on other systems and processes.

It is particularly important to ensure that maximum correction of visual defects has been achieved. Visual examinations to check for disorders of the eye and for changing visual acuity, both of which we know occur more frequently with age, should be conducted by an opthalmologist or optometrist at least every two years. Since we are concerned with optimizing all sources of information, attention needs to be paid to the client's ability to process written as well as spoken words. Excellent lighting conditions should be sought both for reading and for watching people speak. Lubinski (1991b, p. 267) draws attention to the need for large print materials and talking books to provide cognitive stimulation. You need to determine, however, whether a person's hearing is adequate for talking books lest you cause further frustration by their introduction when they are not clearly audible. Lubinski also stresses the importance of being at eye level and close to the person when speaking and of ensuring that all visual materials, pictures, photos, bulletin boards, and so on are placed at a level where they can be seen by people in wheelchairs. These recommendations are particularly important for hearing-impaired persons whose input of general information necessarily is curtailed by the auditory handicap. I would remind you also of the importance of maximizing figure-ground contrast while minimizing glare and shadows.

Spatial and Psychosocial Environments. I am sure that you can see already that there is in fact only one comprehensive environment that, for didactic convenience, we are examining according to different parameters. Spatial and the psychosocial environments are particularly interrelated, both having a direct impact on communication. Social experience in turn is related closely to cognitive experience.

Space exerts a very direct influence upon what we experience. Consider, for example, the differences in the type of activities that can be pursued in a gymnasium, a lounge, a dining room, a reception area or a corridor. Once constructed, space facilitates what it was designed for while inhibiting other activities. Chairs placed appropriately for television viewing often are not situated to allow face-to-face conversation, thus reducing visible speech cues. An oblong dinner table constructed to accommodate six or more people limits the ability to watch the face of a person seated next to the diner, while distance and competing conversation make speaking across the table difficult. In a residential care setting, the arrangement of furniture often seems to be dictated by janitorial rather than by communication needs. Chairs lined up around the wall and tables placed against the wall inhibit communication interaction, while lighting often is poor and furnishings dark.

If communication is to be encouraged and enhanced, space must facilitate social interaction. Large open areas in a building discourage communication and have both a negative auditory and visual effect on people. We like to communicate in small intimate areas; we prefer soft lighting that illuminates well but adds warmth. Bright but not brilliant colors and soft comfortable furnishings encourage conversation. For older persons, not only must the space be easily accessible in terms of distance to walk and absence of stairs, but furniture must be accessible, that is to say, positioned appropriately and easy to sit down in and get up from. Many older clients are wheelchair bound; they too must have easy access to and movement within space intended for social communication. They also may need help getting to and from that area.

A profile of the environment of the older hearing-impaired person will need to be compiled in order to identify the degree of impedance presented to easy communicative social interaction by the various aspects of the physical environment—that is to say, to appreciate the degree of fit. We have discussed what to look for in the auditory and visual environment. Let us look at space now in terms of how well it provides for psychosocial communication needs. Some of these needs we have already discussed. Space is appropriate when

- It is designated for psychosocial interactions.
- It is not used for other activities (e.g., watching TV, occupational therapy).
- It has constant availability to people wishing to use the space.
- Seating arrangement is appropriate with regard to distance between chairs and angle of chairs to each other.
- Ease of changing furniture arrangements is great.
- Flexibility to accommodate dyadic and small group conversation is present.
- Furnishings and lighting are appropriate.

In a family home and in a long-term facility, we need to consider both the individual's personal spatial environment and the shared or public space in terms of how it encourages and facilitates ease of communication.

In senior citizen centers we will be concerned with public space in relation to communication. Lubinski (1991b) in her discussion on environmental consideration for elderly patients includes a Communication/Environment Assessment and Planning Guide which generates both a general environment profile and information identifying personal environment needs. She includes

- Visual environment
- Auditory environment
- Olfactory environment
- Spatial environment
- Psychosocial environment

Her general and personal spatial environment profile derives from answers to the following questions:

GENERAL SPATIAL ENVIRONMENT

1. Do patients have access to a variety of sites to pursue activities and conversations?
2. Is physical accessibility to activities easily available to all patients?
3. Are a majority of activities held on the patient's own floor?
4. Is there a bathroom easily accessible at activity sites?
5. Can furniture be grouped to facilitate communication?
6. Are there private places available for conversations?
7. Are patients' territorial needs respected by caregivers?
8. Do caregivers respect patients' private possessions?

PERSONAL SPATIAL ENVIRONMENT

1. Does the individual have clearly identified personal space?
2. Does the individual personalize his or her personal space?
3. Does the individual's room reflect a personal identity?
4. Is there ample seating available for individual's visitors?
5. Is the individual's room conducive to privacy?

(Lubinski 1991b, p. 276)

MANAGEMENT PROCEDURES

We have focused attention on older persons staying with family and those living in a residential care facility. Thus, when we consider management procedures, we must recognize that the power to implement change rests primarily with family or professional caregivers. In the case of the residential setting, we must work with two layers of staff. The administrator is the person in control; she makes the final decision, but the staff determine how enthusiastically those decisions are implemented. In both family and residential settings, we must work with what the relative, administrator, and staff see as their responsibilities. We can achieve no more than those persons perceive to be appropriate. The following guidelines should help you maximize your chances of success:

- First generate a complete profile of the environment and present needs.
- Provide a concise written summary of conditions and needs.
- Order needs according to priority.
- Recommend actions to reduce problems; these will need to be presented in terms of cost effectiveness.
- Provide information as to how you will attempt to document results of actions.

Your discussion with family members, administrators, and staff should have as the primary focus the need to improve ease of communication for all parties involved. Stress to administrators that the benefits that derive from implementation of your suggestions will accrue to all residents, not just to those you serve. It is reasonable to assume also that the task of the staff will be made easier as a result of the increased independence of the residents. In the family setting you need to express your interest in reducing the communication stress family members experience as the result of their relative's hearing handicap. If you can convince caregivers that you are an advocate *for* them not *against* them on behalf of your client, you may expect a more favorable response. Feasibility and positive and negative implications of suggested changes for other staff and for other functions must be explored. Cost effectiveness will be a paramount factor in achieving your goals.

Inservice Training

I am not enthusiastic about the traditional inservice training program that consists of a lecture on what caregivers need to know and what they should and should not do. Participants often do not pay a great deal of attention and the resultant changes are minimal. Group education sessions, however, are economical in a residential setting. They can be quite successful if conducted as problem-solving seminars dealing with a discussion of the staff members' perceptions of the problems, needs, and behaviors of their hearing-impaired residents. When staff are acknowledged as the key players, when their needs are addressed, when they are part of and party to recommended changes, success is likely.

Koury and Lubinski (1991) in a chapter discussing inservice training draw from Ernst and West's (1983) text to identify three elements essential to the success of inservice training:

1. Identification of the learning needs and objectives of the individuals to be trained
2. Selection and implementation of an appropriate learning experience
3. Follow-up to evaluate whether or not desired outcomes are achieved

The following guidelines should prove helpful:

- Needs must be identified for you by members who represent the group for whom the inservice training is intended.
- Gain further insight into their needs by observing their contacts with those they serve.
- Ask staff to identify the problems they frequently encounter in communicating with residents.

- Use the communication profiles we reviewed in the previous chapter.
- Make sure you identify appropriate, clearly expressed objectives for a specific inservice activity.
- Check in advance that these are appropriate to and needed by participants.
- Select learning experience focused on observing and doing.
- Use situational and case illustrations and role playing activities to facilitate learning.
- Develop an evaluation questionnaire based on your stated goals. Include an assessment of content, organization, and method of training.

If you communicate your seriousness about attempting to help the staff, if you show this by careful preparation and appropriate presentation of information relative to their perception of their needs, your inservice training will be both well received and effective.

Working with the Older Client

Our management of the needs of the individual client must be rooted in a sensitive appreciation of all the effects of the normal aging process that we have discussed in these last two chapters. Furthermore, as the level of dependence of the client increases, we must plan more of our intervention strategies in a manner that accommodates the needs of the caregiver. You will find that a progressive shift toward investment of effort into the improvement of the communication between client and family/staff will prove more effective in most instances than concentrated individual sessions with the client. We have discussed ways to implement a systems management model of intervention. Even so, the client must remain central to our efforts. So in concluding our consideration of the special needs of elderly persons with impaired hearing, we will examine direct therapist-client activities.

Older clients share the same concerns and anxieties about what is happening to them as we do. Their anxieties seldom are crowded out by the demands of daily living; the more dependent they are, the more time they have to worry about their problems. The older we get, the more likely it is that we will experience similar feelings about health problems, communication difficulties, loneliness, and a sense of isolation. This is particularly true of persons in long-term care. Another problem quite common to such environments is how to keep life interesting, how to remain active physically and mentally. It is logical, therefore, that our efforts with the client should aim to address the need for exploration of feelings and for cognitive stimulation. Encompassing each of these two general needs is communication.

Counseling Initially we will wish to establish personal contact with each client. We need him to help us define his needs and wishes as he perceives them. We need also to encourage him to express his feelings about his situation and communication difficulties. Thus our counseling approach will be directed by the same principles we discussed in other chapters. Whenever possible we should seek to have significant family members meet with us in our early talks with the client, though we should not arrange this without the client's approval. In these individual sessions, we will address the need for information counseling and will learn what level of adjustment counseling is needed. Informational counseling must be tailored to address what the client wishes to know. Do not provide a minicourse in audiology and rehabilitative management. Provide only information that the client can absorb and see a use for. Wherever possible illustrate information by analogy; use lay terms for information. Your aim is to explain quite simply to the client why he is experiencing difficulty, why the level of difficulty varies with the situation, why the hearing aid(s) does not solve the problem, what it reasonably can be expected to do, and how the client can get the maximum benefit from it. Your goal is to clear up misunderstandings and build acceptance through confidence. Above all avoid battling for what you want for the client when the client is unable to accept it. Be ready to address underlying fears of the hearing's getting worse, or of becoming deaf, as well as feelings of bitterness and resentment over what has happened, feelings not infrequently directed against family, helping professionals, or residence staff.

Individual sessions should be used to identify and address very individual needs that include adjustment to hearing aids, problems relating to other health matters, personal relations with family, and so on. Whenever possible you should try to work with small groups of hearing-impaired persons. These may be established in a residential facility or, for persons living independently or with family, set up in conjunction with a senior citizen center.

Group Activities. Group work with the older population is desirable because isolation and loneliness are major problems they experience. The environment of the older person tends to become more restricted, providing an increasingly narrow range of experiences without which there is little to communicate, to tell about, to share and react to. Grouping provides for social interaction; it can enrich experience by involving people in shared activity. A group also permits participants to express anxieties, concerns, and problems only to discover that others share the same difficulties, that they are in fact not peculiar to them but to the disability. Groups can provide acceptance and help a person to better understand herself. They provide an opportunity not only to get help but also a sense of usefulness through being able to help others. Clark and Witte (1991) describe the requirements of a group facilitator working with older persons:

> The speech-language pathologist must act as the group's facilitator, must have skills in manipulating turn taking, sustaining the group's interest, knowing when to offer cognitive challenge for eliciting group participation, and maintaining attention in a nonthreatening and nonjudgmental emotional climate. Such an atmosphere fosters positive reinforcement of a patient's participation and establishes an optimal number of communication successes. (p. 245)

Needs. In thinking about group activities with older hearing-impaired persons, do so with the common needs shared by the older population in mind:

- *Enriched experience.* This need results from the limited variability in the things they are involved in.

- *Responsibility.* They are being cared for, thus their responsibilities are minimal. Individuals need the challenge of a position of control.
- *Cognitive, intellectual stimulation.* Their environment makes few demands on their thought process; thus stimulation is a strong need.
- *Motivation.* Lacking in responsibility and stimulation, older persons feel a need for a sense of purpose.
- *Communication.* Without organized activities, a predictable environment generates few new events to warrant conversation.
- *Participation.* Older persons with time on their hands wish to become involved in meaningful activity.

Problems. Recall also the difficulties aging usually gives rise to:

- Poor auditory discrimination
- Comprehension difficulty in noise
- Difficulty with high rates of information
- Difficulty with divided attention
- Reduced memory and recall ability

It is from the needs that we develop our activities and from the problems that we determine strategies.

Activities The activities we choose should be participative in nature. This means that the group becomes involved in a project. The project selected must be one that provokes interest. Think of the kinds of demonstrations that draw a crowd in a department store. For example, you might choose to make muffins, scones, or cookies as a project, or to make pancakes. The project might be spread over two sessions. The first session can revolve around ingredients and recipes. Auditory-visual communication training would be used for relevant vocabulary and phrases. Key words and phrases would be identified and used for discrimination. Ingredients for recipes and the order of instructions can be read to permit auditory memory training. Conversation might be around "some of my favorite recipes" or "foods I hate." Conversational strategies for controlling topic and for repairing communication breakdowns can be demonstrated and practiced. During the second session, the actual activity is carried out, providing for a review of what was learned.

Other activities may arise out of personal interest, for example, "How to pot and force spring bulbs indoors", or "How to make simple drawings." You might use the skills and abilities of one of the older persons, planning the presentation together, or you might invite a guest who has a special skill or hobby. A zoo may be willing to make a presentation involving live animals. Any resident or member of a senior citizen center might attend, but your group would prepare related information and vocabulary prior to the visit and perhaps have a review and discussion session following it. Activities within the center or residence or seasonal events, for example, provide opportunities for the group to accept planning and implementation responsibilities, both of which will require communication skills. A group might wish to take up correspondence with another senior citizen center or residence, writing a periodic group letter that generates communication demands at all levels.

Whenever possible integrate your activities with other professional and staff activities. For example, kitchen staff might be willing to assist in a baking project while occupational therapists might enjoy working with you on a handicraft project.

In the beginning, group activities are difficult to organize. They require very creative planning and a real desire to involve the clients in all stages of the activities. Brainstorm the possibilities available to you. Think of how you might use travel brochures to plan imaginary trips, cookbooks to plan a special dinner, play reading as a tryout for a Broadway play, instruments of the orchestra for fun with music. If you can identify a project that makes you say, "Hey that could be a lot of fun," then you most certainly can adapt it to provide for all your communication enrichment goals. For each project determine ahead of time how you will use it for auditory-visual training for memory and recall and for communication strategies.

The activities you devise will be of interest to you and to the group. They will create experiences and utilize the resources of members of the group, residence or center staff, and people in the community. You will want the activities to actively involve the group members in planning and conducting projects so that they accept responsibility for contributing and you want to get group members talking about an activity common to all of them. The group activities provide for communication that enables you to work on skills such as auditory-visual processing, making predictions about incomplete messages, and utilizing conversational management skills in real-life situations. At the same time you can work on the perceptual processing changes that are associated with the normal aging process and exacerbated by impairment of hearing.

Although such projects will comprise a major part of your communication enhancement efforts, as the group becomes more cohesive, more comfortable in interacting with each other, you will be able to introduce relevant informational counseling. You also will wish to include time for group exploration of anxieties, frustrations, feelings of anger, resentment, and so on arising from being communicatively handicapped.

Elderly people as a group are gravely underestimated and undervalued. They have a wealth of experiences, much courage, and a surprising amount of humor to offer. They are to be enjoyed as company. Your task is to enhance their ability to share with us all the resources they have to offer. Working with this group of people may not have the glamour of working with children; it certainly can afford us equal rewards.

SUMMARY

- Management planning with the older client must occur within a framework broader than the immediate one of the hearing problem.
- The working senior, the retired person living independently, and the person in long-term care each requires different management plans.
- Our goal is to enhance the functions that communication serves. We achieve this using the model we have applied to all age groups.
- Special attention should be paid to the need for assistive listening and alerting devices.
- Every effort should be made to increase the compatibility of the person and the environment.

- The needs of the family and caregivers are particularly important when assisting older persons.
- Wherever possible appropriate modifications should be made in the visual, auditory, spatial, and psychosocial environment.
- Participative inservice experiences will help to gain staff involvement in management.
- Group activities enrich experience, encourage responsibility, stimulate the mind, motivate, provide communication opportunities, and encourage participation.

Conclusion

Handicap management with older clients uses the same basic model used throughout this text. However, certain modifications must be made to accommodate the special circumstances arising from the changing level of independence with increasing age and possible ill health. The need to provide knowledge and practical support to the spouse, family members, or caregivers increases with age of the client. This necessitates that we understand the individual circumstances of each situation and the nature of each environment. We endeavor to increase the compatibility between the individual and the environment and those in it. Because of the limitations often imposed by age, older persons may not share our perception of the value of change. Furthermore, they may feel the effort required exceeds their resources. With older persons, we must make an extra effort to respect their right to choose not to participate in all we would like to arrange for them.

References

CHAPTER 1

AAO-ACO (American Academy of Otolaryngology and American Council of Otolaryngology). Guide for evaluation of hearing handicap. *Jour. Amer. Medical Assn., 241*, 179, 2035–2059.

ERBER., N. Speech perception by hearing impaired children. In eds. Bess, F. Freeman, B. A. and Sinclair, J. *Amplification in Education.* Washington, DC. Alexander Graham Bell Assn. for the Deaf, 1981.

GOFFMAN, E. *Stigma: Notes on the Management of Spoiled Identity.* Englewood Cliffs NJ; Prentice Hall, 1963.

KNAUF, V. H. Language and speech training. In ed. Katz, J. *Handbook of Clinical Audiology.* 2nd ed. Baltimore: Williams and Wilkins, 1978.

LING, D. *Speech and the Hearing Impaired Child: Theory and Practice.* Washington, DC: Alexander Graham Bell Assn. for the Deaf, 1976.

LING, D. and LING, A. H. *Aural Habilitation.* Washington, DC: Alexander Graham Bell Assn. for the Deaf, 1976.

ROSS, M. Definitions and descriptions. In ed. Davis, J., *Our Forgotten Children: Hard of Hearing Pupils in the Schools.* Minneapolis, Univ. of Minnesota Press, 1977.

SANDERS, D. A. Psychological implications of hearing impairment. In ed. Cruickshank, W. M. *Psychology of Exceptional Children and Youth.* Englewood Cliffs, NJ: Prentice Hall, 1980.

SANDERS, D. A. Hearing-aid orientation and counseling. In ed. Pollack, M. *Amplification for the Hearing Impaired.* New York, Grune and Stratton, 1980.

STARK, R. E., ed. *Sensory Capabilities of Hearing-Impaired Children.* Baltimore: University Park Press, 1974.

VERNON, M. and OTTINGER, P. J. Psychosocial aspects of hearing impairment. In eds. Schow, R. L. and Nerbonne, M. A. *Introduction to Aural Rehabilitation.* Baltimore: University Park Press, 1980.

WILLIAMS, D. M. and DARBYSHIRE, J. O. Diagnosis of deafness: a study of family responses and needs. *Volta Review, 84*, 1982, 24–30.

CHAPTER 2

BODE, D. L. Speech signals and hearing aids. In ed. Pollack, M., *Amplification for the Hearing Impaired.* New York: Grune and Stratton, 1975, pp. 287–304.

BOOTHROYD, A. *Hearing Impairments in Young Children.* Englewood Cliffs, NJ: Prentice Hall, 1982.

CONDON, W. S. and SANDER, L. W. Neonate movement is synchronized with adult speech. *Science, 183*, 1973, 99–101.

DANILOFF, R. G. *Normal articulation process.* In eds. Minifie, F. and Hixon, I. J., *Aspects of Speech Hearing and Languages.* Englewood Cliffs, NJ: 1973, pp. 169–209.

FLETCHER, H. *Speech and Hearing in Communication.* New York: D. Van Nostrand, 1953.

GERBER, S. E. Intelligibility of speech. In ed. Gerber, S. E., *Introductory Hearing Science.* Philadelphia: W.B. Saunders, 1974, pp. 238–260.

KAPLAN, E. and KAPLAN, G. The prelinguistic child. In ed. J. Eliot, *Human Development and Cognitive Processes.* New York: Holt, Rhinehart and Winston, 1971.

LEFEVRE, C. A multidisciplinary approach to language and reading: Some projections. In ed. Goodman, K, *The Psycholinguistic Nature of the Reading Process.* Detroit; Wayne State Univ. Press, 1973, pp. 189–312.

LEVITT, H. The acoustics of speech production. In eds. Ross, M. and Giolas, T., *Auditory Management of Hearing Impaired Children.* Baltimore: Univ. Park Press, 1978.

LEVITT, H. Speech as a physical stimulus. In eds. Bess, F. H., Freeman, B. A., and Sinclair, S. J., *Amplification in Education.* Washington, DC: Alexander Graham Bell Assoc. for the Deaf, 1981.

LIBERMAN, A. Some results of research on speech perception. *J. Acoust. Soc. Amer., 29*, 1957, 117–123.

LIBERMAN, A. M., COOPER, F. S., SHANKWEILER, D. P., and STUDDERT-KENNEDY, M. G. Perception of the speech code. *Psychol. Rev., 74(6)*, 1967, 431–461.

LIEBERMAN, P. Intonation and syntactic processing of speech. In ed. Wathen-Dunn, W., *Models for the Perception of Speech and Visual Form.* Cambridge, MA: MIT Press, 1967, pp. 314–319.

537

MARTIN, J. G. Rhythmic hierarchical versus serial structure in speech and other behavior. *Psychol. Rev., 73*, 1972, 487–509.

SANDERS, D. A. *Auditory Perception of Speech—An Introduction to Principles and Problems.* Englewood Cliffs, NJ: Prentice Hall, 1977.

CHAPTER 3

American National Standards Institute, American National Standard for Rating Noise with Respect to Speech Interference, ANSI S3.14, 1977.

BLAIR, J. C. Effects of amplification, speech reading and classroom environment on reception of speech. *Volta Rev., 79*, 1977, 443–449.

BOLT, R. H. and MACDONALD, A. D. Theory of speech masking by reverberation. *J. Acoust. Soc. Amer., 21*, 1949, 577–580.

CRUM, M. A. and TILLMAN, T. W. Effects of speaker-to-listener distance upon intelligibility in reverberation and noise abstract. *ASHA, 15*, 1973, 473.

FINITZO-HIEBER, T. and TILLMAN, T. W. Room acoustic effects on monosyllabic word discrimination ability for normal and hearing impaired children. *J. Speech Hearing Res., 21*, 1978, 440–448.

HOUTGAST, T. Indoor speech intelligibility and indoor noise criteria. Noise as a Public Health Problem. Proceedings of the Third International Congress, *ASHA Reports, No. 10*, American Speech-Language-Hearing Association, Rockville, MD, April 1980, p. 172.

HOUTGAST, T. and STEENEKEN, H. The modular transfer function in room acoustics as a predictor of speech intelligibility. *Acoustica, 28*, 1973, 66–73.

JOHN, J. Acoustics in the use of hearing aids. In ed. Ewing, A. W. G., *Educational Guidance for the Deaf Child.* Manchester, England: Manchester Univ. Press, 1957.

MONCUR, J. P. and DIRKS, D. Binaural and monaural speech intelligibility in reverberation. *J. Speech Hearing Res., 10*, 1967, 186–195.

NABELEK, A. K. and ROBINETTE, L. N. Influence of the precedence effect on word identification by normally hearing and hearing impaired subjects. *J. Acoust. Soc. Amer., 63*, 1978, 187–194.

NIEMOELLER, A. F. Physical concepts of speech communications in classrooms for the deaf. Chapt. 10 in eds. Bess, F., Freeman, B. A., and Sinclair, J. S., *Amplification in Education.* Washington, DC: Alexander Graham Bell Assoc. for the Deaf, 1981, pp. 164–179.

OLSEN, W. O. Acoustics and amplification in classrooms for the hearing impaired. In ed. Bess, F. H., *Childhood Deafness: Causation, Assessment and Management.* New York: Grune and Stratton, 1977.

PEARSONS, K. S. Communication in noise: Research after the 1973 Congress on Noise as a Public Health Problem. In eds. Tobias, J. V., Jansen, J., and Ward, W. D., Proceedings of the Third International Congress on Noise as a Public Health Problem *ASHA Reports No. 10*, Rockville, MD: American Speech-Language-Hearing Assoc., 1980, pp. 165–171.

PEARSONS, K. S., BENNETT, R. L., and FIDELL, S. Speech levels in various noise environments. EPA-600/1-77-025, 1977.

ROSS, M. Classroom acoustics and speech intelligibility. In ed. Katz, J., *Handbook of Clinical Audiology.* Baltimore: Williams and Wilkins, 1978.

ROSS, M. and GIOLAS, T. Effect of three classroom listening conditions on speech intelligibility, *Am. Ann. Deaf, 116*, 1971, 580–584.

RUPF, J. A. Noise effect on passenger communicating in light aircraft. Society of Automotive Engineers, Business Aircraft Meeting, Century II, Wichita, KS, 1977.

SANDERS, D. A. Noise conditions in normal school classrooms. *Exceptional Child, 31*, 1965, 344–353.

THOMAS, H. Architectural acoustics as a fundamental in the design of schools for the deaf. In ed. Ewing, A., *The Modern Educational Treatment of Deafness.* Manchester, England: Manchester Univ. Press, 1960.

CHAPTER 4

BERGER, K. *Speechreading Principles and Methods.* Baltimore: National Educational Press, 1972.

BINNIE, C., JACKSON, P., and MONTGOMERY, A. Visual intelligibility of consonants. A lipreading screening test with implications for aural rehabilitation. *J. Speech Hearing Dis., 41*, 1976, 530–539.

BOOTHROYD, A. Linguistic factors in speech reading. In eds. DeFilippo, C. L. and Sims, D. G. New Reflections on Speechreading, *Volta Rev., 90*, 1988, No. 5.

BRANNON, J. B. and KODMAN, F. The perceptual process in speech reading. *Archives of Otolaryngology, 70*, 1959, 111–119.

COLEMAN, J. C. Facial expression of emotion. *Psychol. Mon., 63*, 1949, 1–36.

DOLANSKI, V. Les aveugles possidentile les sens d'obstacles. *Annee Psychologique, 31*, 1930, 1–51.

FISHER, C. Confusions among visually perceived consonants. *J. Speech Hearing Res., 11*, 1968, 796–804.

FRY, D. E. and WHETNALL, E. *The Deaf Child.* London: William Heinemann Ltd., 1962.

GOFFMAN, ERVING. *Interaction Ritual.* Garden City, NY; Doubleday and Company, 1967.

LESNER, S. and SANDRIDGE, S. Flash-evoked potentials and lipreading in older adults. *J. Acad. Rehab. Aud., 17,* 1984, 97–105.

NITCHIE, E. B. *Principles and Methods of Lipreading,* 1912, mimeographed pamphlet.

PETERS, R. S. *The Concept of Motivation.* London: Routledge & Kegan, Paul, Ltd., 1958.

RUESCH, J. and KEES, W. *Nonverbal Communication.* Berkeley and Los Angeles: Univ. of California Press, 1956.

SHEPHERD, D. C. Visual-neural correlate of speech reading ability in normal-hearing adults: Reliability. *J. Speech Hearing Res., 25,* 1982, 521–527.

SHEPHERD, D. C., DELAVERGNE, R. W., FRUEH, F., and CLOBRIDGE, C. Visual-neural correlate of speech reading ability in normal-hearing adults. *J. Speech Hearing Res., 20,* 1977, 752–765.

UTLEY, J. A. A test of lipreading ability. *J. Speech Hearing Dis., 11,* 1946, 109–116.

WALDEN, B. E., ERDMAN, S. A., MONTGOMERY, A. A., SCHWARTZ, D. M., and PROSEK, R. A. Some effects of training in speech recognition by hearing impaired adults. *J. Speech Hearing Res. 24,* 1981, 207–216.

WALDEN, B. E., PROSEK, R. A., MONTGOMERY, A. A., SCHERR, C. K., and JONES, C. J. Effects of training on the visual recognition of consonants. *J. Speech Hearing Res. 20,* 1977, 130–145.

WOODWARD, M. and BARBER, C. Phoneme perception in lipreading. *J. Speech Hearing Res., 3,* 1960, 212–222.

WOODWARD, M. F. Linguistic methodology in lipreading research. *John Tracy Clinic Research Papers, 4,* December 1957, 1–32.

CHAPTER 5

BERGER, K. W., DEPOMPEI, R. A., and DRODER, J. L. The effect of distance on speech reading performance. *Ohio J. of Speech and Hearing, 5,* 1970, 115–122.

BERGER, K. W., GARNER, M., and SUDMAN, J. The effect of degree of facial exposure and the vertical angle on speech-reading performance. *Teacher of the Deaf, 69,* 1971, 322–326.

BYERS, V. W. and LIBERMAN, L. Lipreading performance and the rate of the speaker. *J. of Speech and Hearing, 2,* 1959, 271–276.

COCCAMISE, F., MEATH-LANG, B. and JOHNSON, D. Assessment and use of vision: critical needs of hearing impaired students. *Amer. Annals of the Deaf, 26,* 1981, 361–369.

DOLANSKI, V. Les aveugles possidentile les sens d'obstacles. *Annee Psychologique, 31,* 1930, 1–51.

ERBER, N. P. Effects of distance on the visual reception of speech. *J. Speech Hearing Res. 14,* 1971, 848–857.

ERBER, N. P. Effects of angle, distance, and illumination on visual reception of speech by profoundly deaf children. *J. Speech Hearing Res. 17*(1), 1974, 99–112.

GREENE, H. Implications of a comprehensive vision screening program for hearing-impaired children. *Volta Rev., 80,* 1978, 467–475.

HARDICK, E. J., OYER, H. J., and IRION, P. E. Lipreading performance as related to measurements of vision. *J. Speech Hearing Res., 13*(1), 1970, 92–100.

JACKSON, P. The theoretical minimal unit for speech perception: visemes and coarticulation. In eds. DeFilippo, C. and Sims, D. New Reflections on Speech Reading, *Volta Review, 90,* No. 5, 1988, Washington, DC: Alexander Graham Bell Assn. for the Deaf.

JOHNSON, D. and SNELL, K. The effect of noncorrectable distance visual acuity problems on the speech reading performance of hearing-impaired adults. Paper presented at the Summer Institute of the Academy of Rehabilitative Audiology, Lake Geneva, WI, 1986.

KANTNER, C. E. and WEST, R. *Phonetics.* New York: Harper & Row, 1941.

KARP, A. Reduced Vision and Lipreading. In eds., DeFilippo, C. and Sims, D. New Reflections on Lipreading, Washington DC: Alexander Graham Bell Assn. for the Deaf, 1988.

KENDLER, H. H. *Basic Psychology.* New York: Appleton-Century-Crofts, 1963.

LARR, A. L. Speechreading through closed circuit television. *Volta Rev., 61,* 1959, 19–21.

MULLIGAN, M. *Variables in the Reception of Visual Speech from Motion Pictures.* Unpublished master's thesis, Ohio State University, 1954.

NAKANO, Y. A. A study on the factors which influence lipreading of deaf children, cited by S. P. Quigley, 1966. Language research in countries other than the United States. *Volta Rev., 68,* 1966, 68–83.

NEELY, K. K. Effects of visual factors on the intelligibility of speech. *J. Acoust. Soc. Amer., 28,* 1956, 1275–1277.

NITCHE, E. B. *Principles and Methods of Lipreading,* 1912 mimeograph pamphlet.

PARASNIS, I. and SAMAR, V. Visual perception of verbal information by deaf people. In *Deafness In Communication,* eds. Sims, D., Walter, G. and Whitehead, R. Baltimore: Williams and Wilkins, 1982.

POLLARD, G. and NEUMAIER, R. Vision characteristics of deaf children, *Am. Ann. Deaf, 119,* 1974, 740–745.

SANDERS, D. A. and GOODRICH, S. J. The relative contribution of visual and auditory components of speech to intelligibility as a function of three conditions of frequency distortion. *J. Speech Hearing Res., 14,* 1971, 154–159.

SUMBY, W. H. and POLLACK, I. Visual contribution to speech intelligibility in noise. *J. Acoust. Soc. Amer., 26,* 1956, 1275–1277.

SUMMERFIELD, A. Q. Audio-visual speech perception. In eds. Luterman, M. E. and Haggard, M. *Hearing Science and Hearing Disorders*. New York Academic Press, 1983.

THOMAS, S. L. *Lipreading as a Function of Light Levels*. Unpublished master's thesis, Michigan State University, 1962.

U.S.W.P.A. Lipreading Project of the Board of Education, New York. USWPA for the City of New York, 1939.

UTLEY, J. A test of lipreading ability. *J. Speech Hearing Dis.*, *11*, 1946, 109–116.

WALDEN, B. E., PROSEK, R. A., MONTGOMERY, A. A., SCHERR, C. K. and JONES, C. J. Effects of training on the visual recognition of consonants. *J. Speech Hearing Res. 20*, 1977, 130–145.

WOODWARD, M. F. Linguistic methodology in lipreading research. *John Tracy Clinic Research Papers, 4*, December 1957.

CHAPTER 6

BERGER, J. *Ways of Seeing*. London: British Broadcasting Corporation, 1986.

BROADBENT, D. E. *Perception and Communication*. New York: Pergamon Press, 1958.

COLEMAN, J. C. Facial expressions of emotion. *Psychol. Mon.*, *63*, 1949, 11–36.

COTZIN, M. and DALLENBACH, M. Facial vision: The role of pitch and loudness in the perception of obstacles by the blind. *Amer. J. Psychol.*, *63*, 1944, 485–515.

FREELANDER, B., Receptive language development in infancy. *Merrill Palmer Quarterly of Behavior and Development, 16*, 1970, 7–51.

HILGARD, E. R. *Introduction to Psychology* (2nd ed.). New York: Harcourt, Brace, and World, 1957.

KOHLER, I. *American Foundation for the Blind Research Bulletin, 4* (14), 1944.

LAWSON, C. A. *Brain Mechanisms and Human Learning*. Boston: Houghton Mifflin, 1967.

LING, D. *Speech and the Hearing-Impaired Child: Theory and Practice*. Washington, DC: Alexander Graham Bell Assoc. for the Deaf, 1976.

MEHLER, J., BERTONICINI, J., BARRIERE, M. et al. Infant recognition of mother's voice. *Perception 7*, 1978, 491–497.

RAMSDELL, D. A. The psychology of the hard of hearing and deafened adult. In eds. Darish, H. and Silverman, S. R., *Hearing and Deafness* (3rd ed.). New York: Holt, Rinehart and Winston, 1970, pp. 435–446.

RICE, C. Human echo perception. *Science, 15S*, February 1967, 656–664.

SANDERS, D. A. Hearing aid orientation and counseling. In ed. Pollack, M. C., *Amplification for the Hearing-Impaired*. New York; Grune and Stratton, 1980, pp. 323–372.

SANDERS, D. A. Psychological implications of hearing impairment. In ed. Cruickshank, W. M. *Psychology of Exceptional Children and Youth*. Englewood Cliffs, NJ: Prentice Hall, 1980.

SENDEN, M. VON. *Space and Sight: The perception of Space and Shape in the Congenitally Blind before and after Operation*. London: Methuen and Co., Ltd., 1960.

SPITZ, R. *The First Year of Life*. New York: International Universities Press, 1965.

SUPA, M., COTZIN, M., and DALLENBACH, M. Facial vision: The perception of obstacles by the blind. *Amer. J. Psychol. 57*, 1944, 142–152.

CHAPTER 7

ABBS, J. H. and SUSSMAN, H. M., Neurophysiological feature detectors and speech perception. A discussion of theoretical implications. *J. Speech Hearing Res.*, *14*, 1971, 23–26.

BERRY, M. F., *Language Disorders of Children*. New York: Appleton-Century-Crofts, 1969.

BJORK, E. L. and HEALY, A. F. Intra-item and extra-item sources of acoustic confusion in short-term memory. In *Communications in Mathematical Psychology*. New York: Rockefeller Institute Technical Reports, April 1970.

BRAZIER, M. A. B. The electrical activity of the nervous system. *Science, 146*, December 1964, 1427.

CROWDER, R. J. and MORTON, J. Precategorical acoustic storage (P.A.S.). *Perception and Psychophysics, 5*, 1969, 356–373.

ESTES, W. K. On the source of acoustic confusions in short-term memory for letter strings. In *Communications in Mathematical Psychology*. New York: Rockefeller Institute Technical Reports, April 1970.

FRENCH, J. D. The reticular formation. *Scientific American, 196*, 1957, 54–60.

HEMDAL, J. F. and HUGHES, A. W. A feature based computer recognition program for the modelling of vowel perception. In ed. Wathen-Dunn, W., *Models for the Perception of Speech and Visual Form*. Cambridge, MA: MIT Press, 1967.

KOHLER, I. American Foundation for the Blind, *Research Bulletin No. 4*, 1944.

LAWSON, C. A. *Brain Mechanisms and Human Learning*. Boston: Houghton Mifflin, 1967.

LIBERMAN, A. M., COOPER, F. S., SHANKWEILER, D. P., and STUDDERT-KENNEDY, M. G. Perception of the speech code. *Psychol. Rev.*, *74* (6), 1967, 431–461.

MILLER, G. A. The magical number 7 ± 2: Some limits on our capacity for processing information. *Psychol. Rev., 63,* 1956, 81–97.

NEISSER, U. Decision time without reaction time: Experiments in visual scanning. *Amer. J. Psychol., 76,* 1963, 376–385.

NEISSER, U. *Cognitive Psychology Century Psychology Series.* New York: Appleton-Century-Crofts, 1967.

SANDERS, D. A. *Auditory Perception of Speech: An Introduction to Principles and Problems.* Englewood Cliffs, NJ: Prentice Hall, 1977.

SANDERS, D. A. and GOODRICH, S. J. The relative contribution of visual and auditory components of speech to intelligibility as a function of three conditions of frequency distortion. *J. Speech Hearing Res., 14,* 1971, 154–159.

SEWARD, J. P. The effect of practice on the visual perception of form. *Archives of Psychol., 20*(130), 1931, 72.

SOLLEY, C. M. and MURPHY, P. *Development of the Perceptual World.* New York: Basic Books, 1960.

STEVENS, K. and HALLE, M. Remarks on analysis-by-synthesis and distinctive features. In ed. Wathen-Dunn, W., *Models for the Perception of Speech and Visual Form.* Cambridge, MA: MIT Press, 1967, pp. 88–102.

UTTLEY, A. M. The classification of signals in the nervous system. *E.E.G. Clin. Neurophysiol., 6,* 1954, 479.

UTTLEY, A. M. Conditional probability computing in a nervous system. In *Mechanization of Thought Processes.* London: Her Majesty's Stationery Office, 1959, pp. 121–147.

UTTLEY, A. M. The transmission of information and the effect of local feedback in theoretical and neural networks. *Brain Res., 2,* 1966, 21–30.

WOODWORTH, R. S. Reinforcement of perception. *Amer. J. Psychol., 60,* 1947, 119–124.

CHAPTER 8

CARRIER, J. K. Application of a non-speech language system with the severely languaged handicapped. In, ed. Lloyd, L., *Communication Assessment and Intervention Strategies.* Baltimore: Univ. Park Press, 1976, pp. 523–547.

CARROLL, J. B. *Language and Thought.* Englewood Cliffs, NJ: Prentice Hall, 1964.

CHERRY, C. *On Human Communication.* New York: John Wiley, 1957.

ENGLEMANN, S. and ROSOV, R. Tactual hearing experiment with deaf and hearing-impaired subjects. *J. Except. Child, 41,* 1975, 243–253.

ERBER, N. and CRAMER, K. Vibrotactile recognition of sentences. *Am. Ann. Deaf, 119,* 1974, 716–720.

EVARTS, E. V. Motor cortex reflexes associated with learned movement. *Science, 179,* 1973, 501–503.

FAIRBANKS, A. Systematic research in experimental phonetics. *J. Speech Hearing Dis., 19,* 1954, 133–139.

FURTH, H. Discussion: language processing and the hearing impaired child. In ed. Stark, R. *Sensory Capabilities of Hearing Impaired Children.* Baltimore: University Park Press, 1974.

LAURIE, P. Your health: The mind, the explorers. London Sunday Times Magazine, March 19, 1967.

LEHITLE, I. The units of speech perception. In ed. Gilbert, J., *Speech and Cortical Function.* New York: Academic Press, 1972.

LIBERMAN, A. The grammars of speech and language. *Cognitive Psych., 1,* 1970, 301–323.

LING, D. *Speech and the Hearing-Impaired Child.* Washington, DC: Alexander Graham Bell Assoc. for the Deaf, 1976.

PREMACK, D. and PREMACK, A. Teaching visual language to apes and language deficient persons. In eds. Schiefelbusch, R. and Lloyd, L., *Language Perspectives—Acquisition Retardation and Intervention.* Baltimore: Univ. Park Press, 1974, pp. 347–376.

SHANNON, C. and WEAVER, W. *The Mathematical Theory of Communication.* Urbana: Univ. of Illinois Press, 1967.

CHAPTER 9

BATESON, A. Cybernetic explanation. *American Behavioral Scientist, 10,* 1967, 29–32.

BOOTHROYD, A. Speech perception and sensorineural hearing loss. Chap. 4 in eds. Ross, M. and Giolas, T. G., *Auditory Management of Hearing Impaired Children.* Baltimore; University Park Press 1978, pp. 117–144.

BOOTHROYD, A. *Influence of Residual Hearing on Speech Perception and Speech Production by Hearing Impaired Children.* Paper presented at the 1976 convention of the American Speech-Language-Hearing Society, Houston, Texas, 1976 cited in eds. Bess, F., Freeman, B. A., and Sinclair, J. S., *Amplification in Education.* Washington, DC: Alexander Graham Bell Assoc. for the Deaf, 1981.

BRONZAFT, A. L. and McCARTHY, D. P. The effects of elevated train noise on auditory discrimination and reading ability in children. *J. Exp. Soc. Psychol., 9,* 1975, 407–422.

COHEN, S., EVANS, A. W., KRANTZ, D. S., STOKOLS, D., and KELLY, S. Aircraft noise and children: Longitudinal and cross-sectional evidence on adaptation to noise and the effectiveness of noise abatement. *J. Pers. Soc. Psychol, 40,* 1981, 330–335.

COHEN, S., GLASS, D. C., and SINGER, J. E. A part noise and discrimination and reading ability in children. *J. Exp. Soc. Psychol., 9*, 1973, 407–422.

ERBER, N. Speech perception by hearing impaired children. Chap. 3 in eds. Bess, F. H., Freeman, B. A., and Sinclair, J. S., *Amplification in Education.* Washington, DC; Alexander Graham Bell Assoc. for the Deaf, 1981.

FINITZO-HIEBER, T. and TILLMAN, T. W. Room acoustic effects on monosyllabic word discrimination ability for normal and hearing impaired children. *J. Speech Hearing Res., 21*, 1978, 440–448.

FLETCHER, H. *Speech and Hearing in Communication.* New York: D. Van Nostrand, 1953.

FRENCH, N. R. and STEINBERG, J. C. Factors governing the intelligibility of speech sounds. *J. Acoust. Soc. Amer., 19*, 1947, 90–119.

FRY, D. B. The role and primacy of the auditory channel in speech and language development. In eds. Ross, M. and Giolas, T. A., *Auditory Management of Hearing Impaired Children.* Baltimore; Univ. Park Press, 1978, pp. 15–42.

FURTH, H. Discussion: Language processing and the hearing impaired child. In ed. Stark, R, *Sensory Capabilities of Hearing Impaired Children.* Baltimore: Univ. Park Press, 1974, pp. 173–196.

GELFAND, S. A. and HOCHBERG, I. Binaural and monaural speech discrimination under reverberation. *Audiology, 15*, 1976, 72–84.

GODFREY, J. J. Linguistic structure in clinical and experimental tests of speech recognition. Chap. 10, in *Speech Recognition by the Hearing Impaired.* ASHA Reports No. 14, American Speech-Language Hearing Association, Rockville, MD, October 1984, pp. 52–56.

HAMBRICK-DIXON, P. J. *The Effects of Subway Extraneous Noise on Children's Psychomotor, Cognitive and Perceptual Performance.* Program of the American Acoustical Soc., Los Angeles, CA, November 1980.

HAMBRICK-DIXON, P. J. *Subway Noise and Children's Visual Vigilance Performance: A Developmental Perspective.* Program of the American Psychological Association, Washington, DC, 1982.

LENNEBERG, E. H., *Biological Foundations of Language.* New York: John Wiley, 1967.

LEVIN, H. B. What the child knows about speech. In eds. Kavanagh, J. F. and Mattingly, I. A., *Language by Ear and by Eye.* Cambridge, MA: MIT Press, 1972.

LING, D. *Speech and the Hearing Impaired Child: Theory and Practice.* Washington, DC: The Alexander Graham Bell Assoc. for the Deaf, 1976.

LING, D. and LING, A. H., *Aural Habilitation.* Washington, DC: The Alexander Graham Bell Assoc. for the Deaf, 1978.

LUKAS, J. S., DUPREE, R. B., and SWING, J. W. Effects of noise on academic achievement and classroom behavior. Calif. Dept. of Transportation Report No. FHWA/CA/DOHS 81/01, 1981.

MCNEILL, D. The capacity for language acquisition. *Volta Rev., 68*, 1966, 17–33.

MILLER, G., HEISE, G., and LICHTEN, W. The intelligibility of speech as a function of the context of the test materials. *J. Exp. Psychol., 41*, 1951, 329–335.

MILLER, G. A. and NICELY, P. E. An analysis of perceptual confusions among some English consonants. *J. Acoust. Soc. Amer., 27*, 1955, 338–352.

MORSE, P. A. The discrimination of speech and non speech stimuli in early infancy. *J. Exp. Psychol., 14*, 1972, 477–492.

MORSE, P. A. Infant speech perception. In Sanders, D. A., *Auditory Perception of Speech.* Englewood Cliffs, NJ: Prentice Hall, 1977, 161–176.

NABALEK, A. K. and PICKETT, J. M. Reception of consonants in a classroom as affected by monaural and binaural listening noise, reverberation and hearing aids. *J. Acoust. Soc. Amer., 56*, 1974a, 628–639.

NABALEK, A. K. and PICKETT, J. M. Monaural and binaural speech perception through hearing aids under noise and reverberation with normal and hearing impaired listeners. *J. Speech Hearing Res., 17*, 1974b, 724–739.

NORLIN, P. F. The language development of hearing impaired children: Constructing inferences from depleted contexts. In eds. Bess, F., Friedman, B., and Sinclair, J. *Amplification in Education.* Washington, DC: Alexander Graham Bell Assoc. for the Deaf, 1981.

PETERSON, A. E., and BARNEY, H. L. Control methods and the study of vowels. *J. Acoust. Soc. Amer., 24*, 1952, 175–184.

PISONI, D. B. Speeded classification of natural and synthetic speech in a lexical decision task. *J. Acoust. Soc. Amer., 70* (Supplement No. 1), 1981, S98.

RISBERG, A., AGELFORS, E., and BOBERG, A. Measurements of frequency discrimination ability of severely and profoundly hearing-impaired children. Speech Transmission Lab., *Quarterly Progress and Status Reports, 1975*, 2–3, 40–48.

WACHS, T. D., UZGIRIS, I., and HUNT, J. Cognitive development in infants of different age levels and from different environmental background. *Merrill Palmer Quarterly, 17*, 1971, 283–317.

CHAPTER 10

AAO-ACO (American Academy of Otolaryngology and American Council of Otolaryngology). Guide for evaluation of hearing handicap. *J. Amer. Medical Assn., 241*, 1979, 2035–2059.

SANDERS, D. A. Noise conditions in normal school classrooms. *Exceptional Child, 31*, 1965, pp. 344–353.

SUTER, A. T. Hearing level and speech discrimination in noise. In eds. Tobias, J., Jansen, A., and Ward, D. W., *Noise as a Public Health Problem*, ASHA Reports 10, Rockland, MD: American Speech-Language-Hearing Assn., April 1980.

CHAPTER 11

CORNELISSE, L., GAGNE, J.-P., and SEEWALD, R. Ear level recordings of the long term average spectrum of speech. *Ear & Hearing, 12*(1), 1991, 47–54.

COX, R. and ALEXANDER, A. Acoustic versus electronic modifications of hearing and low-frequency output. *Ear & Hearing, 4,* 1983, 190–196.

HODGSON, W. A. Procedures for fitting a programmable, digitally controlled, multiple memory hearing aid. *Seminars in Hearing, 9*(3), 1988, 231–237.

HODGSON, W. A. and LADE, K. P. Digital technology to provide increased flexibility and control. *Hearing Journal, 41*(4), 1988, 24–26.

JOHNSON, J. S., KIRBY, V. M., HODGSON, W. A., and JOHNSON, L. J. Clinical study of a programmable, multiple memory hearing instrument. *Hearing Instruments, 39*(11), 1988, 42.

KILLION, M. Problems in the application of broadband hearing aid earphones. In eds. Studebaker A, and Hochberg I. *Acoustical Factors Affecting Hearing Aid Performance.* Baltimore: Univ. Park Press, 1980.

LIBBY, E. Achieving a transparent, smooth, wideband hearing and response. *Hearing Instruments, 36*(1), 1985, 30.

SCHNIER, W. R. Practical applications and benefits of digital hearing aid technology. *Hearing Journal,* April 1988, pp. 10–13.

STACH, B. A., SPEERSCHNEIDER, J. M., and JERGER, J. F. Evaluating the efficacy of automatic signal processing hearing aids. *Hearing Journal,* March 1987, pp. 15–19.

WIDIN, G. P. The meaning of digital technology. *Hearing Instruments, 39*(6) 1987, 38–41, 54.

WOLINSKI, S. Clinical assessment of a self-adaptive noise filtering system, *Hearing Journal, 39,* 1986, 29–32.

CHAPTER 12

American Speech-Hearing and Language Association. tech. ed. Snope, T. *Assistive Listening Devices and Systems: Professional Practices,* Rockville, MD, 1985.

Americans with Disabilities Act of 1990, 302(a), 102(b) (5) (A), 1990.

Assistive Listening Devices in Review Hearing Instruments, 36(2), 18–20, 1985.

Clarke School for the Deaf. The Assistive Devices Center for Oral Education, McAlister Building, Round Hill Road, Northampton, MA 10160-2199, Tel: (413) 584-3450.

Cochlear Corporation. Implantation of the Nuclear-22 Channel cochlear implant approved in children. *Clinical Bulletin,* September 1990, pp. 1–5.

ERBER, N. and ALENCEWICZ, C. Audiologic evaluation of deaf children. *J. Speech Hearing Dis., 41,* 1976, 256–267.

Hal Hen Co., Inc., 35-53 24th Street, Long Island City, NY 11106-4416 (1-800-242-5436), NY State Tel. (1-800-336-9786).

OSBERGER, M., MYAMOTO, R., ZIMMERMAN-PHILLIPS, S., KEMINK, J., STROER, B., FIRSZT, J., and NOVAK, M. Independent evaluation of the speech perception abilities of children with the Nucleus 22-Channel cochlear implant device. *Ear & Hearing, 12*(4), 1991, Supplement, 66S–80S.

OSBERGER, M., ROBBINS, A., BERRY, S., TODD, S., HESKETH, L., and SEDEY, A. Analysis of the spontaneous speech samples of children with a cochlear implant or tactile aid. *Am. J. Otol.,* 1991, Supplement, pp. 173–181.

PALMER, C. V. Assistive devices in the audiology practice. *American Journal of Audiology, 1,* No. 2, 1992, 37–57.

PATRICK, J. AND CLARK, A., The Nucleus 22 Channel Cochlear Implant System. *Ear & Hearing, 12,*(4), 1991, 3S–9S.

STALLER, J., DOWELL, R., BEITER, A., and BRIMACOMBE, J. Perceptual abilities of children with the Nucleus-22 Channel Implant. *Ear & Hearing, 12*(4), 1991, Supplement, 34S–47S.

TOBEY, E. and HASENSTAB, S. Effects of a nuclear multichannel implant upon speech production in children. *Ear & Hearing, 12*(4), 1991, Supplement, 48S–54S.

TOBEY, E., PANCAMO, S., STALLER, S., BRIMACOMBE, J., and BEITER, A. Consonant production in children receiving a multichannel cochlear implant. *Ear & Hearing, 12,* 1991, 23–31.

WILLIAM, G. I. Hearing assistance systems technology. *Sound and Video Contractor* ©, January 1984 issue. Overland Park, KS: Intertec Publishing Corporation.

CHAPTER 13

FIEDLER, F. The concept of an ideal therapeutic relationship. *J. Consult. Psychol., 14,* 1950, 239–245.

FREEDMAN, J. L. and DOOB, A. N. *Deviancy: The Psychology of Being Different.* New York: Academic Press, 1968.

GARGIULO, R. M. *Working with Parents of Exceptional Children.* Boston, MA: Houghton Mifflin, 1985.

GOFFMAN, E. *Stigma: Notes on a Spoiled Identity.* Englewood Cliffs, NJ: Spectrum Press, 1969.

KUBLER-ROSS, E. *On Death and Dying.* New York: Macmillan, 1969.

LUTERMAN, D. *Counseling the Communicatively Disordered and Their Families.* Boston: Little, Brown, 1984.

MOSES, K. Effects of the developmental disability on parenting the handicapped child. In ed. Rieff, M., *Patterns of Emotional Growth in the Developmentally Disabled Child.* Morton Grove, IL: Julia S. Molloy Educational Center, 1977, pp. 31–52.

ROLLIN, W. J. *The Psychology of Communication Disorders in Individuals and Their Families.* Englewood Cliffs, NJ: Prentice Hall, 1987.

SELIGMAN, M. *Strategies for Helping Parents of Exceptional Children.* New York: Free Press, 1979.

TYLER, L. A. *The Work of the Counselor* (3rd ed.). Englewood Cliffs, NJ: Prentice Hall, 1969.

WEBSTER, E. Counseling with parents of handicapped children. *Communicative Disorders, An Audio Journal for Continuing Education,* 1976, No. 1.

WEBSTER, E. J. *Counseling with Parents of Handicapped Children.* New York: Grune and Stratton, 1977.

Webster's New World Dictionary of the American Language (Second College Edition), ed. Guaralnik, D. B. New York; Simon & Schuster, 1984.

CHAPTER 14

ALLEN, T. E. Patterns of academic achievement among hearing impaired students, 1974-1983. In eds. Shildroth, A. N. and Karchmer, A. M., *Deaf Children in America.* San Diego, CA: College Hill Press, 1986, pp. 161–206.

ANTHONY, D. *Seeing Essential English Manual.* Annaheim, CA: Annaheim High School District, 1971.

BLOOM, L. Talking, understanding and thinking. In eds. Schiefelbusch, R. and Lloyd, L. *Language Perspectives—Acquisition, Retardation and Intervention.* Baltimore: Univer. Park Press, 1974, pp. 285–311.

BOOTHROYD, A. *Hearing Impairments in Young Children.* Englewood Cliffs, NJ: Prentice Hall, 1982.

BORNSTEIN, H. A description of some current sign systems designed to represent English. *Am. Ann. Deaf, 188,* 1973, 454–463.

BORNSTEIN, H. Systems of sign. In eds. Bradford, L. and Hardy, W., *Hearing and Hearing Impairment.* New York: Academic Press, 1979, pp. 331–361.

BORNSTEIN, H. Signed English: A manual approach to English language development. *Journal Speech Hearing Disorders, 39,* 1974, 330–343.

BROEN, P. A. *The Verbal Environment of the Language Learning Child.* ASHA Monograph, No. 17, 1972.

BROMWICH, R. *Working with Parents and Infants: An Interactional Approach.* Baltimore: Univer. Park Press, 1981.

CORNETT, R. *Cued Speech Parent Training and Follow-up Program.* Washington, DC: Bureau of Education of the Handicapped, *96,* 1972.

CRABTREE, M. *The Houston Test for Language Development.* Houston, TX: The Houston Test Co., 1963.

DECASPER, A. J. and FIFER, W. P. Of human bonding: newborns prefer their mother's voices. *Science 208,* 1980, 1174–1176.

DOWNS, M. P. and AKIN, J. Unpublished research on a comparison between deaf and normal hearing infant vocalizations. Cited in Northern, J. L. and Downs, M. P., *Hearing in Children.* Baltimore: Williams and Wilkins, 1984.

DOWNS, M. The deafness management quotient. *Hearing Speech News,* January-February 1974.

ENGEN, E. and ENGEN, T. *The Rhode Island Test of Language Structure.* Baltimore: Univ. Park Press, 1983.

ERBER, N. and ALENCEWICZ, C. Audiologic evaluation of deaf children. *J. Speech Hearing Dis., 41,* 1976, 256–267.

FRAYER, C. and ROBERTS, N. Mothers' speech to children of four different ages. *J. Psycholinguistic Res., 4,* 1975, 9–16.

GEERS, A. E. and MOOG, J. S. Predicting spoken language acquisition of hearing impaired children. *J. Speech Hearing Dis., 42*(1), 1987, 84–94.

GUSTASON, A., PFETZING, D., and ZOWOLKOW, E. *Signing Exact English.* Silver Springs, MD: Modern Signs Press, 1975.

HEDRICK, D., PRATHER, E., and TOBIN, A. *Sequenced Inventory of Communication Development.* Seattle: Univ. of Washington Press, 1975.

HORTON, K. Infant intervention and language learning. In eds. Schiefelbusch, R. and Lloyd, L., *Acquisition, Retardation and Intervention.* Baltimore: Univ. Park Press, 1974, pp. 469–491.

JOHANSSON, B., WEDENBERG, E., and WESTIN, B. Measurement of tone response by the human fetus. *Acta Otolaryngol, 57,* 1964, 188–192.

John Tracy Correspondence Course for Parents of Preschool Deaf Children. John Tracy Clinic, 806 West Adams Boulevard, Los Angeles CA 90007, 1968.

JOHNSON, R. E., LIDDELL, S. K., and ERTING, C. J. *Unlocking the Curriculum: Principles for Achieving Access in Deaf Education.* Gallaudet Research Institute Working Paper 89-3. Washington, DC: Gallaudet University, 1989.

JORDAN, I. K., GUSTASON, G., and ROSEN, R. Current communication trends in programs for the deaf. *Am. Ann. Deaf, 121,* 1976, 527–532.

LING, D. and LING, A. H. *Aural Habilitation.* Washington, DC: Alexander Graham Bell Assoc. for the Deaf, 1978.

LUTERMAN, D. and CHASIN, J. The deafness management quotient as an indicator of oral success. *Volta Rev., 83,* 1981, 405.

LUTERMAN, D. M. *Counseling the Communicatively Disordered and Their Families.* Austin, TX: Pro-Ed, 1984.

MALISZEWSKI, S. J. The impact of hearing impairment on the family. In ed. Bess, F., *Hearing Impairment in Children.* Parkton, MD: York Press, 1988.

MASCARINEK, A. S., CAIRNES, G. F., BUTTERFIELD, E. C., and WEAMER, R. K. Longitudinal observations of individual infant's vocalizations. *J. Speech Hearing Dis., 40,* 1981, 267–273.

MATKIN, N. Assessment of hearing sensitivity during the preschool years. In ed. Bess, F., *Childhood Deafness Causation and Measurement.* New York: Grune and Stratton, 1977.

McCARTHY, D. *McCarthy Scales of Children's Abilities.* New York: Psychological Corp., 1972.

McCONNEL, F. and WARD, P. *Deafness in Childhood.* Nashville, TN: Vanderbilt Univ. Press, 1967.

MECHAM, M., JEX, J., and JONES, J. *Utah Test of Language Development.* Salt Lake City, UT: Communication Research Associates, 1978.

MILLER, J. and YODER, D. An ontogenetic teaching strategy for retarded children. In eds. Shiefelbusch, R. and Lloyd, L., *Language Perspectives-Acquisition Retardation and Intervention,* Baltimore: Univ. Park Press, 1974, pp. 503–528.

MOOG, J. S. and GEERS, A. *Scales of Early Communication Skills for Hearing Impaired Children.* St. Louis: Central Institute for the Deaf Press, 1983.

MOOG, J. S., KOZAK, V. J., AND GEERS, A. *Grammatical Analysis of Elicited Language.* St. Louis: Central Institute for the Deaf Press, 1983.

NORTHERN, J. L. and DOWNS, M. P. *Hearing in Children* (3rd ed.) Baltimore: Williams and Wilkins, 1984.

PAUL, P. V. *American Sign Language and English: A Bilingual Minority-Language Immersion Program.* CAID-News "N" Notes, Washington, DC: Conference of American Instructors of the Deaf, 1988.

PHILLIPS, J. R. Syntax and vocabulary of mother's speech to young children: Age and sex comparisons. *Child Development, 44,* 1973, 182–185.

QUIGLEY, S. P. and PAUL, P. V. ASL and ESL? *Topics in Early Childhood Education, 3,* 1984, 17–26.

ROSE, D. S. The psychological world of the hearing-impaired child and the family. In ed. Martin, F., *Hearing Disorders in Children.* Austin, TX: PRO-ED, 1987, pp. 81–111.

SLOBIN, D. Imitation and grammatical development in children. In eds. Endler, N. S., Bautter, L. R., and Osser, H., *Contemporary Issues in Developmental Psychology.* New York: Holt Rinehart and Winston. 1968, pp 437–443.

SCHUMAKER, J. *Mother's Expansions: Their Characteristics and Effects on Child Language.* Unpublished doctoral dissertation, University of Lawrence, 1976.

SCHUMAKER, J. and SHERMAN, J. Parent as intervention: From birth onward. In ed Schiefelbusch R. *Language Intervention Strategies.* Baltimore: Univ. Park Press, 1978, pp. 237–315.

SNOW, C. E. Mothers' speech to children learning language. *Child Development, 43,* 1972, 549–565.

STERN, D. Implications of infancy research for clinical theory and practice. *Dialogue, 6,* 1983, 9–17.

STEVENS, R. P. Education in schools for deaf children. In eds. Baker, C. and Battison, R., *Sign Language and the Deaf Community.* Silver Spring, MD: National Association of the Deaf, 1980, pp. 177–191.

STOKOE, W. C., Jr. *Sign Language Structure: An Outline of the Visual Communication Systems of the American Deaf.* (Studies in Linguistics: Occasional Papers 8). Buffalo, NY: University of Buffalo. [Rev. ed., Silver Spring, MD: Linstock Press, 1978.]

STRONG, M. A bilingual approach to the education of young deaf children: ASL and English. In ed. Strong, M., *Language Learning and Deafness.* New York: Cambridge Univ. Press, 1988, pp. 113–129.

THARP, G. T. and GALLIMORE, R. *Rousing Minds to Life: Teaching Learning in Schooling and Social Context.* New York: Cambridge Univ. Press, 1989a.

THARP, G. T. and GALLIMORE, R. Rousing Schools to life. *American Educator, 13*(2), Summer 1989b, 20–25, 46–52.

TUCKER, B. and GOLDSTEIN, B. *Legal Rights of Persons with Disabilities: An Analysis of Federal Law.* Alexandria, VA: LRP Publications, 1990.

TUCKER, B. P. and GOLDSTEIN, B. A. *Legal Rights of Persons with Disabilities.* Hirsham, PA: LRP Publications, An Axon Group Company, 1991.

TURTON, L. Discussion summary—Early language intervention. In eds. Schiefelbusch, R. and Lloyd, L., *Language Perspectives—Acquisition, Retardation and Intervention.* Baltimore: Univ. Park Press, 1974, pp. 493–501.

VYGOTSKI, L. S. *Thought and Language.* Cambridge, MA: MIT Press, 1962.

WEBSTER, E. *Counseling with Parents of Handicapped Children.* New York: Grune and Stratton, 1977.

WILBUR, R. *American Sign Language and Sign Systems.* Austin, TX: PRO-ED, 1979.

WOODWARD, J. Some sociolinguistic problems in the implementation of bilingual education for deaf students. In eds. Caccamise, F. and Hicks, W, *American Sign Language in a Bilingual Bicultural Context.* Proceedings of the Second National Symposium on Sign Research and Teaching. Silver Spring, MD: National Association of the Deaf, 1978, pp. 183–203.

ZIMMERMAN, I., STEINER, V., and EVATT, R. *Preschool Language Manual.* Columbus, OH: C. E. Merrill, 1979.

CHAPTER 15

ALTSCHULER, K. Z. The social and psychological development of the deaf child. *Social and Psych. Development,* August, 1974, 365–376.

BOOTHROYD, A. *Hearing Impairments in Young Children.* Englewood Cliffs, NJ: Prentice Hall, 1982.

BROMWICH, R. *Working with Parents and Infants: An Interactional Approach.* Baltimore: Univ. Park Press, 1981.

CHURCH, J. *Language and the Discovery of Reality.* New York: Random House, 1961.

CORSARO, W. A. The development of social cognition in preschool children: Implications for language learning: *Topics in Language Disorders, 4*(4), 1984, 77–95.

DARBYSHIRE, J. Play patterns in young children with impaired hearing. *Volta Rev., 79,* 1977, 19–26.

FRIEL-PATTI, S. and LOUGEA-MOTTINGER, J. Preschool language intervention: Some key concerns. *Topics in Language Disorders, 5*(2), 1985, 46–53.

GOFFMAN, E. *The Presentation of Self in Everyday Life.* Garden City, NY: Doubleday, 1959.

GREGORY, H. *The Clinician's Attitudes in Counseling Stutterers.* Memphis: Speech Foundations of America, No. 18, 1983.

LING, D. *Speech and the Hearing Impaired Child.* Washington, DC: Alexander Graham Bell Assoc. for the Deaf, 1976.

LUTERMAN, D. M. Counseling parents of hearing impaired children. Chap. 9 in ed. Martin, F. M., *Hearing Disorders in Children.* Austin, TX: PRO-ED, 1987, pp. 303–319.

MASILSZEWSKI, S. J. The impact of hearing impairment on the family. In ed. Bess, F. H., *Hearing Impairment in Children.* Parkton, MD: York Press, 1988.

MATKIN, N. Hearing aids for children. In eds. Hodgson, W. and Skinner, P., *Hearing Aid Assessment and Use in Audiologic Habilitation.* Baltimore: Univ. Park Press, 1979.

McCUNE-NICHOLICH, L. and CARROL, S. Development of symbolic play: Implications for the language specialist. *Topics in Language Disorders, 1*(1), 1981, 1–4.

MEERS, H. *Helping Our Children Talk.* London and New York: Longman, 1976.

MENYUK, P. Cognition and language. *Volta Rev. 78,* 1976, 250–257.

MOELLER, P. Management of preschool hearing impaired children: A cognitive linguistic approach. In ed. Bess, F., *Hearing Impairment in Children.* Parkton, MD: York Press, 1988.

NORTHCOTT, W. H. Normalization of the preschool child with hearing impairment. *Otolaryngology Clinic of North America, 8,* 1975, pp. 195–196.

POLLACK, D. *Educational Audiology for the Limited Hearing Infant.* Springfield, IL: Charles C Thomas, 1970.

ROSS, A. O. *The Exceptional Child in the Family.* New York: Grune and Stratton, 1964.

SCHLESINGER, H. and MEADOW, K. *Deafness and Mental Health: A Developmental Approach.* San Francisco: Langley Porter Neuropsyduatric Institute, 1971.

THARP, A. T. and GALLIMORE, R. Rousing schools to life. *American Educator, 13*(2), Summer 1989, 20–25, 46–52.

WEBSTER, E. J. *Counseling with Parents of Handicapped Children: Guidelines for Improving Communication.* New York: Grune and Stratton, 1977.

WEIKART, D. P., ROGERS, L., ADCOCK, C., and McCLELLEN, D. *The Cognitively Oriented Curriculum.* Urbana: The Univ. of Illinois Press, 1971.

WHITEHURST, M. *Teaching Communication Skills to the Preschool Child, A Manual.* Washington, DC: Alexander Graham Bell Assoc. for the Deaf, 1971.

WOOD, B. *Children and Communication: Verbal and Non Verbal Language Development.* Englewood Cliffs, NJ: Prentice Hall, 1976.

VERNON, M. Sociological and psychological factors associated with hearing loss. *J. Speech Hearing Dis., 12,* 1969, 541–563.

CHAPTER 16

LEVINE, E. Psychological tests and practices with the deaf: a survey of the state of the art. *Volta Review, 76,* 1974, 298–319.

NORTHCOTT, W. *The Hearing Impaired Child in a Regular Classroom.* Washington, DC: Alexander Graham Bell Assn. for the Deaf, 1973.

Your Child's Right to an Education: A Guide for Parents of Handicapped Children in New York State. The State Education Department, Office of Education of Children with Handicapping Conditions, New York: The University of the State of New York, 1978.

SULLIVAN. P. AND VERNON, M. Psychological assessment of hearing impaired children. In ed. Lloyd, L. *Communication Assessment and Intervention Strategies.* Baltimore: University Park Press, 1976.

VERNON, M. The psychological examination. In eds. Berg, F. and Fletcher, S. *The Hard of Hearing Child.* New York: Grune and Stratton, 1970.

VERNON, M. Psychological evaluation of hearing impaired children. In ed. Lloyd, L. *Communication Assessment and Intervention Strategies.* Baltimore: University Park Press, 1976.

VERNON, M. AND BROWN, D. A guide to psychological tests and testing procedures in the evaluation of deaf and hard of hearing children. *J. Speech Hearing Dis., 29,* 1964, 414–423.

CHAPTER 17

ALTSCHULER, K. Psychiatric considerations of the adult deaf. *Am. Ann. Deaf, 107,* 1962, 560–561.

BANGS, T. E. *Vocabulary Comprehension Scale.* Boston, MA: Teaching Resources, 1975.

BATES, E. *Language and Context: The Acquisition of Pragmatics.* New York: Academic Press, 1976.

BERRY, M. and ERICKSON, J. Speaking rate: Effects on children's comprehension of normal speech. *J. Speech Hearing Res., 16,* 1973, 367–374.

BESS, F. H. The minimally hearing impaired child. *Ear and Hearing, 6,* 1985, 43–47.

BLAGDEN, C. and McCONNELL, N. *Interpersonal Language Skills Assessment.* Moline, IL: Lingui Systems, 1983.

BLOOM, L. and LAHEY, M. *Language Development and Language Disorders.* New York: John Wiley, 1978.

BLOOM, L., LIGHTBOWN, P., and HOOD, L. Structure and variation in child language. *Monogr. Soc. Res. Child Develop., 38*(2), 1975.

BOEHM, A. E. *Boehm Test of Basic Concepts.* New York: The Psychological Corporation, 1971.

BOHANNAN, J. The relationship between syntax and discrimination and sentence imitation in children. *Child Devel., 46,* 1975, 441–451.

BRANNON, J. Linguistic word classes in the spoken language of normal, hard-of-hearing and deaf children. *J. Speech Hearing Res., 11,* 1968, 279–287.

BRANNON, J. B. and MURRAY, T. The spoken syntax of normal, hard-of-hearing and deaf children. *J. Speech Hearing Res., 9,* 1966, 604–610.

BROWN, R. *A First Language: The Early Stages.* Cambridge, MA: Harvard Univ. Press, 1973.

BUNCH, G. *Test of Expressive Language Ability.* Toronto: G. B. Services, 1978a.

BUNCH, G. *Test of Receptive Language Ability.* Toronto: G. B. Services, 1978b.

CALVERT, D. R. and SILVERMAN, S. R. *Speech and Deafness.* Washington, DC: Alexander Graham Bell Assoc. for the Deaf, 1975.

CARROW-WOOLFOLK, E. *Test for Auditory Comprehension of Language* (rev. ed.). Allen, TX: DLM Teaching Resources, 1985.

CRABTREE, M. *The Houston Test for Language Development,* Part I and Part II. Houston, TX: The Houston Test Co., 1958, 1963.

DAVIS, F. B. Psychometric research on comprehension in reading. *Reading Research Quarterly, 7*(4), 1972, 628–678.

DONNELLY, J. and BRACKETT, D. *Conversational Skills of Hearing-Impaired Adolescents: A Simulated TV Interview.* Paper presented at the Convention of the American Speech-Language-Hearing Assoc., Toronto, Canada, 1982.

DUCHAN, J. Language assessment of hearing-impaired children: Influences from pragmatics. *J. Acad. Rehab. Aud.,* Monograph Supplement XXI, 1988, 19–40.

DUNN, L. *Peabody Picture Vocabulary Test.* Circle Pines, MN: American Guidance Service, 1965, revised 1981.

ENGEN, E. and ENGEN, T. *Rhode Island Test of Language Structures.* Baltimore: Univ. Park Press, 1983.

ENGLEMAN, S., ROSS, D., and BINGHAM, V. *Basic Language Concepts Test.* Tigard, OR: C.C. Publications, 1982.

ERBER, N. *Auditory Training.* Washington, DC: Alexander Graham Bell Assoc. for the Deaf, 1982.

ERBER, N. and GREER, C. Communication strategies used by teachers at an oral school for the deaf. *Volta Rev., 75,* 1973, 480–485.

FISHER, B. The social and emotional adjustment of children with impaired hearing attending ordinary classes. *Brit. J. Educ. Psychol., 36,* 1966, 319–321.

FOSTER, R., GIDDAN, J., and STARK, J. *Assessment of Children's Language Comprehension: Manual.* Palo Alto, CA: Consulting Psychologists Press, 1973.

FREEDMAN, J. L. and DOOB, A. N. *Deviancy: The Psychology of Being Different.* New York: Academic Press, 1968.

GARDNER, M. *Expressive One Word Picture Vocabulary Test.* Novato, CA: Academic Therapy Publications, 1981.

GEFFNER, D. S. and FREEMAN, L. R. Assessment of language comprehension of six year old deaf children. *J. Comm. Dis., 13,* 1980, 455–470.

GERMAN, D. J. *Test of Word Finding.* Allen, TX: DLM Teaching Resources, 1966.

GIVENS, G. and GREENFIELD, D. Revision behaviors of normal and hearing-impaired children. *Ear & Hearing, 3,* 1982, 274–279.

GOETZINGER, C., HARRISON, C., and BAER, C. Small perceptive hearing loss: Its effect on school-age children. *Volta Rev., 66,* 1964, 124–131.

GOLDMAN, R. and FRISTOE, M. *Test of Articulation.* Circle Pines, MN: American Guidance Service, 1969.

HASKINS, H. A. *A Phonetically Balanced Test of Speech Discrimination for Children.* Masters thesis, Northwestern University, 1949.

HOOD, R. B. and DIXON, R. F. Physical characteristics of speech rhythm of deaf and normal hearing speakers. *J. Comm. Dis., 2,* 1969, 20–28.

JERGER, S., LEWIS, S., HAWKINS, J., and JERGER, J. Paediatric speech intelligibility Test I. Generation of test materials. *International J. Paediatric Otorhinolaryngology, 2,* 1980, 217–230.

KATZ, D. and ELLIOT, L. Development of a new childrens' speech discrimination test. Paper presented at the Convention of the American Speech Language-Hearing Assn., Chicago, IL, 1978.

KENNY, K. and PRATHER, E. *The Coarticulation Assessment in Meaningful Language.* Tucson, AZ: Communication Skills Builders, 1984.

KENNY, K. and PRATHER, E. Coarticulation testing of kindergarten children. *Language Speech and Hearing Services in Schools, 17,* 1986, 285–291.

KRETSCHMER, R. and KRETSCHMER, L. *Language Development and Intervention with the Hearing Impaired.* Baltimore: University Park Press, 1978.

LARR, A. and STOCKWELL, R. A. A test of speech intelligibility. *Volta Rev. 61,* 1959, 403–407.

LEE, L. Developmental sentence types: A method for comparing normal and deviant syntactic development. *J. Speech Hearing Dis., 31,* 1966, 311–330.

LEE, L. L. *Northwestern Syntax Screening Test.* Evanston, IL: Northwestern Univ. Press, 1969, 1971.

LEE, L. *Developmental Sentence Analysis.* Evanston, IL: Northwest Univ. Press, 1974.

LEE, L. L. Reply to Arndt and Byrne Letters to the Editor. *J. Speech Hearing Dis., 42,* 1977, 323–327.

LEREA, L. Assessing language development. *J. Speech Hearing Res., 1,* 1958, 75–85.

LEVINE, E. *Youth in a Soundless World: A Search for Personality.* New York: New York Univ. Press, 1956.

LING, D. *Speech and the Hearing Impaired Child: Theory and Practice.* Washington, DC: Alexander Graham Bell Assoc. for the Deaf, 1976.

LING, D. and LING, A. H. *Aural Habilitation.* Washington, DC: Alexander Graham Bell Assoc. for the Deaf, 1978.

LUND, N. and DUCHAN, J. *Assessing Children's Language in Naturalistic Contexts* (1st ed.). Englewood Cliffs, NJ: Prentice Hall, 1983.

LUND, N. and DUCHAN, J. *Assessing Children's Language in Naturalistic Contexts* (2nd ed.). Englewood Cliffs, NJ: Prentice Hall, 1988.

MAGNER, M. E. *A Speech Intelligibility Test for Deaf Children.* Unpublished Masters thesis, Northhampton, MA: Clark School for the Deaf, 1972.

MARKIDES, A. The speech of deaf and partially hearing children with special reference to factors affecting intelligibility *British Journal of Disorders of Communication, 5,* 1970a, 126–140.

MARKIDES, A. Ratings related to the speech of deaf and partially deaf children. *Teacher of the Deaf, 68,* 1970b, 323–330.

MARKIDES, A. Whole-word scoring versus phoneme scoring in speech audiometry. *British Journal of Audiology, 12,* 1978, 40–50.

MCCARTHY, D. The language development of the preschool child. *Institute of Child Welfare Monograph Series, No. 4,* Minneapolis: Univ. of Minnesota Press, 1930.

MCCARTHY, D. *McCarthy Scales of Children's Abilities.* New York: Psychological Corporation, 1972.

MCDONALD, E. T. *A Deep Test of Articulation.* Pittsburgh: Stanwix House, 1964.

MEACHAM, M., JEX, J., and JONES, J. D. *The Utah Test of Language Development.* Salt Lake City, UT: Communication Research Associates, 1963.

MEADOW, K. and SCHLESINGER, H. The prevalence of behavioral problems in a population of deaf school children. *Am. Ann. Deaf, 116,* 1971, 346–348.

MILLER, J. *Assessing Language Production in Children.* Baltimore: Univer. Park Press, 1981.

MILLER, J. and CHAPMAN, R. Length variables in sentence imitation. *Language and Speech, 16,* 1975, 35–41.

MOELLER, M. P. Developmental approaches to communication assessment and enhancement. In ed. Cherow, E., *Hearing Impaired Children and Youth with Developmental Disabilities.* Washington, DC: Gallaudet College Press, 1985, pp. 171–199.

MONSEN, R. B. A usable test for the speech intelligibility of deaf talkers. *Am. Ann. Deaf, 71,* 1982, 845–852.

MOOG, J. and GEERS, A. *Grammatical Analysis of Elicited Language.* St. Louis, MO: Central Institute for the Deaf, 1979.

MOOG, J. and KOZAK, V. *Teacher Assessment of Grammatical Structures.* St. Louis, MO: Central Institute for the Deaf, 1983.

MUMA, J. *Language Handbook; Concepts Assessment Intervention.* Englewood Cliffs, NJ: Prentice Hall, 1978.

NEWCOMER, P. and HAMILL, D. *Test of Language Development.* Austin, TX: Empire Press, 1977.

OLSEN, W. O. and MATKIN, N. D. Speech audiometry. In ed. Rintelmann, W. F. *Hearing Assessment.* Baltimore: University Park Press, 1979.

PASCOE, D. An approach to hearing aid selection. *Hearing Instruments, 29,* 1978, 12–16.

PENN, J. P. Voice and speech patterns of the hard of hearing. *Acta Orolaryngologica,* Supplement No. 124, 1955.

PRUTTING, C. A. Pragmatics and social competence. *J. Speech Hearing Dis. 47,* 1982, 123–134.

QUIGLEY, S., STEINCAMP, M., POWER, D., and JONES, B. *Test of Syntactic Ability.* Beaverton, OR: Dormac, 1978.

REICH, C., HAMBLETON, D., and HOULDIN, B. The integration of hearing impaired children in regular classrooms. *Am. Ann. Deaf, 122,* 1977, 534–543.

RICHARDS, D. L. *Telecommunications by Speech: The Transmission Performance of Telephone Networks.* New York: John Wiley, 1973.

RIPICH, D. and SPINELLI, F. *School Discourse Problems.* San Diego, CA: College Hill Press, 1985.

ROSS, M. *Hard of Hearing Children in Regular Schools.* Englewood Cliffs, NJ: Prentice Hall, 1982.

ROSS, M. and LERMAN, J. A picture identification test for hearing impaired children. *J. Speech Hearing Res., 13,* 1970, 44–53.

SANDERS, D. A. *Auditory Perception of Speech.* Englewood Cliffs, NJ: Prentice Hall, 1977.

SEEWALD, R. C. *The Interrelationships Among Hearing Loss, Utilization of Auditory and Visual Cues in Speech Reception and Speed Production Intelligibility in Children.* Unpublished Ph. D. dissertation, University of Connecticut, Storrs, 1981.

SHRINER, T. A review of mean length of response as a measure of expressive language development in children. *J. Speech Hearing Dis., 34,* 1969, 61–68.

SIMMONS, A. A comparison of the type-token ratio of spoken and written language of deaf and hearing children. *Volta Rev., 64,* 1962, 117–121.

SIMON, C. *Evaluating Communicative Competence: A Functional-Pragmatic Procedure.* Tucson, AZ: Communication Skill Builders, 1984a.

SIMON, C. Functional-pragmatic evaluation of communication skills in school-aged children. *Language Speech and Hearing Services in the Schools, 15,* 1984b, 83–97.

SMITH, F. *Comprehension and Learning.* New York: Holt, Rinehart and Winston, 1975.

STARK, R. E. and LEVITT, H. Prosodic feature reception and production in deaf children. *J. Acoust. Soc. Amer., 55, Supplement,* 1974, p 63.

STEWART, L. Problems of severely handicapped deaf: Implications for educational programs. *Am. Ann. Deaf, 116,* 1971, 362–368.

STONE, P. *Blueprint for Developing Conversational Competence: A Planning/Instruction Model with Detailed Scenarios.* Washington, DC: Alexander Graham Bell Assoc. for the Deaf, 1988.

SUBTELNY, J. D., ORLANDO, N. A., and WHITEHEAD, R. L. *Speech and Voice Characteristics of the Deaf.* Washington, DC: Alexander Graham Bell Assoc. for the Deaf, 1981.

TEMPLIN, M. C. *Certain Language Skills in Children.* Institute of Child Welfare Monograph Series, No. 26. Minneapolis: University of Minnesota Press, 1957.

THIES, T. and TAMMEL, J. Development and implementation of the auditory skills instructional planning system. In eds. Hochberg, J., Levitt, H., and Osberger, M., *Speech of the Hearing Impaired.* Baltimore: Univ. Park Press, 1983, pp. 349–367.

TILLMAN, T. W. and CARHART, R. An expanded test for speech discrimination utilizing CNC monosyllabic words. Northwestern University Auditory Test No. 5, Technical Report, SAM-TR-66-55, USAF School of Aerospace Medicine, Brooks Airforce Base, Texas, 1966.

TRUAX, R. R. Reading and language. In eds. Kretschmer, R. R. and Kretschmer, L. W., *Language Development and Intervention with the Hearing Impaired.* Baltimore: Univer. Park Press, 1978, pp. 279–310.

TYACK, D. and GOTTSLEBEN, R. *Language Sampling, Analysis, and Training: A Handbook for Teachers and Clinicians.* Palo Alto, CA: Consulting Psychological Press, 1974.

VAN RIPER, C. and EMERICK, L. *Speech Correction: An Introduction to Speech Pathology and Audiology.* Englewood Cliffs, NJ: Prentice Hall, 1990.

WEBER, S. and REDDELL, R. C. A sentence test for measuring speech discrimination in children. *Aud. Hearing Educ.,* August-September, 1976, 25–30.

WILBUR, R. An explanation of deaf children's difficulty with certain syntactic structures in English. *Volta Rev., 79,* 1977, 85–92.

YUKER, H. and BLACK, J. *Challenging Barriers to Change: Attitudes Toward the Disabled.* Albertson, NY: Human Resources Center, 1979.

CHAPTER 18

ALPINER, J. G. Evaluation of adult communication function. In eds. Alpiner, J. G. and McCarthy, P. A., *Rehabilitative Audiology: Children and Adults.* Baltimore: Williams and Wilkins, 1987, Appendix 3C.

BITTER, G. and JOHNSON, J. *Systems O.N.E.* Salt Lake City: University of Utah Educational Media Center, 1974.

BOEHM, A. E. *Boehm Test of Basic Concepts.* New York: The Psychological Corporation, 1971.

BOOTHROYD, A. Discussion and summary: Auditory training. In eds. Ross, M. and Giolas, T. G., *Auditory Management of Hearing Impaired Children.* Baltimore: Univ. Park Press, 1978, pp. 295–339.

COHEN, O. P. The deaf adolescent: "Who am I?" In eds. Nehers, A. and Austin, G., *Deafness and Adolescence: A Monograph. Volta Rev., 80,* 1978, 265–274.

FITCH, J. Orientation to hearing loss for educational personnel. *Language, Speech and Hearing Services in the Schools, 13*(4), October 1982, 252–259.

FLEXER, C., WRAY, D., and IRELAND, J. Preferential seating is not enough: Issues in classroom management of hearing impaired students. *Language, Speech and Hearing Services in Schools, 20*(1), January 1990, 11–20.

FRY, D. The role and primacy of the auditory channel in speech development. In eds. Ross, M. and Giolas, T. *Auditory Management of Hearing Impaired Children.* Baltimore: Univ. Park Press, 1978, pp. 15–43.

GILDSTONE, P. Do's and don'ts for the classroom teacher. In ed. Northcott, W., *The Hearing Impaired Child in a Regular Classroom.* Washington, DC: Alexander Graham Bell Assoc. for the Deaf, 1973.

GOFFMAN, G. *Stigma: Notes on the Management of a Spoiled Identify.* Englewood Cliffs, NJ: Prentice Hall, 1963.

GREENBERG, B. L. and WITHERS, S. *Better English Usage: A Guide for the Deaf.* Indianapolis: The Bobbs-Merrill Co., 1965.

HINE, W. D. The attainments of children with partial hearing. *Volta Rev., 66,* 1970, 124–131.

KIDDER, T. *Among Schoolchildren.* Boston: Houghton Mifflin, 1989.

KODMAN, F. Educational status of hard-of-hearing children in the classroom. *J. Speech Hearing Dis., 28,* 1963, 297–299.

LAUGHTON, J. and HASENSTAB, S. *The Language Learning Process.* Rockville, MD: Aspen Publishers, 1986.

LIBBY, S. *Attitudes Toward Communication of "Mainstreamed" Hearing-Impaired Adolescents.* Unpublished master's thesis, Boston University, Department of Special Education, 1978.

LING, D. *Speech and the Hearing Impaired Child.* Washington, DC: Alexander Graham Bell Assoc. for the Deaf, 1976.

LING, D. Auditory coding and recoding: An analysis of auditory training procedures for hearing impaired children. In ed. Ross, M., *Auditory Management of Hearing Impaired Children: Principles and Prerequisites for Intervention.* Baltimore: Univ. Park Press, 1978, pp. 181–218.

LUND, N. and DUCHAN, J. *Assessing Children's Language in Naturalistic Contexts* (2nd ed.). Englewood Cliffs, NJ: Prentice Hall, 1988.

MARTIN, F., BERNSTEIN, M. E., DALY, J., and CODY, J. Classroom teachers' knowledge of hearing disorders and attitudes about mainstreaming hard-of-hearing children. *Language, Speech and Hearing Services in the Schools, 19,* 1988, 83–95.

MCCARR, D. *Vocabulary Building Exercises for the Young Adult.* Beverton, OR: Dormac, 1978.

MENYUK, P. That's the "same" "another" "awful" way of it. *J. of Special Education, 158,* 1976, 25–28.

NOBER, L. *Hearing Impaired Formal Inservice Program.* Northhampton, MA: North East Regional Media Center for the Deaf, 1975.

QUIGLEY, S. P. and THOMURE, R. E. Some Effects of Hearing-Impairment on School Performance. Urbana: Univ. of Illinois, Institute of Research on Exceptional Children, 1968.

RINGALEBEN, R. and PRICE, J. Regular classroom teachers' perception of mainstreaming effects. *Exceptional Children, 47,* 1981, 302–303.

ROSS, M. *Hard of Hearing Children in Regular Schools.* Englewood Cliffs, NJ: Prentice Hall, 1982.

ROSS, M. *Aural Habilitation.* Austin, TX: PRO-ED Publishers, PRO-ED studies in Communication Disorders, 1986.

SEARLE, J. Indirect speech acts. In eds. Cole, M. and Morgan, J., *Syntax and Semantics* (Vol. 3). New York: Academic Press, 1975, pp. 55–82.

STONE, P. *Blueprint for Developing Conversational Competence: A Planning/Instruction Model with Detailed Scenarios.* Washington, DC: Alexander Graham Bell Assoc. for the Deaf, 1988.

TRUAX, R. R. Reading and language. In eds. Kretschmer, R. R. and Kretschmer, L. W., *Language Development and Intervention with the Hearing Impaired.* Baltimore: Univ. Park Press, 1978, pp. 279–310.

WALSVIK, O. *Suggestions and a General Plan for Therapy for the Hard of Hearing Child.* Madison, WI: Bureau of Handicapped Children, 1966.

CHAPTER 19

ALPINER, J. *Handbook of Adult Rehabilitative Audiology.* Baltimore: Williams and Wilkins, 1978.

ALPINER, J. Evaluation of adult communication function. In eds. Alpiner, J. and McCarthy, P., *Rehabilitative Audiology: Children and Adults.* Baltimore: Williams and Wilkins, 1987, pp. 44–114.

ALPINER, J. G., CHEVRETTE, W., GLASCOE, G., METZ, M., and OLSEN, B. The Denver Scale of Communication Function. Unpublished study, Univ. of Denver (1974) cited in eds. Alpiner, J. and McCarthy, P., *Rehabilitative Audiology: Children and Adults.* Baltimore: Williams and Wilkins, 1987, p. 47.

BILGER, R., NUETZEL, J., RABINOWITZ, W., and RZECZKOWSKI, W. Standardization of a test of speech perception in noise. *J. Speech Hearing Res., 27,* 1984, 32–48.

BILGER, R., RZECZKOWSKI, C., NUETZEL, J., and RABINOWITZ, W. Evaluation of a test of speech perception in noise (SPIN). Paper presented at Annual Convention, American Speech Language Hearing Assn., Atlanta, 1979.

BINNIE, C. and ALPINER, J. A Comparative Investigation of Analytic versus Synthetic Methodologies in Lipreading. Paper presented at the annual convention of the American Speech and Hearing Association, Chicago, 1969.

BRAINERD, S. and FRANKEL, B. The relationship between audiometric and self-report measures of hearing handicap. *Ear & Hearing, 6,* 1985, 89–92.

DAVIS, H. The articulation area and the social adequacy index for hearing. *Laryngoscope, 58,* 1948, 761–778.

DAVIS, H. and SILVERMAN, S. R. *Hearing and Deafness.* New York: Holt, Rinehart and Winston, 1970.

GIOLAS, T. G. *The Measurement of Hearing Handicap: A Point of View.* Maico Audiological Library Series, *8,* Minneapolis, MN: Maico Hearing Instruments, 1970.

GIOLAS, T. G., OWENS, E., LAMB, S. H., and SCHUBERT, E. D. Hearing performance inventory. *J. Speech Hearing Dis., 44,* 1979, 169–195.

HAIVES, N. and NISANDER, P. Comparison of revised Hearing Performance Inventory with audiometric measures. *Ear & Hearing, 6,* 1985, 93–104.

HIGH, W. S., FAIRBANKS, A. and GLORIG, A. Scale for self-assessment of hearing handicap. *J. Speech Hearing Dis., 29,* 1964, 215–230.

JERGER, S. and JERGER, J. Quantifying auditory handicap: A new approach. *Audiology, 18,* 1979, 225.

KALIKOW, D. N., STEVENS, K. N., and ELLIOTT, L. L. Development of a test of speech intelligibility in noise using sentence materials with controlled word probability. *J. Acoust. Soc. Amer., 61,* 1977, 1337–1351.

LAMB, S. H., OWENS, E., and SCHUBERT, E. D. The revised form of the hearing performance inventory. *Ear & Hearing, 4,* 1983, 152–159.

McCARTHY, P. and ALPINER, J. The McCarthy-Alpiner Scale of Hearing Handicap. Unpublished study (1980) cited in eds. Alpiner, J. and McCarthy, P., *Rehabilitative Audiology: Children and Adults.* Baltimore: Williams and Wilkins, 1987, p. 52.

NEWBY, H. *Audiology.* New York: Appleton-Century-Crofts, 1964.

NOBLE, W. A. and ATHERLEY, G. R. The Hearing Measurement Scale. *J. Aud. Res., 10,* 1970, 229–250.

NOBLE, W. A. The hearing measurement scale as a paper-pencil form: Preliminary results: *J. Amer. Aud. Soc., 5,* 1979, 95–106.

O'NEILL, J. and OYER, H. Aural rehabilitation. In ed. Jerger, J., *Modern Developments in Audiology.* New York: Academic Press, 1973.

OWENS, E. and SCHUBERT, E. Development of the California Consonant Test. *J. Speech Hearing Res., 20,* 1977, 463–474.

OYER, H. J., FREEMAN, B., HARDICK, E., DIXON, J., DONNELLY, K., GOLDSTEIN, D., LLOYD, L., and MUSSEN, E. Unheeded recommendations for aural rehabilitation. *J. Acad. Rehabil. Aud., 9,* 1976, 20–30.

ROSSI, J. and HARFORD, E. An analysis of patients and reactions to a clinical hearing and selection process. *ASHA, 10,* 1968, 283–290.

SANDERS, D. A. Hearing-aid orientation and counseling. In ed. Pollack, M., *Amplification for the Hearing-Impaired.* New York: Grune and Stratton, 1975.

SANDERS, D. A. *Aural Rehabilitation.* Englewood Cliffs, NJ: Prentice Hall, 1982.

SCHOW, R. and NERBONNE, M. Hearing handicap and Denver Scales: Applications, categories, interpretation. *J. Acad. Rehab. Aud., 13(2),* 1980, 66–77.

SCHOW, R. and NERBONNE, M. Communication screening profile: Use with elderly clients. *Ear & Hearing, 3,* 1982, 135–147.

SCHOW, R. L. and TANNAHILL, C. Hearing handicap scores and categories for subjects with normal and impaired hearing sensitivity. *J. Amer. Aud. Soc., 3,* 1977, 134–139.

SCHWARTZ, D. and SURR, R. Three experiments on the California Consonant Test. *J. Speech Hearing Dis., 44,* 1979, 61–72.

CHAPTER 20

BINNIE, C. A. Attitude changes following speech reading training. *Scandinavian Audiology, 6,* 1977, 13–19.

CASTANADA, C. *Journey to Ixtlan: The Lessons of Don Juan.* New York: Pocket Books, a Simon & Schuster Division of Gulf & Western Corp., 1972.

DAVIS, J. M. and HARDICK, E. J. *Rehabilitative Audiology for Children and Adults.* New York: John Wiley, 1981.

EDGERTON, B. J. and DANHAUER, J. *Clinical Implications of a Speech Discrimination Test Using Nonsense Stimuli.* Baltimore: Univ. Park Press, 1979.

GARSTECKI, D. C. Audiovisual training paradigm for hearing-impaired adults. *J. Acad. Rehab. Aud., 14,* 1981, 223–228.

GIOLAS, T. G. A sample eight-week aural rehabilitation program. In Giolas, T. J., *Hearing Handicapped Adults.* Englewood Cliffs, NJ: Prentice Hall, 1982, pp. 108–116.

GIOLAS, T. G. Sample 8-week adult aural rehabilitation group outline. In eds. Schow, R. L. and Nerbonne, M. A., *Introduction to Aural Rehabilitation* (2nd ed.). Austin, TX: PRO-ED, 1989, pp. 577–586.

HARDICK, E. J. Aural rehabilitation programs for the aged can be successful. *J. Rehab. Aud., 10,* 1977, 51–67.

LARSON, L. L. *Consonant Sound Discrimination.* Bloomington: Indiana Univ. Press, 1950.

LEVITT, H. and RESNICK, S. Speech reception by the hearing-impaired. Methods of testing and the development of new tests. *Scandinavian Audiology, 6,* Supplement No. 1, 1978, 107–130.

LIEBERTH, A. K. The effects of acquired hearing loss. *The Voice,* January-February 1986, p. 13.

LUTERMAN, D. *Counseling the Communicatively Disordered and Their Families.* Boston: Little, Brown, 1984.

LUTERMAN, D. Audiological counseling and the diagnostic process. *ASHA, 32,* 1990, 35–37.

McCARTHY, P. and CULPEPPER, N. B. The adult remediation process. In eds. Alpiner, J. and McCarthy, P., *Rehabilitative Audiology: Children and Adults.* Baltimore: Williams and Wilkens, 1987, pp. 305–342.

McCARTHY, P. A., CULPEPPER, N. B., and LUCKS, L. Variability in counseling experiences and training among E.S.B. accredited programs. *ASHA, 28,* 1987, 49–52.

MONAT-HALLE, R. Speech-language pathologists as counselors and sex educators. *ASHA, 29,* December 1987, 35–36.

NABALEK, A. K. and NABALEK, I. V. Room acoustics and speech perception. In ed. Katz, J., *Handbook of Clinical Audiology.* Baltimore: Williams and Wilkins, 1985.

NETT, E. M., DOEFLER, L. G., and MATTHEWS, J. *The Relationship Between Audiological Measures and Handicap.* Unpublished manuscript, Vocational Rehabilitation Administration Project 167, 1960.

OYER, H. J. *Auditory Communication for the Hard of Hearing.* Englewood Cliffs, NJ: Prentice Hall, 1966.

REITER, R. Romance, sexuality and hearing loss. *ASHA 29,* December 1987, 29–33.

STONE, J. R. and OLSWANG, L. B. The hidden challenge of counseling. *ASHA, 31,* 1989, 27–31.

VAN RIPER, C. *A Career in Speech Pathology.* Englewood Cliffs, NJ: Prentice Hall, 1979.

WEBSTER, E. J. *Counseling with Parents of Handicapped Children: Guidelines for Improving Communication.* New York: Grune and Stratton, 1977.

CHAPTER 21

ALPINER, J. and BAKER, B. Communication assessment procedures in the aural rehabilitation process. *Seminars in Speech, Language and Hearing, 2,* No. 3. 1981, 189–204.

ALPINER, J. and McCARTHY, P. *Rehabilitative Audiology: Children and Adults.* Baltimore: Williams and Wilkins, 1987.

BENGSTON, V. L. *The Social Psychology of Aging.* Indianapolis: Bobbs Merrill, 1973.

BENJAMIN, B. J. Changes in speech production and linguistic behaviors with aging. In ed. Shadden, B. B., *Communication Behavior and Aging: A Sourcebook for Clinicians.* Baltimore: Williams and Wilkins, 1988, pp. 162–181.

BERGMAN, M., BLUMFIELD, V. A., CASCADO, D., DASH, B., LEVITT, H., and MARGUILES, M. Age related decrement in hearing for speech. *J. Gerontology, 31,* 1976, 533–538.

BOTWINICK, J. *Aging and Behavior.* New York: Springer-Verlag, 1973.

BOWLES, N. L. and POON, L. W. Aging and retrieval of words in semantic memory. *J. Gerontology 40,* 1985, 71–77.

BRAZIER, M. The electrical activity of the nervous system. *Sciences, 146,* December 1964, 1427.

CLARK, L. W. and WITTE, K. Nature and efficiency of communication management in Alzheimer's Disease. In ed. Lubinski, R., *Dementia and Communication.* Philadelphia: B. C. Decker, 1991, pp. 238–256.

COMALLI, P. E., WAPNER, S., and WERNER, H. Interference effects of Stroop color word test in childhood, adulthood and aging. *J. Genetic Psychol., 100,* 1962, 47–53.

CANESTRARI, R. E. Paced and self-paced learning in young and elderly adults. *J. Gerontology, 18,* 1963, 165–168.

CORSO, J. F. Age and sex differences in pure-tone thresholds. *Archives of Otolaryngology, 77,* 1963, 53–73.

ELIAS, M. F. and ELIAS, P. K. Motivation and activity. In eds. Birren, J. and Schaie, K., *Handbook of the Psychology of Aging.* New York: Van Nostrand Rheinhold, 1977.

FOZARD, J. L., WOLF, E., BELL, B., McFARLAND, R., and PODOLSKY, S. Visual perception and communication. In eds. Birren, J. E. and Schaie, K. W., *Handbook of Psychology of Aging.* New York: Van Nostrand Rheinhold, 1977, p. 497.

GELFAND, S. A., PIPER, N. and SILMAN, S. Consonant recognition in quiet and noise with aging among normal hearing listeners. *J. Acoust. Soc. Amer., 80,* 1986, 1589–1598.

GLORIG, A. and NIXON, J. Hearing loss as a function of age. *Laryngoscope, 27,* 1962, 1596–1610.

GLORIG, A., WHEELER, D., QUIGGLE, R., GRINGS, W., and SUMMERFIELD, A., 1954 Wisconsin State Fair Hearing Survey, Monograph, American Academy of Opthalmology and Otolaryngology, 1957.

GRIMES, A. Auditory changes. In ed. Lubinski, R. *Dementia and Communication.* Philadelphia: B. C. Decker, 1991, pp. 47–69.

HARBERT, F., YOUNG, I. M., and MENDUKE, H. Audiologic findings in presbycusis. *J. Aud. Res., 6,* 1966, 297–312.

HARDICK, E. J., OYER, H. J., and IRION, P. E. Lipreading performance as related to measurements of vision. *J. Speech Hearing Res., 13,* 1970, 1, 92–100.

HERON, A. and CHOWN, S. M. *Age and Function.* London: Churchill, 1967.

HOWARD, D. V., LASAGA, M. I., and McANDREWS, M. P. Semantic activation during memory encoding across the adult life span. *J. Georontology, 35,* 1980, 884–890.

KALIKOW, D. N., STEVENS, K. N., and ELLIOTT, L. L. Development of a speech intelligibility test in noise using sentence materials with controlled word predictability. *J. Acoust. Soc. Amer., 61,* 1977, 1337–1351.

KAPLAN, H., FEELEY, J., and BROWN, J. A modified Denver Scale: Test-retest reliability. *J. Acad. Rehab. Aud., 11,* 1978, 15–32.

KASTEN, R. N. and MILLER, W. E. Modifications of hearing and evaluation of fitting procedures for elderly clients. In ed. Hull, R., *Rehabilitative Audiology*. New York: Grune and Stratton, 1982.

KAUSLER, D. H. *Experimental Psychology and Human Aging*. New York: John Wiley, 1982.

KAUSLER, D. H. Cognition and aging. In ed. Shadden, B. B., *Communication Behavior and Aging: A Sourcebook for Clinicians*. Baltimore: Williams and Wilkins, 1988, pp. 79–106.

KAUSLER, D. H. and HAKAMI, M. K. Memory for topics of conversation: Adult age differences and intentionality. *Exp. Aging Res., 9*, 1983, 153–157.

KENNEY, R. A. Psychology of aging. In ed. Shaddon, B. B., *Communication Behavior in Aging: A Sourcebook for Clinicians*. Baltimore: Williams and Wilkins, 1988, pp. 58–78.

KIMMEL, D. C. *Adulthood and Aging*. New York: John Wiley, 1974.

KIRCHNER, W. K. Age differences in short term memory of rapidly changing information. *J. Exp. Psychol., 55*, 1958, 352–358.

KITE, M. E. and JOHNSON, B. T. Attitudes toward older and younger adults: A meta-analysis. *Psych. Aging, 3*, 1988, 233–244.

KONKLE, D., BEASLEY, D., and BESS, F. Intelligibility of time-altered speech in relation to chronological age. *J. Speech Hearing Res., 20*, 1977, 108–115.

KORIAT, A., BEN-ZUR, H., and SCHEFFER, D. Telling the same story twice: Output monitoring and age. *J. Memory Language, 27*, 1988, 23–39.

LAWSON, C. A. *Brain Mechanisms and Human Learning*. Boston: Houghton Mifflin, 1967.

LIGHT, L. L. and CAPS, J. L. Comprehension of pronouns in young and older adults. *Dev. Psychol., 22*, 1986, 580–585.

LUBINSKI, R. Learned helplessness: Application to communication of the elderly. In ed. Lubinski, R., *Dementia and Communication*. Philadelphia: B. C. Decker, 1991, pp. 142–151.

MARSHALL, L. Auditory processing in aging listeners. *J. Speech Hearing Dis., 46*, 1981, 226–240.

MCCARTHY, P. Rehabilitation of the hearing impaired geriatric client. In ed. Alpiner, J., and McCarthy, P. *Rehabilitative Audiology: Children and Adults*. Baltimore: Williams and Wilkins, 1987, pp. 370–427.

MCPHERSON, B. D. *Aging as a Social Process*. Toronto: Butterworths, 1983.

National Center for Health Statistics. Prevalence of Selected Impairments, United States, 1977, Vital Health Statistics, *10*, No. 134, Pub. No. (PHS), 1981, 81–1562.

OBLER, L. K., NICHOLAS, M., ALBERT, M. L., and WOODWARD, S. On comprehension across the adult lifespan. *Cortex 21*, 1985, 273–280.

PARKINSON, S. R., LINDHOLM, J. M., and INMAN, V. W. An analysis of age differences in immediate recall. *J. Gerontology, 34*, 1982, 533–539.

POON, L. W. and FOZARD, J. L. Speed of retrieval from long term memory and lateness of information. *J. Gerontology, 33*, 1978, 711–717.

QUILTER, R. E., GIAMBRA, L. M., and BENSON, P. E. Longitudinal age changes in vigilance over an eighteen year interval. *J. Gerontology, 38*, 1983, 179–186.

RABBITT, P. An age decrement in the ability to ignore irrelevant information. *J. Gerontology, 20*, 1965, 233–238.

RABBITT, P. Talking to the old. *New Society, 55*, 1981, 140–141.

RAIFORD, C. A. Modifications in hearing assessment procedures for older adults. In ed. Shadden, B. B., *Communication Behavior and Aging: A Sourcebook for Clinicians*. Baltimore: Williams and Wilkins, 1988, 227.

RANKIN, J. L. and COLLINS, M. Adult age differences in memory elaboration. *J. Gerontology, 40*, 1985, 451–458.

ROLLIN, W. J. *The Psychology of Communication Disorders in Individuals and Their Families*. Englewood Cliffs, NJ: Prentice Hall, 1987.

RYAN, E. B. Normal aging and language. In ed. Lubinski, R., *Dementia and Communication*. Philadelphia: B. C. Decker, 1991, pp. 84–97.

SALTHOUSE, T. A. *Adult Cognition: An Experimental Psychology of Human Aging*. New York: Springer Publishing, 1982.

SALTHOUSE, T. A. Speed of behavior and its implications for cognition. In eds. Birren, J. E. and Schaie, K. W., *Handbook of Psychology of Aging* (2nd ed.). New York: Van Nostrand Rheinhold, 1985, p. 176.

SALTHOUSE, T. A. Effects of aging on verbal abilities: Examination of the psychometric literature. In eds. Light, L. L. and Burke, D. M., *Language, Memory and Aging*. Cambridge: Cambridge Univ. Press, 1988, pp. 17–35.

SALTHOUSE, T. A., The role of processing resources in cognitive aging. In eds. Howe, M. L., Brainerd, C. J., *Cognitive Development in Adulthood: Process in Cognitive Developmental Research*. New York: Springer-Verlag, 1988, p. 185.

SCHOW, K. L. and NERBONNE, M. A. Assessment of hearing handicaps by nursing home residents and staff. *J. Acad. Rehab. Aud., 10*, 1977, 2–12.

SHOOP, C. and BINNIE, C. A. The effect of age upon the visual perception of speech. *Scandinavian Audiology, 8*, 1979, 3–8.

SOLLEY, C. M. and MURPHY, P. *Development of the Perceptual World*. New York: Basic Books, 1960.

SOMBERG, B. L. and SALTHOUSE, T. A. Divided attention abilities in young and old adults. *J. Exp. Psychol., 8*, 1982, 651–663.

TRAP, E. P. and SPATZ, T. Considerations for the practitioner with older clients. In ed. Shadden, B., *Communication Behavior and Aging.* Baltimore: Williams and Wilkins, 1988, pp. 219–226.

VENTRY, I. and WEINSTEIN, B. The hearing handicap inventory for the elderly. *Ear & Hearing, 3,* 1982, 128–134.

WEINSTEIN, B. Management of the hearing impaired elderly. In ed. L. Jacobs-Condit, *Gerontology and Communication Disorders.* Rockville, MD: American Speech-Language-Hearing Assoc., 1984, p. 244.

WINGFIELD, A., STINE, E. A., LAHAR, C. J., ABERDEEN, J. S. Does the capacity of working memory change with age? *Exp. Aging Res. 4,* 1988, 103–107.

WRIGHT, R. E. Aging, divided attention and processing capacity. *J. Gerontology, 36,* 1981, 605–614.

ZARNOCH, J. M. and ALPINER, J. A. The Denver Scale of Communication Function for Senior Citizens Living in Retirement Centers. Unpublished study (1977) cited in eds Alpiner, J. and McCarthy, P., *Rehabilitative Audiology: Children and Adults.* Baltimore: Williams and Wilkins, 1987, pp. 370–427.

CHAPTER 22

ALPINER, J. The psychology of aging. In ed. Henoch, M., *Aural Rehabilitation for the Elderly.* New York: Grune and Stratton, 1979.

CLARK, L. W. and WITTE, K. Nature and efficacy of communication management in Alzheimer's disease. In ed. Lubinski, R., *Dementia and Communication.* Philadelphia: B. C. Decker, 1991, pp. 238–256.

CUMMING, E. and HENRY, W. H. *Growing Old.* New York: Basic Books, 1961.

ERNST, N. S. and WEST, H. L. *Nursing Home Staff Development: A Guide for Inservice Programs.* New York: Springer Publishing, 1983.

JOHNSON, C., DANHAUER, J., and EDWARDS, R. The "hearing aid effect" in geriatrics—fact or fiction? *Hearing Instruments, 10,* 1982, 10–24.

KALISH, R. A. *The Later Years.* Pacific Grove, CA: Brooks/Cole Publishing, 1977.

KOURY, K. and LUBINSKI, R. Effective in-service training for staff working with communication-impaired patients. In ed. Lubinski, R., *Dementia and Communication.* Philadelphia: B. C. Decker, 1991, pp. 279–289.

LAWTON, M. P. *Environment and Aging.* Pacific Grove, CA: Brooks/Cole Publishing Co., 1980.

LUBINSKI, R. Learned helplessness: Application to communication of the elderly. In ed. Lubinski, R., *Dementia and Communication.* Philadelphia: B. C. Decker, 1991a, 142–151.

LUBINSKI, R. L. Environmental considerations for elderly patients. In ed. Lubkinski, R., *Dementia and Communication.* Philadelphia: B. C. Decker, 1991b, 257–278.

MAURER, J. F. Auditory impairment and aging. In ed. Jacobs, B., *Working with the Elderly.* Washington, DC: The National Council on Aging, 1976.

WEINSTEIN, B. E. Auditory testing and rehabilitation of the hearing impaired. In ed. Lubinski, R., *Dementia and Communication.* Philadelphia: B. C. Decker, 1991, pp. 223–237.

An Epilogue: Looking Back–Looking Forward

We have considered so many types of information relevant to hearing impairment and its management that beginning students may feel overwhelmed. The size and complexity of the needs created by hearing impairment can be bewildering. It is true that to understand the problems involved requires a strong basic knowledge of communication sciences. This you bring to the task from other studies. What you now must do is apply selective parts of that knowledge to understanding what impairment of hearing imposes on the development and function of the communication process and how you can use the relevant knowledge in ameliorating the problem. Beyond the fundamental information which applies to the population of hearing-impaired persons at large, the application of knowledge becomes highly individualized. For each client you must identify the specific problems and demands and circumstances which create them. You must determine how the person is meeting the demands, whether the use of existing resources can be improved and which additional resources can be marshalled. It is reassuring to remember that the same problem-solving model applies to each person regardless of age or lifestyle, only the values fed into the model vary with the individual. Once you understand the management model and the questions that generate the required information, you will begin to feel comfortable.

As you anticipate assuming management responsibilities, keep constantly in mind the knowledge that this is a co-operative task, a partnership, not only with the hearing-impaired child or adult but also with immediate family and significant others. A hearing impairment causes others also to experience communication breakdown and its related anxieties and emotional reactions. Thus, you do not have to have all the answers, it is not your responsibility to provide solutions. Your role is to provide information, to explore individual circumstances, to offer suggestions for consideration, and to provide encouragement and support. You have the necessary knowledge to begin being a partner with your clients. As you work with them you quickly will become adept at soliciting, listening to, and being guided by their information. Although I have provided you with much information, my emphasis has been on helping you to conceptualize the task. Remember your greatest resource is your ability to think independently and creatively and your courage to do so.

Author Index

556

Dallenbach, M., 69
Daly, J., 385
Danhauer, J., 491, 522
Daniloff, R., 25
Darbyshire, J., 12, 294
Dash, B., 503
Davis, F., 330
Davis, H., 435, 446
Davis, J., 497
DeCasper, A., 71
DeLavergne, R., 48
DePompei, R., 56
Dixon, J., 429
Dixon, R., 367
Doeffler, L., 485
Dolanski, V., 44, 69
Donnelly, J., 363
Donnelly, K., 429
Doob, A., 219, 374
Dolanski, V., 69
Dowell, R., 210
Downs, M., 230, 247–248, 257
Droder, J., 56
Duchan, J., 349, 357, 361–363, 406
Dunn, L., 352
Dupree, R., 138

Edgerton, B., 491
Edwards, R., 522
Elias, M., 500
Elias, P., 500
Elliott, L., 341, 446, 509
Engen, E., 249, 356
Engen, T., 249, 356
Engleman, S., 97, 354
Erber, N., 6, 54–56, 97,
        126, 211, 249, 342, 363
Erdman, S., 48
Erickson, J., 350
Ernst, N., 531
Erting, C. 251–252
Estes, W., 85
Evans, A., 137
Evarts, E., 114
Evatt, R., 231

Fairbanks, A., 113, 436
Feeley, J., 511
Fiedler, F., 219
Fifer, W., 71
Finitzo-Heiber, T., 35, 133–134
Firszt, J., 210
Fisher, B., 373
Fitch, J., 385
Fletcher, H., 29
Flexer, C., 385
Foster, R., 353
Fozard, J., 502, 505
Frankel, B., 433
Frayer, C., 255
Freedman, J., 219, 374
Freelander, B., 72
Freeman, B., 429
Freeman, L., 367–368
French, J., 87
French, N., 122
Friel-Patti, S., 266, 274

Fristoe, R., 368
Frueh, F., 48
Fry, D., 44, 131–132, 400
Furth, H., 198, 132

Gagne, J., 174
Gallimore, A., 268
Gallimore, R., 240, 268
Gardner, M., 352
Gargiulo, R., 220
Garner, M., 56
Garstecki, D., 491
Geers, A., 248–249
Geers, A., 355–356
Geffner, D., 367–368
Gelfand, S., 135, 501
Gerber, S., 28
German, D., 352
Giambra, L., 503
Giddan, J., 353
Gildstone, P., 386
Giolas, T., 33, 436, 439, 485, 495, 497
Givens, G., 363
Glascoe, A., 438
Glass, D., 137
Glorig, A., 436, 501
Godfrey, J., 128, 130
Goffman, E., 5, 42, 219, 294, 420
Goldman, M., 368
Goldstein, B., 234
Goldstein, D., 429
Goodrich, S., 59, 88
Goetzinger, C., 373
Gottsleben, R., 347
Greenberg, B., 405
Greene, H., 51
Greenfield, D., 363
Greer, C., 363
Gregory, H., 303
Grimes, A., 501
Grings, W., 501
Gustason, A., 251

Hakami, M., 506
Halle, M., 77, 88
Hambleton, D., 373
Hambrick-Dixon, P., 137
Hamill, D., 353
Harbert, F., 50
Hardick, E., 52, 429, 495, 497, 502
Harford, E., 428
Harrison, D., 373
Hasenstab, S., 211, 401, 404
Haskins, H., 341
Hawkins, J., 342
Healy, A., 85
Hedrick, D., 231
Hemdal, J., 83
Henry, W., 518
Heron, A., 500
Hesketh, L., 210–211
High, W., 436
Hilgard, E., 70
Hine, W., 385
Hochberg, I., 135
Hodgson, W., 163

Sedey, A., 210, 211
Seewald, R., 174, 370
Seligman, M., 220
Senden, von M., 69, 71
Seward, J., 88
Shankweiler, D., 24, 88
Shannon, C., 98, 101
Shepherd, D., 48
Sherman, J., 258
Shoop, C., 502
Shriner, T., 245
Silman, S., 501
Silverman, S., 367, 446
Simmons, A., 346
Simon, C., 360–361
Singer, J., 137
Slobin, D., 258
Smith, F., 372
Snell, K., 53
Snow, C., 255
Solley, C., 76–78, 81, 87, 503
Somberg, B., 504
Spatz, T., 499
Spitz, R., 71
Speerschneider, J., 162
Spinelli, F., 361
Stach, B., 162
Staller, J., 205, 210–211
Stark, J., 353
Stark, R., 7, 367
State of New York, 321
Steeneken, H., 36
Steinberg, J., 122
Steincamp, M., 356
Steiner, V., 231
Stern, D., 253
Stevens, K., 77, 88, 446, 509
Stevens, R., 252
Staller, J., 205, 210–211
Stewart, L., 373
Stockwell, R., 370
Stokoe, W., 250
Stokols, D., 137
Stone, J., 473, 475
Stone, P., 344, 361–364, 408
Stroer, B., 210
Strong, M., 252
Studdert-Kennedy, M., 24, 88
Subtelny, J., 367
Sudman, J., 56
Sullivan, P., 315, 323–325
Sumby, W., 59
Summerfield, A., 501
Supa, M., 69
Surr, R., 446
Sussman, H., 87
Suter, A., 143–144
Swartz, D., 446
Swing, J., 138

Tannahill, C., 436
Templin, M., 346–347
Tharp, G., 240, 268
Tharp, R., 258
Thomas, H., 35
Thomas, S., 54
Thomure, R., 385

Tillman, J., 35, 133–134
Tobey, E., 211
Tobin, A., 231
Todd, S., 210–211
Trapp, E., 499
Truax, R., 371, 390
Tucker, B., 234
Turton, L., 255
Tyack, D., 347
Tyler, L., 219, 222

University of the State of New York, 32
USWAPA, 58
Utley, J., 48, 52
Uttley, A., 87
Uzgiris, I., 137

Van Riper, C., 470
Ventry, I., 511
Vernon, M., 12, 300, 314–315, 323–325
Vygotsky, L., 240

Wachs, J., 137
Walden, B., 48, 60
Walsvik, O., 386
Wapner, H., 504
Ward, D., 228
Weamer, R., 257
Weaver, W., 98, 101
Weber, S., 342
Webster, E., 219–220, 236, 470, 495
Wedenberg, E., 71
Weikert, D., 264
Weinstein, B., 510–511, 523
Werner, S., 504
West, H., 531
West, R., 61
Westin, B., 71
Wheeler, D., 501
Whetnall, E., 44
Whitehead, R., 367
Whitehurst, M., 280
Widin, G., 162
Wilbur, R., 250, 372
Williams, D., 12
Williams, G.L., 192
Withers, S., 405
Witte, K., 513, 533
Wolf, E., 502
Wolinski, S., 162
Wood, B., 294–295
Woodward, J., 252
Woodward, M., 47–48, 60
Woodward, S., 505
Woodworth, R., 81, 84
Wray, D., 385
Wright, R., 500

Yoder, D., 254
Young, I., 501
Yuker, H., 374

Zarnoch, J., 514
Zimmerman, I., 231
Zimmerman-Phillips, S., 210
Zowolkow, E., 251

560

Subject Index

564